# LET'S COOK IT RIGHT

*GOOD HEALTH COMES*
*FROM GOOD COOKING*

ADELLE DAVIS, B.A., M.S.

## Let's Cook It Right

## by Adelle Davis

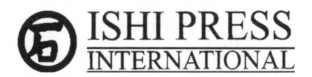

ISHI PRESS
INTERNATIONAL

# Let's Cook It Right

# by Adelle Davis

First Published in 1947

## ISBN  4-87187-958-5
## 978-4-87187-958-3

Ishi Press International
1664 Davidson Avenue, Suite 1B
Bronx NY 10453-7877
USA
1-917-507-7226
samhsloan@gmail.com

Printed in the United States of America

## *Introduction by Sam Sloan*

## Let's Cook It Right

## by Adelle Davis

## Introduction by Sam Sloan

Adelle Davis is an incredibly famous and popular author and this book, **Let's Cook It Right**, is the book that made her famous.

Here is one of the most popular, helpful, and widely praised cookbooks ever published. Dedicated to the principle that foods can be prepared to retain their delightful flavors, as well as their rewarding nutrients, Adelle Davis, a well-known nutritionist, has completely reviewed the recipes in this edition, added dozens of new ones, rewritten old ones, deleted little used ones. and changed hundreds to keep pace with recent scientific findings. In addition to nearly four hundred basic recipes for preparing every type of food, she has supplied thousands of easy-to-fix variations of them. A major change in this new edition has been to reduce solid fats to a minimum and to increase the use of vegetable oils. thus minimizing dangers from a high level of cholesterol in the blood. Adelle Davis has also attempted to eliminate any ingredients that contain possible cancer-producing additives, such as those found in chemicals used in certain colorings, preservatives, bleaches, artificial sweeteners, flavorings, and dyes. She also warns against food contaminations from lacquers, enamels, waxes, and some widely used insecticide sprays.

Easy-to-follow, concise, and complete, this new edition will be warmly welcomed by every homemaker who wishes to maintain her family's maximum physical and emotional well-being.

Her name and whose books have reached the household

word status. Her recommendations are followed by millions today. She is the leading spokesperson for the organic foods movement. She is known for popularizing the phrase "You Are What You Eat". When you see organic food stores all over and special organic foods shelves in supermarkets, think of Adelle Davis as the person who popularized all of this.

She was born in Lizton, Indiana on February 25, 1904. Her first book was Optimum Health published in 1935. This book did not have a publisher. The first book to make her famous was this cook book published in 1947: *Let's Cook it Right*. This was followed by **Let's Have Healthy Children** (1951) and **Let's Eat Right to Keep Fit** (1954).

Her movement became popular because of the increased use of pesticides, chemicals, additives and fertilizers to increase food production.

Davis wrote a series of four books, starting with a cookbook in 1947, that ultimately sold over 10 million copies in total. Although her ideas were considered somewhat eccentric in the 1940s and 1950s, the change in culture with the 1960s brought her ideas, especially her anti-food processing and food industry charges, into the mainstream in a time when anti-authority sentiment was growing. She also contributed to, as well as benefited from, the rise of a nutritional and health food movement that began in the 1950s, which focused on subjects such as pesticide residues and food additives, a movement her critics would come to term food faddism. During the 1960s and 1970s, her popularity continued to grow, as she was featured in multiple media reports, variously described as an "oracle" by the New York Times, "high priestess" by Life and was compared to Ralph Nader, the popular consumer activist, by the Associated Press. Her celebrity was demonstrated by her repeated guest appearances on

### *Introduction by Sam Sloan*

The Tonight Show Starring Johnny Carson, as she became the most popular and influential nutritionist in the country.

Let us say that her works have not been without criticism. Critics state that there is no scientific proof for some of her claims, especially her claims that non-organic foods are a significant health risk. She is also criticized recommending for large doses of Vitamin A and Vitamin D. However, her nutritional ideas such as the need for exercise, the dangers of vitamin deficiencies as well as the need to avoid hydrogenated fat, saturated fat and excess sugar consumption remain relevant to even mainstream nutritionists.

Her followers were shocked when Adelle Davis developed cancer at age 70. She was shocked too as she had contended that almost any disease could be prevented by proper diet. When she contracted the cancer that later killed her, she maintained that it did not invalidate her theories about proper diet. She attributed the illness to the junk food she had eaten at college. She wrote:

> "I think that I am sympathetic with the people who are quite annoyed with the fact that I have cancer. When I was told I had it I could not believe it either. I thought this was for people who drink soft drinks, who eat white bread, who eat refined sugar and so on."

However, then she realized that her diet had changed when she went to Purdue University at age 19. From 1924 to the early 1950 she ate "Commercial Junk Food". She blamed this plus her heavy work load and a series of Xray examinations on the fact that he had cancer.

Adelle Davis died on 31 May 1974 in Los Angeles, having gone there to die knowing that her life was at its end.

## *Introduction by Sam Sloan*

Adelle Davis' book is a simple. sound and above all practical guide to the principles of nutrition. "Nutrition is a personal matter," says Miss Davis, "as personal as your diary or income tax report. Your nutrition can determine, how you look, act, and feel; whether you are grouchy or cheerful, homely or beautiful, whether you think clearly or are confused, enjoy your work or make it a drudgery."

Let's Eat Right To Keep Fit is designed to help any normal adult find his or her way to maximum fitness through proper diet. The book discusses the sixty or more nutrients needed by the body to build health, and tells what foods supply these nutrients in the most concentrated form. The essential vitamins and minerals are dealt with in detail, and their function in the body analyzed according to the most up-to-date medical information. Miss Davis then makes specific recommendations for a balanced diet supplying-adequate quantities of all these vital substances. In a final section, the author discusses the general aspects of the nutrition problem, and tells what the individual can do to help build national health.

ADELLE DAVIS was a consulting nutritionist in Los Angeles. She studied at Purdue University, Columbia, the University of California, and U.C.L.A., and had a Master of Science degree from the University of Southern California Medical School. She served as a dietitian at Bellevue Hospital in New York City, and as Supervisor of Health Education in the public schools of Yonkers, New York.

**Sam Sloan**
**Bronx, New York**
**USA**
**September 2, 2013**

# PREFACE

The application of nutritional knowledge in the kitchen has lagged decades behind the progress made in nutritional research. It is in the hope of helping to rectify such a deplorable situation that this book has been written. Only when nutrition is applied in planning and preparing meals day after day can ideal health be attained. To achieve this end this complete cookbook has been prepared.

The author wishes to express her thanks to the many friends and students who have contributed to this book, aided in testing recipes, and offered valuable criticisms of the manuscript. Outstandingly helpful have been Mrs. Leah D. Widtsoe, Mrs. Mabel Garvey, Dr. Gladys Stevenson, Mrs. Susan Crawford Moore, Mrs. Horace J. Smith, Dr. Harry J. Deuel, Jr., Mrs. Iris Albert, Mrs. Harriett Sabey, Mrs. Frances Locus, Mrs. Gertrude Kendall, Mrs. Hazel Gough, Mrs. Gladys Lindberg, Miss Berta Strauch, Mrs. Ruth Conrad Norbury, Mrs. Anne Mihaylo, Miss Olive Burchfiel, and Mr. and Mrs. Carl Pudlich.

The author also wishes to thank the following companies for materials and equipment used in testing recipes: the Century Metalcraft Corporation for the Guardian Service cooking utensils; the Luer Packing Company for meats; the Golden State Milk Company of San Francisco for powdered milk; the Ocean Foods Corporation for fish and sea foods; the Converted Rice Company of Houston, Texas, for all-vitamin rice; the El Molino Mills of Alhambra, California, for wheat germ, rice polish, soy grits, and many varieties of flours; the Southern California Gas Company; and the General Electric Company for the use of their appliances.

ADELLE DAVIS LEISEY

# CONTENTS

# CHAPTER 1

## GOOD HEALTH COMES FROM GOOD COOKING

If nutrition is to be successfully applied, the homemaker must be able to prepare delicious foods which appeal to the eyes and nostrils as well as to the taste buds. It is a popular belief that anything which builds health tastes like witches' brew and looks like baby spinach. Exactly the reverse; foods which retain their greatest nutritive value also have the best flavor, texture, and color.

Whenever methods of preparing foods are discussed, one hears women remark, "My recipe book says—"and they invariably outline methods apparently designed by gremlins to destroy or throw away nutritive value. If one examines critically most of the countless recipe books on the market, one appears to be reading, not recipe books, but directions telling how to remove vitamins and minerals from foods. Millions of these books are used daily as a guide in producing the health of our nation. The cookbooks containing much glib chit-chat about saving nutrients often give the same cooking methods as the books written before the science of nutrition existed.

For example, if a food is rich in vitamins and minerals which will dissolve in water, most cookbooks are likely to say to soak the food overnight and to throw the water away. If a vegetable contains valuable minerals in the skin, it is to be peeled and the minerals tossed into the garbage. If the vitamins in a food are destroyed by the addition of soda, these books say to add soda. If the nutritive value of a food is decreased by long cooking, one is instructed to turn the heat low and let the food simmer throughout the day. If the incorporation of air destroys the vitamins, directions say to beat with an eggbeater until fluffy. A comprehensive recipe book usually has two or three pages given to preparing vegetables other than potatoes, yet gives two hundred pages or more to the preparation of pastries, breads, cakes, pies, jams, jellies, and candies,

3

made, of course, with white flour and refined sugar. One would be led to assume that only food faddists and crackpots would dare believe that foods can be delicious and still be prepared in such a way as to retain the maximum nutritive value put there by nature.

Most recipe books appear to have only one designed purpose: to bring about the physical degeneration of the race at all possible speed. It is little wonder that our national health record is something to be ashamed of. Such books are supposedly written for the Epicurean, although it is questionable whether a true Epicurean could enjoy foods prepared by the methods they recommend; in any case, said Epicurean would, at the age of fifty if not sooner, be food for Epicure worms. Would it not be better for him to have enjoyed such foods as could enable him, at the age of ninety, to pick up the table over which he had frequently leaned, and carry it into the garden for a pleasant breakfast in the sunshine?

The intelligent, informed person of today demands that food be delicious and that it build health. Although one who greatly enjoys food may scoff at individuals who eat for health's sake, at least he wants to remain healthy enough to continue to enjoy eating.

Thousands of housewives have studied nutrition, but they are usually bewildered as to how to apply their knowledge. The teachings of nutrition classes, articles in women's magazines, and directions in recipe books give varying advice. Not infrequently a conscientious mother feels she has failed her family because she has cooked by methods which she later learns are destructive to nutritive value. Therefore, I feel that a need exists for a book which shows how nutrition can be applied in the kitchen, together with recipes which give, according to present knowledge, scientific procedures designed to save maximum nutritive value.

Definite policies have been followed throughout the book. For example, I have given much space to meat cookery for the following reasons: Americans particularly enjoy meats; menus are largely built around them; they are the most expensive items on the food budget; thousands upon thousands of dollars are wasted because of improper cooking methods; and anyone can cook delicious meats, provided the principles of meat cookery are once learned and carefully applied.

Instead of grouping menu suggestions separately, I have put

them with recipes of meat dishes around which dinners are planned. I have matched the cooking time of the foods suggested; if meat requires 10 minutes to cook, the vegetable likewise can be cooked in 10 minutes. A housewife following these menu suggestions thus knows approximately how long it will take to prepare a meal and can plan her week's menus according to her activities. These suggestions contain much purposeful repetition of foods of outstanding nutritive value.

I have included an unusually large number of recipes for cooking vegetables. Many a culinary crime is committed in preparing vegetables, and few recipes are known for making them appetizing.

Each recipe has been checked with the idea of keeping dirty dishes to a minimum; in fact I have emphasized this point so much that several friends have nicknamed me One-dish Adelle. When flavor or color, however, can be retained better by cooking foods separately and then combining them, this procedure has been recommended. The ingredients have been listed in the order in which they should be added. All measurements are level and have been made by standard measuring equipment; whenever possible, those which can be easily halved or doubled have been used. Since the average American family has 3.8 members, all recipes have been planned for a family of four. In testing I have kept the preparation of all meals to a half hour of working time, but not necessarily of cooking time.

Recipes have been simplified and procedures shortened; if foods are to retain their nutritive value, little work is involved in their preparation. If a woman spends much time cooking for a family of four, she is probably using poor equipment and obsolete methods which destroy nutritive value.

It has been my purpose to show how easy cooking can be, especially for the working girl, the professional woman, and the young mother. These people often prepare sketchy meals because they believe cooking is difficult. By the time a woman has cooked enough to discover how amazingly easy it is, she usually enjoys promoting the illusion that cooking is an art achieved by long years of experience Although I have had almost thirty years of cooking experience, I have found it detrimental many times because faulty habits are difficult to break.

There are only four fundamental recipes: those which tell you how to stew, fry, broil, and bake. All other recipes are combinations of these four, varying largely through suggestions for seasoning. Steaming, boiling, French frying, sautéing, pan-broiling, and roasting are only variations of stewing, frying, broiling, and baking. When once you have cooked by these four methods, you know the fundamentals of food preparation. There is no reason why a beginner cannot prepare as delicious meals the first day she cooks as a person who has cooked for fifty years.

It may appear that the recipes are designed for ill persons who wish to rebuild their health. Quite conversely, I wish my major emphasis to be upon the healthy person and upon keeping him healthy. When one learns to recognize minor deviations indicating that health is below par, or when one has a conception of what radiant rather than mediocre health can mean to him individually, he quickly discovers that it is almost impossible to find a "healthy" person. It has often been said that if one eats a "well-balanced diet," he will get all the nutrients he needs. That statement is as true as saying that if a person works hard, he will earn a million dollars.

I have attempted to make this book sufficiently comprehensive to serve the beginner in case she does not happen to own another book which gives cooking procedures. On the other hand, hundreds of well-known recipes have been purposely omitted because their object appears to be the destruction of nutritive value.

I have used basic recipes and given instructions for varying them. Since such recipes differ from the old block-style recipes with their endless repetition, you may not like them at first. On using them, however, you will find that they offer many advantages. If you study only the basic recipes, you should be able to prepare foods without further effort. By using a basic recipe repeatedly, varying only a seasoning, an amateur should become an accomplished cook in a short time. Such recipes give detailed directions desired by some, yet allow flexibility for the person who enjoys being creative. These recipes save time because you need not read dozens of recipes before choosing one to follow; I find that to decide upon a particular cookie recipe, for example, is usually as difficult as buying a tie for my husband. By using the variations of the basic recipes, you can avoid monotony; you may substitute one ingredient for another which may be disliked or not available or of greater or different nutritive value. Thus the food you prepare can meet the health needs of your individual family.

The recipes present a number of foods which are not commonly used, though such a policy may limit the value of the book when it is first purchased. For example, I have suggested the frequent use of fresh pimentos and paprika peppers, although they are not sold in many markets. However, when people find how delicious and sweet these peppers are—the Hungarians serve them for dessert—and come to appreciate their outstanding nutritive value, I hope that these peppers will be grown in every home garden. Powdered milk is also a food which few people use. Even dried skim milk makes cream soups and milk drinks taste as if they were made of cream. It improves the flavor of breads, waffles, and many other foods, besides supplying protein, vitamin $B_2$, and calcium. Therefore, it should become a household item.

Recipes designed to increase the nutritive value of foods often appear to be masterpieces of faddism, especially to persons unaware of the part which sound nutrition plays in maintaining their own appearance, vitality, and general well-being. As though by some perversity of nature, foods having the greatest concentration of vitamins, minerals, and proteins are frequently those which Americans rarely eat. The use of almost any unfamiliar food is at first labeled a fad, regardless of how valuable that food may be. A fad, however, is defined as a passing whim or fancy, pursued for a short time with undue zeal. Such foods as yogurt (a Bulgarian-culture milk) soybeans, and tampala, a green leafy vegetable of outstanding nutritive value, have been eaten for thousands of years. Their value was proved before the food analyst lived. Your grandmother and grandmother's grandmother were brought up on black molasses. Such foods, therefore, are scarcely passing fancies. The use of any food which can contribute to your youthfulness and zest for life is not a fad, even though it be so labeled.

Although each recipe in this book has been tested repeatedly, the most thorough testing does not assure that you will enjoy the food prepared by that recipe. No two people exist who have the same tastes. I expect you who use this book to alter the recipes or to choose the variation your families will enjoy the most.

Nor does careful testing assure that the food prepared by the recipe will be a success. A women's magazine conducted an experiment in which a cake recipe was prepared in its testing kitchen. The result was a delicious cake, even and light in texture; the instructions were considered so easy to follow as to be foolproof. The recipe was then submitted to ten housewives known to be excellent and experienced cooks, and each was asked to prepare a cake. No two cakes were alike and only one was a success. Some of the women had failed to cream the fat and sugar sufficiently and the cake had a coarse texture; others had omitted an ingredient; still others had allowed their oven temperatures to be either too high or too low, and so on.

Time and again, I have been discouraged by failures of friends—excellent cooks—who have helped me test recipes. A soufflé fell, obviously undercooked, though surely everyone knows that soft-cooked eggs have a habit of lolling about in a relaxed manner. The cake was dry; although the thermostat had been set at the temperature specified, the oven temperature had not been checked and the thermostat was 45° F. higher than it should have been. No doubt many recipes in this book will be considered worthless and much good food will be wasted because busy women do not follow instructions accurately.

Perhaps I have stressed thrift and economy in foods to the point of appearing ridiculous. For example, because a large part of American garbage is bread, it seems wise to use bread crumbs more often than cracker or cereal crumbs. Since the customary American breakfast consists of bacon or ham, I believe that the drippings, which contain B vitamins, should be used. Luxury foods, such as porterhouse steaks, caviar, lobster, or even butter and cream, have not been emphasized. Butter and cream may be used instead of the fats suggested. I feel, however, that the butter-and-cream enthusiast needs little help in being shown how to use these foods, whereas persons who cannot afford them or who wish to avoid their calories will appreciate learning about substitutes.

I have tried to give recipes which fit present-day conditions. Most people today take little exercise; hence fewer calories are needed than were required a generation ago. Many recipes still in use have been handed down from the past when high-calorie foods were essential because people did vigorous work. The continued use of such recipes has caused many people to become harmfully overweight. Moreover, research indicates that the diet of even a slender person should be moderately low in calories, yet rich in proteins, vitamins, and minerals. Such a diet has been fed to thousands of animals by Dr. McCay of Cornell University. These "underfed" animals retained their characteristics of youth to a late age; their degree of health throughout life was unusually high; and their life span was the equivalent of 150 human years. It has long been known that overeating causes poor health and early death in humans. I have, therefore, planned menus and recipes lower in calories than those given in most cookbooks, although I doubt that this fact will be obvious to the reader; in many foods concentrated calories cannot be avoided.

No space has been given to artistic flower arrangements, attractive table settings, linens, dishes, crystal, and silver, all excellently dealt with in women's magazines and numerous recipe books. This lack of emphasis does not mean that I consider beauty unimportant. The surroundings in which you eat have a tremendous bearing upon your health. The more attractive the surroundings, the more you enjoy the meal and the more relaxed you will probably be; these factors are conducive to the abundant flow of digestive juices and to the absorption of nutrients into the blood. For these reasons I urge you to dine rather than merely to eat, and to believe that beauty has health value worth considerable effort and expense.

One point which in my opinion has been insufficiently stressed is the health value of graciousness in the home. Dr. Pavlov, the great Russian scientist, proved that a happy atmosphere is conducive to normal digestion; that anger and other distressing emotions stop the flow of digestive juices and may seriously interfere with health. It is futile for a mother to go to great effort to prepare foods properly if during the meal she allows unpleasantness to occur which can stop the digestion and absorption of those carefully prepared foods. Too often children are rudely corrected at the table, and too frequently disturbing problems are discussed. The health of the family can be proportional to the degree of cheerfulness during meals. These recipes, if used, can contribute to graciousness because as nutrition is improved, quarreling, bickering, irritabilities, and anxieties brought on by malnutrition quickly disappear. Co-operativeness and cheerfulness surge forward.

This book is not intended to be merely a cookbook. A cookbook has as its sole purpose showing how delicious foods may be prepared; my purpose is to help build health through applied nutrition which, if successfully applied, makes good cooking a necessity. Although the size of this book does not permit nutrition to be dealt with fully, I have tried to give the fundamentals of nutrition as they apply to cookery.

To get the greatest value out of this book, you should treat it with disrespect; mark the recipes used and any ingredients varied, and add your comments. I want you thus to avoid monotonous menus and to become acquainted with many nutritious foods by trying each recipe in the book.

I urge that your goal as an intelligent person be to see that the food you eat daily supplies as a necessity the ideal amounts of each vitamin, each mineral, and each of the many other body requirements; that, with the exception of calories, you strive to obtain as a luxury as much more of each requirement as you can. The nutritive needs of the body are many, and several requirements are most difficult to obtain from the American diet. I believe that these recipes, designed to build health, will help meet such needs.

Although we live in an era of vitamin capsules and mineral tablets, good health must still come from good cooking.

## CHAPTER 2

## EXPAND YOUR FOOD HORIZONS

Food serves a threefold purpose: to bring delight to the senses of taste, smell, and sight; to produce health; and to provide opportunity for artistic expression. Music serves but one purpose, to delight the sense of hearing; and art, the sense of sight. Totally aside from the health-building value of foods, life is made rich by a discriminating and highly developed sense of taste as well as by an appreciation of Beethoven and Rodin.

Consider your own favorite foods, and contrast the pleasure you derive with that of a person who enjoys only meat, bread, potatoes, and pie. Is he not missing a great deal? One usually assumes that an unfamiliar food will be disliked; yet hundreds of such foods would be enjoyed immediately. Examples are the delightful Chinese vegetables, such as leeks, cabbage, mustard, and celery, each of which is sweeter, more delicious, and more tender than our corresponding varieties, yet tasting much the same. Lettuce, our favorite leafy vegetable, was given us by China. There is a fifty-fifty chance that you will enjoy any new food. Do not rob yourself by being afraid to widen your food horizons. Set out to cultivate a taste for all good foods.

If a flavor is entirely new, it may not be enjoyed until the food has been tasted several times. Every food you now enjoy was once new and strange to you; the eleventh olive did the trick. One learns to enjoy food only by eating it.

Any new food may be introduced pleasantly by a few Golden Rules: combine it with a familiar food; make this strange food particularly appetizing by using favorite seasonings; serve tiny amounts, minced to distribute the flavor, until the new taste becomes familiar; increase the amounts gradually but keep the servings small until the flavor is enjoyed; disguise a particularly disliked food beyond all possible recognition and give it the name of a

11

similar food which is enjoyed; if the food is especially important in building health, persist with a sort of geological time-sense even though you must hide it a hundred times; and probably the most important, maintain the silence of the moon. You can always win the game if you play it well; you can no more win it by force than you can thus win respect or love.

Let us suppose you are introducing mustard or similar greens; a few tender leaves are finely shredded and added to a favorite salad; a few leaves may be cooked with chopped parsley and spinach and seasoned with diced bacon and minced garlic. An unpopular root vegetable can be chopped and added to a soup, stew, or soufflé. If a fruit such as the guava is being introduced, a single chopped guava may be added to a fruit gelatin or cocktail. If brain is disliked, it may be steamed, chopped with large amounts of parsley and mixed herbs, called "deviled eggs," and added to soufflés, stuffed peppers, tossed salads, or any number of dishes. Yogurt may be beaten with an eggbeater and served as "buttermilk." Should you wish to emphasize black molasses, the family's taste might be refreshed by gingerbread or spice cookies; small amounts of molasses may later be used to sweeten caramel milkshakes and caramel custard.

Even after a new food becomes familiar, progress can be instantly ruined if amounts of it are increased too rapidly. The servings should be kept small until larger ones are requested; a clever homemaker gives herself a chance to be flattered by being asked for a second helping. In case a new food, when served alone, is not eaten, it should be prepared with other foods for a while longer.

Let us suppose that a person hates the food being introduced, as many people do liver or brain; unless this food is disguised or hidden and unless silence is maintained, the best recipe in the world will probably not entice him to eat it. Often the hated food has never been tasted; an unpleasant emotional association causes it to be avoided. If the emotional attitude is not overcome, the food may be eaten once under protest and never tasted again. It is far better that a taste be developed gradually and enjoyed for a lifetime. Since no two persons have identical dislikes, each housewife must adjust the amount of any ingredient to that which she can wisely use.

Psychologists say that children are trained in bad food habits and are taught to dislike health-building foods by mothers who use bribery, or the reward-and-punishment system, to persuade the children to eat. These well-meaning mothers, underestimating the intelligence of their children, base their theory on the assumption that health-building foods are disliked and desserts are invariably greeted with enthusiasm. Actually the child may enjoy the juicy roast beef and the buttered baked potato more than the dessert his mother holds as his reward. The minute anything goes wrong, however, he expresses his rebellion against parental control by refusing the meat and vegetables, which he actually wants, and distresses his mother by demanding dessert, which he knows she thinks he wants.

If such a situation continues long, the mother in most cases decides in desperation that the child "will starve if he doesn't eat," and gives him the dessert. Since one comes to enjoy the taste of foods by eating them, the child is actually taught to prefer desserts. Moreover, children quickly adopt the attitudes of their parents. If such a faulty behavior pattern is repeated throughout the years, the health-building foods naturally come to be disliked and desserts are tremendously overemphasized. A mother should realize that a child, like herself, may eat heartily at one meal and little at another; that if only foods which go to make up an adequate diet and to build health are served at each meal and midmeal, and if vitamin D is supplied, the child will probably achieve excellent health with no further effort on the mother's part.

A mother should at least attempt to treat her children as if they were her guests, remembering that guests are not coaxed, bribed, scolded, forced to eat, or sharply corrected for mistakes in table manners. If given a chance, children pick up good manners by imitating their parents. The mother should be quick to praise a child, especially when he eats foods not too well liked. Such praise soon teaches him that attention is gained by eating health-building foods. A mother should no more think of discussing food at the table than she would of discussing sex meal after meal.

Good food habits often become tremendously important during illness. For example, if a half teaspoon of brewers' yeast is put into a quart of milk or fruit juice daily, the amount is insignificant to health even though yeast is perhaps the most nutritious of all known foods. If that amount is gradually increased as the taste comes to be enjoyed, it soon becomes of great value in maintaining health. During a severe illness, the fact that the health-building food is enjoyed can be the determining factor between life and death.

For example, suppose there occurs a severe reaction to sulfa drugs, caused by a lack of B vitamins which are destroyed by these drugs. If yeast, which is like no familiar food in taste, odor, appearance, or texture, has never been tasted and is forced on the ill person, he will probably be unable to retain it; but if the taste is already enjoyed, he will take it in quantities sufficient to ensure a speedy recovery. Similarly, if a child with a severe cold or bronchitis coughs until his body is racked with pain, what could ease his mother's anxieties more quickly than his enjoyment of black molasses, the basis for cough syrups since time began? If the taste had not been developed, he would probably refuse it. In the same way, dozens of outstanding foods are of value during illness.

The greatest single cause of sickness is undoubtedly dislike for health-building foods. The mother determines the food likes and dislikes of her family. If she serves only health-building foods, her family soon come to enjoy these foods most. The reverse is equally true.

Just as the father is responsible for the financial support of the family, so is the mother responsible for their health. She may produce any degree of health she desires.

# CHAPTER 3

## PLAN YOUR MENUS WISELY

If ideal health is to be attained, it is not enough to prepare food so that it be delicious, that little of its nutrients be lost, and that its ingredients offer the greatest health value possible. Your daily menus must supply foods needed to meet your family's vitamin, mineral, and protein requirements; and this food must be distributed throughout the day in such a way as to provide maximum efficiency.

For example, if you wish to feel your best, you cannot afford to go without breakfast, although the meal need not be large. The breakfast found to produce the most buoyant feeling of well-being and the ability to think most clearly is one in which half the calories are supplied by protein and the other half by fat and carbohydrate. The time-honored breakfast chiefly of ham or bacon and eggs has passed its scientific test and come through with blue ribbons.

Experiments have shown that people who omit breakfast or who eat a breakfast supplying too concentrated sweets or supplying no starches and sugars at all suffer from weakness, hunger, foggy thinking, and fatigue throughout the morning. Whether too little or too concentrated carbohydrates are eaten, the resulting symptoms, caused by a decrease in blood sugar, are the same. When no carbohydrate is eaten, the blood sugar falls because there is insufficient stored sugar to replenish it. When too concentrated carbohydrates, such as jam, sugar, or syrup, are eaten, the flow of insulin, which helps to store sugar as glycogen, or body starch, is so stimulated that too much sugar is changed into glycogen, and relatively too little is left in the blood. When a high-protein breakfast containing some carbohydrate is eaten, the flow of insulin is not overstimulated, yet the blood sugar is replenished. For this reason whole-grain cereals, supplying protein and carbohydrate in the form of starch which digests slowly and releases sugar gradually

15

into the blood, are excellent for breakfast.

If you wish to feel your best, eat a breakfast of fruit or fruit juice and cereal or eggs, bacon, or ham, or dark bread and milk. Take little or no sugar with cereals, coffee, or tea. It is well to avoid jam, jelly, honey, sweet rolls, coffee cake, doughnuts, and the usual variety of hotcakes with syrup. If you are willing to deviate from the conventional breakfast pattern, try eating melted cheese on toast when time does not permit preparing other protein foods. Should you prefer to take only fruit juice, at least stir into it a heaping tablespoon of the miracle food, brewers' yeast, which contains more protein than does an egg.

With the exception of box lunches, present-day lunches are usually better planned than other meals. The excellent feature is that lunch is customarily a light meal with egg, cheese, fish, or meat added perhaps to a soup or salad. Like breakfast, lunch must supply protein and some carbohydrate if a feeling of well-being is to be maintained throughout the afternoon. Milk, buttermilk, or yogurt should be drunk, and if dessert is eaten, fruit would be preferable to any other. You women whose husbands and children are gone for the day are usually the worst offenders about omitting lunch. Even if you do not wish to sit down to eat, at least have a glass of milk, perhaps a hard-cooked egg or a piece of cheese and a raw carrot or other fresh vegetable.

Dinners have become far too elaborate. So much food is usually prepared that persons often overeat. Food is frequently left uneaten; it may be used as leftovers at a sacrifice of flavor and nutritive value, but too often it is thrown away. Such a large meal is more expensive than dinner need be. Moreover, when many foods are served, the same ones frequently appear several times in the course of a week; menus become deadly monotonous, especially when the variety of vegetables is limited.

Large dinners require so much time and work to prepare that many women have been driven to the excessive use of a can opener. Too many dirty dishes and cooking utensils accumulate and have to be washed when one is most fatigued and desirous of relaxation. Worse still, both the meal preparation and dishwashing come at the most pleasant time of day when puttering in the garden, visiting with one's children, playing tennis or badminton, or peacefully enjoying the twilight is so inviting that it is unfair to be shut indoors with a hot stove and dirty dishes.

The chief reasons for overelaborate dinners are that too little food is eaten earlier in the day and that popular nutrition education has stressed the serving of meat or a meat substitute, one or two cooked vegetables, a salad, milk, dark bread, and a simple dessert. These excellent recommendations are made in an attempt to influence people to eat foods which meet the needs of the body. As long as this requirement is fulfilled, a person wishing to eat a "dinner" of dark bread and milk or raspberries and yogurt would have the blessings of any nutritionist.

Even if the recommendations of health authorities are followed to the letter, they can be met simply. The meat and cooked vegetables can be combined in the form of a soup, a stew, or a casserole dish; the salad need be nothing more than carrot sticks or fresh pepper strips; raw or canned fruit is ideal for dessert. Moreover, the recommendations are intended to be flexible. Only one cooked vegetable need be served, provided it is green or yellow and is enjoyed sufficiently that fairly large portions will be eaten. Or the cooked vegetables may be waived and larger amounts of nutrients obtained from a salad containing many vegetables. If the other meals are adequate, there is no need of serving a large variety of foods for dinner; strive for variety but get that variety in the course of a day or week.

The pattern for dinner menus might well be as follows: fish or fruit appetizer, fruit or vegetable juice, or soup; meat or meat substitute; one cooked vegetable aside from potato, which need not be served; salad or raw vegetable; milk and dark bread. The dessert, like the appetizer or soup, should be optional. No two foods should be similar in taste, appearance, or composition. For example, dry beans, rice, macaroni, noodles, or corn should not be served with white potatoes, nor should two white vegetables, as turnips and cauliflower, be served together.

Breakfast, lunch, and dinner should supply approximately three-fourths of the food intake for the day. The remaining fourth should be eaten in the form of midmeals, or snacks. Studies have shown that persons who eat between meals are more efficient, think more clearly, have greater endurance and energy, and suffer less from fatigue than those who fail to eat between meals. Since energy is produced from sugar supplied by the blood, the purpose of the snack is to replenish the blood sugar so that energy can be maintained at a high level. The ideal midmeal should contain a small amount of sugar such as that found in fruits, vegetables, or milk, which gives a quick pick-up, and some starch which digests slowly and therefore gives a sustained pick-up. The concentrated sugar of candy bars and soft drinks is likely to overstimulate the flow of insulin, cause a drop in blood sugar, and decrease efficiency. No snack should be so sweet or eaten so late that the appetite for the next meal is ruined.

Fruit and milk are the best snacks for children and women who are at home. Laborers, office workers, teachers, and business people should have snacks which can be slipped into a pocket, purse, or desk drawer; dried fruits, a few nutritious crackers or cookies, nuts, cheese snacks (p. 253), or homemade candy containing powdered milk (p. 550) would be excellent. Cheese and crackers, a warm milk drink, yogurt, or other food supplying calcium which relaxes the nerves and makes for sound sleep, form ideal bedtime snacks.

In planning your menus, try to see the day as a whole. Instead of planning merely a dinner menu, think of dinner as a part of a unit consisting also of breakfast, lunch, and snacks, the sum total of which must, without oversupplying calories, furnish adequate amounts of all vitamins, all minerals, proteins, and other requirements necessary for abundant health. When the foods cannot furnish these needs, then turn to the excellent vitamin and mineral supplements now available. On the days when you cannot work enough citrus juices, tomatoes, or green peppers into the menus to supply adequate vitamin C, supplement those menus with inexpensive vitamin C tablets. Unless you and your family have spent an hour or more in midday summer sunshine, supplement the diet with fish-liver-oil capsules or concentrates furnishing at least 1000 units of vitamin D. Keep these food supplements in an attractive container on the table; consider them part of your daily menus and their cost part of your food budget.

Menu planning often involves a special problem, such as consideration of a member of the family who wishes to reduce. In this case, foods should be prepared principally for the overweight person. Meats should be broiled, roasted, or braised without rich sauces. Skim milk, strained buttermilk, or yogurt prepared from skim milk should be provided. Vegetables should be cooked with little or no fat, and large amounts of raw vegetables, particularly tomatoes, should be served. The other members of the family can add butter and mayonnaise at the table. Food need not be uninteresting merely because it is low in calories. When well-seasoned appetizers, delicious jellied bouillons, soups thick with lean meat and vegetables, attractive gelatin aspics, and perfectly cooked meats are served, one need scarcely be aware that he is eating a low-calorie diet.

Cooking for a very young child involves almost no extra menu planning, provided you customarily serve your family foods which build health. When glandular meats and quick-cooked vegetables are on the menu, part of them can be chopped for the child in a small chopping bowl sold for mincing herbs. If the child's mealtime does not coincide with the preparation of the foods, the meat and vegetables can be quickly frozen in compartments of an ice tray. Such a tray can hold 20 frozen cubes of food, ready to be reheated at a moment's notice or to be carried frozen whenever the child is to be left with its grandmother for the day. Surely no more flagrant violation of the Golden Rule could be found than the practice of feeding a child only overcooked, colorless, tasteless, unappetizing canned vegetables day after day. Use such vegetables when convenience demands but not to the exclusion of all others.

There is no reason why a baby should not be given many nutritious foods which are now considered taboo: foods well seasoned with herbs; salad containing onions and garlic, provided they are minced or chopped; quickly cooked cabbage; or most raw fruits. What foods could be better for cutting teeth than raw carrots, turnips, or green peppers? Yogurt should be introduced early, and black molasses should supply the iron most children lack. Many outstanding pediatricians now recommend that blackstrap molasses be used in the baby's formula instead of refined corn syrup and that several teaspoons of brewers' yeast also be added. Mixing these excellent foods with milk should be continued indefinitely.

Many mothers find it difficult to plan menus for box lunches. Every box lunch should contain some protein food: eggs, meat,

cheese, nuts, or peanut butter. These foods may be used as sandwich fillings; or the hard-cooked eggs, cubes of cheese, slices of
meat, or celery stuffed with peanut butter, cheese, or liver paste
(p. 232) may be taken separately. Milk, buttermilk, yogurt, a
cream soup, or a hot-milk drink should be carried in a thermos
bottle. Fresh vegetables or finger salads (p. 273) should always be
included.

Sandwich fillings should contain 1 or 2 tablespoons each of powdered milk and ground or finely chopped parsley, watercress,
young spinach, or other green leaves. Try chopped watercress,
cream cheese, bits of crisp bacon, and powdered milk; or shredded
spinach, chopped egg, pimento, and powdered milk, each spread
moistened with mayonnaise or fresh milk. Bell peppers and fresh
pimentos make excellent containers and may be filled with cottage
cheese, liver paste, cole slaw, shredded carrot salad, or other salad.

Canned fruits or fruit or vegetable salads can be carried in cottage cheese cartons. Fresh and dried fruits, cheese snacks (p. 253),
nutritious cookies (p. 538), soy nuts (p. 549), peanuts, and canned
juices are all excellent for box lunches. The lunch should also contain food for morning and afternoon midmeals. The overweight person who wishes to avoid sandwiches can have a palatable lunch of
hard-cooked eggs, low-fat cheeses or meats, skim milk and/or
canned juices, raw vegetables, and fresh fruits.

Many ideas concerning menus for guest dinners are about as
obsolete as a feather bed. Often housewives who customarily serve
milk and nutty, full-flavored dark bread feel that when entertaining they must substitute ice water and white bread having little
more taste than mattress stuffing. The amount of butter added to
vegetables, mayonnaise to salads, and cream to desserts is often
doubled or tripled for guest dinners. So much food is served that the
guests have the unpleasant choice of hurting their hostess's feelings
by refusing it or of overeating and becoming uncomfortable. Since
blood is drawn away from the brain to the digestive tract after a
heavy meal, the evening's conversation, despite efforts to the contrary, is often as boring as that following Thanksgiving and Christmas dinners. The build of the guests is usually completely disre-
garded. Persons who hate their obesity have high-calorie foods
forced upon them; they often go home discouraged, thinking that if

they are to reduce, they must refuse all dinner invitations. There is no reason why one should serve more food or higher-calorie food to guests than to the family. A gracious hostess serves at least a few foods which may be eaten generously by overweight guests without fear of gaining. Make it a rule to ask your guests at the end of the main course if they would not prefer eating dessert later. Many women enjoy having unexpected guests take potluck with the family more than other types of entertaining. Why should not all guest dinners be like that? How much more often people could see and enjoy their friends if women would stop feeling that they must be clever, unusual, or fancy about guest dinners! A guest dinner should certainly be colorful, delicious, and nutritious, but every dinner should meet these qualifications.

For large gatherings or late suppers, nothing is more delightful than a Dutch lunch, buffet, or smörgåsbord. The plates of cheeses, cold meats, jellied fish, vegetable aspics, tossed salads, olives, and pickles can be largely prepared in advance, leaving the hostess free to enjoy her guests. The guests have the advantage of being able to choose any food they find enticing and to omit foods they care little for. People who plan men's luncheons and church suppers would do well to substitute a buffet for the waterlogged mashed potatoes, overcooked canned peas, white rolls, and lukewarm meat and gravy so often served on such occasions.

And holiday dinners! How many wives can love their relatives or feel thanksgiving in their hearts or good will toward men when Thanksgivings and Christmases are spent year after year in hours of cooking and dishwashing? The husband of a friend of mine set his firm but considerate foot down after a year or two of scarcely seeing his wife on holidays and declared, "This nonsense has to stop." Since then this couple serves a hot holiday dinner on Thanksgiving and Christmas Eves. Dinner the following day is served as a buffet on attractive paper plates. The husband and wife are now happy, and the guests love it. No longer are they first starved and then stuffed; they simply eat at intervals from the time they walk in the door until they leave.

Other menus which are badly in need of modernizing are those arranged for children's parties, such as the early birthday parties. Children often become ill after such parties, largely because excitement inhibits the flow of digestive juices to such an extent that foods cannot digest. Since fat retards digestion and causes food to be retained in the stomach longer than does either protein or carbohydrate, the refreshments should contain little or no fat. Instead of serving rich cake and ice cream, have a meringue cake with colorful icing, ice milk, sherbet, or an attractive gelatin dessert containing little except water or fruit juices.

Older children should be allowed to prepare their own refreshments as a part of entertaining their guests. The atrocious prepared drinks of sugar, flavoring, and coloring to which water is added have become popular because children can make these drinks themselves. Fruit ades, punches, malted milk, milkshakes, ice creams, and sherbets can easily be prepared by small children. Any number of simple spreads for potato chips, whole-grain crackers, and sandwiches can be made by children with little or no help from an adult. The 4-H Club groups have been outstanding in preparing delicious and nutritious foods. The preparation of wholesome refreshments should be part of the training of other such groups.

During adolescence high-calorie foods are needed, and youngsters' appetites can easily tax the budget for entertaining. Inexpensive but filling foods such as chili beans, whole-wheat macaroni, wieners or pigs in blankets, powdered-milk drinks, and salted soy nuts can be served to advantage. If such food is not provided for informal entertaining, the youngsters often fill up on soft drinks, hamburgers, or other foods none too wholesome. Today when delinquency is a problem of large proportions, entertaining at home can scarcely be overemphasized. Parents must often compete with cocktail bars, roadhouses, and night clubs. And youngsters, now as always, enjoy bringing their friends home when they know delicious food is to be served.

Not only is much of the charm of entertaining built around the deliciousness of the food served, but the charm of everyday living is also enhanced by excellent food. If you modernize your menus, you will certainly enjoy your cooking more; and you can have ample time to see the sunsets and to watch the twilights change into night.

# CHAPTER 4

## DO NOT UNDERESTIMATE SEASONINGS, COLORINGS, AND FLAVORINGS

It is as impossible to be a good cook without knowing and using seasonings as it is to be a good skater without ever having been on skates. The charm of seasonings, flavorings, and colorings lies in the fact that with a mere flick of the fingers, cooking changes from a monotonous routine to a creative art; an uninteresting dish becomes a delightful one; an ordinary cook, a chef par excellence. The more attractive health-building foods are, the more appetizing their aromas, and the more delicious their taste, the more they are enjoyed; thus the use of these substances may determine whether the family is in optimum health or in mediocre health. The cost of seasonings, flavorings, and colorings pays for itself in greater vitality and youthfulness and by saving dental and medical bills. Do not underestimate their health value.

A search of the medical literature reveals no basis for the popular belief that colorings and seasonings, particularly vinegar and condiments, are "bad for you." The acetic acid in vinegar is weak compared with the hydrochloric acid in a healthy stomach; acid is essential before proteins can be digested or alkaline minerals absorbed. Acetic acid is carried in the blood only as a neutral salt, such as sodium acetate; it is eventually used to produce energy. Far from being harmful, vinegar is beneficial.

Vegetable food colorings are as harmless as the proverbial kitten; for example, yellow coloring is sometimes almost pure vitamin A, or carotene; red coloring comes largely from the root of the herb borage. Even salt has been considered harmful; yet people have died on hot days from lack of it. Peppers, although often condemned, are among the richest known sources of vitamin C when fresh. Alarmists threaten with internal blisters all persons who eat black pepper, horseradish, dry mustard, and similar condiments. The entire digestive tract of a healthy person is covered with a protective coating of thick mucus; thus such condiments cannot touch delicate membranes; they reach the blood only as simple sugars, fats, and amino acids. Any seasoning which brings delight to the taste buds is justified unless a physician asks that it be omitted. Since pleasant aromas and delectable flavors stimulate the flow of digestive juices, seasonings are beneficial even in feeding invalids and babies.

Flavorings have health value in that if the amount is doubled, sugar can usually be decreased to half without being noticed. The chief difference between tiny cookies which sell for 80 cents a pound and the cheaper varieties lies in the kind and amount of flavoring used. If peaches are of poor quality, yet too good not to use, their taste can be enhanced by peach flavoring. Do not be discouraged if you find fruit flavorings which are not satisfactory; simply purchase another brand. I have used an orange flavoring, for example, which is atrocious, but have now found a brand more delicious than fresh oranges. Money can be saved by buying flavorings of known quality by the quart. If you wish to prepare food for a queen's taste, buy dried vanilla beans from a druggist and grate them into your desserts.

Add colorings not only to desserts but to any foods which can thus be made enticing. At expensive restaurants you pay dearly for infinitesimal amounts of red coloring in a tomato-juice cocktail, green in split-pea soup, and yellow in chicken à la king. Colorings can improve the appearance of food so much, to say nothing of their contribution to the fun of cooking, that my idea of a careless cook is one who fails to keep herself supplied with them. The trick of adding concentrated colorings to food is to use a medicine dropper, purchased for 5 cents at any drugstore.

If you want to enjoy cooking, get acquainted with all the seasonings available and use each one. The stalk and leaves of celery root, which taste like those of celery, are especially delightful; they may be dried in a slow oven if not needed for immediate use. There are many excellent sauces on the market such as dill, soy, Tabasco, A-1, and Worcestershire. Sweet dill sauce is particularly delicious; don't miss it. I have to restrain myself to keep from adding dill sauce to everything I cook, and I have not found one person who dislikes it. Butter-flavoring added to cooking fats gives the delightful odor, color, and taste of butter. It is largely coloring and butyric acid which occurs naturally in butter and is added commercially to butter and margarine. I use it constantly and would never be without it. Smoke-flavoring enhances beans, lentils, split-pea soup, and many gravies and stews; it may be purchased as a liquid, powder, or salt.

Many delightful seasonings, all of which are available and should be kept on hand, have been listed on pages 28 to 30. Do not overlook cassia buds, which are the buds of the cinnamon tree and taste like red cinnamon candies. Keep freshly ground horseradish in the refrigerator. Buy ground paprika by the pound and use it as a seasoning as well as a garnish; sprinkle it generously on any food you wish to brown without submitting to high heat. Form the habit of using peppercorns rather than commercially ground pepper; they are less hot and the flavor is far more delightful. They must, however, be well crushed. I use twice the amount of peppercorns I have dared to suggest in the recipes. Concentrate on receiving a pepper grinder for Christmas; a good one, though expensive, lasts for generations whereas a cheap one is usually valueless.

For the more sophisticated taste, dry wines are excellent for seasoning; the alcohol they contain evaporates in a few minutes of cooking but the flavor is well retained. Their acid content makes them valuable in tenderizing meat and dissolving calcium from bones. Wine, herb, and cider vinegars are valuable as seasonings. When it is desirable that vinegar be used in cooking and yet no taste of it remain, white, or distilled, vinegar should be used.

Herbs and seeds are almost as essential to good cooking as is salt. Fresh herbs are to dried ones as a fresh rose is to dried petals; grow herbs if you possibly can. Since fresh herbs are not often available, in the recipes I have suggested dried ones, feeling sure that you who have fresh herbs will use them instead. Almost every variety of dried herbs and seeds can be purchased or ordered at any large grocery in packages which cost only 10 cents; the amount in each package is often enough to last 2 years. By adding basil to tomatoes, savory to meat sauces, anise to fish, and thyme to chicken gravy, delightful flavors can be produced. Fresh dill does something indescribable to potato salad, and orégano changes a recipe containing onions and peppers from a mediocre dish to an inspired one. The person who has not tasted eggs scrambled with delicious Chinese garlic, or cheese mixed with caraway seeds, or tiny new potatoes rolled with fresh minced herbs has surely not enjoyed life to its fullest.

Garlic and onions contain a strong germicide, acrolein. Garlic is reported to benefit persons suffering from digestive disturbances and gas formation. Experiments have shown that most mouths are sterile after onions and garlic are chewed; hence eating these foods may be important in preventing tooth decay. Medical journals have given credit to garlic for the fact that digestive diseases, appendicitis, and colitis are almost unknown among Italians. When garlic is cooked gently in foods, acrolein passes into them and the benefits may be obtained without eating garlic itself. In the recipes, therefore, I have used onions and garlic and, because of their outstanding vitamin C content, fresh peppers whenever possible. Anyone who wishes may omit them or any other seasoning suggested.

The substances which give the delightful taste to seasonings are known as aromatic oils. With a few exceptions, they are not true oils but are largely alcohols and similar substances which volatilize, or evaporate, extremely easily. The trick of seasoning food well lies in keeping these oils in the seasoning until they are to be used, and then extracting them in the food without letting them escape. Making coffee and tea are processes of extracting aromatic oils; extracting oils from seasonings is similar and should be done with equal care.

Whole seasonings, like unground coffee, may keep fresh for years. Many of the aromatic oils are lost in grinding. Most ground herbs are as stale as last year's cigar butt; avoid them and purchase the dried, whole leaves. All seasonings should be kept airtight. When they no longer have a delightful odor, discard them and replenish your supply. Just as coffee must be ground before the oils can be extracted, so must peppercorns be crushed; fresh herbs should be minced or mashed; dried ones pulverized; and onions, peppers, and celery should be chopped. Seeds should usually be soaked or simmered. When seasonings are added to hot foods, they must be given time to steep; when added to cold foods, as chives to cottage cheese, a half hour or more should be allowed for the oils to pass into the food.

Since the aromatic oils readily escape, or soak out, onions should not be sliced under water. If one stands between an open door and window, onions can be chopped or ground without a tear. If they are grated or shredded directly into hot foods, the steam carries the acrolein upward and prevents it from reaching the eyes. Onion juice may be obtained by salting slices of onion and scraping off the juice which is drawn out.

When seasonings are cruelly subjected to high temperatures or long cooking, the aromatic oils flee like bunnies before a forest fire. Whenever appetizing odors come from foods during cooking, these oils are being driven off. It is as impossible for them to remain in such foods as for water to remain in a teakettle that has boiled dry. Boiled coffee made when camping is famous for odor but not for taste. Most seasoning should therefore be added to foods during cooking only 10 to 15 minutes before they are done.

The taste for any unfamiliar seasoning, like that of unfamiliar food, music, or art, must be cultivated to be enjoyed. New seasonings should be introduced in extremely small amounts, and these amounts only gradually increased. The purpose of seasoning is to bring out the flavor of the food. Overseasoning is the mark of an amateur; careful seasoning, the mark of an artist. Even if you are a herb-lover, season only one or at most two dishes a meal with herbs.

There is no reason why Americans cannot become as famous for excellent seasoning as are the French, Scandinavians, Italians, and Spanish. The great American gesture of reaching for the salt and pepper before foods are tasted is mute testimony to the need for improvement. Books on etiquette should point out that when the food is well seasoned, this gesture is a direct insult to the person who has prepared it. A chef of a French king is said to have committed suicide when he saw the king reach for salt.

When you learn to use and to enjoy all seasonings, monotony in taste disappears forever. Cooking is a science only up to a certain point; after that it becomes an art. The person who seasons food delightfully and makes it appetizing with enticing aromas and colors is an artist. The means by which you can instantly become an artist in this respect, however, may be stated simply: add only a small amount of seasoning, extract the volatile oils without letting them escape, then taste the food; repeat the process if necessary, and taste again. If you are not delighted, continue until perfection is attained.

### SUMMARY OF FLAVORINGS, COLORINGS, AND SEASONINGS

If you would be a good cook, check over the following list and purchase each item which you do not already have on hand.

**Butter-flavoring.**

**Colorings:** red, yellow, orange, brown, green; medicine droppers to apply them.

**Condiments:** ground horseradish, dry mustard, curry powder, cayenne, paprika, chili pepper; white and black peppercorns.

**Flavorings:** peach, banana, pineapple, strawberry, peppermint, winter-green, rum, brandy; extracts of vanilla, lemon, orange, almond, maple; dry vanilla beans; dry rinds of lemon, orange, and lime.

**Fresh seasonings to be grown in garden:** paprika, cayenne, pimento, bell peppers, chili tepines, large and small chili peppers; garlic, Chinese garlic, chives; red, yellow, and white onions; leeks; green multiplying onions, or shallots; parsley and other fresh herbs; unbleached celery stalks and leaves; celery root for leaves and stalks.

**Ground spices for baking:** ginger, cloves, allspice, cinnamon, nutmeg.

**Herbs especially recommended:** chives, Chinese garlic, mint, burnet, marjoram, dill, basil, savory, rosemary, orégano, bay, thyme, sage; try to have chervil, cumin, tarragon, fennel, costmary, anise, and rose-scented geranium.

**Seeds:** anise, cardamom, cumin, mustard, caraway, celery, coriander, sesame, and poppy.

**Smoke-flavoring:** powder, liquid, or salt.

**Whole peppers, dried:** cayenne, large and small chilis, and chili tepines.

**Whole spices:** preserved or candied ginger; cloves, allspice berries, whole nutmeg, cinnamon stick, cassia buds; whole mixed spices, or pickling spices.

### A GUIDE FOR USING HERBS, SEEDS, AND OTHER SEASONINGS

A teaspoon of minced fresh herbs, measured after mincing, or ⅛ teaspoon of dried herbs, is usually sufficient for four servings of food. Err on the side of adding too little rather than too much.

Be particularly careful to use smaller amounts if you change from long cooking of herbs to short.

Before adding seeds and peppercorns to food, crush them well with a hammer. The trick of crushing peppercorns without having them roll around the kitchen is to wrap them in a piece of paper before hitting them vigorously with a hammer. Mince fresh herbs with the scissors, or mash them thoroughly with the fingertips. Pulverize dried herbs by rolling them between the palms of the hands. Add herbs and seeds to cooked foods 10 minutes before serving; to uncooked foods, a half hour. Peppercorns and whole cloves should be steeped longer than other seasonings; their oils volatilize less readily. The following foods are usually considered to be made delicious by addition of the herbs, seeds, or other seasonings suggested.

**Beef:** savory, basil, marjoram, rosemary; orégano if tomatoes and fresh peppers are also used.

**Bread:** butter-flavoring; poppy, cardamom, anise, caraway, sesame, and cumin seeds; mix in the dough or moisten top of loaf and press seeds into it; rosemary, parsley, and other herbs may be added to biscuits and muffins.

**Butter-flavoring:** add to shortening to be used in making breads, cakes, pastry, and cream sauce, or for sautéing or French frying; measure accurately with a medicine dropper 10 drops of butter-flavoring to 1 cup of oil or soft, warmed shortening; beat into shortening with an eggbeater.

**Capers:** fish, fish cocktails, lamb, mutton, cold tongue, heart; potato salad, tossed salads.

**Cheese, American:** fresh basil, chives, sage, caraway seeds, dill stalk or dill sauce; add to shredded or grated cheese, moistened to make a paste.

**Cheese, cottage:** Chinese garlic, chives, fresh basil, dill, parsley, burnet; caraway seeds; multiplying onions, or shallots.

**Cheese, Swiss:** cumin, caraway, sesame, dill, or cardamom seeds; dill sauce; basil, chives, or sage for spreads.

**Chicken gravy and stuffing:** savory, tarragon, basil, chives, thyme, marjoram, parsley, sage, or rosemary for gravy; all except chives, basil, and tarragon for stuffing.

**Cookies:** anise, cumin, caraway, poppy, sesame, and cardamom seeds.

**Eggs:** Chinese garlic, capers, chives, basil, savory, tarragon, thyme, multiplying-onion tops, or dill sauce; if dried herbs are used, they should be added to the milk to be used in preparing scrambled eggs or omelets or to the mayonnaise used in preparing deviled eggs.

**Fish:** capers, fresh fennel, marjoram, thyme, basil, fresh dill or dill sauce; crushed fennel, dill, or anise seeds.

**Fruit:** rose or mint geranium added to applesauce and discarded after steeping; fresh fennel, mint, and lemon balm for fruit salads; cumin, caraway, or anise seeds in applesauce; caraway seeds served with raw apples.

**Italian dishes:** savory, orégano, basil, rosemary, marjoram, thyme, bay; cumin seeds.

**Lamb gravy, sauces, and stuffing:** capers, rosemary, savory, chervil, marjoram, fresh dill or dill sauce, mint for sauce.

**Pork gravy and stuffing:** savory, basil, sage, thyme, chives, Chinese garlic, multiplying-onion tops, parsley; smoke-flavoring for gravy.

**Potato salad:** fresh dill, dill seeds, dill sauce, caraway seeds, capers.

**Rabbit gravy and stuffing:** capers, savory, basil, thyme, marjoram, parsley, chives.

**Soups and stews:** savory, thyme, basil, marjoram, rosemary, chervil, orégano, parsley; grated lemon rind; smoke-flavoring for bean, lentil, and split-pea soups; anise, fennel, and dill seeds for fish bisques.

**Spanish dishes:** orégano and marjoram; fresh large and small chilis; chili tepines; cumin and coriander seeds.

**Veal gravy and stuffing:** marjoram, savory, rosemary, basil.

**Vegetable-juice cocktails:** basil, marjoram, orégano, tarragon, thyme, savory, chives, Chinese garlic, multiplying-onion tops, parsley.

**Vegetables, cooked:** fresh dill with potato salad; a tiny amount of mint with peas, carrots, or new potatoes; chives with potatoes, string beans, and steamed celery root; basil with tomatoes prepared in any manner; orégano with dried beans, lentils, and vegetable dishes with onions and peppers as seasoning; mustard seed with green beans; curry powder or smoke-flavoring with lentils or soybeans; basil or savory with zucchini and summer squash; smoke-flavoring with beans and dry peas.

**Vegetable salad:** every variety of seed or fresh herb may be added to salad vegetables; dried herbs should be steeped in vinegar to be used for salad dressings.

This guide should be merely a beginning. Develop your own specialties by sprinkling bits of any herbs or seeds into any soup, salad, sauce, or gravy; then use combinations of herbs and seeds. It is this zeal for adventure which makes cooking a creative art.

# CHAPTER 5

## EQUIP YOUR KITCHEN FOR HEALTH

The health of your family can depend on such "insignificant" items as 10-cent pieces of kitchen equipment. For example, copper destroys vitamin C the instant it comes in contact with it; yet copper is exposed at the surface of almost all kitchen spoons, knives, peelers, colanders, shredders, eggbeaters, chipped enamel utensils, iron frying pans, iron Dutch ovens, and many other pieces of equipment which are not well tinned, chrome-plated, or made of stainless steel, glass, or aluminum. Most of the vitamin C in raw foods and often all of this vitamin in cooked food is destroyed when housewives use copper-containing equipment. If a woman fails to equip her kitchen so that she can prepare fruits and vegetables quickly, these foods soon reach room temperature and much vitamin C is destroyed by oxygen.

The housewife who is careless about the equipment she uses is duplicating in her home the procedure of a scientist in the laboratory when he puts experimental animals on a diet undersupplied in vitamin C. The scientist knows full well that ill-health will be the inevitable result. The lack of vitamin C causes susceptibility to infections and slow recovery from them; it causes bones to break easily, teeth to decay, and any healing to be retarded. Such a deficiency is a causative factor in allergies, pyorrhea, infections of the gums, arthritis, tuberculosis, and any number of other infections. The mother whose kitchen is poorly equipped, therefore, sooner or later produces some form of ill-health in herself, her husband, and her children.

Vitamin C is only one nutrient which most housewives unwittingly destroy. If a mother fails to buy a 10-cent vegetable peeler which would ensure thin parings, she probably removes so much of the iron stored near the surface of many vegetables that she produces anemia in herself and her children. If she prepares foods con-

31

taining vitamin $B_2$, or riboflavin, in glass utensils admitting light which quickly destroys this vitamin during cooking, she can produce defective vision; she may be responsible for grandmother's cataracts. If she fails to purchase utensils with tight-fitting lids, her principal method of cooking vegetables is probably by boiling them. Maybe she drains the cooking water down the sink, thereby throwing away more than half of the minerals and vitamins C, P, and the many B vitamins the food contained. By her failure to equip her kitchen wisely, she thus produces illness in her family as surely as the scientist produces it in experimental animals.

Regardless of what standard one uses to judge equipment, hundreds of thousands of housewives whose budgets are not limited have poorly and meagerly equipped kitchens. In thousands of these same kitchens there are beautiful ranges which cost perhaps two hundred dollars or more. With the most expensive range available and poor equipment, nutritive value of foods is destroyed or thrown away and ill-health results. With the cheapest range sold and good equipment, most of the nutrients in foods may be saved and health improved and maintained. The combination of expensive ranges and meager and worse-than-valueless equipment tells its pitiful story of lack of health education; of unsatisfied psychological cravings for recognition which drive one to great expense to keep up with the Joneses. It is understandable that 40 per cent of the young men of America, at the very height of their physical development, were found during World War II to be physically unfit, even though extremely low standards were used to judge their health.

Excellent pieces of equipment are usually thought of as labor-saving devices. Even in this respect equipment has health value aside from preventing fatigue. If the work of cooking tires the person who prepares the meal, she probably does not feel like making the few seconds of effort needed to add a drop of coloring or a pinch of herbs, or to grind fresh peppercorns which could give the food an appetizing appearance, a delectable taste, and a delightful aroma. Unattractive foods which have neither a delicious taste nor an appetizing aroma are not eaten in quantities needed to maintain health, even though they are rich in nutrients.

Of all kitchen equipment, thermometers probably save the most time, energy, and food and add the greatest satisfaction to cooking.

A number of home economists and friends who read this book in manuscript have insisted that I was making a mistake in recommending thermometers. "You simply don't understand," they explained patiently, "that average housewives won't use thermometers. They're too dumb." This remark makes me see red. I'm an average housewife and you probably are. And we certainly are not too dumb to read numbers between 10 and 400. If we do lack intelligence, that is all the more reason why we should cook with thermometers. One has to be an intelligent person to be a good cook by the old guess-and-hope methods, but thermometers take the guesswork out of cooking. As for women refusing to use them, have you heard of women once accustomed to an oven thermostat, which approximates a thermometer, refusing to use it? Although two of my thermometers cost 30 cents each and the most expensive one only $1.39, I would part with my silver before I would with my thermometers. I predict that you will feel the same after you have used them.

Check the accuracy of your thermometers occasionally by putting them into boiling water. If they do not register 212° F. or whatever the boiling point is at the altitude at which you live, make your corrections accordingly. For example, my oven thermometer registers the boiling point at 202° F., which is 10 degrees too low; when I wish the oven temperature to be 325° F., I know this thermometer will register 315° F.

Thermometers and other good equipment can help you prepare meals with minimum nutritive loss and minimum effort, with maximum pleasure and maximum flavor. If your budget is limited, buy one or two items each week. Much excellent equipment costs little. Take justified pride in having your kitchen equipped for health Look upon your kitchen as your workshop or your chemical laboratory where the health of your family is largely determined.

The use of many items in the list of equipment which follows will become clear as the book is read and used. I have tried to list essentials rather than all equipment which might be convenient. Make a shopping list of the items you can use but do not have. Discard the articles destructive to your family's health and replace them with safe equipment.

**Alarm clock:** keep where conveniently seen from the range; use the alarm whenever cooking should be timed.

**Apple corer:** well tinned.

**Baking dishes and casseroles:** heat-resistant so that it can be used over the direct heat; attractive enough to be used for serving; unbreakable so that chilled foods can be put into extremely hot utensils; aluminum alloys are most satisfactory; terra cotta breaks easily; glass may "explode" and fly in every direction.

**Baking sheets, or cookie sheets:** 2 or more different sizes; those used for broiling vegetables and baking yeast breads may be wiped with paper towels instead of washed; use for trays and general carrying; cover with napkins and use for buffet suppers if needed.

**Bean slicer and stringer.**

**Biscuit and cookie cutters:** fancy cutters for cookies and candies for children; large cutters with handles removed and bent into oblong shape for poaching eggs.

**Bread knife:** sawtooth, sharp.

**Bread pans:** 1 muffin pan; 1 biscuit pan; pans for baking yeast breads with a minimum of crust.

**Brushes:** 1 or 2 for cleaning vegetables; 1 for cleaning cooking utensils; 1 steel brush, long prongs, for cleaning cooking utensils; 1 brush or mop for washing dishes.

**Butter paper such as butchers use:** cheaper than wax paper; keep open on working surface in attractive container sold for facial tissue.

**Cake-cooling racks:** 2 or more; use for cooking meats; select size to fit into pans used for Swiss steak and pot roast.

**Canisters:** loose lids like those of cookie jars but not admitting light; have a variety of sizes; square or rectangular ones take the least space; paint them attractively and make them part of your kitchen decorations; keep them at the back of working surface. Have canisters for brewers' yeast, rice polish, wheat germ, and each type of flour used frequently. On purchasing flour, sift it directly into canister.

**Can opener:** rotary variety permanently attached.

**Cardboard-box tops:** from heavy corrugated boxes; keep in reserve for baking fish; use as trays for assembling ingredients.

**Cheese grater:** like a miniature meat grinder.

**Cheese slicer:** of wire for slicing soft cheese.

**Chopping board:** label one side of the breadboard and use for chopping such foods as onions and garlic. Do not wash unnecessarily; water splits wood and dirt gets into cracks; soap stays in pores of wood.

**Chopping bowls:** preferably 1 large and 1 small; one about 6 inches in diameter, sold for chopping herbs, is invaluable if cooking for a baby or an invalid who must have a smooth diet.

**Chopping knives:** chrome-plated, stainless-steel, or plastic blades. Sharpen them frequently on soapstone.

**Cleaver or hatchet:** for chopping bones; a hardwood board which can be mistreated.

**Colander:** aluminum or well tinned; cone-shaped with large wooden mallet usually most satisfactory. Food mill may be used but mashes food too badly to be valuable in making tomato juice and fruit juices.

**Cooking forks:** stainless steel, chrome-plated, or plastic; several sizes. One with 4 or 6 slanting, firm prongs to use for scraping and beating.

**Cooking utensils:** must have tight-fitting lids; of thick lightweight material; must not admit light. Buy at least 2 or more, preferably an entire set designed for "waterless" cooking which distributes heat evenly to sides and lid, thus cooking foods from all directions. Aluminum alloys are preferable and distribute heat much better than does stainless steel. Such utensils pay for themselves in saving fuel, to say nothing of medical bills. Test when possible before buying; heat a flat utensil thoroughly and move until only one edge is over heat; bake a pancake on the edge over heat and another on the edge farthest from heat. If it is a good utensil, both pancakes will brown in the same time. Buy no cooking utensils of iron or enamel; iron contains copper; enamel cracks and exposes copper. The new type of pressure cooker with adjustable lid is excellent for use in high altitudes, for women who must cook foods quickly, and for cooking vegetables, if it is in the hands of a perfectionist with one eye on a stop watch.

**Dipper or ladle:** well tinned, stainless steel, or chrome-plated.

**Double-boiler:** must not admit light; several sizes if used for cooking vegetables; do not wash the bottom unnecessarily. If it is used frequently with hard water, put 1 tablespoon of vinegar in the bottom to prevent deposition of scale.

**Eggbeater:** a double-action variety similar to two eggbeaters put together.

**Electric mixer:** if you have one, keep it in a convenient spot and use all the attachments. Buy new attachments if nickel plating is worn off.

**Flour sifter:** triple-action with 3 layers of wire screening.

**French-frying equipment:** the utensil should not be of iron; preferably of thick but lightweight aluminum; wire basket should be well tinned; utensil shaped like top of double boiler requires least fat.

**French whip:** similar to an eggbeater, but with a handle which goes up and down; excellent for making thickenings, whipping ice cream without removing from tray, and mixing powdered milk and brewers' yeast in liquids.

**Frying pans:** 1 large, preferably of aluminum, with tight-fitting lid; not made of iron or tinned metal; tin wears off quickly; iron pans contain copper and do not distribute heat; clean with absorbent paper; avoid washing whenever possible. Small pans are not needed if a grill is available.

**Garbage pail:** foot lever for opening; rustproof bucket.

**Garbage tray:** perforated; throw away rusty ones which stain the sink.

**Grapefruit and fruit knife:** sawtooth; stainless steel or chrome-plated.

**Grater, shredder, and slicer:** a combined grater, shredder, and slicer; or a set of 4 or an adjustable one called a kraut cutter; well tinned, stainless steel, or chrome-plated.

**Greiser:** a meat-grinder type of utensil for shredding vegetables; 4 different sizes of knives; easily washed; permanently set up. Well worth the investment.

**Grill or griddle:** a "must" in a well-equipped kitchen; made of thick but lightweight aluminum; a tight-fitting dome-shaped lid; must distribute heat evenly; get the reversible variety with one side designed for general frying and sautéing, the other for pan-broiling with depression for collecting fat; use for general frying and for eggs, meat, fish, and fried or sautéed vegetables. Avoid washing whenever possible; clean with soft paper.

**Grinder for peppercorns.**

**Hammer:** for crushing peppercorns, seeds, and whole spices.

**Knife holder:** hang on the wall at the most convenient spot.

**Knife sharpener and soapstone:** use both frequently.

**Knives:** 2 or more paring knives, 1 large butcher knife, 1 medium-sized meat knife, 1 carving knife. All of chrome-plated steel, stainless steel, or plastic. Spend money on these and get varieties which will stay sharp. Keep as sharp as razors.

**Liquefier or blender:** especially valuable if cooking for a baby, an elderly person, and one who must stay on a smooth diet. May be used instead of electric mixer in a small family.

**Measuring cups:** 1 cup measure of glass and another of aluminum with lips for pouring; 1 pint measure; a set for measuring ¼, ⅓, ½, and 1 cup.

**Measuring spoons:** variety with ¼, ½, and 1 teaspoon and 1 tablespoon measures together on ring; hang on inside of deep drawer.

**Meat grinder:** buy type with cutting knives instead of grinding apparatus and with detachable cylinder which opens to allow easy washing. Have grinder permanently attached if possible. Make a nightcap for it of material sold for shower curtains. Keep knives sharp on soapstone. Have 4 or more sizes of knives.

**Meat tenderer:** purchase the variety which has different sizes of cleats on each side of mallet.

**Mixing bowls:** have 4 or 5 sizes, attractive colors, which are fun to use and clean; lips for pouring. Keep conveniently placed.

**Molds:** have a heat-resistant ring mold which can be used for baking; have other molds for gelatin if needed.

**Orange squeezer:** glass, with a large, sharp center; throw away any tin ones.

**Pancake turner:** stainless steel or chrome-plated.

**Paper:** such as toilet paper or other soft paper; hang over working surface; use for cleaning dishes and dirty utensils, draining bacon, crushing peppercorns, etc. Saves expense for paper towels, and incalculable time.

**Paper plates:** use for sifting flour; keep with flour sifter.

**Paper towels:** keep on rack above working surface.

**Pastry brushes:** 1 for general purposes such as brushing pastry sheet, grill used for sautéing, surface of meats, dough, and bread; keep in fat in the refrigerator; 1 for fish, 1 for applying molasses, and 1 for buttering toast. Label each, wrap in soft paper, and keep in refrigerator during hot weather.

**Pie pans:** with levers to loosen crust; of tin or lightweight aluminum which will cool quickly.

**Putty knife:** purchase at a hardware store; use for removing dried meat juices from dripping pans, for general prying and scraping.

**Range:** if you are seriously considering a range, look for one with a broiler compartment with adjustable low-heat unit; one you don't have to stand on your head to look into; a broiler tray which is easy to wash; a broiler door which remains open when the tray is inside. A simmer burner is a "must"; check it before purchasing a range by heating water, taking the temperature, and see that it remains at 180 to 185° F. I have used several ranges which, when turned to the heat marked simmer, have kept water at a rip-roaring boil. Warming oven and/or pilot light which can maintain a heat of 160 to 165° F. Oven equipped with glass door, preferably with a light inside. The clocks, bells, automatic turner-oners, and beautiful enamel have their value, but look for essentials first.

**Refrigerator jars:** glass dishes or wide-mouth glass jars of various sizes; square dishes with flat lids require the least space; metal or glass covers desirable.

**Refrigerator pan, or hydrator:** glass or enamel; must have tight-fitting lid. Tray for refrigerator pan, similar to trays sold with turkey roaster, should stand about ¼ inch above bottom of pan.

**Rolling pin:** do not wash unnecessarily; when rolling dough, fasten wax paper around rolling pin with rubber bands or cover with a child's white stocking.

**Scissors:** at least 2 pairs, 1 large, 1 small; chrome-plated, stainless steel, or well nickeled; bone scissors for dressing fowl or rabbit.

**Scoops:** have 1 for each canister.

**Scraper, or pusher:** rubber or rubber substitute; for cleaning dishes, emptying bowls, and general use.

**Scratch pad with pencil:** hang at a convenient place; use for memoranda and a continuous shopping list.

**Shelf for herbs and spices:** have above working surface, away from heat of range. When possible, keep all seasoning in attractive airtight bottles or tiny jars. Label each and keep in alphabetical order. Half the trick of seasoning foods well is to have the seasonings conveniently placed.

**Spatulas:** have sizes to fit each mixing bowl and use instead of spoons; stainless steel or chrome-plated.

**Spoons:** 2 or 3 wooden ones of different sizes; 1 chrome-plated or stainless steel with open slits for draining; 1 or more stainless-steel spoons for tasting.

**Steel wool:** use instead of a dishcloth for washing cooking utensils; keep on a wire rack for quick drying or dry above pilot light.

**Strainers:** 2 or more sizes; different sizes of wire mesh; discard any not well tinned.

**Thermometers:** 1 meat thermometer; 1 upright oven thermometer; 1 dairy thermometer for making yogurt and/or cottage cheese; 1 cooking thermometer variously spoken of as a jelly, candy, or French-frying thermometer; should be enclosed in unbreakable glass and should register between 10 and 350° F.; should have adjustable clasp to hold thermometer to edge of utensil. Buy these without fail.

**Toothpicks:** hardwood; use when trussing fowl or roast.

**Turkish towels:** old and absorbent, for drying smooth root vegetables.

**Utility bags:** make several sizes; use attractive material sold for shower curtains, not oiled silk; close with drawstrings. Have 1 small for pie dough; 1 slightly larger for yeast dough for rolls; 1 large for melons; 1 long for celery; 2 or 3 for general purposes, such as saving parings for soup; to supplement the hydrator. These bags are easily washed, take no space when empty, can be put into a crowded space in the refrigerator; drawstrings are more flexible than zippers, which rust or break.

**Vegetable peeler:** to ensure thin parings; discard any not well tinned.

**Wax paper and holder:** hang above the working surface.

**Whirling bag:** use for drying leafy vegetables; make of cheesecloth or other thin cloth. About a half yard long and a foot wide. Top open without drawstrings.

**Wire pastry cutter, or blender.**

**Wire whip or whisks:** for mixing thickenings, gravies, and for general stirring; chrome-plated or stainless steel.

**Wooden salad bowl:** an absolute "must"; do not wash; water splits wood, and soap gets into the pores; clean with soft paper.

The amount of money anyone believes he can afford to spend is usually more closely related to the value he places on the purchase under consideration than to the amount he has. Many a housewife has spent twenty dollars for a dress she did not really need; yet she continues to use a stained 10-cent knife and a dull one at that. Regardless of how much you try to "economize," sooner or later you must spend a certain amount of money in one of two ways: to pay your physician, dentist, and druggist or to buy nutrient-saving equipment. You, as an intelligent homemaker, must choose the way you consider the wiser.

# CHAPTER 6

## ORGANIZE YOUR KITCHEN FOR EFFICIENCY

The speed with which you prepare meals without sacrificing deliciousness or charm of serving depends upon how efficiently you organize your work. Since people are more efficient in pleasant surroundings and women spend much time in the kitchen, thought should be given to making the room attractive.

Planning dinner menus for at least three or four days in advance is essential before anyone can enjoy cooking to the greatest extent or hope to guard the family's health. Making out the menus need take only a few minutes. Jot down meats or meat substitutes, vegetables to be cooked; fill in soups or appetizers, salads or raw vegetables, and add pickles and sauces if desired. Whole-grain breads and milk should be served at each dinner; they need not be listed unless you wish to make fresh bread or a milk drink. Desserts may be added or omitted. A glance will tell you whether the colors and color combinations will be attractive and whether the cooking time will fit your working hours and social plans.

If you have studied nutrition, quickly calculate the fourth-grade arithmetic necessary to make sure that each dinner supplies more than a third of the body requirements estimated to meet the individual needs of each member of your family. Be particularly careful to see that 25 grams of protein or more are supplied for each person; if the needs are not met, adjust your menus accordingly. These few minutes of planning will probably save an hour of worry later.

If the family eats lunch at home, another 5 minutes should go to planning lunch menus. Excellent breakfasts can usually be arranged on the spur of the moment.

Unless you are cooking a roast or similar meat or planning an elaborate dessert, a half hour should be sufficient for preparing dinner. Spend the first minute or two thinking through what you expect to do. Could you shorten any procedure? Use one utensil less?

40

Cut out any unnecessary steps? Put away one utensil or dish as you reach for another?

Perhaps the most efficient method of preparing dinner is to prepare the meat or meat substitute first; then set the table, check the flower arrangement, and put out but do not uncover the bread and butter; next prepare the appetizer or soup in case either is to be served, and combine the salad, putting it into the refrigerator until time to toss it or add dressing. Unless a utensil is greasy, wash it as soon as you have finished using it. Only when the family have gathered should most vegetables be put on to cook. Preparing a meal need be no more difficult than that. A delightful meal can be prepared in so short a time, however, only when the kitchen work is organized efficiently.

The trick of preparing meals quickly is to save time by having foods ready in advance. A business firm would not consider allowing small tasks to be done each day if they could be combined and time saved. Washing vegetables just before using them, for example, wastes hours in the course of a single month. Since housewives often market only once or twice a week, time should be set aside after coming from market for washing vegetables and for preparing foods when such work can be done in advance. Market whenever possible in the morning when the produce is still fresh. If you are working throughout the day, the advance preparation may be done in the evening. The following list is made up of suggestions only, many of which will not be clear until the remainder of the book is read.

> Pick over and wash vegetables; wipe or whirl dry; store in covered refrigerator pan; wash and/or store fruits.
>
> Make soup stock (p. 309) or vegetable-cooking water (p. 328); prepare hard-cooked eggs in such stock.
>
> Blend butter-flavoring with cooking fat or oil (p. 29).
>
> Mix yeast bread, rolls, or waffles (p. 423).
>
> Grate cheese; grind parsley and other greens; grind bread crumbs.
>
> Sharpen knives; fill salt shakers.
>
> Prepare salad-seasoned vinegar (p. 293), French dressing, mayonnaise (p. 294), and sauces (p. 160); prepare

cream sauce; set gelatin salads or aspics (p. 285); cook
and marinate vegetables to be served cold.

Set yogurt (p. 452).

Tenderize and/or season meats (p. 104).

Cook fish or meats to be served cold, in salads, box
lunches, or aspics (p. 187).

Make sandwich fillings for box lunches.

Study the week's menus and see if any other foods can
be prepared in advance.

By such a program you can make your housework into a whirl
of efficiency with several foods cooking while a gelatin cools and
crumbs are zipped through the meat grinder.

During hot weather much the same routine in miniature may
take place each morning when all foods needed throughout the
day, including snacks and beverages, can be prepared at one
time. Women who use this routine tell me they have cut in half
their working time in the kitchen and that they wish they had
started such a program years sooner.

# CHAPTER 7

## YOU NEED HAVE NO FAILURES
## IN COOKING MEATS

Since meat is the most expensive item on the food budget and since protein deficiencies are widespread, it is more important to know how to cook meat than any other food. Menus are planned around meats or meat substitutes. Should a housewife learn nothing more about cooking than how to prepare meats well, she would know enough to be a passable cook.

The secret of cooking meats successfully is to remember that a high temperature makes proteins tough. This statement explains a thousand cooking failures and is the basis of dozens of household rules. It explains why a milk bottle rinsed first in hot water is difficult to wash; why a blood-stained handkerchief remains stained if put into boiling water; why baking in a hot oven makes a soufflé shrink and toughens an angle-food cake. It explains why eggs fried in smoking fat might be used for vulcanizing tires and why cheese browned under the broiler usually resembles chewing gum. Thousands of dollars' worth of tender, delicious meats have been ruined, many a guileless steer blamed, and many an innocent butcher cursed because housewives have not realized that high temperatures make proteins tough. Meats need not be ruined if one merely glances at a thermometer and controls the heat.

Research in meat cookery has been carried on by the National Live Stock and Meat Board, the United States Department of Agriculture, and the Departments of Home Economics of many state universities. More than 20,000 cuts of meat have been cooked under experimental conditions. Meats have been measured before and after being cooked by different methods, and the percentage of shrinkage has been computed. The escaped juices have been collected and weighed, and the amounts compared. The toughness or tenderness of the cooked meats has been tested by the pounds of force needed to tear the meat fibers. The meats have been tasted by thousands of people whose opinions as to the best flavor and the tenderest and juiciest meat have been pooled and analyzed statistically. The findings of this tremendous amount of research can be summarized in a single sentence: *Meats should be cooked at low temperatures.*

Actually every piece of meat successfully cooked since the legendary shack burned down with a pig in it has been cooked at low temperature. Often, however, the heat has been kept high, and effort, money, and fuel have been wasted to achieve the low temperature. A housewife may fry or broil meat with a high heat, but by turning the meat frequently she may allow one side to cool before it has time to heat through, a useless sort of reducing exercise. Broiling is often done with a high heat and the meat put many inches from it, as wasteful a process as if a furnace were turned on full tilt and the windows opened. Since cold fat conducts heat slowly, people pay high prices for meats streaked with fat which will cook at a low internal temperature even when the cooking temperature is high.

There are many advantages in cooking meats at low temperatures. The least tender cuts may be roasted and served rare, an accomplishment formerly thought to be impossible. There is no danger of meat burning or becoming tough. Meats cook evenly throughout with the same degree of rareness or doneness from surface to center; when high temperatures are used, the outside may be burned while the inside is raw. At low temperatures meats shrink little and are more attractive; they are juicier and more delicious. Studies have shown that the fuel consumption is less during several hours of low-temperature cooking than during an hour of cooking at high temperature; thus money is saved. Since the meats need little watching when cooked at low temperatures, almost no work is involved; the method, therefore, allows social advantages.

The principles of meat cookery are clear when you understand that lean meat is muscle tissue. Muscles are made of long fibers such as those seen in the stringy meat of overcooked stew. In raw meat, the protein in the fibers is delicate and soft, like the proteins in a raw egg. Since muscles must be strong, the soft fibers are given strength, held together, and bound into bundles by a tough yet elastic substance known as connective tissue from which gelatin is made. Although the sheets of connective tissue are thin in tender cuts of meat, in meats sold for soup they are so thick that they look like strips of tough gelatin, or gristle. The meat juices, containing flavor, vitamins, and minerals, are held in and around the muscle fibers by these sheets of connective tissue. A bundle of muscle fibers, therefore, is somewhat like fresh, moist stems of a corsage of violets held together by Scotch tape.

When meat is cooked at low temperatures, the proteins of the muscle fibers, like those of a gently cooked egg, merely become firm. The sheets of connective tissue, which keep the meat from being tender, gradually soften. The softening is brought about because some of the connective tissue when heated changes to gelatin. Since tender meats contain little connective tissue, they need to be cooked only a short time. The less tender cuts, which contain much connective tissue, must be cooked slowly for a long time so that the connective tissue will have time to soften. When meat has been cooked to doneness at low temperature, the softened connective tissue continues to hold the meat fibers together so that the meat slices evenly without tearing apart; it continues to hold the juices, flavor, and nutritive value in the meat; the meat is therefore juicy and its flavor delicious.

When meats are cooked at high temperatures, the heat causes the proteins to contract, shrivel, and become hard, dry, and tough. The effect of heat is usually seen when bacon is fried until crisp. The protein, or lean part, may contract until the fat is gathered into a ruffle; the lean meat is so hard and dry that if it were thick, it would not be edible. The high temperature causes the connective tissue surrounding the meat fibers to break down and split; part of it changes completely to liquid gelatin. The contracting proteins act like a hand squeezing water from a sponge; they squeeze the delicious meat juices through the holes split by the heat in the sheets of connective tissue. If you ever attempted to brown ground meat, you probably noticed this squeezing process. Heat penetrates such tiny pieces of meat almost immediately. You found that the more you tried to brown the meat, or the higher the temperature you used, the more the juices poured out, the tougher the meat became, and the more stubbornly it refused to brown.

These processes are less noticeable when you cook large cuts of meat, because heat penetrates them gradually. The same changes nevertheless take place whenever meat is heated to high temperature. As the proteins contract and juices are squeezed out, the meat shrinks. A large attractive cut which you thought would be enough to serve six or eight people may become small, shriveled, ugly, and may be scarcely enough to serve four persons. When meats are broiled or roasted, telltale juices in the dripping pan show the unnecessary dryness of the meat and the loss of flavor and nutritive value. When meats are fried, the temperature is often so high that spilled juices evaporate immediately and cannot be noticed.

Everyone agrees that well-cooked meat should be delightfully tender. It is equally important, however, that the connective tissue should remain firm. Only then are juices and flavor held in the meat. Whenever connective tissue is allowed to break, the meat becomes less delicious and will not slice evenly without pulling apart.

In cooking meats, you must keep two temperatures clearly in mind: the temperature inside the meat, or the internal temperature; and the temperature outside the meat used for cooking it. The inside temperature can be known only by using a meat thermometer. The outside temperature, or the cooking temperature, usually ranges between 185° F., or that of simmering water used for stewing and steaming, to 350° F., sometimes used for broiling and roasting. How long it takes the inside of the meat to heat depends on how high the cooking temperature is, how large the cut is, and what kind of heat is used. The moist heat of water or steam penetrates meat twice as quickly as the dry heat of the oven or broiler at the same temperature.

Think of the connective tissue throughout meat as being tough gelatin, and of cooking meat as a process of softening such gelatin. If you put a set gelatin into a warm oven, it becomes softer. How quickly it becomes soft depends on how large and tough it is and how warm the oven is. If left in a warm oven for a certain time, it will become soft throughout without becoming liquid. If put into a hot oven, it will become liquid quickly. In cooking meat, the "gelatin" must be softened without being allowed to change to liquid.

Like a gelatin, the connective tissue throughout meat softens as heat penetrates the inside of the cut. Little softening occurs until the internal temperature reaches 120° F. The longer meat cooks, the more tender it becomes even at this low internal temperature. If the heat outside the meat is increased, tenderness can be developed more rapidly. The catch in heating meat quickly is that the connective tissue near the surface heats first and breaks down before that in the center has had time to become tender. The change to gelatin is slow at first, but juices are lost rapidly after the temperature reaches 170° F., the point at which proteins start to become tough. If you want meats to be juicy, tender, and delicious, to shrink as little as possible, and to slice as well as commercially cooked ham, you must give the connective tissue sufficient time to become tender largely between the internal temperatures of 120 and 160° F. The entire trick of roasting, broiling, pan-broiling, and sautéing, or the so-called dry-heat methods of cooking meats, lies in maintaining this range of temperature inside the meat until it becomes tender.

When meats are ground, the cut connective tissue does not need to be softened by heat. If it is not to become tough and dried out, such meat should be allowed to heat only to 170° F. or less. Unless ground meat is packed into a firm loaf, as in meat loaf, heat penetrates it especially rapidly. Ground meat added to boiling soup, for example, is cooked well done in less than a minute. Pounding meat breaks down part of the connective tissue and softens the remaining part. A well-pounded but less tender cut should be cooked as if it were a tender one containing little connective tissue. Such meats, therefore, should be cooked for a relatively short time even at low temperature.

If the external and internal temperatures at which meats are cooked are known and controlled so that the meats can become delightfully tender without reaching the point where connective tissue breaks down and proteins become tough, one need have no failures in cooking meat. These temperatures, therefore, should be carefully checked with thermometers whenever possible. During one's lifetime, inexpensive thermometers can save hundreds of dollars' worth of meats. The use of thermometers changes hit-and-miss methods into exact ones; it puts the amateur on a par with the experienced cook. To prepare meats by methods handed down from

one's great-great-grandmother is comparable to cooking as she did
on an open hearth.

## KEEP THE JUICES IN THE MEAT

Even if meats are cooked carefully at low temperatures, juices
may be drawn out in other ways. Just as salt in a shaker attracts
water during rainy weather, salt sprinkled on the surface of meat
draws out juices. Several days after meat is salted, the salt has not
penetrated it more than half an inch. There are no empty spaces
inside meat or forces to push salt into it; therefore unless meat is
soaked in brine for a long period, as is corned beef, salt cannot season the interior of the cut. Moreover, all meat juices are salty
because the animal from which meat came had to eat salt to live.
If the juices are drawn out, the meat is robbed not only of moisture
and flavor but also of salt. It tastes so flat that much salt must be
added to make it palatable. In making stew or frying chicken, it is
desirable to draw out juices by adding salt to give flavor to the
gravy or browned crust. Although salt is necessary to health and
generous amounts should be eaten, meat should be salted only at
the table if juiciness and delicious flavor are desired. Many cookbooks state that salting meat brings out its flavor. How right they
are! Salt brings it out into the dripping pan.

Seasonings other than salt do not bring out juices, but their
aromatic oils are largely lost if the meat is to be cooked a long time.
Seasonings cannot penetrate meat any more than can salt. The
flavor of garlic slipped into meat is not distributed, and someone
invariably gets the garlic in his mouth, to his disgust. Onions, peppers, and celery quickly overcook and their flavor becomes stale.
When seasonings are added shortly before serving, the freshness of
a spring garden is served with the gravy or sauce. If thin cuts of
meat, to be cooked only a short time, are allowed to stand with the
seasonings until the aromatic oils penetrate the meat, they may be
seasoned before cooking without loss of flavor.

When meats are broiled or roasted, loss of juices through evaporation is often a serious problem. Evaporation may best be prevented by brushing the lean meat carefully with oil or melted fat.
Moisture cannot penetrate a layer of fat. Meat streaked with fat
stays juicy after it is cooked, because melted fat coats the meat

fibers and prevents evaporation. Unless carefully brushed with fat, a flat roast loses more moisture through evaporation than does a cube-shaped one, because much surface is exposed to heat. Tying a roast compactly decreases evaporation. A roast should be set with the fat side up so that melted fat will drip over it as the meat cooks.

Contrary to public opinion, basting dries out meat; it washes off the fat and increases evaporation. If you like to hover lovingly over meat as it cooks, baste it with a pastry brush dipped in melted fat.

The old belief was that juices could be held in by searing, or browning, meat at high temperature. When meat is submitted to high temperature, part of the protein breaks down chemically and develops the delightful "browned-meat" flavor and appetizing color. Far from being held in, juices are spilled as the proteins contract, but they evaporate too quickly to be noticed. Although searing is justified as a means of developing flavor, if you want meat to be delightfully juicy, brown it with the aid of flour, crumbs, molasses, paprika, or sweetened fruit juices which brown easily. Red meat, such as roast beef or broiled steak, does not need to be seared but will brown by the time it is ready to serve.

If you want juices drawn out for soup or gravy, sear the meat and salt it before cooking. If you want the meat to be juicy, sear it very quickly if at all, and salt it just before it is to be eaten.

### COOK YOUR MEATS TO RETAIN MAXIMUM NUTRITIVE VALUE

Both fat and protein of meat supply calories. The principal contribution meat makes to health, however, is the protein of lean meats. The human body is built of protein supplied by foods. The health of the muscles, internal organs, hair, nails, blood cells, antibodies, and hormones, each made of protein, is limited by the kind and amount of protein eaten. An extensive survey made by the United States Department of Agriculture indicates that nine out of every ten Americans suffer from protein deficiencies.

Proteins are not harmed when meats are cooked at low temperatures; at high temperatures, some of the essential amino acids are broken apart by heat, and their health-promoting value is decreased. Overcooking can also harm the proteins. Try not to cook any meat longer than is necessary to make it tender.

Energy production, or every movement of a muscle, whether animal or human, requires the aid of many and perhaps all of the B vitamins. Since meats are muscles, they are therefore rich sources of these vitamins. With the possible exception of folic acid, the anti-pernicious-anemia vitamin, the B vitamins are not harmed even by long cooking at low temperature except at the surface of the meat. Above the boiling point, the destruction of several B vitamins increases in proportion to the temperature.

All the B vitamins and the minerals supplied by meat, iron, copper, and phosphorus, dissolve in water and can be lost if meats are soaked or boiled and the cooking water not used, or if juices are allowed to escape and are not used. Juices which seep from frozen meats during thawing should be saved and added to the gravy. If juices are lost in the broiling pan, they should be used in gravy or added to soup stock. Try to make only the amount of gravy which will probably be eaten at a meal; use leftover gravy in sauces, soups, dressings, and meat loaf.

You can increase the nutritive value of meats containing bone by soaking or cooking them with a little acid, as tomatoes, vinegar, or sour cream. The acid dissolves some of the calcium from the bones into the gravy or sauce. If the cut does not contain bones, purchase bone to cook with any meat to be braised or stewed. A single serving of pickled pigs' feet has been found to supply as much calcium as 3 quarts of milk. Since calcium deficiencies are widespread, it has often been pointed out that more value is sometimes obtained by chewing the bones of fried chicken than by eating the meat. It is unfortunate that culture-vultures frown on such a health-building practice.

When uncooked meat and bones are soaked with a small amount of vinegar for 48 hours, the cooking time is often decreased by a third to a half. The meat, however, must be no thicker than 1 inch, so that the acid can penetrate it. Acid softens connective tissue. Tomatoes, sauerkraut juice, sour cream, blackstrap molasses, and cooking wines may be used, but the acids they contain are less concentrated than is the acetic acid of vinegar. If any trace of vinegar remains, it can be evaporated off before the gravy is made.

The high temperatures used when meats are fried, boiled, or cooked in a pressure cooker are particularly destructive to the health-promoting value of the protein. Moreover, the proteins are toughened before the connective tissue has time to soften. The meat must be overcooked until the proteins change chemically and again become soft; by this time much connective tissue has broken down, juices have been squeezed out, and the meat is usually hard, dry, or stringy. When meats are boiled, so much water is used that both the meat and the gravy lack flavor. If any of the cooking water is discarded, as it often is after ham or tongue is boiled, much of the vitamin and mineral content of the meat is lost.

To fry meat means to cook it in the heat of fat, which can soar quickly to extremely high temperatures. What housewife has not fried bacon which seemed to be progressing well one minute and burned the next? The heat under the frying pan did not suddenly become hotter and burn it. When meats are protected by flour or batter, the high temperatures of hot fat are excellent for browning, but such a method requires continuous attention. Hot fat does not sputter unless moisture is added to it; the inevitable sputtering of frying meat tells that juiciness and flavor are being lost. I wish to make it perfectly clear, however, that I do not imply that fried meats are "hard to digest"; for years I have tried to find what is hard on what, why, and how.

### A 10-MINUTE METHOD FOR LEARNING THE CUTS OF BEEF

Innumerable housewives buy meat year after year, often spending hundreds of dollars, without any conception of why one roast or steak is delicious and another a failure. When they learn the cuts of meat and can tell the approximate age of the animal, such hit-and-miss results can be eliminated.

If you are willing to make yourself utterly ridiculous, you can learn the cuts of meat in a few minutes and forever afterward have a basis for buying and preparing each cut. The trick is more fun when done with others but is usually interrupted by everyone rolling on the floor with laughter. Get down on all fours, imagine you are a steer, try to imitate the movements a steer would make, and notice which muscles you use. The lean meat of the frequently used muscles will have the most flavor; the least used will be most tender.

By now you should be chewing cud, a peaceful exercise but one you persist in. The large muscles in your cheeks may be used for soup meat, hamburgers, or chicken-fried steak. If you wiggle your ears, you find there are muscles attached to them and to the skin of your scalp, used for head cheese. Your brain is little valued but is nevertheless excellent food. Your tongue is a much-used muscle without bone or fat.

You are a curious animal, often turning, lowering, and raising your head; the muscles of your neck will be rich in flavor. Your legs and arms get much use; the muscles of your fore quarters are smaller and cut into less attractive steaks and roasts than those of your hind quarters. You occasionally wiggle the muscles on either side of your backbone to frighten away a fly; certainly they will be tender. The muscles around the rump are used in walking and swishing the tail; they will be flavorsome. In general, the muscles across your back are the most tender, and flavor increases in the order of shoulders, hind legs, front legs, neck, and jaw muscles.

You may now lie down in a shady spot and ponder morbidly over how you will be butchered. You will first be quartered by being cut lengthwise along your backbone and breastbone and crosswise around your waist, the cut slanting in front to well below your ribs. The sections from your hands to elbows and from feet to knees are sold as soup bones. Your elbows and knees, including some of the muscles and bone above them, are your fore and hind shanks. The upper part of your arms, your shoulders, shoulder blades, the first six ribs, and the back of your neck are collectively called the *chuck*, usually sold for pot roasts. The large muscle over your shoulder blade is the *clod*.

Between your shoulder blades and your waist, the large muscles and ribs are usually cut into *roasts*. The ribs may be cut off, leaving a boned *rib roast*, or the meat rolled into a rolled rib roast. If the ribs are tied into a circle giving the appearance of a crown, it becomes a *crown roast*, but if nothing is done to the roast, it is called a *standing rib roast*. The muscles over the last rib at your waist are the most tender; a roast including this rib is spoken of as a *prime rib roast*. The ribs and muscles may be cut into *rib steaks;* if the bones are removed, rib steaks become *Spencer steaks.*

The front of your chest, from your neck to just above your waist and from the cut along your breastbone to your shoulders, is the *brisket*. This cut includes the upper chest bones, the muscles which move your chest in breathing, and other muscles which pull your head grassward; such muscles are rich in connective tissue and flavor. The wall of your upper abdomen and lower chest is a flat, platelike cut known as the *plate*. The ribs under your arms, between the plates and rib roasts, are cut only 5 to 7 inches long and are called *short ribs*, delicious when barbecued.

In the hind quarters, the lower part of your back below your waist is the *loin* section, usually cut into steaks which become larger and slightly less tender as they near the rump. Uppermost are the small *club steaks*. Next are the *T-bones*, which contain short bones protruding from the backbone in semblance to a T. Following the T-bones are the still larger *porterhouse steaks*, named for a certain Mr. Porter who served them frequently years ago in his hotel, or "house," in England. Finally come the large *sirloin steaks*, which include the muscles to the side of the hips. The sirloin steaks nearest the porterhouse steaks are spoken of as the *top sirloin*. The sirloin may be left uncut and cooked as a roast.

The large, frequently used muscles of the buttocks are cut as a *rump roast*, usually boned and rolled. The tail, sold as *oxtail* regardless of the sex of the animal, contains flavorful muscles and much cartilage; it surpasses other cuts for making delicious soup.

The muscular wall of the abdomen is the *flank*. It is a thin layer of flavorful muscles with fibers running lengthwise. The flank may be cut into steaks or rolled as a roast.

Surrounding the thigh bones are round clumps of muscles customarily cut into steaks known as the *upper*, or *top*, *rounds*, the *middle rounds*, and the *bottom rounds*. These well-exercised muscles are usually prepared as Swiss steaks or chicken-fried steaks. Between the bottom round and the hind shank is the heel of the round which contains so much connective tissue that it is customarily used for stews. The round steaks become progressively smaller and less tender as they near the shank.

A muscle which must contract before you can lean forward runs along the inside of the backbone. Since steers infrequently bend their backs into semicircles, this muscle is tender regardless of the animal's age. It may be sliced directly across the grain into a small steak known as a *filet mignon;* filet means boneless and mignon means delicate, lovable, and pleasing. In case this delicate, lovable, boneless pleasure is cut diagonally, larger steaks result known as *New York cuts.* The term New York cut, however, is sometimes used to refer to a top sirloin or a boned porterhouse steak.

You have now learned the cuts of beef. Has it taken 10 minutes?

If you cannot remember the name of a cut, look at the size and shape of the muscles and bones. Where in your body are bones and muscles of comparable shape? A cut with a small round bone must be a leg. A rib you readily recognize. Large chunks of muscles and flat bones must be shoulder or rump. It is easy, once you think about it.

When the cuts of beef are known, cuts of other meat are easily learned. Veal is cut into *fore shank, breast, shoulder, rib, loin,* and *round.* The shoulder may be sold as *roasts* or *blade* and *arm steaks;* the rib section, as *roasts* or *rib steaks.* The loin is cut into *kidney chops,* followed by *loin chops,* and lastly, *sirloin steaks. Veal cutlets* are sliced from the thighs and are comparable to the round steaks of beef. The breast includes the entire under part of the body, the chest bones and muscles and the abdominal wall; it may be rolled as a roast or cut into riblets, stew meat including the riblets, or ground meat for veal patties. In other respects the cuts are similar to those of beef.

Lamb is cut in the same manner as veal. The rib section along the backbone, comparable to the rib roasts of beef, is known as the *rack.* Both the rack and loin may be sold as roasts or cut into chops. The thigh, or *leg of lamb,* includes the rump; although it is usually left whole, it may be cut as small roasts and steaks. Mutton cuts are similar to those of lamb and veal.

People in general are familiar with the cuts of pork. The shoulder and fore leg may be cut together and sold as a *fresh pork roast* or cured as a *picnic ham.* The ribs and loin section are sold as *fresh pork roasts* or *pork chops.* The *spareribs* include all the chest bones of the under part of the body. The abdominal walls are cured as *bacon* or *salt pork.* The muscle along the inside of the backbone, comparable to the filet mignon of beef, is the *tenderloin;* when cured, it becomes *Canadian bacon. Ham* includes muscles of the rump and the pelvic bones at the larger, or butt, end; the smaller,

# STANDARD LAMB CUTS

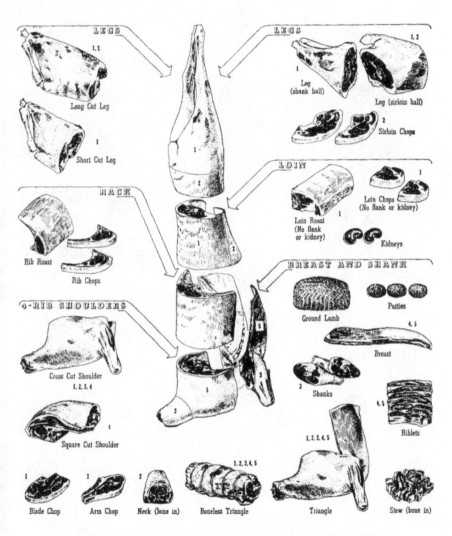

PRIMAL (WHOLESALE) LAMB CUTS AND THE RETAIL CUTS MADE FROM EACH

# STANDARD VEAL CUTS

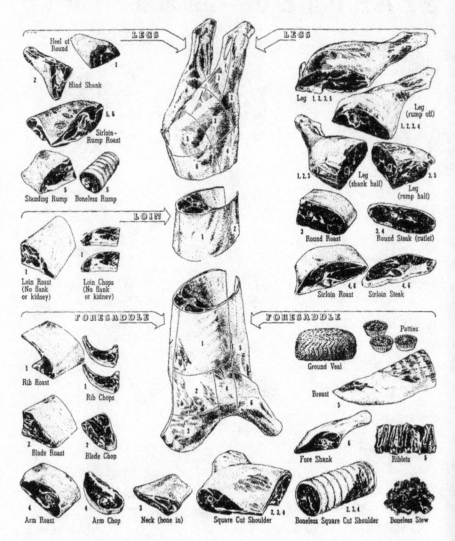

Heel of Round · Hind Shank · Sirloin-Rump Roast · Standing Rump · Boneless Rump

LEGS · LEGS

Leg 1, 2, 3, 5 · Leg (rump off) 1, 2, 3, 4 · Leg (shank half) 1, 2, 3 · Leg (rump half) 3, 5 · Round Roast · Round Steak (cutlet) 2, 4 · Sirloin Roast 4, 6 · Sirloin Steak 4, 6

LOIN

Loin Roast (No flank or kidney) · Loin Chops (No flank or kidney)

FORESADDLE · FORESADDLE

Rib Roast · Rib Chops · Blade Roast · Blade Chop · Arm Roast · Arm Chop · Neck (bone in) · Square Cut Shoulder 2, 3, 4 · Boneless Square Cut Shoulder 2, 3, 4 · Boneless Stew · Ground Veal · Patties · Breast · Fore Shank · Riblets

PRIMAL (WHOLESALE) VEAL CUTS AND THE RETAIL CUTS MADE FROM EACH

# STANDARD BEEF CUTS

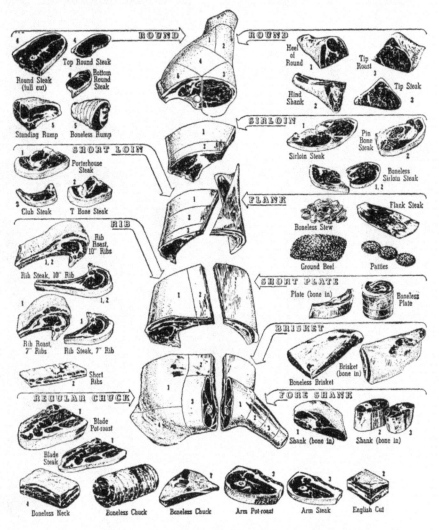

PRIMAL (WHOLESALE) BEEF CUTS AND THE RETAIL CUTS MADE FROM EACH

# STANDARD PORK CUTS

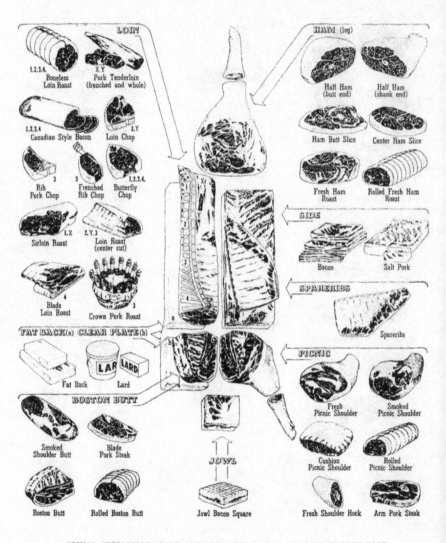

**LOIN**

1.2.3.4. Boneless Loin Roast
X.Y Pork Tenderloin (trenched and whole)

1.2.3.4 Canadian Style Bacon
2.Y Loin Chop

3 Rib Pork Chop
3 Frenched Rib Chop
1.2.3.4. Butterfly Chop

1.X Sirloin Roast
2.Y.3 Loin Roast (center cut)

4 Blade Loin Roast
3 Crown Pork Roast

**FAT BACK (a) CLEAR PLATE (b)**

Fat Back
Lard

**BOSTON BUTT**

Smoked Shoulder Butt
Blade Pork Steak

Boston Butt
Rolled Boston Butt

**JOWL**

Jowl Bacon Square

**HAM (leg)**

Half Ham (butt end)
Half Ham (shank end)

Ham Butt Slice
Center Ham Slice

Fresh Ham Roast
Rolled Fresh Ham Roast

**SIDE**

Bacon
Salt Pork

**SPARERIBS**

Spareribs

**PICNIC**

Fresh Picnic Shoulder
Smoked Picnic Shoulder

Cushion Picnic Shoulder
Rolled Picnic Shoulder

Fresh Shoulder Hock
Arm Pork Steak

PRIMAL (WHOLESALE) PORK CUTS AND THE RETAIL CUTS MADE FROM EACH or shank, end includes the large bones and cartilage of the knee joint.

### HOW TO DETERMINE THE TENDERNESS, FLAVOR, AND JUICINESS OF MEAT BEFORE BUYING IT

When you buy meat, you have a definite flavor in mind which you want it to have after it is cooked. Certainly you want it to be tender and juicy. You can easily learn to tell the tenderness, flavor, and juiciness of meat merely by looking at it provided you have some idea of the age of the animal from which it came.

In general, tender meats are muscles which have been used little because life was short or used little during a long life. Tenderness is also determined by the amount of fat throughout the meat. Fat is deposited in the connective tissue and divides it into thin sheets as it is in tender meats. Meats streaked with fat can be depended upon to be tender. The lack of fat allows very lean veal and other meats to be quite tough, even though the muscle has been used during a short life.

Little-used muscles or meat from young animals have a milder and more delicate flavor than frequently used muscles or meat from older animals. Tender beef from a young steer, for example, may resemble veal rather than stew meat. The more a muscle is used and the older the animal becomes, the more pronounced is the flavor of the lean meat.

It is the fat which gives the characteristic flavor to the meat of each species. Just as you can disguise tuna as creamed chicken if you wash off the oil and cook it with chicken fat, so you can change the flavor of any meat by removing the fat and preparing the meat with fat of another species. This principle is used in preparing liver with bacon and in cooking mutton chops, trimmed free of fat, with butter or oil. Aside from the flavor of the lean meat, the amount of flavor in any cut of meat is in proportion to the quantity of fat throughout the meat fibers.

. When meats are served hot, much of the so-called juice is actually melted fat. Fat also makes for juiciness by preventing evaporation. The juiciest meats are those from mature young animals and from less frequently used muscles; such meat has high moisture as well as high fat content, hence are the most expensive.

Just as veal differs in color from stew meat, so does all meat vary in color in proportion to age. The meat of a young steer is a light or cherry red; that of an old animal is dark red, or purplish red.

Meat fibers become larger with use. The small fibers of young animals cause a cut surface to have the velvety appearance seen in veal chops. Because of the large fibers of older animals, a cut surface is somewhat rough like that of beef cut for stew.

If you compare veal bones with soup bones, you will notice that they are different in appearance. Relatively few minerals are deposited in the bones of young animals. Such bones contain a large proportion of connective tissue which is white and shiny. Since growing bones must be well supplied with blood, a cut surface of these bones has a pinkish cast and a smooth, glossy appearance. The bones of older animals contain much larger amounts of minerals, and no blood vessels can be seen; such bones have a yellowish-gray color, and a sawed surface is rough and grainy.

Young animals, such as calves, are so active that they store little fat. As the animal becomes well developed, fat is usually stored throughout the little-used muscles. The meat of a young, fattened steer will show much fat throughout such a muscle and around it. Since streaks of fat through the dark lean give the appearance of marble, such meat is spoken of as "well marbled." When older animals are fattened, they are like fat women without the benefit of girdles; they bulge in funny places. The meat may show no marbling but be surrounded by fat an inch thick or more.

The color of fat depends largely on the presence or absence of carotene, the yellow pigment which is changed into vitamin A in the body. The fat of a young animal is white because there was little time to store carotene, and requirements for vitamin A are high during growth. If the animal's diet is adequate, carotene is stored in proportion to the length of time it lives; the older the animal, the more carotene stored in the fat and the deeper yellow the color. Jersey and Guernsey cattle, however, store carotene more efficiently than do other breeds; certain feeds cause the fat to be yellow; and an animal of any age, when fed dry feed, quickly uses up stored carotene, and its fat becomes white; hence the color of the fat can serve as only a rough guide.

If a cut is cherry-red, has a velvety surface, contains pink and white bones, and is marbled with white fat, you may be sure that it comes from a young animal, will be tender and juicy, and will have much flavor of fat. If the cut is rough and dark red, the sawed bone is grainy and yellowish-gray, and the meat shows no marbling but is surrounded by a thick layer of yellow fat, it comes from an older animal. Between these extremes lie all degrees of variations.

When you know the cut of meat and the approximate age of the animal, not only can you buy the cut with the flavor you desire but also you know, by looking at the meat, how to cook it. If the meat is a less tender cut from an older animal, you know that you can make it tender by grinding, pounding, or cooking it a long time at low temperature. The less fat and more connective tissue it contains, the longer it must be cooked and the lower the cooking temperature must be. If the meat comes from a young animal and has a mild flavor, you can add flavor by browning it in flour or crumbs or serving it with a highly seasoned sauce. If the meat is lean and you enjoy the flavor of fat, you can add this flavor by grinding the meat with fat, by browning it in fat, or by cutting it into small pieces and serving it in a gravy rich in fat. If the meat is well marbled and comes from a mature animal, you know that it has a delicious flavor of both fat and protein and can be broiled or roasted without any seasonings added to it. If the meat comes from a much-used muscle of an old animal, you know it will make delicious stew or soup.

Prepare your meat to have the flavor you most enjoy. Add flavor, leave it alone, or divide the flavor with the gravy.

### WHAT YOU GET FOR YOUR MONEY WHEN YOU BUY FIRST-GRADE BEEF

Many magazine articles and recipe books advise you to buy only first-grade beef. Since the price of meat is proportional to the grade, you should know what you are getting for your money. If less expensive meats can be purchased, a higher degree of health can be maintained.

Housewives often believe that the poorer grades of meat are not as carefully handled or inspected for disease as the better grades. All government-inspected meats, regardless of grade, are examined for disease and are handled with equal care under the same sanitary conditions.

Meats are graded by three standards known as conformation, finish, and quality. Conformation in feminine terms means a good figure, but contrary to feminine standards, the highest grade of beef as judged by conformation has a prize-fighter neck, bulging shoulders, back, hips, and legs, and big ankles. Finish refers largely to the color and amount of fat throughout the meat. The highest grade of beef as judged by finish shows abundant marbling with white fat; the fat surrounding the cut must be no more than ¾ inch thick. Quality has to do with firmness of muscle fibers and the amount of connective tissue the meat contains. Judged by quality, the highest grade of beef has small muscle fibers and a velvety cut surface, and contains little connective tissue; the desirable color is cherry-red. Such beef obviously comes from a young but mature animal; the meat, if properly cooked, will be tender and juicy.

The official United States grades of beef are divided into prime, choice, good, commercial, utility, cutter, and canner grades. The grade is shown on the purple government stamp. In general, the grades range from young animals to older ones, from fattened to lean, and from chunky to angular. Prime meat is from a young steer of heavy build and shows more marbling than other grades. Choice and good grades are both from high-quality young steers or heifers, but the cuts in each grade are slightly smaller and less marbled than in prime grade. Cutter and canner grades are largely from older cows or poorly fed young animals which are rangy, angular, and thin. Meats from bull carcasses are usually not sold on the retail market.

When you buy prime meat, for the higher price you obtain greater tenderness and juiciness and a more pronounced flavor of fat. If you use low cooking temperatures, allow the connective tissue time to soften, and prevent evaporation, you can develop tenderness and retain a fair amount of juiciness in any cut of any grade. You can prepare a well-marbled chuck roast or shoulder clod of choice or good grade to be a fair imitation of a prime-grade rib roast. If you wish to serve the roast cold, one of commercial, utility, or even cutter or canner grade may be as satisfactory as prime or choice grade. If you use low temperature, you can certainly broil a tender steak of choice or good grade to be as delicious as a similar steak of prime grade. For broiling I prefer well-marbled tender steaks of commercial or utility grade to any others.

If the meat is to be ground with fat and then broiled or made into hamburger or meat loaf, the lean meat of utility, cutter, or canner grades will be a better buy than prime or choice grades. If the flavor of fat is to be added by browning, as in Swiss steak or chicken-fried steak, the leaner and more flavorful meat would again be preferable. If the flavor of the lean meat is to be diluted and shared with the gravy, cutter and canner grade would be superior to all others. When I want delicious stews, I buy meat from animals which would possibly have died of old age if they had not reached the slaughterhouse in the nick of time. Decide on the flavor you desire and the method you intend to use in preparing your meat, and buy the grade accordingly.

Pork, veal, and lamb are also graded. Pork is tender and flavorful by virtue of its fat content. Veal and lamb are relatively uniform because there is little variation in age when they are marketed. The grades of these meats, therefore, are less important to you than are the grades of beef.

### COOK PORK CAREFULLY

You have been repeatedly cautioned to cook pork thoroughly in order to destroy any possible trichinae. You have probably been told not to broil pork for fear that it may be eaten undercooked. As a result, women who are aware of trichinosis usually overcook pork until it loses much flavor, juiciness, and nutritive value. Trichinae are destroyed when pork is cooked for an hour at 122° F. (50° C.) or a few minutes at 131° F. (55° C.).* Even rare beef is customarily not served under an internal temperature of 140° F.

Pork is richer in B vitamins than is any other meat. A single serving of lean pork, or 100 grams, can, if properly cooked, supply more than a third of the minimum daily requirement of an adult in vitamin $B_1$, almost a third of the vitamin $B_2$, and three-fourths of

* Ransom, B. H., and B. Schwartz, "Effects of Heat on Trichinae," *Journal of Agricultural Research*, 17:201–221 (1919).

niacin, the vitamin which can make the difference between a blue
Monday and a pleasant day. Pork is also rich in vitamin $B_6$, needed
to keep nerves relaxed, the three anti-gray-hair vitamins, and the
anti-bald-head vitamin, inositol, as well as biotin and cholin. Unnecessary overcooking of pork causes destruction of considerable
amounts of many of these vitamins and has undoubtedly contributed to the widespread deficiencies which exist, particularly in dis-
tricts where pork is the principal meat used.

Just as overcooking should be avoided, so should undercooking
be avoided because of the possibility that trichinae are present.
Trichinosis is caused by a parasite which is transmitted from pork
to humans. Almost all pork is infected with it. The trichinae hatch
in the human body and burrow into the muscles and tendons. The
body forms capsules of calcium around the parasites, making itself
the oyster in which they are the pearls. These walled capsules eventually cause pain whenever the infected person moves about. When
the diet is inadequate in calcium or in vitamins C or D, the capsules
break, the trichinae migrate elsewhere, multiply rapidly, and burrow into other muscles and tendons. Although trichinosis is difficult to diagnose, autopsies indicate that 20 per cent of all persons
are infected with it; that millions of people spend years of their lives
feeling below par from this one cause alone. It is likely that much of
the "rheumatism," "neuritis," and "arthritis" suffered by persons
who have eaten carelessly prepared pork is caused by trichinosis.

This infection is the result of carelessness and ignorance. Women
sometimes taste uncooked pork sausage when seasoning it. Tenderized hams are frequently undercooked because housewives confuse them with precooked hams. The protein-digesting enzymes in-
jected into the hams to tenderize them do not destroy trichinae.
Roadside hamburger stands have long been considered the worst
offenders in spreading trichinosis. During World War II an epi-
demic believed to be largely from this source reached nation-wide
proportions; because of the labor shortage and difficulty in ob-
taining beef, hamburgers containing much pork were prepared by
persons unaware of trichinae or careless in cooking. Since the law
requires that wieners be cooked before being sold, parents are wise
to influence their children to choose wieners instead of hamburgers
when eating out.

With a few exceptions, all pork should be cooked with a meat thermometer which can show the temperature at which trichinae will have been destroyed and can also prevent overcooking to the extent that flavor and nutrients are lost. Since pork has changed from pink to light gray by the time the internal temperature is 150° F., the absence of pink can serve as a guide when the thermometer cannot be used.

### BROILING CAPTURES THE CAMPFIRE FLAVOR

There are only three basic methods of, or recipes for, cooking meats: broiling, roasting, and braising, or steaming. Other methods are only variations of these three. The easiest method, and the one many people enjoy most, is broiling.

The authors of recipe books often confuse broiling, or cooking by direct heat, with roasting, or cooking by dry heat surrounding the meat. Recipes often advise you to heat the broiler before using it, to keep the temperature high during broiling, and to have the broiler door closed. Naturally the meat dries out, shrivels, curls, and toughens; juices pour from the contracting protein and burn on the broiler pan; the kitchen often resembles a smoke barrage. Unless you are as agile as a monkey and grab the meat at the instant it is done, it is ruined.

When you go camping or perhaps deer hunting and broil steaks, you do not cook them with the high temperatures of the flames but with the low heat of glowing coals. Only the side of the meat exposed to the coals is cooked at one time. The other surface is possibly bathed with wind or snow; no heat surrounds the meat which could dry it out. The steaks to be served to persons wishing them well done are cooked longer than those for persons who enjoy rare steaks; well-done and rare steaks alike are cooked by low temperature. To duplicate this method in the kitchen is simplicity itself.

You can broil meat perfectly 100 per cent of the time if you do not preheat the broiler compartment, if you keep the heat low, if you leave the broiler door open, and if you watch the internal temperature with a meat thermometer. The "wind and snow" are essential in preventing the meat from being dried out. If you are using a gas range in which the heat can be easily controlled, set the broiler rack on the top ledge. The tiny flames, intensely hot at the tips, slowly brown the meat, yet give off too little heat to toughen it. Once you adjust the heat, you need not glance at the meat until you turn it, or until half the calculated cooking time has expired. A few glances at the thermometer tell you exactly when the meat is ready to serve. It is juicy, beautifully browned, and delicious; the broiler pan is not burned; no wisp of smoke and almost no juices have escaped; and you, as a cook, rank with the experts.

Since the thermostat on a broiling compartment controls the temperature only when the door is closed, disregard the thermostat and adjust the heat by hand. If you have a strange broiler door which snaps shut when the rack is pushed inside, find a mechanically talented child to tear it apart. If you have no low-heat broiler unit on your electric range, your only choice is to place the meat 5 or 6 inches from the heat. When the temperature becomes high, use stored heat for a short time.

Just as broiling over a campfire is the same whether you broil fish, venison, or beef, so is broiling at home the same regardless of whether you cook chicken, steak, or ham. It is particularly important for you who are amateurs at cooking to realize that if you can broil one steak successfully, you can broil any meat successfully.

### COOKING TIMES AND TEMPERATURES FOR BROILING, PAN-BROILING, AND SAUTÉING MEATS

Refer to the following table each time before broiling, pan-broiling, or sautéing meat; the information is not repeated in each recipe.

Adjust estimated cooking time to characteristics of meat. Use figures for shorter cooking time when meat shows little marbling, contains bone, or has been frozen. Use figures for longer cooking time when meat is well marbled or contains no bone

COOKING TIMES AND TEMPERATURES FOR BROILING, PAN-BROILING, AND SAUTÉING MEATS

| Type of Meat | The Cut, or Thickness of Slice | Broiling Temperature at Surface of Meat | Internal Temperature at Which to Be Served | Approximate Cooking Time in Minutes |
|---|---|---|---|---|
| Bacon | | Very low | | 12–15 |
| Beefsteaks, less tender | 1 inch | Very low | Rare, 135° F. | 35–40 |
| | | | Medium, 150° F. | 45–50 |
| | | | Well done, 160° F. | 50–55 |
| Beefsteaks, tender | 1 inch | Low | Rare, 140° F. | 25–30 |
| | | | Medium, 155° F. | 35–40 |
| | | | Well done, 165° F. | 40–45 |
| Brains | ¾ inch | Low | 175–185° F. | 15–20 |
| Chicken, fryer or young broiler | Quartered or halved | Low | 165–170° F. | 45–50 |
| Ham or shoulder, tenderized | 1 inch | Low | 150–155° F. | 20–30 |
| | 1½ inches | Low | 150–155° F. | 35–40 |
| Ham or shoulder, not tenderized | 1 inch | Low | 165–170° F. | 40–45 |
| | 1½ inches | Low | 165–170° F. | 55–60 |
| Kidneys | ½ inch | Very low | 140–155° F. | 12–16 |
| Lamb chops, patties, or steaks | 1 inch | Low | 140–160° F. | 20–30 |
| | 2 inches | Low | 140–160° F. | 40–45 |
| Liver, beef, veal, or lamb | ¾ inch | Low | 140–155° F. | 12–18 |
| Liver, pork | ¾ inch | Low | 155–160° F. | 18–22 |
| Milt | Uncut | Low | 140–155° F. | 15–18 |
| Pork chops or steaks | 1 inch | Low | 165–170° F. | 30–35 |
| | 1½ inches | Low | 165–170° F. | 40–45 |
| Rabbit, young fryer, 2 pounds, dressed | Quartered | Low | 165–170° F. | 45–50 |
| Veal cutlets | 1 inch | Low | 175–180° F. | 30–35 |
| Wieners | | Very low | 130–140° F. | 8–10 |

## BROILED BEEFSTEAK

Select steaks cut approximately 1 inch thick; they may be club, T-bone, Spencer, rib, sirloin, porterhouse, or filet mignon.

If steaks are of prime or choice grade, use the cooking time and temperature for tender steaks; if a flank steak, or one of good, commercial, or utility grade, use the cooking time and temperature for less tender steaks.

Allow meat to heat to room temperature before starting to broil it, or remove from refrigerator about ½ hour before cooking. Trim off fat, leaving ⅛ inch to prevent evaporation.

Carefully insert punch for meat thermometer, holding it parallel to the surfaces of the meat, and making a hole in the center of the thickest portion; avoid bone or fat; withdraw punch and insert thermometer.

Estimate cooking time. At the calculated number of minutes before time to serve the meat, put it on the broiler rack with the reading of the meat thermometer down. Brush all surfaces of the meat lightly with oil.

If heat can be controlled, put broiler rack on upper ledge about 2 inches from heat; turn heat on low; if using an electric range without a low-heat unit, set rack 5 or 6 inches from heat. See that the part of the steak holding meat thermometer gets no more heat than any other.

When half the estimated cooking time has passed, turn the meat; the thermometer should now be facing up.

Check reading of the meat thermometer frequently; remove meat when reading is 135 or 140° F. for rare, 150 or 155° F. for medium, 160 or 165° F. for well done.

Sprinkle steaks with **freshly ground peppercorns** and dot with **herb butter** (p. 167) or serve with meat sauce (p. 166) as desired. Salt at the table.

After orange-apricot appetizer (p. 259), serve with French-fried white or sweet potatoes (p. 398), salad of tomatoes, cucumbers, and leeks.

*Variations:*

Just before serving, rub surface of meat lightly with mashed garlic.

If broiling only 1 steak, broil on cake rack set over a pie pan.

If heat is to be so low that probably no juices will be lost, save dishwashing by covering dripping pan with heavy paper to catch melted fat.

*In the following variations the procedure is identical with that outlined in the recipe for broiling beefsteak, referred to as the basic recipe. When preparing other meats, mentally substitute for steak the name of the meat you plan to cook; follow this basic recipe in broiling all meats.*

**Bacon:** If no more than 5 strips of bacon are to be broiled, place on a cake rack set over a pie pan; omit oiling and thermometer. If bacon curls, the heat has been allowed to become too high. Cooking bacon on a rack in a slow oven is a most satisfactory substitute for broiling it.

**Brains:** Use 1 pound of uncooked beef, lamb, pork, or veal brains; remove membranes under running water; dry on paper towels, slice, and place on oiled baking sheet; oil and sprinkle generously with **paprika**; proceed as in basic recipe. After tomato-juice appetizer (p. 258), serve with raw creole sauce (p. 167), steamed shredded carrots (p. 346), head lettuce with Thousand Island dressing.

**Chicken:** Cut broilers (1½ to 2 pounds) into halves along backbone and breastbone; insert thermometer in center of breast muscle, making sure it does not touch bone. Brush all surfaces well with **oil or melted fat,** and sprinkle generously with **paprika** before broiling. If a young chicken weighs 3 to 4 pounds, cut into quarters, one piece including leg, thigh, and lower back, and the other including breast and wings; before serving remove thermometer from breast and check temperature of large thigh muscle. After artichoke appetizer (p. 339), serve with mushroom gravy seasoned with basil (p. 151), edible-pod peas (p. 351), stuffed pimento, bell pepper rings (p. 275). It is regrettable that only an occasional housewife broils chickens; they are delicious.

**Hamburger steaks:** Use 1½ pounds of ground hamburger or round steak; season with **freshly ground black peppercorns, sautéed onions, and/or pinch of savory, basil, or marjoram;** *do not salt;* form into firm cakes 1¼ inches thick or pack firmly into cardboard milk carton; slice meat through cardboard before removing it; broil as a tender beefsteak; insert thermometer when turning. After lentil soup (p. 326), serve with steamed watercress (p. 379), cole slaw with onions and yogurt dressing.

*Meat patties:* Prepare meat patties (p. 136) and broil as hamburgers.

**Kidney:** Use 1 to 1½ pounds beef, lamb, or veal kidneys; slice beef or veal kidneys into ½-inch slices; cut lamb kidneys in half lengthwise; remove all white tissue; lay on baking sheet and brush both sides lightly with **vinegar,** then with **oil.** Before serving, rub well with **garlic;** serve lamb kidneys with tart mint sauce (p. 169), beef and veal kidneys with marjoram-flavored butter or margarine (p. 167). Serve with quick-steamed carrots (p. 346), corn on the cob (p. 408), sliced leeks and cucumbers, chilled yogurt.

*Pork kidney:* Broil to internal temperature of 155° F.; after removing from heat, rub with **mashed garlic** and sprinkle with **ground mustard, freshly ground peppercorns,** and ground parsley.

**Lamb chops, steaks, or patties:** Mix 1 teaspoon dill seeds with 1 pound ground lamb for patties; broil as in basic recipe. Serve with eggplant (p. 352), frozen mint sherbet (p. 509), shredded carrot and apple salad (p. 277).

**Liver:** Use baby beef, veal, or lamb liver sliced ¾ inch thick; brush with **bacon drippings;** before serving, rub with **mashed garlic** and sprinkle with **freshly ground peppercorns.** After cream of onion soup (p. 320), serve with raw creole sauce (p. 167), steamed Chinese cabbage (p. 384), salad of watercress and grapefruit (p. 290), rye bread (p. 424).

*Pork liver:* Before oiling sprinkle with **caraway seeds** and press into surface; broil slowly to internal temperature of 155° F.; if slices are too thin to hold thermometer, test temperature by inserting thermometer for a moment diagonally to surface. This is a delicious recipe. After jellied consommé (p. 312), serve with zucchini patties (p. 370), shredded carrot salad with avocado (p. 277), spiced pimentos (p. 365).

**Pork chops or steaks:** Do not broil without a meat thermometer; trim off fat; sprinkle both sides generously with **paprika** before broiling.

*Stuffed pork chops:* Buy chops 2 inches or more thick; cut pocket by inserting knife into side and rotating to edge of lean meat. Fill with **1 cup of crumb, fruit, or vegetable stuffing** (p. 155); broil as in basic recipe. Serve with baked yams (p. 394), steamed New Zealand spinach (p. 377), Bibb lettuce salad with Thousand Island dressing (p. 294).

**Pounded steaks:** Choose a Swiss steak about 1 to 1½ inches thick, cut from young animal; pound well and cut into serving sizes; broil as tender steak; brush with **fat** when steaks are turned. Serve with butter or margarine, zucchini and onions (p. 367), sautéed bananas (p. 406), salad of grated beets in gelatin (p. 286).

**Tenderized steaks:** choose moderately tender steaks; rub with **garlic** or sprinkle with **minced garlic;** cut into individual servings, put in refrigerator dish and pour **1 tablespoon lemon juice or French dressing** over each serving; let stand in refrigerator 24 hours. Broil as a less tender steak. Serve with country gravy seasoned with savory (p. 150), sautéed rutabagas (p. 392), steamed kale (p. 376), finger salads (p. 273).

**Sweetbreads:** Clip off elastic tissue with kitchen scissors; cut into serving sizes; broil as brains. Serve with baked sweet potatoes (p. 394), pineapple aspic (p. 289) on bed of watercress with French dressing.

**Veal cutlets:** Brush with **oil** before broiling and when turning; broil on an oiled baking sheet; after broiling rub with **mashed garlic** and sprinkle with **ground white peppercorns.** Serve with cooked tomatoes seasoned with basil (p. 368), French-fried yams (p. 399), tossed green salad (p. 298), raised bran muffins (p. 431).

**Wieners:** You need not oil; otherwise broil as in basic recipe. After cream of pea soup (p. 322), serve with steamed sauerkraut seasoned with caraway seeds (p. 390), apple-celery salad with mayonnaise.

## PAN-BROILING

Pan-broiling is a variation of broiling, or of cooking by direct heat. The utensil used to hold the meat is not greased; it serves only as a rack and dripping pan. The ideal utensil for pan-broiling is a reversible grill surrounded by a groove into which the fat drains as it is rendered out. The method is confined to cooking well-marbled steaks and meats having a sufficiently high fat content so that they will not stick to the pan during cooking; the meats must also have flat surfaces. At the beginning of cooking, pork chops, bacon, sausage, and ham are customarily pan-broiled. As the fat is rendered out, the meat fries, or is cooked by the heat of the fat, which almost invariably becomes so hot that flavor and juices are lost. If the fat drains off or is poured off as it is rendered out, the cooking temperature can easily be kept low; the meat does not dry out, shrivel, curl, burn, or need careful watching.

Pan-broiling, like broiling, is similar to cooking over glowing coals: the temperature is low; unless searing is desired, the utensil used should be cold; the meat is not covered at any time. If the meat is covered, the temperature becomes too high, juices seep out and heat quickly to boiling temperature; the meat curls, shrivels, and becomes tough. Any fat rendered from the meat should be poured off before it has time to soar to a high temperature. When you understand the procedure of pan-broiling, you can cook meat by this method without failure.

Since many people do not have good equipment for pan-broiling and since heat cannot always be kept low, it is sometimes difficult to brown meat satisfactorily without searing it first. In this case, the grill or pan is heated until extremely hot before the meat is put on it. The meat is then allowed to sear so short a time that the high temperature does not penetrate the interior of the cut. Immediately after searing the heat should be turned off or, if electricity is used, the utensil moved and the meat allowed to cook only from the heat of the utensil until it has cooled to moderate temperature. The meat

**Pork steaks:** Use steaks cut from a fresh pork leg or shoulder; cook as in basic recipe. Serve with country gravy (p. 150), yellow squash (p. 415), turnip tops (p. 380), carrot sticks.

**Lamb chops, steaks, or patties:** Pan-broil as in basic recipe; insert thermometer in patties when nearly done. Serve with beet tops cooked in milk (p. 379), zucchini, tomato aspic (p. 287).

**Mutton chops:** Select 2-inch chops; trim off fat; cut pocket in side and stuff with **prunes or sautéed onions;** pan-broil, allowing 50 minutes for cooking. Serve with string beans (p. 356), spiced purple cabbage (p. 386), lettuce with Roquefort-cheese dressing.

**Pork sausage:** Mold sausage into firm cakes; proceed as in basic recipe; insert meat thermometer when sausage is nearly done. After vegetable purée soup (p. 315), serve with tomato gravy seasoned with basil, fresh soybeans (p. 413), salad of sliced cucumbers, leeks, and ripe pepper rings.

**Link sausage:** Pierce casings of 1 pound of link sausages in several places with fork so that steam can escape; omit thermometer; pan-broil for 12 to 15 minutes. Serve in casserole over creamed potatoes (p. 397), tampala with vinegar sauce (p. 380), raw kohlrabi sticks.

**Venison, elk, or bear steaks, or steaks from other big game:** Choose rib or loin steaks; proceed as in basic recipe. Serve with vinegar sauce (p. 165), fried rice (p. 205), spiced apples (p. 459), broiled tomatoes (p. 369), tossed salad (p. 298).

## SAUTÉED MEATS

Although sautéing is frequently confused with frying, it is a variation of broiling; the food is cooked by direct heat, not by the heat of fat. The utensil is merely brushed with fat to prevent the food from sticking to it; otherwise the method is identical with pan-broiling. The advantages of sautéing over frying are that the heat can be easily controlled, the meat requires little watching, and there need be no danger of the temperature becoming so high as to dry out the meat or rob it of flavor.

The meats which are sautéed rather than pan-broiled are those which are low in fat. Since they lack the prominent flavor of fat, flavor is added by dredging them in flour or crumbs.

As in pan-broiling, the temperature should be kept low except for a few minutes of searing. A flat grill surrounded by a ½-inch rim, or the reverse side of the utensil used for pan-broiling, is best for sautéing. Such a utensil allows room for the meat thermometer to be inserted into one serving. The cooking times and temperatures are the same as those used for broiling (p. 63).

Unless the taste of fat meat is actually enjoyed, meats to be dipped in flour, crumbs, or batter should be carefully trimmed. After expecting a delicious bite of beautifully browned meat, I for one hate to discover that my mouth is full of fat; there is something deceitful about hiding it under the crust.

Meats to be sautéed are salted before cooking; the juices are caught and held in the flour, crumbs, or batter, and thus add flavor to the crust.

## SAUTÉED VEAL CUTLETS

Trim undesired fat from cutlets; mix on wax paper:

**3 tablespoons whole-wheat pastry flour   1 teaspoon salt**

Dredge cutlets, insert thermometer into thickest portion, and sear 2 or 3 minutes on each side on hot grill brushed with fat; lower heat and continue cooking slowly until brown on both sides, taking 25 to 30 minutes; *do not cover at any time.*

When internal temperature reaches 175 to 180° F., put veal on serving platter; heat in drippings:

**½ cup vegetable-cooking water          dash of salt**
**2 tablespoons minced chives            freshly ground peppercorns**

Pour sauce over veal. Serve with broiled tomatoes (p. 369), hash-browned potatoes (p. 403), romaine lettuce with Roquefort-cheese dressing (p. 293).

*Variations:*

Dredge veal and pound well with meat tenderer; cook at moderate temperature 10 minutes on each side.

Dip cutlets in egg stirred with 2 tablespoons milk, 1 teaspoon salt, a generous pinch of savory; dredge in sifted whole-wheat-bread crumbs; after removing cutlets heat 1 cup tomato sauce (p. 166) in a grill and serve over meat.

Put veal on rack after browning; prepare country gravy (p. 150) seasoned with marjoram or savory.

Dip veal in **batter** (p. 183) and sauté; insert thermometer before dipping in batter.

*In the following variations, the procedure is the same as that outlined in the recipe for sautéing veal cutlets, referred to as the basic recipe. Follow this recipe when preparing other meats, merely substituting the name of the meat for veal cutlets. Refer to tables (p. 63) for cooking times and temperatures.*

**Beef Stroganoff:** buy 1 or 1½ pounds round steak cut ½ inch thick; dredge, pound well, and cut with scissors into strips ½ inch wide; dredge again, sear 1 minute, and sauté slowly until tender, or about 8 minutes; add **1 cup sour cream or commercial yogurt;** salt and sprinkle with **freshly ground black peppercorns;** serve as soon as heated through. Vary by sautéing mushrooms with beef; or instead of sour cream add 1 can condensed mushroom soup, 1 tablespoon lemon juice or vinegar, ¼ cup milk. Serve with steamed wheat or buckwheat (p. 407), broccoli (p. 383), tossed salad of watercress, romaine, tomatoes (p. 298).

*Beef paprika:* Prepare beef as in preceding recipe; sauté with beef **1 finely chopped onion;** when tender, put beef in serving dish and prepare **2 cups country gravy;** add **1 to 3 teaspoons paprika;** stir beef and onions into gravy to reheat before serving. After fruit appetizer, serve with kale (p. 380), crookneck squash (p. 366), salad of cottage cheese and pears.

**Brains with chives:** Remove membranes from uncooked lamb, veal, or beef brains while holding under running water; cut into ½-inch slices; dredge with **fine whole-wheat-bread crumbs,** sprinkle with **paprika** and **salt,** and sauté; before serving sprinkle generously with **chives.** Serve with mustard greens (p. 374), spiced beets (p. 343), cucumber and bell pepper salad (p. 278).

**Chicken-fried steak:** Trim, dredge, pound, and brown ½-inch slices of round steak in rendered suet, allowing 25 to 30 minutes for total cooking time. Serve with country gravy (p. 150) seasoned with sage, hash-browned potatoes (p. 403), steamed chard (p. 380), lettuce salad with mayonnaise.

**Chicken-fried venison, elk, or bear meat:** Dredge and pound thoroughly; sauté as in basic recipe. Serve with country gravy seasoned with a pinch each of savory, marjoram, sage; rutabagas (p. 390), string beans (p. 356), bread-and-butter pickles, finger salads (p. 273).

**Lamb chops or steaks:** Sauté as in basic recipe or dip in **egg or milk and crumbs.** Serve with dill or caper sauce (p. 163), asparagus (p. 341), sautéed rutabagas (p. 392), mixed-fruit salad (p. 283).

**Liver:** Use lamb, baby beef, veal, or pork liver cut into ½-inch slices; sear no longer than 2 minutes on each side; sprinkle generously with **freshly ground black peppercorns.** Serve with raw creole sauce (p. 167), spiced purple cabbage (p. 386), stuffed tomato salad (p. 281).

*With bacon:* Cut strips of bacon in half and pan-broil before sautéing liver; drain on paper; after liver is browned, put bacon above liver to reheat; serve at once.

*With onions:* Chop fine **2 cups sweet onions;** sauté in bacon drippings 8 to 10 minutes before sautéing liver, using same utensil; put on serving dish; just before serving, add onions to liver and reheat. After lentil soup (p. 326) serve with creamed spinach seasoned with nutmeg (p. 373), mixed-vegetable salad set in aspic (p. 286).

**Pork:** Use pork chops, tenderloin, or steaks; trim off fat and sauté as in basic recipe or dip in **egg** mixed with **2 tablespoons milk** and then in **crumbs.** Serve with country gravy (p. 150) seasoned with sage, purple-plum purée (p. 470), steamed leeks, eggplant with tomatoes (p. 353), apple and grape salad (p. 275).

**Quick Swiss steak:** Since Swiss steak is pounded, it should be cooked as a tender cut of meat; the *utensil should not be covered* at any time. Purchase a Swiss steak about 1 to 1½ inches thick; dredge with **whole-wheat flour** and pound thoroughly; sauté in **3 tablespoons fat** rendered from suet; cook slowly to an internal temperature of 140 to 165° F., or about 30 minutes. Meanwhile steam together in another utensil **1 or 2 each quartered onions, unpeeled potatoes, carrots, turnips;** when vegetables start to be tender, add **1 cup fresh or frozen peas.** When steak is done, put on serving platter and prepare brown or tomato gravy (p. 151). Season gravy with **salt, crushed black peppercorns, basil, savory;** combine vegetables and gravy and pour over meat. Serve with frozen apricot purée and tossed green salad. This type of Swiss steak in my opinion is far more delicious than the overcooked variety.

## THE PERSON WHO WORKS AT ROASTING RUINS THE MEAT

To roast meat means to cook it with dry heat. Meat to be roasted is set on a rack above a dripping pan, brushed with oil to prevent evaporation, and allowed to cook until the meat thermometer indicates the degree of doneness most enjoyed. What else can you do without ruining the meat? If you salt it, sear it in a preheated oven, or baste it, juices are drawn out or lost by evaporation, and the meat is left drier. If you cover the meat with a lid, it is steamed instead of roasted. If you set it on a pan instead of a rack, the lower surface is first steamed, eventually rests in melted fat, fries, and becomes tough. If you want delightfully roasted meat, let it alone and honor its privacy.

Meats cooked in a covered "roaster" are not roasted, even though cooked in an oven. A so-called pot roast is really a "pot steam." If a "roaster" is not used for cooking on top of the range, it should be planted with herbs or converted into a baby's bathtub.

When roasting meat, set an upright oven thermometer on the rack beside the roast. A thermostat, or heat control, can give nothing more than a general indication of the oven temperature. Every woman knows that heat rises and causes a cake to brown more quickly at the top of an oven than at the bottom. The temperature in one part of an oven is often 360° F. and in another part, 275° F. Moreover, thermostats are rarely accurate. I have checked oven temperatures of ranges of perhaps two dozen of my friends and have yet to find a thermostat which, when turned to 300° F., for example, is not 25 to 50 degrees too high or too low. Unless the cooking temperature is known, there is no way of determining whether the meat will be done an hour before dinnertime or 2 hours later.

The tables giving the estimated cooking times and temperatures should be referred to before roasting any meat. Although these tables are worked out to help you know when to put the meat on to cook, they can be nothing more than a rough guide. Unless you carefully consider the characteristics of each individual roast, you may have eggs for dinner or meat for dessert.

Roasts with certain characteristics cook slowly; those which contain no bones or only short, compact bones; cube-shaped or rolled roasts which have relatively little surface through which heat can penetrate; and a well-marbled roast, since fat is a poor conductor of heat. On the other hand, meats which show no marbling heat through rapidly. Long, slender bones conduct heat readily; a crown roast often cooks in half the time needed for the same amount and cut of meat made into a rolled roast. Meats which have been frozen and thawed cook more quickly than fresh meats. A large flat roast, cut like a pot roast, may cook in half the time required for a thicker roast which weighs less. In terms of minutes per pound, a large roast cooks much more quickly than does a small one. Putting a preheated stuffing into a roast also shortens the cooking period. Consider all of these factors and allow yourself plenty of time. If the roast gets done before time to serve, take it from the oven when it is 5 degrees below that of desired doneness; it will continue cooking from its own heat for an hour or more.

As in broiling, if you have successfully roasted one meat, you can roast any meat. The only variations lie in the cooking times and temperatures and the preparation of the meat before it is put into the oven.

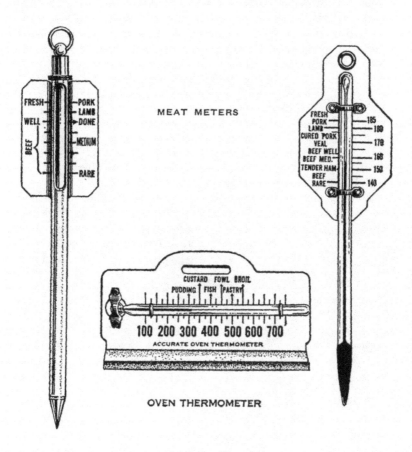

MEAT METERS

OVEN THERMOMETER

## COOKING TIMES AND TEMPERATURES FOR ROASTING OR BARBECUING MEATS WITH MODERATE HEAT

In calculating time when meat is to be put on to cook, use figures for shorter cooking time if the roast shows little marbling, contains long, slender bones, has been frozen and thawed, has a relatively large surface area, is flat, weighs 4 pounds or more, or is stuffed with preheated dressing. Use the figures for longer cooking time when meat is well marbled, contains no bones or has short, compact bones, is rolled or cube shaped, or weighs less than 4 pounds.

| Type of Meat | Approximate Cooking Time in Minutes per Pound | External Temperature of Upright Oven Thermometer | Degree of Doneness | Internal Temperature at Which Meat Is Served |
|---|---|---|---|---|
| Beef, less tender cuts | 45–50 | 225–250° F. | Rare | 135° F. |
| | 55–60 | | Medium | 150° F. |
| | 60–70 | | Well done | 160° F. |
| Beef, tender cuts | 18–20 | 300° F. | Rare | 140° F. |
| | 20–25 | | Medium | 155° F. |
| | 27–30 | | Well done | 165° F. |
| Chicken, roasting | 35–45 | 300° F. | | 185° F. |
| stewing | 60–70 | 225–250° F. | | 185° F. |
| Duck, young | 25–30 | 300° F. | | 185° F. |
| Goose, young | 25–30 | 300° F. | | 185° F. |
| Ham, home cured | 25–30 | 300° F. | | 165–170° F. |
| tenderized | 20–25 | 300° F. | | 150–155° F. |
| Lamb, leg | 25–30 | 300° F. | | 155–160° F. |
| shoulder | 40–45 | 275° F. | | 155–160° F. |
| Liver, uncut | 15–20 | 300° F. | | 145–160° F. |
| Mutton, leg or shoulder | 60–70 | 225–250° F. | | 180–185° F. |
| Pork roast | 35–40 | 300° F. | | 165–170° F. |
| Rabbit | 30–35 | 300° F. | | 180° F. |
| Spareribs | 30–35 | 300° F. | | 180–185° F. |
| Turkey, large | 15–18 | 300° F. | | 180–185° F. |
| small | 20–25 | 300° F. | | 180–185° F. |
| Veal, standing roast | 40–45 | 275° F. | | 180–185° F. |
| rolled | 45–50 | 275° F. | | 180–185° F. |

## ROAST BEEF, LESS TENDER CUTS

Select roast weighing 3 pounds or more cut from chuck, clod, round muscles, or rump of prime or choice grade or from rib or loin section of good, commercial, utility, or canner grade.

Allow meat to reach room temperature, or allow about ½ hour per pound if taken from refrigerator. If it is frozen, put over dripping pan to thaw.

Estimate cooking time, considering characteristics of meat (p. 76).

Trim off fat, leaving ½ inch for self-basting.

If desired, use **vegetable, fruit, or crumb stuffing** (p. 155); if roast is not compact, tie with heavy strings 1 inch apart to prevent evaporation.

Carefully pierce hole for meat thermometer, inserting punch into center of thickest part of roast and being careful not to touch fat, bone, or dressing; insert meat thermometer.

Put meat on broiler rack above broiler pan or on similar rack above dripping pan; brush all lean surfaces with **oil or melted fat**; set roast on rack with fat side up and put into cold oven; *do not salt or season in any way.*

Adjust thermostat to 225 or 250° F.; turn on heat. Set oven thermometer on rack beside meat.

After 15 minutes read oven thermometer and adjust heat or thermostat accordingly; if adjustment is necessary, check reading and readjust heat again in 15 minutes.

As end of calculated cooking time approaches, take reading of meat thermometer.

Make gravy when meat is 10 degrees or more below the temperature desired for serving. Season gravy with savory and marjoram.

Serve meat when internal temperature, shown by meat thermometer, is 135° F. for rare, 150° F. for medium done, and 160° F. for well done.

Serve with baked onions (p. 388), plum sherbet (p. 470) or spiced peach pickles (p. 487), tossed salad of chicory, romaine, mustard greens (p. 298).

*Variations:*

If meat is to be served cold, subtract 10 degrees from desired temperature of doneness; turn off heat and let meat cool in oven.

*In the following variations, the meats are roasted in the same manner outlined in the recipe for less tender beef roast, referred to as the basic recipe. Regardless of the type of meat you wish to roast, follow the basic recipe, merely substituting for beef the name of the meat.*

**Beef, tender cut:** Roast as in basic recipe except at higher temperature and shorter cooking time (p. 76). After tomato-juice appetizer, serve with baked potatoes, watercress salad.

**Chicken:** Salt chicken inside if desired; fill with stuffing (p. 156). Brush with oil and proceed as in basic recipe, inserting thermometer into thickest part of thigh muscle next to body; set chicken on broiler rack breast side up. Serve with clear gravy (p. 151), peas, frozen apricot purée (p. 470), green salad of New Zealand spinach, new mustard greens, and tomatoes, hot yeast rolls (p. 425).

**Duck and goose, domestic:** Stuff with **apple, onion, or buckwheat stuffing** (p. 157); insert thermometer into thigh muscle next to body; roast as in basic recipe. After fruit appetizer (p. 260), serve with browned gravy (p. 151), Brussels sprouts (p. 383), cottage cheese and spinach salad (p. 282).

**Ham, whole or half, home cured or tenderized:** Wash well if home-cured; trim, leaving ½ inch of fat; save trimmings for seasoning; leave skin over shank, or more pointed end, cutting skin with kitchen shears into star-shaped or semicircular border; score fat into diamonds by cutting diagonally across surface; brush with **black molasses** and put **clove** in center of each diamond; roast or bake as in basic recipe. Serve with mustard and horseradish sauce (p. 163), quick-baked yams (p. 394), steamed beet tops (p. 379), pickled crabapples or apple sherbet (p. 470), and cucumber and pimento salad.

**Lamb:** Select leg, shoulder, loin, rack, or breast; bone and stuff leg if desired; or bone, stuff, and roll breast; or make pocket between bones and meat in breast or shoulder roast for stuffing. Do not remove thin membrane covering leg or shoulder. Proceed as in basic recipe; garnish platter with sprigs of **fresh mint.** Serve with brown gravy (p. 151), spiced red apples (p. 459), sautéed parsnips (p. 363), lettuce and green onion salad.

**Liver:** Buy 2 pounds or more of unsliced baby beef, veal, lamb, or pork liver; make pocket in center of liver, stuff with **onion dressing** (p. 157), or roast without stuffing; cut **2 or 3 slices of bacon** in half and put over top, holding them securely with toothpicks; roast as in basic recipe. Serve with tomato or creole sauce (p. 166), broiled sweet potatoes (p. 396), creamed mustard-spinach (p. 373), tossed salad (p. 298).

**Mutton:** Buy leg, shoulder, rack, or loin roast; ask butcher to remove oil gland from leg. Cut off all mutton fat and cover with **slices of bacon** held in place with toothpicks. Roast as in basic recipe. Garnish roast and platter with **fresh mint.** Serve with tart mint aspic (p. 235), steamed spinach (p. 380), baked banana squash (p. 414), radishes and assorted vegetable sticks (p. 273).

**Pork:** Select fresh shoulder, leg, loin, or tenderloin; bone and stuff shoulder or leg (p. 153) if desired; proceed as in basic recipe. Serve with pineapple rings sautéed in pork drippings, corn on the cob (p. 408), tossed green salad (p. 298).

**Rabbit:** Select a mature rabbit; stuff with **rice and tomato dressing** (p. 157); insert meat thermometer into thigh muscle next to body; roast as in basic recipe. Garnish platter with **sprigs of parsley.** Serve with country gravy seasoned with basil (p. 150), lentils (p. 199), green asparagus (p. 341), carrot-celery salad (p. 277), hot wheat-germ rolls (p. 425).

**Roast suckling pig:** Should weigh 9 to 12 pounds; clean thoroughly, wipe with cloth, fill half the pig with **rice or buckwheat stuffing** (p. 158), and half with **onion dressing** (p. 157); tie front legs together and pull backward; tie hind legs together and bring forward, as if the pig were lying down; tie all four legs together securely. Prop mouth open with small **raw potato.** Insert thermometer in top of hip muscles; set with back up. Brush with **oil** and roast as in basic recipe at 350° F. for 5 hours or more, or until internal temperature is 165 to 170° F. Put on serving platter, place a **small red apple** in pig's mouth, **fresh cranberries** in eyesockets, and a wreath of **parsley** around neck. Make brown cream gravy seasoned with sage and savory. Serve with frozen spiced apple purée (p. 470), string beans (p. 356), purple cabbage salad (p. 277).

**Spareribs:** Select 2 or 3 pounds of meaty spareribs; cut pocket between meat and bones and stuff with **onion dressing** or fill with **sauerkraut** seasoned with **caraway seeds;** or put dressing between two matching sections. Serve with shredded hash-browned potatoes (p. 403), tossed green salad, wheat-germ bread (p. 425).

**Turkey:** Stuff with **giblet dressing** (p. 156); insert thermometer into thigh muscle next to body, being careful not to touch bone; roast as in basic recipe. Serve with scalloped onions (p. 389), cranberry aspic (p. 291), fresh celery.

**Veal:** Select breast, leg, loin, rib, or shoulder roast; bone, stuff, and roll if desired; make sure thermometer does not touch dressing if any is used; cover with ¼-inch layer of **kidney fat** if there is no fat on meat. Proceed as in basic recipe. Serve with tomato gravy seasoned with basil and marjoram (p. 151), edible-pod peas (p. 351), fresh pepper and cabbage salad (p. 277), warm rye bread (p. 424).

**Venison, elk, moose, buffalo, bear, or other big game:** Roast as a less tender cut of beef, cooking to medium or well done. Serve with highly seasoned gravy (p. 152), tart plum sauce, mashed rutabagas (p. 392), vegetable-gelatin salad (p. 287).

**Wild duck, grouse, pheasant, wild turkey, prairie chicken, or squab:**
Stuff with **buckwheat, wild rice, or apple stuffing** (p. 157). Insert meat
thermometer into thigh next to body. Roast duck to 140° F., other wild
fowl to 185° F. Follow cooking time for chicken, depending on age and
probable tenderness of meat. Roast as in basic recipe. After yellow-tomato-
juice appetizer (p. 262), serve with milk or tomato gravy seasoned with
sage and/or basil (p. 151), creamed Brussels sprouts (p. 383), celery-
carrot salad (p. 277).

## SLOW ROASTING

In experiments where identical roasts were cooked at different
oven temperatures to the same degree of doneness, roasts cooked
for 26 to 32 hours were preferred in 100 per cent of the taste tests to
roasts cooked in 3 hours or less. Although the cooking time seems
startling at first, the meat is so amazingly delicious, juicy, and
tender, slices so beautifully, and shrinks so little that meats cooked
at higher temperatures no longer taste good to you.

In slow roasting, the oven temperature is set approximately at
the temperature you want the meat when it is done. Just as meat
taken from a refrigerator will warm to room temperature, so will
meat put into such an oven heat to oven temperature. It cannot
burn; it needs no watching; vitamins and proteins cannot be
harmed at such low heat; almost no fuel is needed to cook it. One
might say that it cooks itself. Many warming ovens are adjusted so
that a pilot light maintains a constant temperature of 165° F.,
which is ideal for this type of roasting.

Probably you often buy a roast the day before you plan to cook
it. If you wish to use this method, instead of putting the meat in
the refrigerator, simply brush it with oil, insert the meat thermometer, set it in the oven, adjust the heat, and forget about it. The
longer it cooks, the more tender it becomes. A top chuck roast cut
from the neck muscles or a heel of the round, perhaps the least
tender of all roasts, becomes so tender that it can be cut with a fork
when cooked for 24 hours at a temperature of 150 to 160° F.

Although the pasteurization point at which bacteria are killed
is 140° F. and bacteria cannot penetrate the interior of meat any
more than can salt, the variation of slow roasting which I use to
make sure that all bacteria are killed is to heat the meat for an hour

at 250° F. before reducing the temperature to that of desired doneness. After this period of preheating, the cooking time is approximately three times that of moderate-temperature roasting, although there is considerable variation between different roasts. In using the method, estimate the time needed to cook the roast at moderate temperature (p. 76), multiply by three, and add the hour of preheating.

Slow roasting is an ideal method if persons must be away throughout the day and have warming ovens, adjustable oven pilot lights which can reach slow-roasting temperatures, or well-insulated ovens which can maintain low temperatures at almost no cost. The chief advantage of a knowledge of slow roasting is that you can cook your meat at a temperature which most suits your convenience. Combine moderate-temperature roasting with slow roasting or use any cooking temperature between 140° F. and the temperature recommended in the tables on page 76 for the type of meat you wish to cook. Within this range, the lower the temperature used in cooking, the more delicious the meat will be, particularly if the cut is a less tender one. Since the lower temperature requires longer cooking, its use must depend on when you wish to serve the meat. You might have a roast which could be cooked at moderate temperature in 3 hours; yet you wish to be away from home for 6 hours. You could cook the roast at moderate temperature for a short time while you are at home, decrease the temperature to that of desired doneness when you must be away, and if the meat is not done when you get home, increase the temperature again. Thus your roasting can be adjusted entirely to your convenience.

At first the objection to using variation of temperatures appears to be that you cannot tell when the meat will be done. If you cook it at a temperature of desired doneness, or 160° F. or below, the connective tissue softens but breaks down little or none, even if the meat is cooked longer than necessary; hence the exact cooking time is less important than when higher temperatures are used. Remember only that the lower the cooking temperature, the longer the meat must be cooked. Allow yourself plenty of time when using low temperatures and let your meat thermometer be your guide to the degree of doneness you desire.

## BARBECUING IN THE KITCHEN

When meat is barbecued over an open fire or charcoal flames, a revolving spit allows it to broil on one surface while the other surfaces cool; the flames some distance away cause the meat to be surrounded by dry heat as if it were in a slow oven; thus barbecuing is a combination of broiling and roasting. Barbecuing at home can be done by cooking meat in a broiler compartment with the door closed. If carefully cooked, the meat is delicious indeed. Since the temperature of both the direct and accumulated dry heat can be controlled, turning the meat more than once is unnecessary.

An advantage of barbecuing rather than roasting is that the surface becomes beautifully browned; yet the low direct heat cannot penetrate far into the meat. The meat therefore shrinks much less than if it were browned to the same degree in a closed oven. On ranges where one unit heats both the broiling compartment and the oven, the oven is left free for other cooking. During the summer, food to be served cold can be prepared for several meals at one time. The method is especially well adapted for cooking meat with flat surfaces, as a chuck roast cut as a thick pot roast. As in roasting, the meat should be tied tightly to make it compact and thus prevent evaporation from occurring between the muscles of the meat. The size of the meat to be barbecued is limited only by the size of the broiling compartment.

The procedure of barbecuing differs from roasting in that the meat is turned when half the estimated cooking time has passed. The fat side of the meat should be placed down during the first half of barbecuing, and turned to the direct heat for the remainder of the cooking time. Fowl, tied so that their legs and wings are held close to the body, are laid breast side up during the first half of the cooking period. The surface of the fowl or meat should be brushed with oil at the beginning of cooking and again at the time it is turned. If barbecue sauce is to be poured over the meat, it should not be applied until 15 minutes before the meat is served.

Since the procedure for barbecuing meat is so nearly the same as that for roasting, only one basic recipe is given. Any meat which can be roasted may be barbecued by following this basic procedure.

The cooking times and temperatures to be used are the same as those used for roasting (p. 76).

Still lower temperatures may also be used, and the meat will be even more delicious. If the meat is barbecued on a gas range, it may be placed so that the top surface is 3 inches from the flames; if electricity is used, the top surface should not be nearer than 5 inches. Persons with electric ranges seem particularly enthusiastic about this method of cooking meat.

Do not try to barbecue meat without using thermometers; your chances are ten to one that you will ruin the meat.

## BARBECUED LEG OF LAMB

Select leg of lamb of desired weight; if mild lamb flavor is preferred, ask butcher to remove oil gland.

Estimate cooking time at 25 to 30 minutes per pound.

Wash thoroughly and dry; trim off undesired fat, leaving ¼ to ½ inch; *do not remove membrane over lean meat.*

Put on broiler rack, lean side up, and brush lean surface with **oil or melted fat.** Press punch into thickest part of lean meat, withdraw, and insert thermometer.

Place in broiling compartment so that top surface is 3 inches below gas heat or 5 inches below electric heat. Set oven thermometer on rack beside meat; turn on heat and adjust thermostat to 300° F.

After 15 minutes read oven thermometer; adjust heat if necessary.

Turn meat fat side up after it has cooked for half the estimated cooking time; brush surfaces with **oil** or **melted fat.**

Cook until meat thermometer shows internal temperature of 155 to 160° F.

Serve with caper sauce (p. 162) or gravy seasoned with dill (p. 152), green asparagus (p. 341), browned potatoes (p. 398), tomato salad.

*Variations:*

Bone leg of lamb and stuff with **onion dressing** (p. 157).

Barbecue beef, chicken, duck, ham, fresh pork, or other meat by same procedure. For preparing meats, follow directions given under roasting.

### THE MOIST-HEAT METHODS OF COOKING MEAT

The methods of meat cookery discussed thus far, broiling, roasting, and their variations, are known as the dry-heat methods. Since dry heat penetrates meat slowly and is easy to control, meats properly cooked by these methods lose so little flavor and are so delicious that no seasonings are needed. When meats are cooked by moist heat, or by hot water or steam, the internal temperature used is so high that much flavor is lost; therefore such meats are usually served well seasoned.

A myriad of recipes exist for cooking meats with moist heat. They may be called braised, smothered, potted, fricasseed, baked (in a covered utensil), or half a dozen other terms. They run the gamut of all the less tender cuts of meat of all sizes and from all the animals commonly used as food. These recipes include almost every known vegetable and seasoning and combinations of vegetables and seasonings. As a result they are so confusing and their number so appalling as to convince an amateur that she will never learn to cook, to say nothing of driving an author of a cookbook to insanity.

Meat cookery becomes simplified when you understand why thousands of so-called separate recipes exist. In past centuries, when few vegetables and fruits were known, meat was the chief food. It spoiled easily, yet had to be eaten to prevent starvation. The spoiled meats were highly seasoned with spices and herbs to make them palatable. Thousands of lives were lost in the search for trade routes to obtain spices; and America was discovered because of spoiled meat. Through generation after generation, thousands of ideas for seasoning meats have been written down into what are now considered to be different recipes. The person who originated each idea was probably no more intelligent than you; his ideas are probably no better than yours.

Aside from seasonings, there are really only four variations in recipes for cooking meat by the moist-heat methods: the method of browning; the vegetables cooked with the meat; the amount of moisture used in cooking; and the type of gravy prepared. The meat may be browned by frying, sautéing, pan-broiling, or roasting; it may be seared or dipped in flour, crumbs, or batter. The vegetables used, like the seasonings, will depend on what your family happens to enjoy and which ones you have on hand. The gravy may be clear, brown, or made with milk or tomatoes. Stripped of their excess baggage, the thousands of recipes may be reduced to two recipes, or methods—braising and stewing.

Nothing has clarified meat cookery so much for me as this realization. I believe it will also simplify cooking for the amateur. If you are aware of these variations and can cook one meat successfully by a moist-heat method, you can cook all meats with equal success. Moreover, you can throw away all other recipes (including mine) and make up your own. When the principles of cookery are known, the only value of recipes is to suggest ideas which you may not have thought of at the moment.

### BRAISE MEATS TO RETAIN THEIR FLAVOR

According to schools of cookery, to braise meat means to cover it during cooking. The covering may be hot coals or stones, the lid of a utensil, or a browned crust. Regardless of its type, the covering holds steam around the meat so that it is cooked by steam.

When meat is cooked in liquid, much of the meat flavor passes into the liquid. If meat from a young animal or a muscle which has been little used is stewed, almost no flavor is left in the meat, and the gravy is unworthy of the name. If the meat is steamed, or cooked on a rack standing ¾ inch above the bottom of the pan, the loss of flavor is largely prevented. Since the rack allows steam to surround all surfaces of the meat, they are evenly heated and the cooking time is shortened by a third or more.

Steam held in a utensil stays at exactly the same temperature as the water below it. It is extremely important that the water used not be allowed to go above simmering temperature, or 185° F. Even this temperature quickly toughens the protein. Although connective tissue starts to break down below 185° F., the less tender cuts used for braising contain thick sheets of connective tissue which soften and break down slowly. If the water (hence the steam) does reach boiling temperature, the connective tissue breaks down more rapidly, but the proteins become so tough that much flavor is lost and the cooking time must be prolonged an hour or more before the proteins become tender again. When braising meat, turn the heat as low as you can get it; check the temperature of the water with the cooking thermometer. If the heat cannot be turned low enough to maintain simmering temperature, set the utensil to one side so that it covers only half or a third of the heating unit. Since steam heat penetrates rapidly, the meat cooks at an internal temperature of 185° F. and a meat thermometer is rarely needed.

Such meats as pot roast and Swiss steak are often cooked by steam formed only from meat juices, no water being added. Since most cooking utensils allow some steam to escape, the meat shrinks more and is less moist than if water is added at the beginning of cooking. As the meat nears doneness, however, the water may be allowed to evaporate off and the meat juices browned by the melted fat in the utensil to ensure rich, luscious gravy.

Most meats to be braised should not be salted until ready to serve. Meats cooked by this method are less tender cuts already low in moisture; they are usually served with a sauce or gravy, which may be generously salted.

Since vinegar and other acids tenderize meat and shorten the cooking time, use them in all braising. If the meat does not contain bone, buy a small amount of bone and cook it in the water and acid used for steaming; thus calcium and a delightful flavor are added to the gravy or sauce.

Braised meats are frequently overcooked. The test of a well-cooked meat is that it will slice evenly without pulling apart. If it is stringy, flavor has been lost which cannot be recaptured.

The simplest form of braising is that which serves as a substitute for boiling, a criminal means of cooking meat. Not only is flavor lost in boiling, but valuable nutrients are discarded when the liquid left from cooking such meats as tongue or ham is thrown away.

## BRAISED, OR STEAMED, CHICKEN

Select stewing chicken; wash outside thoroughly; disjoint or leave whole. If disjointed, put neck and wing tips in the bottom of the utensil. Set a rack standing ¾ inch high over bones; place chicken on rack and add:

½ to 1 cup water                    1 tablespoon white vinegar or white
                                    wine for each pound of chicken

Cover utensil and set over simmer burner or extremely low heat; after 10 minutes check temperature of water with cooking thermometer; if it is greater than 185° F., adjust heat or set utensil to one side of burner. No bubbles should be bursting on the surface of the water.

Cook until tender when pierced with a fork, or about 2 to 2½ hours. Use chicken in making soufflé (p. 210), chicken loaf (p. 230), chicken salad (p. 235), or creamed chicken (p. 216).

*Variations:*
*Although the types of meat in the following variations differ widely, they are steamed in the same manner outlined in the recipe for steamed chicken, referred to as the basic recipe. Merely substitute for chicken in the basic recipe the name of the meat you wish to prepare.*

**Corned beef:** Prepare as in basic recipe, using **vinegar** and steaming 3⅓ to 4 hours; 10 minutes before serving, set meat on platter, skim off excess fat from drippings, and steam sauerkraut or shredded cabbage in same utensil; add **1 to 4 teaspoons caraway seeds.** After mixed-fruit appetizer, serve with sautéed parsnips (p. 363), sliced tomatoes, raised cornbread (p. 430).

**Ham:** Steam as in basic recipe, allowing 20 minutes per pound for large ham, 30 for small, half, or picnic ham; save drippings for seasoning. Serve hot or cold with baked beans (p. 199), applesauce (p. 460), tossed green salad (p. 298).

**Heart:** Use half a beef heart, 1 veal or pork heart, or 4 lamb hearts; wash well and clip out tough membranes; score (p. 97); steam as in basic recipe, allowing 3½ hours for beef heart, 2½ hours for pork, veal, or lamb hearts. Slice meat while hot, serving beef heart with celery or curry sauce (p. 163), pork with caraway or horseradish sauce (p. 163), lamb with caper or dill sauce (p. 162); or slice and serve cold with chilled sauces (p. 168). If more convenient, cook beef or veal heart while making meat soup or stock. After tomato-juice appetizer (p. 258), serve with beet greens, steamed carrots, sliced tomatoes and cucumbers.

*Stuffed heart:* Select whole heart which has not been cut; steam as above; prepare 1½ **cups fruit, celery,** or **crumb stuffing** for beef or veal heart; **cornbread stuffing** for pork heart; **rice stuffing** seasoned with 1 teaspoon **dill seeds** for lamb hearts. As soon as meat is tender, heat stuffing thoroughly in drippings; pack into heart, sprinkle dressing generously with **paprika,** and brown under broiler. Don't miss this recipe; it makes an excellent inexpensive entree. Serve with steamed spinach (p. 376), mixed vegetable salad in aspic (p. 286), chilled yogurt.

**Liver:** Use unsliced lamb, pork, or baby beef liver; insert meat thermometer and steam about 8 minutes for each inch of thickness; take up when internal temperature is 155° F.; slice and serve hot or cold with creole sauce (p. 167). Prepare liver in this way for persons who must use a reducing or fat-free diet. After jellied bouillon (p. 312) serve with New Zealand spinach, assorted finger salads (p. 273).

**Tongue:** Use 1 fresh, pickled, or smoked beef, veal, or pork tongue or 6 to 8 lamb tongues; wash thoroughly and steam 1 hour per pound; remove skin while hot; slice diagonally. Serve beef, veal, or pork tongue hot or cold with horseradish sauce (p. 169), lamb tongues with caper sauce. Serve with steamed kohlrabi (p. 359), rhubarb chard, tossed salad.

*Creamed lamb tongues:* Steam 1 pound of lamb tongues as above; prepare 2 cups caper or dill sauce; cut tongues into fingers and add to sauce 5 minutes before serving. After fruit appetizer (p. 260), serve with steamed broccoli (p. 383), mint aspic (p. 235) or sherbet (p. 509), tomato and cottage cheese salad.

### BRAISED MEATS BROWNED IN THE OVEN

Large tender cuts of meat which are usually served well done, such as turkey, ham, or a leg of lamb, can be steamed until almost tender and then browned in the oven. This method is a delightful, fast, and economical substitute for roasting. When steamed, these meats cook in about half the time required for roasting, shrink less than when cooked by dry heat, and stay moist and juicy. The oven temperature must be kept the same as that used for roasting, and browning is done with the aid of substances which brown quickly. In using this method, calculate the cooking time required for roasting (p. 76) and divide by 2.

This is my pet method for "roasting" turkey, chickens, and ham. Each Thanksgiving when other housewives spend hours hovering over a turkey, mine cooks in 2 or 3 hours over a simmer burner, and instead of being dry, juices pour from it when it is sliced.

### BRAISED TURKEY BROWNED IN THE OVEN, OR MOCK ROAST TURKEY

Singe, remove any pin feathers with tweezers, and wash the outside thoroughly; dry.

If brown gravy (p. 150) is desired, keep out a small amount of fat.

Loosen skin over breast and fill breast and inside with hot giblet stuffing (p. 156); fasten skin securely with string and hardwood toothpicks.

Estimate cooking time for roasting (p. 76) and divide by 2.

Chop neck; put in bottom of large turkey roaster or steamer; add small amount of fat and sear until light brown to develop flavor; set turkey on rack over bones; add 1 to 2 cups water and 1/4 cup vinegar.

Bring water to simmering, and simmer for 2 to 3½ hours, or until meat is almost tender when pierced with a fork.

Lift rack with turkey to lid of steamer or set over broiler tray; remove any moisture from surface with paper towel and brush thoroughly with a paste of **4 tablespoons melted margarine, butter, or drippings mixed with 2 tablespoons whole-wheat flour, 1 teaspoon paprika.** Put turkey into preheated moderate oven at 350° F. until golden brown, or about 35 minutes.

If any odor of vinegar remains in cooking liquid, boil it a few minutes; make gravy (p. 151); season with a pinch each of sage and savory.

Serve with broiled whole onions (p. 388), cranberry sherbet or aspic (p. 291), mixed finger salads of celery, carrot sticks, olives, radishes.

*Variations:*

Fill inside of turkey with giblet dressing; fill neck with dressing of fried rice (p. 205) or steamed buckwheat.

Chill turkey, glaze (p. 234), and serve cold for buffet.

*In the following variations, proceed as in recipe for steamed turkey, referred to as the basic recipe. When cooking other meats, merely substitute for turkey the name of the meat. Calculate the cooking time for roasting (p. 76) and divide by 2.*

**"Baked" ham or cured shoulder:** Use cured or tenderized ham or shoulder; trim off part of the fat, leaving ½ inch thick; steam as in basic recipe; brush surface with mixture of **2 tablespoons each dry mustard and black molasses;** brown until golden. If desired, decorate before browning by pushing into fat thin rings of green pepper and slices of stuffed olives or half rings of orange peel with slices of maraschino cherries set in center; omit molasses and sprinkle generously with **paprika.** Serve with brown gravy, baked yams (p. 394), spiced whole apples (p. 459), watercress and grapefruit salad.

**Mock roast chicken:** Select an old stewing chicken; prepare, stuff, cook, and brown as in basic recipe, steaming 2½ to 3 hours. Chicken cooked in this manner is usually more delicious than a roasting chicken. Serve with mashed potatoes (p. 399), cream gravy (p. 150), green asparagus (p. 341), sliced tomatoes.

*Glazed chicken:* Stuff and cook as above; chill and glaze (p. 234). Serve cold with chilled celery root marinated in French dressing, peach pickles, sliced cucumbers, leeks, and green-pepper rings.

**Mock roast lamb:** Steam a leg or shoulder roast without removing membrane; brush with oil, sprinkle generously with **paprika,** and brown. Breast or shoulder of lamb may be stuffed with **1½ cups of any dressing** (p. 155) and then steamed and browned. Vary by steaming lamb with meat thermometer to 145° F.; brown to 155° F. Serve with apricot sherbet (p. 470), baked yams (p. 394), tossed green salad (p. 298).

## BRAISED MEATS BROWNED BY FRYING

Strange though it may seem, fried chicken and other meats which are dipped in flour or batter and browned in fat are cooked by the heat of steam, or are actually braised. The browned crust serves the same purpose as does the lid of a utensil, holding in steam formed from meat juices. If chicken were fried without the protective coating, the meat would be so dry and tough you could not eat it.

The chief purpose of frying is to utilize the heat of fat not merely to brown the crust but to carry heat into curves and contours of meat which cannot lie flat on the surface of a utensil. The only meats which should be browned by frying are those which have irregular surfaces. In braising tender meats which cook in a relatively short time, it is important that the utensil not be tightly covered. If steam is held in even for a few minutes, it is quickly heated by the hot fat to boiling temperature; the meat becomes tough and must be overcooked, it is less juicy, and much delightful flavor is lost.

Before home canning of meats or refrigeration for farm homes was heard of, I lived on a farm where we ate delicious fried chicken at almost every breakfast, dinner, and supper from the time spring chickens were large enough to eat until it was cold enough to butcher hogs without danger of the meat spoiling. Being an optimist, I have persistently ordered fried chicken in restaurants over a period of twenty years and in almost every state, but like a homesick New Englander who orders Boston baked beans and finds them cooked with tomatoes, I leave the restaurant a sadder person. The way you can depend on getting delicious fried chicken is to ask a genuine farmer's wife to fry one for you; these women are gracious and wholehearted and will not let you down. If you are lucky enough to find one like Mrs. Johnson, who lives on our farm near Lizton, Indiana, along with the fried chicken and country gravy you will be served creamed peas, new potatoes, sliced tomatoes, corn on the cob, homemade cottage cheese golden with rich cream, a pitcher of milk, home-canned peaches, and fresh berry pie; and your hostess will apologize because she did not get around to baking a cake.

Although everyone who enjoys fried chicken has his own standards as to the way it should be cooked, most people would probably agree that every bit of surface should be an even and golden brown, that the crust should be crisp but tender, and that the meat should not be dried out. These standards we met quite accidentally years ago. It was difficult to urge the old wood stove to produce efficient heat; hence the surface of the meat was browned at moderate temperature, flour which dropped from the meat was not burned, and the meat was not dried out. Since there were usually huge jars of lard in the cellar, we used a generous amount in browning the chicken; curved surfaces which could not touch the bottom of the skillet were thus browned as golden as the flat surfaces. We did not own a lid which fitted the frying pan; hence steam could not be held in to make the crust soggy or to reach a temperature which could overcook or toughen the meat. To prepare delicious fried chicken, these conditions should be duplicated.

## CRISP FRIED CHICKEN, INDIANA STYLE

Allow approximately ¾ hour for frying a 3-pound chicken and 1 hour for a 4-pound chicken.

If you dress the chicken, disjoint so that each piece will be as flat as possible; cut lower back into 2 pieces; crack and flatten ribs along upper spine; wash quickly and dry immediately.

Before frying, mix in a paper bag:

| | |
|---|---|
| 3 or 4 tablespoons whole-wheat flour | ½ teaspoon freshly ground peppercorns |
| 1 teaspoon salt | |

Dredge chicken by shaking 2 or 3 pieces at a time; lay on wax paper and allow 10 minutes for the flour to be dried on the surfaces; dredge a second time if a thick crust is desired.

Meanwhile heat in a frying pan:

½ cup lard, butter-flavored cooking fat, or bacon drippings

When fat is moderately hot, or 300° F., carefully shake off any excess flour from chicken as it is put into pan; place larger pieces in center of pan over source of heat, put smaller pieces around edge, or brown them later. Keep out liver and brown it 10 minutes before serving.

See that fat is sufficiently deep to reach into all curves of the lower surfaces of the meat; add more fat if needed. Leave frying pan uncovered, or set lid to one side, allowing steam to escape. Maintain heat at moderate temperature and allow crust to brown slowly; there should be no smoking fat or sputtering.

As soon as lower surfaces are deep golden brown, turn and brown other surfaces; when all surfaces of a piece are completely browned, pile it on top of those browning so that it can cook at low temperature; continue browning slowly until all surfaces are golden.

When browning is complete, lower heat and cook until meat is tender, keeping lid well to one side; pour off excess fat, leaving 2 tablespoons for each cup of gravy desired; make country gravy (p. 150) seasoned with a pinch of sage.

Serve with fresh peas, cole slaw with sour-cream dressing (p. 295), hot wheat-germ rolls (p. 425).

*Variations:*

If several chickens are to be browned at one time, use deeper fat and heat to 325° F. to hasten browning; when each piece is well browned, set chicken in a moderate oven at 300° F. on a flat pan or broiler rack. Do not cover pan. Roast until tender, or for 15 to 30 minutes.

**Chicken fried in batter:** Make a batter by beating together ½ cup each milk and whole-wheat flour, 1 teaspoon salt, 1 egg, ¼ teaspoon freshly ground white peppercorns, pinch of sage, dash of cayenne; dip the chicken in batter and fry as in basic recipe, or in deep fat at 300° F. Serve with dandelion greens (p. 375), sautéed parsnips (p. 363), carrot and pineapple salad (p. 277).

**Chicken fried in crumbs:** Beat 1 egg slightly with 3 tablespoons milk, 1 teaspoon salt, ⅛ teaspoon each paprika and freshly ground black peppercorns; dip chicken in egg, then in sifted whole-wheat-bread crumbs; fry as in basic recipe. Serve with tomato gravy seasoned with basil (p. 150), brown rice (p. 202), edible-pod peas (p. 351), beets in raspberry aspic (p. 291).

**Chicken paprika:** Brown chicken as in basic recipe; drain fat, leaving about 4 tablespoons; add 2 or 3 chopped onions or leeks and sauté as chicken continues to cook; pile chicken to one side and stir in 2 tablespoons whole-wheat flour; cook slowly 10 minutes; put chicken on serving tray; add to flour and onions ½ teaspoon salt, 1 to 2 teaspoons paprika, 2 cups sour cream or yogurt; stir well and heat through. Pour the sauce over the chicken. Serve with brown rice or whole-wheat noodles (p. 202), New Zealand spinach (p. 377), tossed salad of tomatoes and endive (p. 298).

**Chicken, Spanish style:** When chicken is browned, add 1 minced clove garlic, ½ cup each chopped onions, celery, green peppers and/or pimentos; set chicken on top of vegetables; keep heat low and simmer 15 minutes; put chicken on serving platter; add to vegetables and heat quickly 2 cups tomatoes, 1 teaspoon salt, dash of cayenne; pour sauce over chicken. Serve with summer squash (p. 367), savoy cabbage (p. 384), citrus-fruit salad (p. 284) with French dressing.

**Fried duck, goose, guinea hen, and other fowl:** Choose a young fowl and fry as in basic recipe, allowing ¾ to 1 hour for cooking time. Serve with country gravy seasoned with a pinch of sage, baked potato, shredded beets (p. 342), endive salad.

**Fried rabbit:** Choose a young rabbit weighing 3 to 4 pounds. Prepare as in basic recipe or any variation of fried chicken, cooking about 45 minutes. Serve with mustard greens cooked in milk (p. 379), banana squash (p. 415), tomato aspic (p. 287).

**Fried roasting chicken:** Choose a young roasting chicken and disjoint; brown at moderate temperature as in basic recipe; set on rack above dripping pan and roast in moderate oven at 300° F. until tender, or about ½ hour. Serve with country gravy, carrots (p. 346), eggplant (p. 355), head lettuce salad.

**Fried turkey:** Select a young turkey, preferably weighing between 8 and 10 pounds; disjoint and cut into pieces approximately the size of those of chicken prepared for frying; split thighs into 2 parts along bone; cut breast into 6 or 8 pieces, upper back into 3 or 5, and lower back into 4. Proceed as if frying several chickens at one time, setting browned pieces on a rack in a moderate oven at 300° F. and cooking until tender, or from 25 to 40 minutes; or pile browned turkey in large baking dish, add 1 cup cream, and finish cooking in oven. Serve with baked yams (p. 394), salad of celery, pimento, apple (p. 276). If you haven't eaten fried turkey, you haven't really lived.

When mature rabbits, stewing chickens, and other less tender meats with irregular surfaces are browned by frying and then braised, the procedure is identical with that of frying chicken except that the cooking time is longer, the utensil is tightly covered, the meat is placed on a rack above water, and usually a highly seasoned gravy or sauce is prepared. Since these meats are lean, the purpose of browning is to add the flavor of fat as well as that of browned flour or crumbs. These meats, which are low in moisture, should not be salted until ready to serve.

Many cookbooks advise that meats to be braised be "baked" in a covered utensil in the oven for several hours. Since the cover holds in steam and baking means to cook with dry heat surrounding the food, to follow such advice is obviously impossible. Steaming in the oven is recommended because oven heat penetrates slowly and can easily be controlled; there is less danger of the steam reaching boiling temperature than when meat is carelessly cooked on top of the range. Such a procedure, however, is extremely extravagant. My simmer burner over which I cook turkeys, hams, and any meat to be stewed or braised, has 6 outlets for gas; my oven has 120. Even if you haven't a simmer burner, you use 10 to 15 times more fuel and obtain less heat when you braise meats in an oven than over a surface burner.

## BRAISED CHICKEN

Select a stewing chicken weighing 4 to 5 pounds; singe, wash, disjoint, and dredge in **whole-wheat pastry flour**; follow procedure for frying chicken (p. 91), allowing 30 minutes to brown all surfaces to a deep golden. Pour off fat not needed for gravy; *do not salt.*

Set all chicken except wing tips and neck on rack standing ¾ inch above bottom of utensil; add:

| | |
|---|---|
| ½ cup water | 1 tablespoon white vinegar for each |
| ¼ cup dry white wine or | 2 pounds of chicken |

Cover utensil; put over simmer burner or extremely low heat; in 10 minutes check temperature of water with cooking thermometer and see that it is 185° F.; steam chicken until starting to be tender, or about 2 to 2½ hours.

Lift rack holding chicken to serving platter; increase heat, boil a few minutes if any odor of vinegar remains, and add:

| | |
|---|---|
| 1 cup vegetable-cooking water | 3 or 4 diced unpeeled carrots |
| pinch of thyme or sage and basil | 2 to 4 diced green onions with tops |
| ¼ teaspoon crushed white peppercorns | 1 teaspoon salt |

Shake together until smooth:

**4 tablespoons whole-wheat flour      ½ cup vegetable-cooking water**

Add thickening slowly to sauce, stirring well; boil 2 or 3 minutes, put tray of chicken over sauce; cover utensil and simmer until chicken and vegetables are tender.

Before serving add **2 tablespoons ground parsley.**

Taste for seasonings; put chicken on platter, sprinkle with salt, and pour sauce over it.

Serve with edible-pod peas (p. 351), watercress and tomato salad with French dressing.

*Variations:*

Before browning dip chicken in 1 egg stirred with 3 tablespoons milk; roll in whole-wheat-bread crumbs.

Instead of carrots and onions cook in sauce any of the following combinations of vegetables; 1 cup fresh or frozen peas, 3 or 4 fresh or canned pimentos; celery, carrots, zucchini; 1 cup each mushrooms, diced carrots, leeks; cauliflower and string beans seasoned with basil; green peppers, chopped onions, carrots.

**Braised chicken with spinach:** Omit vegetables, seasoning, and thickening of basic recipe; when chicken is almost tender, set aside on rack; add **1 minced clove garlic, 1 bunch shredded spinach, ½ bunch shredded parsley;** stir well and cook greens until tender, or about 6 minutes; **salt;** put greens on serving platter with chicken in center; sprinkle chicken well with salt. Prepare any other greens in the same way. Serve with steamed carrots (p. 346), tomato and cucumber salad.

**Braised chicken with sour cream:** Omit seasonings, thickening, and vegetables of basic recipe; when chicken is tender, evaporate broth to ¼ cup and add **salt, peppercorns, 2 tablespoons each chives and parsley, 2 cups sour cream or commercial yogurt.** Vary by adding seasonings suggested for sour-cream sauces (p. 169). Serve with chard and beet-gelatin salad (p. 286).

**Braised chicken with cream sauce:** Instead of sauce in basic recipe prepare **2 or 3 cups caper, celery, dill, mushroom, mock Hollandaise, or olive sauce** (p. 162), using **chicken broth** instead of part of the fresh milk. Place chicken on serving platter, pour sauce over it; garnish with **parsley and paprika.** After melon appetizer (p. 261), serve with broccoli (p. 382), cottage cheese and apricot salad (p. 290).

**Braised chicken with tomato sauce:** Instead of sauce in basic recipe prepare 2 or 3 cups tomato sauce (p. 166); pour over chicken. Serve with steamed brown rice (p. 204), sautéed carrots (p. 344), Bibb lettuce with French dressing.

**Braised duck:** Prepare as in basic recipe or any variation for braised chicken, steaming 3 to 3½ hours. Serve with steamed chard (p. 373), apple sherbet (p. 470), shredded carrot and raisin salad (p. 277).

**Braised duck with sauerkraut:** Braise as directed above; set tray of duck aside when tender; add to broth 1 or 2 teaspoons caraway seeds, 3 or 4 cups sauerkraut; steam 10 minutes; put sauerkraut on serving platter with duck in center; sprinkle meat well with salt and paprika. Duck prepared in this way is truly delicious. Serve with spiced apples (p. 459), watercress in tomato aspic (p. 287).

**Braised goose, guinea hen, and other tame fowl:** Braise like chicken, steaming 2½ to 3 hours; season sauce with sage, tarragon, or basil. Vary by making sauce of 2 cups orange juice; salt and thicken as in basic recipe, mixing flour with orange juice; add 2 teaspoons grated orange rind. Omit other seasonings.

**Braised squab:** Cut in half along breastbone and backbone 2 or more squabs; flatten pieces and brown as in basic recipe; set aside on rack; bring to boiling 2 cups vegetable-cooking water, add slowly 1 cup brown rice, ¼ to ½ teaspoon crushed black peppercorns; set tray of squab over rice and steam 40 minutes; season rice with 1 teaspoon salt, 2 chopped pimentos. After fruit appetizer (p. 263), serve with steamed parsley and spinach (p. 376), cole slaw with onions and sour-cream dressing (p. 295).

**Braised rabbit:** Use a 3- to 5-pound stewing, or old, rabbit; braise as in basic recipe or any variation for chicken. Serve with broiled whole onions (p. 388), rhubarb chard, assorted finger salads.

**Curried chicken:** Braise as in basic recipe; when meat is tender, prepare in same utensil 2 or 3 cups curry sauce (p. 163); pour over chicken. Serve with steamed all-vitamin rice (p. 204), carrot and pineapple salad (p. 277).


## BRAISED MEATS BROWNED BY SAUTÉING

Meats which have flat surfaces, such as Swiss steaks and pot roasts, should be browned by sautéing rather than frying. The heat can be easily controlled, and there is far less danger of toughening or drying out the meat. When meat contains fat, as does a pot roast, the fat melts during cooking and the gravy becomes greasy if much fat has been used for browning. Meats browned by sautéing may be browned with or without being dredged in flour or crumbs, depending on the flavor you desire.

Whenever meat to be braised contains so little bone that a knife can penetrate it readily, the meat should be scored thoroughly. Scoring shortens the cooking, thus allowing a more delightful flavor to be retained. The modern method of scoring is to use a sharp-pointed knife and push it through the meat at ½-inch intervals, being particularly careful that the blade is at a right angle to the meat fibers. If the knife is ½ inch wide, a ½-inch cut alternates with ½ inch which is not cut. Although stabbed full of holes, the meat itself remains intact; the cut holes quickly seal over during cooking so that juices are not lost.

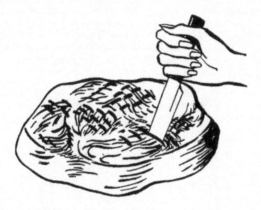

A friend who read this manuscript wrote on the margin, "This type of scoring sounds goofy to me." Actually, it is extremely easy, takes only a moment, and works like a charm. The usual method of scoring, or cutting the surface of the meat diagonally to the fibers to the depth of ¼ to ½ inch does not cut the connective tissue in the center of the meat. Hence tenderness is increased but little, especially when the cut is thick. Moreover, so much surface is exposed that many juices are lost and the meat becomes dry and lacks flavor. My butcher likes to torture a flank steak in this atrocious manner, which to my way of thinking is analogous to ruining it.

## POT ROAST OF BEEF

Select pot roast weighing 3 pounds or more; purchase bone if it contains none. Score meat by pushing knife through it at a right angle to meat fibers and at intervals of ½ inch in rows 1 inch apart; turn and score the other side, making slits between those already made.

Put on wax paper and dredge meat well with:

#### 4 to 5 tablespoons whole-wheat flour (optional)

Render fat from suet; brown meat well on both sides, sear bone; keep heat moderate, taking 15 to 20 minutes. Lift meat and set rack under it, leaving bone in bottom of utensil; add:

| | |
|---|---|
| ½ cup vegetable-cooking water | 1 tablespoon white vinegar for each |
| ¼ cup dry red wine or | 2 pounds of meat |

Cover utensil, put over simmer burner or extremely low heat; after 10 minutes tip utensil and check temperature of water with cooking thermometer; if above 185° F., set utensil to one side of burner. Simmer until almost tender, or about 3 hours.

When meat is almost tender, set lid of utensil to one side; let moisture evaporate and meat juices cook in fat until a rich brown; set rack of meat over serving platter and make **2 cups brown gravy or tomato gravy** (p. 151); add and cook in gravy:

| | |
|---|---|
| 2 or 3 unpeeled carrots cut into quarters lengthwise | 1 diced bell pepper or fresh pimento or paprika |
| 2 or 3 unpeeled turnips cut into quarters | 1 minced clove garlic |
| 1 or 2 potatoes, preferably unpeeled, cut into quarters | 1 or 2 sliced onions, leeks, or green onions with tops |
| ¼ to ½ teaspoon crushed black peppercorns | ½ crushed bay leaf |
| | pinch of basil or savory |
| | 1½ teaspoons salt |

Cover utensil and boil 5 to 6 minutes until vegetables are heated through; lower heat to simmering; return tray holding meat, cover utensil, and simmer 10 or 15 minutes, or until vegetables are tender; sprinkle meat with salt. Taste gravy for seasonings.

Serve with tossed green salad (p. 298) and sour rye bread.

*Variations:*

Omit vegetables suggested and add fresh or frozen peas, cauliflower, string beans, zucchini, kohlrabi, or other vegetables in time for them to be tender by the time meat is ready to serve.

Make gravy with milk; cook in gravy diced carrots, green peas, 2 or 3 diced pimentos; season with a pinch of thyme.

Omit vegetables, bay, and basil; prepare brown gravy; 5 minutes before serving spread meat with dry or prepared mustard or freshly ground horseradish; or simmer 3 tablespoons finely diced preserved ginger in gravy. The flavor is super with preserved ginger.

*Unless otherwise stated, the meats in the following variations are prepared as in the recipe for pot roast, referred to as the basic recipe. Follow this recipe, merely substituting for pot roast the name of the meat you wish to cook.*

**Braised beef brisket:** Select 3 or 4 pounds of fresh brisket; remove bone to cook under rack; score meat, brown, cook, and season as in basic recipe or any variation, steaming 2½ to 3 hours. Vary by cooking in gravy ½ cup each diced onion, carrots, celery, green peppers. Serve with mixed-green vegetables set in tomato aspic (p. 287).

**Braised brisket with wheat:** Omit vinegar; score and brown brisket and set aside on rack; heat 2½ **cups vegetable-cooking water** to boiling and add 1 **cup unground wheat or dry lima beans;** place rack of meat on top and simmer until tender; season with ½ **teaspoon crushed black peppercorns,** 1½ **teaspoons salt,** omitting gravy, vegetables, and seasonings of basic recipe. Serve with broccoli cooked in milk (p. 383), tossed green salad (p. 298). Beef brisket with wheat is an Argentina recipe and is delicious.

**Braised flank:** Select 2 pounds or more of beef flank; score; prepare 1 **cup cereal, vegetable, or fruit stuffing** (p. 159) and spread on flank; fold ends over and pin edges together with toothpicks, making a roll so that meat can be sliced across the fibers; lace securely with string. Dredge and brown surface of roll; steam as in basic recipe 1½ to 2 hours. Serve with spinach (p. 376), brown gravy, sautéed turnips (p. 392), fruit-gelatin salad (p. 290). This is one of my pet recipes; it is especially delicious with apple or prune stuffing.

**Braised pork roast:** Select fresh pork roast weighing 3 pounds or more; if shoulder roast is used, stuff with **prune or apple dressing** (p. 158); trim off excess fat; braise as in basic recipe 2½ to 3 hours. Serve with brown gravy, steamed green cabbage (p. 384), citrus-fruit salad (p. 284).

**Braised lamb or mutton:** Select shoulder roast weighing 3 pounds or more; score and braise as in basic recipe, allowing 1½ hours for lamb, 2½ to 3 hours for mutton. Add or omit vegetables or use vegetables suggested under variations. Serve with baked yams (p. 394), steamed collards, carrot sticks.

**Braised rump roast:** Select boned and rolled rump roast; score, cook, and season as in basic recipe or any variation. Serve with citrus-fruit salad (p. 284), French dressing.

**Braised veal roast:** Select shoulder or rump roast weighing 3 pounds or more; braise as in basic recipe or any variation, steaming 1½ to 2 hours. Serve with French-fried yams (p. 399), stuffed tomato salad (p. 281).

**Heart pot roast:** Select beef heart and bone from shank sawed into 1-inch pieces; wash heart, trim tough membranes, and cut so that meat lies flat; score, cook, and season as in basic recipe or any variation, simmering 3½ hours. Serve with tampala or other greens (p. 377), marinated raw cauliflowerlets (p. 273).

**Pot roast with sour cream:** Cook pot roast as in basic recipe; instead of gravy, vegetables, and seasonings, add **2 cups chopped onions, ½ cup chopped celery, ½ teaspoon paprika, 1 teaspoon salt, 1 or 2 cups sour cream or commercial yogurt;** simmer 5 minutes and serve with sauce poured over meat; the onions should still be crisp. Serve with broiled yams (p. 396), zucchini (p. 367), spinach and cottage cheese salad (p. 282).

**Stuffed breast of lamb or veal:** Select veal or lamb breast weighing 3 or 4 pounds; make pocket between meat and ribs for **crumb, vegetable, cereal, or fruit stuffing** (p. 155); omit scoring; prepare as in basic recipe, steaming 1½ to 2 hours. Add vegetables suggested in basic recipe or variations, or cook in gravy **½ cup each chopped celery, onions, pimentos, 1 teaspoon dill seeds.** Serve with applesauce, assorted finger salads.

**Swiss steak:** See page 73; score or pound Swiss steak well after dredging; prepare and season as in basic recipe, simmering 2 to 2½ hours. After fruit cocktail serve with spiced peaches and tossed green salad (p. 298).

The following braised meats, which are browned by sautéing, are prepared in exactly the same manner as are Swiss steaks and pot roasts. The only essential difference is that the cuts are smaller.

## BRAISED LAMB OR VEAL SHANKS

Select 4 lamb or veal shanks; ask butcher to saw 1 inch of bone from smaller ends; score meat from all sides by jabbing a knife into it at intervals of ½ inch in rows ½ inch apart.

Heat in utensil:

**2 or 3 tablespoons fat rendered from suet**

Sear meat until brown on flat surfaces, with or without first dredging in whole-wheat pastry flour; sear small bones; set shanks on rack, leaving bones in bottom of utensil; add:

½ cup vegetable-cooking water        ¼ cup vinegar or cooking wine

Cover utensil, put over simmer burner or extremely low heat; after 10 minutes tip utensil and check temperature of water with cooking thermometer; if above 185° F., set utensil to one side of burner. Simmer 1½ to 2 hours.

When meat is almost tender, set lid of utensil to one side; let moisture evaporate and meat juices cook in fat until a rich brown. Set rack of meat over serving platter and make **2 cups brown gravy or tomato gravy** (p. 151); season gravy with:

1 or 2 minced cloves garlic          1¼ teaspoons salt
¼ crushed bay leaf                   pinch each of marjoram, basil, and/
¼ to ½ teaspoon crushed black          or savory
   peppercorns

Simmer gravy with seasonings 10 minutes. Serve shanks in gravy or in separate dish.

Serve with fresh lima beans (p. 413), Chinese cabbage (p. 384), carrot and pineapple salad (p. 277).

*Variations:*

Cook in gravy of basic recipe or any variation 2 or more of the following: onions, bell pepper, pimento, paprika, celery, carrots, potatoes, turnips, kohlrabi, string beans, cauliflower, zucchini, fresh lima beans, or other vegetables. Be particularly careful to add vegetables only in time for them to become tender when the meat is ready to serve. Leave vegetables whole or halve, quarter, dice, or cut into fingers.

Omit herbs; add 1 teaspoon dill seeds.

*Prepare the meats in the following variations as outlined in the recipe for braised lamb shanks. Merely substitute for lamb shanks in the basic recipe the name of the meat you wish to cook. Achieve variety by following herb guide (p. 28) in seasoning gravy.*

**Braised beef brisket:** Select 2 pounds or more of brisket, cut into serving sizes; braise 2½ to 3 hours as in basic recipe, removing part of the bone to cook under rack; or cook diced **carrots, celery, and onions** in gravy. Serve with sautéed rutabagas (p. 392), salad of apples and oranges (p. 284), raised muffins (p. 430).

**Braised lamb or mutton breast:** Select 2 pounds or more of lamb or mutton breast, cut into serving sizes; cut off 2 or 3 bones to cook under rack; braise as in basic recipe, steaming lamb 1½ hours, mutton 2½ to 3. If taste of mutton is undesirable, remove as much fat as possible, marinate in ¼ cup **French dressing** for 24 hours; sear in **bacon drippings or beef suet.**

**Braised oxtail:** Select 2 pounds of oxtail; let 1 or 2 smaller pieces cook under rack; braise and season as in basic recipe, cooking 2½ hours; or cook in gravy **2 each chopped onions and diced carrots, 1 cup tomatoes, ½ cup chopped celery, 3 cloves;** add **bay, garlic, salt, and peppercorns.** Serve with steamed potatoes, tossed salad (p. 298).

**Braised short ribs of beef:** Select 2 pounds or more of meaty short ribs cut into serving sizes; remove 2 or 3 bones to cook under rack; braise as in basic recipe, steaming 2½ to 3 hours. After shrimp cocktail (p. 265) serve with steamed kohlrabi (p. 359), sautéed pineapple slices, celery and olives.

**Braised veal or lamb riblets:** Select 2 pounds or more of meaty veal or lamb riblets; remove bones to cook under rack; braise as in basic recipe, steaming 1½ to 2 hours. Serve with buttered beets (p. 343), spiced crab-apples, salad of sliced tomatoes, green pepper rings, cottage cheese.

**Curried lamb, beef, or veal:** Use 2 pounds or more of lamb, beef, or veal shoulder cut into 2-inch pieces; remove bone to cook under rack; sear without dredging in flour; braise as in basic recipe, cooking lamb or veal 1½ hours, beef 2½ to 3; prepare **brown gravy,** omitting all the seasonings of basic recipe except salt. Add ½ to 2 teaspoons **curry powder and ¼ cup of one or more of the following: raisins, diced apple, crushed pineapple, diced banana, shredded coconut.** Cook no longer than 10 minutes after curry and fruit are added. Don't miss this recipe. I put an entire fruit salad in my curry, and even curry-haters agree that it is delicious. Serve with steamed brown or all-vitamin rice (p. 204), carrot and celery salad.

**Lamb or veal stew:** Select 2 pounds or more of lamb or veal stew meat cut into 2-inch pieces; purchase bone or remove bone to cook under rack; braise 1½ hours and season as in basic recipe; cut **carrots, potatoes, onions, green peppers, and celery** in 1-inch chunks and cook in **brown or tomato gravy,** adding each vegetable only in time to become tender. Immediately before serving combine lamb or veal with gravy and vegetables. Above all, do not cook these meats in water. Lamb or veal stew is especially delicious with fresh or frozen peas or fresh lima beans; use any vegetables suggested under variations. Serve with salad of mixed vegetables set in lemon aspic (p. 287), wheat-germ rolls (p. 425).

### SLOW BRAISING

Probably every person with a discriminating taste would agree that meats which are broiled or roasted, or cooked at low internal temperatures, are more delicious than braised meats which are cooked at the internal temperature of 185° F. or above. Since meats which are braised are the more flavorful cuts, the reverse should be true. Simmering temperature, however, is so high that proteins toughen and much flavor is lost. Commercially "boiled" ham, certainly one of the most delicious of all meats cooked with moist heat, is usually cooked at a temperature of 160 to 165° F. The water used for steaming it is not allowed to go above this temperature at any time. The proteins do not toughen; the connective tissue does not break down; the delicious flavor is retained, and the meat, although delightfully tender, slices beautifully without tearing apart. There is no reason why meats which you braise at home cannot be equally delicious.

If you are fortunate enough to have a low simmer burner, a vigorous pilot light, a burner known as a coffee warmer, a warming oven, or an oven pilot light, set a pan of lukewarm water over the source of heat, let it heat for an hour or more, and check the temperature with the cooking thermometer. If a temperature of 160 to 165° F. can be maintained, you can prepare delicious meats without effort and almost without fuel cost by braising them slowly. Actually, lower temperatures can also be used. I have even cooked a turkey over a pilot light which maintained the water under the rack at 140° F. Although it took 24 hours, I have never tasted more delicious fowl.

Meats to be braised slowly are browned and seasoned in the same manner as when braised at simmering temperature. After browning them, or before, if they are to be browned by roasting, you simply cover the utensil, set them over the source of heat, and forget about them. Hours later you return to find them tender and delicious indeed. The cooking time varies widely with the particular cut of meat, but is roughly three times that required for braising at simmering temperature, or from 8 to 12 hours. This method, which I recommend heartily, is ideal for the person who must be away from home during the day. As in slow roasting, one of its principal advantages lies in being able to combine ordinary braising with slow braising to suit your activities.

Since the purpose of stewing meat is to extract flavor, there is no point in preparing stews at low temperature.

## ONLY THE MOST FLAVORFUL CUTS SHOULD BE STEWED

Stewing is a variation of braising. The only difference is that enough water is added to make the amount of gravy desired and the meat is cooked in the liquid. The purpose of stewing meat, aside from developing tenderness, is to prepare delicious gravy and add the flavor of fat. Only the well-exercised muscles of mature animals have sufficient flavor to share with the gravy. Shank, brisket, neck, or oxtail of cutter or canner grade is preferable to other cuts and grades of beef.

Stew meats may be seared without being dredged in flour, or dredged and seared, or not seared at all, depending on what flavor you prefer. If meat of prime or choice grade is used, dredging and searing are needed to develop flavor. Salt should be added at the beginning of cooking to bring out juices desired for the gravy. One or more bones should be cooked with the meat to supply calcium and add flavor. Whenever time permits, soak the meat and bones overnight or longer in vinegar or other acid to shorten the cooking and to increase the calcium content of the gravy. Be particularly careful not to overcook stew; although the meat should be tender enough to cut with a fork, it should not fall apart.

Although only conventional recipes for stews have been included, if your family happens to enjoy meats that are sweet, fruits can make delightful additions to stews. Here is one of my favorites: Brown the meat well, cook it until it starts to become tender, and then cook prunes in the gravy. Chunks of sliced pineapple are even more festive. Diced firm apples, raisins, cling peaches, or any assorted fruits, even including bits of preserved ginger, may be used. Whenever fruits are added, herbs and vegetables are of course omitted.

Recipes for stewed lamb and veal are purposely omitted. Such meats are so much more delicious when braised that there is no excuse for stewing them.

## BEEF STEW

Select 1½ pounds stew meat of canner or cutter grade, a small piece of suet, and ½ pound of bone cut from shank; ask butcher to saw bone into 1-inch pieces.

Cut meat into 1-inch cubes; put bones and meat into a refrigerator dish; add and stir well:

2 to 3 tablespoons vinegar
¼ cup vegetable-cooking water or red cooking wine

1 to 3 teaspoons blackstrap molasses
2 teaspoons salt

Set in refrigerator for 12 to 48 hours; if meat has soaked 48 hours, put on to cook 1 hour before serving; if soaked 12 hours, put on 2¼ hours before serving; if not soaked, allow 3 hours for cooking.

Render fat from suet; shake moisture from meat, dredge with flour if desired, and sear meat and bones; keep heat moderate, searing 10 to 15 minutes; lift marrow from bones and mash with a fork; add:

liquid left from tenderizing meat
3 cups vegetable-cooking water or tomato juice

¼ to ½ teaspoon crushed black peppercorns

Cover utensil and simmer until meat is almost tender; discard bones and suet; add the following chilled vegetables:

2 or 3 unpeeled carrots, cut into halves lengthwise
1 quartered potato
2 quartered turnips, rutabagas, or kohlrabi

2 onions or leeks cut into quarters
1 minced clove garlic
pinch each of savory and marjoram

Cover utensil, heat vegetables quickly, and simmer 10 minutes; shake to a smooth paste and add slowly:

½ cup vegetable-cooking water
4 tablespoons whole-wheat flour

more water or tomato juice if needed

Stir well and simmer 10 minutes. Taste for salt. Stir in 3 tablespoons parsley.

After tomato-juice appetizer (p. 258), serve with tossed green salad (p. 298), rye bread, chilled yogurt.

*Variations:*

Vary stews by adding one or more of the following vegetables only in time to become tender before serving: fresh asparagus, cauliflower, zucchini, string beans, green onions, celery, broccoli, green or red bell peppers, pimentos, fresh lima beans, cabbage, fresh or frozen peas, mushrooms, tomatoes, summer squash, celery root.

Vary stews by seasoning with Worcestershire, lemon juice, paprika, 1 or 2 chili tepines, 1 whole cayenne, or 3 to 6 whole cloves; or follow herb guide (p. 28).

**Beef and kidney pie:** Use a heat-resistant casserole and prepare stew as in basic recipe with 1 pound beef. Omit turnips; dice other vegetables and add **1 cup fresh or frozen peas;** season with **thyme and basil;** prepare **wheat-germ biscuit** dough (p. 432) and bake on a pie pan the size of casserole or cut into biscuits. Remove white tissue from **1 beef kidney, 2 veal kidneys, or 3 lamb kidneys;** dice; 5 minutes before serving, add kidneys and **1 tablespoon Worcestershire** to stew; put crust or biscuits on top. Serve with lettuce and Roquefort-cheese dressing (p. 294).

**Beef paprika:** Prepare beef as in basic recipe, dredging in flour and simmering with **1 cup vegetable-cooking water** until tender; add **1 cup sour cream, 1 teaspoon paprika;** omit vegetables and other seasonings.

**Beef stew with wheat:** Prepare as in basic recipe, using **4 cups vegetable-cooking water;** omit vinegar or wine; add and cook with meat **1 cup unground wheat;** 15 minutes before serving add **¼ cup each chopped onions, celery, green peppers;** add **herbs, parsley, garlic;** omit vegetables. Serve with creamed watercress (p. 373), shredded carrot salad with Roquefort-cheese dressing.

**Heart stew:** Select a beef heart, wash, trim, and cut into cubes; tenderize, stew, and season as in basic recipe. Serve with salad of fruit set in lemon aspic (p. 469), cucumber pickles, raised cornbread (p. 430).

**Hungarian goulash:** Prepare stew as in basic recipe; omit turnips and herbs; add **carrots, onions, garlic, potatoes, 1 cup canned or fresh tomatoes, 3 chopped fresh or canned pimentos, 1 or 2 teaspoons powdered paprika.** Serve with salad of purple cabbage, cucumbers, leeks with yogurt dressing (p. 295).

**New England boiled dinner:** Cut into cubes and stew 3 hours without tenderizing or searing **2 pounds corned beef or fresh brisket;** about 20 minutes before time to serve, add **small whole carrots, turnips, potatoes cut in half, small cabbage cut into sixths;** add vegetables in order of size and time required for cooking, being careful that none overcooks; thicken gravy, season with **salt and white peppercorns.** After tomato-juice appetizer (p. 258), serve with green salad (p. 298).

Stewed beef with dumplings: Sear meat and bones thoroughly to develop flavor; add 1½ quarts vegetable-cooking water; when meat is almost tender, prepare dumplings (p. 108); omit potatoes and turnips. Bring liquid to boiling; add carrots, onions, garlic, herbs; drop in dumplings, cover utensil, and cook 15 minutes without removing lid. Thicken gravy. Serve with sliced tomatoes and green pepper rings.

## STEWED CHICKEN

Select a stewing chicken, dress, disjoint; put into utensil with:

| | |
|---|---|
| 3 cups vegetable-cooking water | ½ teaspoon crushed peppercorns |
| 3 tablespoons white vinegar | 2 teaspoons salt |

Simmer for 2½ to 3 hours, or until nearly tender; if odor of vinegar can be detected, remove the lid of the utensil during the last ½ hour of cooking; skim off excess fat.

Combine and shake or beat until smooth:

| | |
|---|---|
| ½ cup vegetable-cooking water | 4 tablespoons whole-wheat flour |

Stir thickening into sauce and add:

| | |
|---|---|
| 1 to 2 tablespoons chopped fresh sage or ⅛ teaspoon dry sage | 1 or 2 drops yellow coloring |

Simmer 10 minutes.

Serve with string beans, watercress in lemon-gelatin salad (p. 290), hot wheat-germ rolls (p. 425).

*Variations:*

Add 10 minutes before serving fresh peas, diced carrots, potatoes, asparagus, leeks, lima beans, celery, or onions.

Instead of sage season with fresh or dried savory, tarragon, thyme, or basil.

Shake flour for thickening with 1 cup fresh milk, ½ cup powdered milk.

Spanish chicken: Prepare as in basic recipe, using 2 cups water; when nearly tender, add 1 cup tomatoes, ½ cup each chopped onions, carrots, celery, 2 diced pimentos, 1 minced clove garlic, pinch of basil or orégano, drop of red coloring, thickening; garnish with chopped parsley. Serve with steamed celery root (p. 348), frozen apricot purée (p. 470), salad of romaine with French dressing.

**Chicken pie:** Stew chicken as in basic recipe in heat-resistant casserole; cook 1 cup each fresh or frozen peas and diced carrots in gravy. Prepare wheat-germ biscuits (p. 432), bake dough on pie pan the same size as the casserole; put baked crust over chicken. Serve with steamed beet roots and tops (p. 379), lettuce with Roquefort-cheese dressing.

**Chicken with dumplings:** Stew chicken in 1½ quarts vegetable-cooking water; when it is almost tender, make dumplings of 1 cup whole-wheat flour, ⅓ cup powdered milk, ½ teaspoon salt, 2½ teaspoons baking powder, 1 beaten egg, ⅓ cup cooled chicken broth; put chicken on serving platter; drop dumplings from teaspoon into hot broth; cover tightly and cook 15 minutes without removing lid; remove dumplings and add sage, coloring, and thickening. Serve with edible-pod peas (p. 351), carrot and pineapple salad (p. 277).

**Chicken with noodles:** Stew chicken in 5 cups vegetable-cooking water; make noodles by stirring together 2 eggs, ⅓ cup powdered milk, 1 teaspoon salt, enough whole-wheat pastry flour to make a stiff dough; knead and roll ¹⁄₁₆ inch thick; let dry 30 minutes and cut into strips ¼ inch wide; put chicken on serving platter, increase broth to a rolling boil, drop in noodles so slowly that boiling does not stop; reduce heat, add coloring, sage; cover utensil and simmer 10 minutes. After fruit appetizer, serve with chard (p. 373), carrot and raisin salad (p. 277).

**Chicken with paprika:** Prepare as in basic recipe; omit sage, add 2 or 3 chopped fresh paprika peppers or canned pimentos and 1 or 2 teaspoons ground paprika; mix ½ cup powdered milk with thickening. Serve with baked yams, tossed green salad.

**Curried chicken:** Prepare as in basic recipe; omit sage; mix 1 to 2 teaspoons curry powder with thickening; just before taking up, add 3 tablespoons shredded coconut, ½ cup crushed pineapple, and/or 1 small diced banana. After melon appetizer, serve with summer squash (p. 367), assorted finger salads (p. 273).

**Chicken stew with vegetables:** 15 minutes before chicken is ready to serve, add ½ cup each baby lima beans, diced carrots, chopped onions or leeks, celery, bell pepper or pimento. Season with pinch each of sage, basil, thyme. Serve with salad of lettuce, avocado, grapefruit (p. 276).

**Chicken with mushrooms and olives:** Follow basic recipe; add 1 small can button mushrooms and ¼ cup sliced stuffed olives. Serve with steamed celery root (p. 348), spiced purple cabbage (p. 386), sliced tomatoes and cucumbers.

**Chicken with pineapple:** Omit sage; just before serving add 1 cup diced fresh unsweetened pineapple or broken slices of well-drained canned pineapple.

**Chicken with rice:** Stew chicken as in basic recipe, using 4 cups vegetable-cooking water; 45 minutes before serving, add 1 cup brown rice; 10 minutes before serving, add ¾ cup each fresh peas, diced carrots. Omit thickening. After apricot appetizer (p. 263), serve with tossed green salad.

**Stewed rabbit:** Use an old rabbit; disjoint and prepare as in basic recipe or any variation for chicken.

### EAT THE SUPERIOR MEATS MOST OFTEN

The meats most important nutritionally are liver, kidney, brain, spleen (milt), thymus (sweetbreads), and heart. The liver is the storage place, or the "savings bank," of the body. If there is an excess of protein, sugar, vitamins, and any mineral except calcium and phosphorus, part of the excess is held in the liver until it is needed. Vitamins C, P, and the many B vitamins dissolve in water; since water is not stored in the body, they cannot be stored. If an excess is available, however, they are held in greater concentration in the liver juices than in other body fluids. Liver is, therefore, nutritionally the most outstanding meat which can be purchased.

Brain, which is one of the richest sources of the B vitamin cholin, and milt and kidney rank close to liver in nutritive value. Milt is an outstanding source of iron. It resembles liver in taste and delicacy of texture. Pancreas, used in the production of insulin, is not sold on the retail market, but if obtainable after home slaughtering, it should be prepared by recipes given for liver, milt, or sweetbreads. The thymus, or sweetbread, is a gland in the chest of young animals which disappears, or atrophies, at maturity.

The function of these meats in the living animal is to carry on vital life processes; therefore, they contain proteins of the most superior quality and larger quantities of many vitamins and minerals than do muscle meats. Although brain and kidney are not glands, these meats are collectively spoken of as glandular meats in contrast to muscle meats, which are cut from muscles into chops, steaks, and roasts.

The heart is a group of muscles and in flavor resembles other muscle meats. Since it must work continuously from the animal's birth, it has an abundance of excellent protein and the B vitamins necessary to produce energy. Animals, like people, die quickly when their heart muscles are undersupplied with these nutrients. Although heart is not a glandular meat, it is grouped with these meats because of its nutritive value.

Muscle meats, such as steaks, chops, and roasts, have an amino-acid make-up similar to that of human muscles. Their amino acids, however, are combined into proteins totally different from those of the glandular organs. The protein intake of a cannibal would be nutritionally the best obtainable because the amino-acid make-up of the protein eaten is identical with that of the protein in his own body. Although I do not suggest that anyone eat his great Aunt Nettie or his mother-in-law, I wish to point out that the best protein a non-cannibal can obtain is that of glandular meats. The vital organs make up a large percentage of the body weight, and the number and kind of amino acids in the glandular meats are similar to the amino-acid content of the human brain, kidneys, and glands.

It has been assumed that the amino acids needed to build and repair the vital organs can be equally well supplied by any adequate protein; but this assumption has not been proved. The health of the vital organs may be far better maintained by carefully chosen proteins. In an experiment, a number of children were given brain daily over a 5-year period starting in infancy. They were allowed no other meat. When they entered school, it was found that each ranked in the genius class and that the group had the highest intelligence quotients ever recorded in the school they attended. Although the number of children was too small to be statistically significant, the experiment quite possibly indicates that the health of the human liver can be best maintained by eating liver, brain by eating brain, and kidneys by eating kidneys. The person who conceived the idea that fish was excellent brain food must have had an inferiority complex.

Since glandular meats are especially rich in the B vitamins, all of which quickly dissolve in water, they should not be touched unnecessarily with water. Before niacin, the vitamin which prevents and cures pellagra, was available in pure form, the standard treatment for pellagra was to administer the vitamin-rich water in which some glandular meat had been soaked. The mouths of pellagrins became so sore that solid food could not be eaten; hence water was poured over liver, brain, or kidney, allowed to stand, then drained off, and given the patient. Although such patients were often raving insane and near death, they quickly recovered when this liquid teeming with B vitamins was given them. When foods are washed slowly or soaked, they lose iron, copper, and other minerals as well as the B vitamins.

Glandular meats spoil quickly unless refrigerated; they are so outstanding in nutritive value that they support the growth of many more bacteria than do other meats. Before refrigeration was known, they spoiled so quickly that they were considered impure. This old attitude, passed on by early conditioning from parents to children, still exists to cause thousands of people to have emotional dislikes for glandular meats. The mother today who conditions her children against these meats is acting like the mother of early New England who believed in witches and taught her children to fear them.

There is almost no connective tissue in glandular meats. Except when they are seared, they should not be submitted to high temperatures. Since these meats cook quickly, with the exception of salt they may be seasoned before cooking.

The housewife who wishes to maintain maximum health in her family is wise to serve glandular meats at least twice a week; perhaps once as an entree and at other times in an appetizer, soup, salad, or sandwich filling. These meats are more economical than any other meat because they give more health value for money spent and contain no waste. The mother who wishes to build beautiful children could do no better than to serve only glandular meats.

Since glandular meats are so frequently disliked, I have tried to work out recipes especially for those persons who sincerely wish to develop an enjoyment of these nutritious foods.

## YOU CAN GET OVER IT IN FIVE MINUTES

I can claim no virtues when it comes to eating brains. Like thousands of other people, for years I reacted emotionally to the thought and sight of them. Since I believe that one should enjoy all nutritious food, I have attempted to eat brains, but only occasionally. Both Mrs. Kendall, my assistant, and I dreaded testing brain recipes.

When the actual testing began, both of us found that this feeling disappeared almost immediately. After the membrane is slipped off, the attractive white meat looks like sweetbread, which is five times as expensive. The first recipe we tested was brains baked with bacon. The taste is not only surprisingly good; it is absolutely delicious. Although I play safe and speak of brains as sweetbreads, I have recently served them to many guests who claim they hate brains; without exception, every person has exclaimed about the delightful flavor.

Future research may show that brains are of greater health value than is now appreciated. In an experiment on the self-choice of foods by infants conducted by Dr. Clara M. Davis, the favorite meat of all the children was raw calves' brains. These children ate brains in amazing quantities, often more than a pound at a meal. The mothers of children whose diets I supervise frequently give the same report. It is uncanny how a child whose appetite is not perverted by sweets will select foods of outstanding nutritive value.

I am convinced that people usually dislike cooked brains not because of the taste but because of the soft, somewhat greasy texture when undercooked. The secret of making brains enjoyable is to cook them to the temperature at which proteins become quite firm or even slightly tough.

## BAKED BRAINS IN BACON RINGS

Select 1 pound of veal, pork, lamb, or beef brains; remove all membrane while holding under running water; dry on paper towels.

Make **6 bacon rings,** overlapping ends of bacon strips and fastening each with a toothpick; place rings on oiled baking sheet; cut brains into 6 portions and drop into rings; sprinkle generously with **paprika** and dot with ½ **teaspoon bacon drippings.**

Bake in moderate oven at 350° F. for 20 minutes, or until bacon is crisp and brains, when pierced with meat thermometer, have reached 185° F. Garnish with **parsley or chopped chives.**

Serve with fresh peas, mashed banana squash (p. 415), apple and banana salad (p. 276).

*Variation:*

Broil under moderate heat about 12 minutes on each side.

## CREAMED BRAINS

Select 1 pound of veal, pork, lamb, or beef brains; remove all membrane while holding under running water; dry on paper towels and dice into ¾-inch cubes.

Prepare **2 cups medium cream sauce** (p. 161); when boiling, drop in brains, piercing 1 cube with meat thermometer and making sure tip of mercury is in center of cube. Simmer until temperature of brains reaches 185° F., or about 7 minutes. Stir in:

| | |
|---|---|
| **1 teaspoon salt** | **3 tablespoons chopped parsley** |
| **2 tablespoons lemon juice or sherry** | |

Serve over whole-wheat toast with steamed whole leeks (p. 389), avocado and tomato salad (p. 276).

*Variations:*

Use ½ pound of brains; add to creamed sweetbreads, creamed ham, tuna, chicken, shrimp, fish, or other creamed meats. If it is desirable to disguise the brains, this is the way to do it.

Prepare brains as in basic recipe, using any cream sauce (p. 162); they are particularly delicious when cooked in the following sauces: cheese, caraway, curry, dill, egg, mock Hollandaise, mushroom, olive, or pimento.

Cook brains as in basic recipe, using any brown sauce (p. 162), well-seasoned leftover gravy, tomato sauce (p. 166), or tomato cream sauce (p. 162).

## SAUTÉED BRAINS

Select 1 pound of veal, pork, lamb, or beef brains; remove all membrane while holding under running water; dry on paper towels and cut into serving sizes. Dip in:

| | |
|---|---|
| **1 egg stirred with** | **1 teaspoon salt** |
| **2 tablespoons milk and** | |

Dredge with **sifted whole-wheat-bread crumbs**

Sauté in **bacon drippings or butter-flavored fat** until golden brown on both sides, or about 20 minutes over moderate heat; pierce with meat thermometer and serve when temperature reaches 185° F. Garnish with **parsley**.

Serve with radish greens (p. 376), broiled yams (p. 396), salad of purple and green cabbage (p. 277) with yogurt dressing.

*Variations:*

Dip in batter (p. 183) and sauté as in basic recipe; or cut into half-size servings, dip in batter, and fry in deep fat at 260° F. until internal temperature reaches 185° F. and crust is a deep golden.

**Mock oysters:** Prepare brains as directed and cut into 1-inch cubes; dip in **egg and crumbs** or in **batter** (p. 183); sauté as in basic recipe or fry in deep fat at 300° F. to an internal temperature of 185° F.; or use leftover steamed brains and fry at 340° F. until golden brown, or about 3 minutes. Serve with tartar sauce (p. 169), baked potatoes, tossed salad (p. 298).

**With scrambled eggs:** Cut brains into ½-inch cubes; sauté with or without crumbs until firm; add **eggs** and scramble (p. 240); or use diced steamed brains. Serve with steamed broccoli (p. 383), stuffed tomato salad (p. 281).

**With sour cream or yogurt:** Dice brains into ¾-inch cubes and prepare as in basic recipe; when golden and well done, add **1 cup sour cream or commercial yogurt, 1 teaspoon salt, 2 tablespoons each diced pimentos and chopped chives.** After purée of spinach soup (p. 316), serve with steamed all-vitamin rice, assorted finger salads (p. 273).

**With sautéed tomatoes:** Prepare brains as in basic recipe, cutting into slices ½ inch thick; dip firm slices of tomatoes in **egg and crumbs** and sauté; serve brains over or between tomato slices. Vary by sautéing with eggplant slices (p. 354). Serve with creamed tampala or other greens (p. 373), pear and cottage cheese salad.

**With vegetables:** Cut brains in 1-inch cubes and sauté as in basic recipe; sauté with brains **1 each finely chopped onion, carrot, pimento, stalk celery;** sprinkle with **salt and freshly ground peppercorns.** Serve with hash-browned potatoes (p. 403), apple and orange salad with fruit dressing (p. 292).

## BRAINS IN CASSEROLE

Select 1 pound veal, pork, lamb, or beef brains; remove all membrane while holding under running water; drain and cut into ½-inch cubes. Mix with brains:

| | |
|---|---|
| **2 cups medium cream sauce or left-over gravy** | **1 teaspoon salt** |
| **1 grated onion** | **¼ teaspoon freshly ground peppercorns** |
| **2 tablespoons ground parsley** | **1 cup cubed American cheese (optional)** |
| **¼ cup wheat germ** | |

Pour into flat baking dish brushed with oil; sprinkle with **whole-wheat-bread crumbs**; bake at 350° F. for 35 minutes, or until the temperature, taken by inserting meat thermometer, reaches 185° F. Serve with steamed parsley and chard (p. 380), sautéed carrots (p. 344), apple-celery salad (p. 276).

*Variations:*

Add any diced leftover meat, such as chicken, ham, liver, lamb, tuna, shrimps, or fish.

Omit cheese; add 2 tablespoons lemon juice, 1 teaspoon grated lemon rind.

**Brain loaf:** Omit cream sauce; add **1 egg, ½ cup fresh milk, ⅓ cup powdered milk, pinch each of basil and thyme;** chop onion and sauté lightly with **1 stalk celery, 1 diced bell pepper or pimento;** combine ingredients, form into loaf in flat baking dish; sprinkle generously with **paprika.** Bake as in basic recipe. Serve with potato fingers, steamed until heated through and then baked around loaf, steamed cabbage (p. 384), finger salads (p. 273).

**Brain croquettes:** Instead of medium sauce use **1 cup thick cream sauce;** add **1 teaspoon dill or caraway seeds;** include **cheese;** combine all ingredients, form into croquettes, roll in sifted **whole-wheat-bread crumbs,** and fry in shallow fat or in deep fat at 260° F. to an internal temperature of 185° F.; or use leftover steamed brains, fry in deep fat at 350° F. until golden. Serve with celery root cooked in milk (p. 348), tossed green salad (p. 298).

**Peppers stuffed with brains:** Prepare as brain loaf, omitting green pepper from stuffing; use **nippy cheese,** such as Cheddar; fill peppers, sprinkle with **paprika,** and bake as in basic recipe for 20 minutes; or use leftover steamed brains, bake 10 to 12 minutes, and serve with peppers hot but crisp. Don't miss this recipe; it is delicious. Use brains prepared in this way for stuffing cucumbers, zucchini, tomatoes, or onion shells. Serve with broiled yams (p. 396), avocado, tomato, and leek salad (p. 276).

## BRAIN SALAD

Select 1 pound of veal, pork, lamb, or beef brains; remove all membrane while holding under running water; put into utensil with tight-fitting lid and add:

**2 to 4 tablespoons water**          **1 tablespoon vinegar**

Steam 15 minutes, or until internal temperature, tested with meat thermometer, is 185° F. Chill, dice, and add:

¼ cup French dressing                     ¾ teaspoon salt
4 tablespoons ground parsley

Stir well; be sure to retain any moisture left from steaming; let brains chill in moisture and French dressing ½ hour or longer. Add:

1 or 2 diced hard-cooked eggs             2 diced pimentos
1½ cups diced celery and leaves           2 tablespoons or more mayonnaise

Combine and serve on lettuce or watercress. Serve with sliced tomatoes and green pepper rings, cottage cheese, chilled yogurt, rye bread. Brains prepared in this manner are usually assumed to be hard-cooked eggs.

*Variations:*

Cut steamed brains into fingers like shoestring potatoes; mix with parsley and dressing; add to tossed salad or any vegetable salad.

Add with parsley one or more of the following: 1 grated onion or chopped leek; 1 finely diced pimento or green pepper; 1 or 2 teaspoons dill or caraway seeds or commercial dill sauce; ¼ to 1 teaspoon curry powder; freshly ground horseradish or dry or prepared mustard; 2 tablespoons chives or Chinese garlic; 1 minced clove garlic. Use these seasonings when it is desirable to disguise flavor of brains.

**Brain appetizer:** Steam as in basic recipe, using ½ pound of brains; omit seasonings except salt; prepare as appetizer (p. 266).

**Brain sandwich spread:** Use ½ pound of brains; steam and dice fine; decrease celery to 3 tablespoons finely diced; use or omit French dressing; add any seasonings suggested under variations; use for sandwich spread on rye bread.

**Brain sausage:** Steam as in basic recipe; pass through meat grinder; omit seasonings except salt; add **fresh or dried sage, freshly ground black peppercorns, ¼ cup each wheat germ and powdered milk;** mold into patties, dredge with **whole-wheat flour,** and fry until golden brown. Add brains prepared in this manner to meat loaf, hamburgers, pork sausage, or other foods.

**Brains with sour cream or yogurt:** Prepare and season as in basic recipe; stir into **1 or 2 cups sour cream or thick commercial yogurt;** garnish with **parsley sprigs and paprika;** serve chilled for buffet. Vary by omitting seasonings of basic recipe and fold into any sour-cream or yogurt sauce (p. 168); especially delicious with dill, caper, onion, or curry sauce. Serve with sliced Swiss cheese, marinated parsnips, tossed green salad.

## SWEETBREADS

Sweetbreads can be prepared by any recipe given for brains (p. 112). They are particularly delicious when creamed, sautéed, baked in bacon rings, or served in salad. If you wish to be especially elegant, sauté them and serve them topped with sautéed mushrooms on toasted bread rings. *In preparing sweetbreads, follow the recipes for brains, merely substituting the word sweetbreads for brains.* Sweetbreads need not be cooked beyond the internal temperature of 160° F.

Sweetbreads are held together by elastic connective tissue. Although it is customary to steam sweetbreads before removing this tissue, I find it quicker and equally satisfactory to snip it off with the kitchen scissors. If serving sizes are desired, the sweetbreads can then be held together with toothpicks until they are cooked. When sweetbreads are to be cooked in a cream sauce, small pieces can easily be pulled free from the elastic tissue. If to be served in salad, they should be steamed with vinegar to prevent the meat from darkening.

Since sweetbreads are so expensive and such a delicacy, when serving them in salad or cream sauce I would recommend that you use half sweetbreads and half brains. I have served them together many times and none of the persons eating them could tell which was which.

## KIDNEYS CAN BE DELICIOUS

Few recipes need revising as much as do the old recipes for preparing kidneys. Generally the recipes were written without a knowledge of anatomy or physiology. When an intelligent housewife once understands the structure and function of the kidney, her dislike for this excellent food usually disappears. Around the outer layer, or cortex, of a kidney are several million tiny knots of capillaries. The walls of these capillaries, laid flat, are estimated to cover more than a square mile. Through this tremendous surface the force of the blood pressure pushes blood plasma, which is chemically almost identical with the juices of meats universally considered delicious. The blood plasma flows through tiny tubes surrounding the knots of capillaries into collecting tissue which is white and can be seen easily against the dark background of the kidney. It is only when the plasma reaches this white tissue that it takes on the composition of urine. In preparing kidneys, therefore, the cook should let no water touch them until the white tissue is snipped away with the kitchen scissors.

Another reason kidneys are often disliked is that when they are cooked at too high temperature or overcooked, the odor of ammonia can be detected. Since ammonia occurs in urine, an untrained person assumes that the odor of improperly cooked kidney proves that the meat is saturated with urine. All proteins and the products into which used proteins are changed contain nitrogen. Much nitrogen is converted by enzymes in the kidney into ammonia which readily dissolves in water; in this way nitrogen which is no longer needed by the body can be thrown off. Heat accelerates enzyme action, or the production of ammonia, and also causes ammonia to evaporate. Although this odor does not indicate that urine is in the kidney tissues, a little vinegar should be added to neutralize the ammonia. When kidneys are not cooked too long, no odor of ammonia can be detected.

One of my greatest thrills in writing this book was to work out kidney recipes from a knowledge of chemistry and meat cookery and to find on testing them that they were genuinely delicious. Although my assistant and I spent 2 entire days cooking kidneys, not once could a trace of ammonia be detected by odor or taste.

In preparing any recipe in which kidneys are to be cooked in a sauce, it is important that the sauce be sufficiently thick to take up the juices squeezed from the meat as it cooks. I have sometimes thinned the sauce before adding the meat only to find it too thin later. If more thickening must be added, the meat either overcooks or a raw-flour taste lingers in the sauce.

### KIDNEY CREOLE

Cut lengthwise 1 beef kidney, 2 pork or veal kidneys, or 4 lamb kidneys; remove all white tissue; dice into ¾-inch cubes and mix well with **2 teaspoons vinegar;** put into a paper bag and shake with:

**3 tablespoons whole-wheat pastry**       **2 tablespoons powdered milk**
   **flour**

Insert meat thermometer into one cube, making sure tip of mercury is in center; sear kidneys about 3 minutes in **bacon drippings**, or until temperature reaches 140° F.; turn onto paper towel. Sauté 5 minutes in same utensil:

| | |
|---|---|
| 1 chopped onion | 1 minced clove garlic |
| 1 diced pimento or green pepper | 1 chopped stalk celery with leaves |

Add:

| | |
|---|---|
| 1 cup tomato purée or canned to-matoes | ¼ teaspoon freshly ground pepper-corns |
| 1 teaspoon salt | pinch each of basil, savory, thyme |

Simmer 10 minutes; add kidneys and reheat to 155° F. Serve over steamed brown or all-vitamin rice with tossed green salad.

*Variation:*

**Kidney hash:** Sauté with vegetables of basic recipe **1 finely diced carrot;** omit tomatoes; prepare kidneys as directed and cut into ⅛-inch slices; when vegetables are tender, add kidneys, **salt, pepper, 3 drops Tabasco;** stir, heat 3 minutes, and serve. After tomato-juice appetizer serve with string beans and salad of watercress, grapefruit, and avocado (p. 276).

## KIDNEY PATTIES

Slice lengthwise 1 beef kidney, 2 pork or veal kidneys, or 4 lamb kidneys; remove all white tissue, chop in a chopping bowl until fine; add and mix well:

2 teaspoons vinegar

Sauté lightly in bacon drippings:

| | |
|---|---|
| 1 chopped onion or leek | 1 minced clove garlic |

Meanwhile add to kidneys:

| | |
|---|---|
| ¼ cup powdered milk | 1 egg |
| ¼ cup wheat germ | 4 drops Tabasco |
| ¼ cup fresh milk | sautéed vegetables |
| 1 teaspoon salt | |

Drop onto hot grill brushed with bacon drippings; shape with spoon into patties; brown on both sides, or to internal temperature of 155° F.

Serve with fresh or frozen peas, stewed purple cabbage (p. 385), apple and orange salad (p. 284).

*Variations:*

Instead of kidneys use chopped raw liver, brain, or sweetbreads.

Shred 1 chilled unpeeled potato and brown with high heat before adding onions and garlic; add to other ingredients with 2 teaspoons chopped fresh dill, dill seeds, or dill sauce; mix together thoroughly. Vary by omitting garlic and cooking 1 or 2 teaspoons caraway seeds with potato.

Omit onion and garlic and add 3 chopped fresh or canned pimentos or ½ cup lightly sautéed sliced mushrooms.

## KIDNEYS WITH SOUR CREAM

Remove all white membrane from 1 beef, 2 veal or pork, or 4 lamb kidneys; cut into fingers ½ inch thick and mix with:

1 tablespoon vinegar

Shake kidney in paper bag with:

| | |
|---|---|
| 3 tablespoons whole-wheat pastry flour | ½ teaspoon paprika |
| | ¼ teaspoon freshly ground black |
| 2 tablespoons powdered milk | peppercorns |
| 1 teaspoon salt | |

Insert meat thermometer into one piece; brown quickly in bacon drippings or oil, cooking to temperature of 150° F.

Lower heat and stir in:

| | |
|---|---|
| 1 cup sour cream or thick yogurt | 1 small can mushrooms (optional) |

When heated to 155° F., serve with steamed broccoli (p. 383), sautéed turnips (p. 392), tomato and cucumber salad.

*Variations:*

Omit sour cream and mushrooms; pour 1 cup cream sauce over browned kidneys; when sauce is hot, add ½ teaspoon each paprika and salt; simmer 3 minutes before serving. Vary by adding 1 cup cucumbers sliced paper-thin.

**Kidneys with onion:** While kidneys are browning, cook with them 1 or 2 grated or shredded onions, ¼ crushed bay leaf, generous sprinkling of nutmeg; serve with or without sour cream.

**Kidneys with tomato sauce:** Omit sour cream and mushrooms; when kidneys have browned, add 1 cup tomato purée, ⅛ teaspoon basil, 5 drops Tabasco, salt, peppercorns. Vary by adding any tomato sauce (p. 166).

## SAUTÉED KIDNEYS

Cut 1 beef or 2 veal or pork kidneys into ½-inch slices; snip out all white tissue with scissors; brush surfaces with **vinegar;** fasten together into serving-size rings with toothpicks; dredge in **whole-wheat pastry flour** and sear in **bacon drippings** 2 or 3 minutes on each side, or to internal temperature of 155° F.

Serve with herb butter (p. 167) or creole sauce (p. 167), steamed carrots, avocado and grapefruit salad (p. 276).

*Variations:*

Marinate sliced kidneys in 2 tablespoons French dressing or mayonnaise for ½ hour or longer before sautéing.

Mix together 1 egg, 2 tablespoons each powdered milk and fresh milk, 1 teaspoon salt, and 2 teaspoons minced fresh dill or dill seeds; dip kidney slices in egg mixture and then in sifted whole-wheat-bread crumbs; sauté as in basic recipe.

## KIDNEY STEW

Mince 2 or 3 tablespoons of fresh or leftover beef and brown well in **bacon drippings** to develop a pronounced meat flavor; add:

½ cup soup stock
1 or 2 unpeeled potatoes cut into quarters

2 or 3 carrots cut into quarters lengthwise
1 quartered onion or 2 leeks
1 or 2 quartered turnips or kohlrabi

Cover utensil and cook 10 to 12 minutes; add:

2 cups brown stock or tomato juice
¼ teaspoon crushed black peppercorns
pinch each of savory, marjoram, thyme

1½ teaspoons salt
5 tablespoons whole-wheat flour shaken with
½ cup stock or tomato juice

Cook until thick and vegetables are tender, or 6 to 8 minutes. If sour tomato juice is used, add **2 teaspoons black molasses.**

Meanwhile remove white membrane from 1 pound of beef, veal, or lamb kidneys and cut into ¾-inch cubes; pierce one cube with meat thermometer; 3 minutes before serving, stir kidneys into stew and heat until temperature reaches 155° F.; add **2 tablespoons ground parsley.** Taste for seasonings.

After cream of celery soup (p. 320), serve with tossed salad (p. 298).

## BAKED LIVER WITH SOUR CREAM

Cut 6 or 8 small pockets in sides of:

1 or 2 pounds of unsliced baby beef, lamb, or veal liver

Place in each slit:
1-inch piece of bacon

Place in flat baking dish and put over top:

| | |
|---|---|
| 1 minced clove garlic | 1 cup sour cream or thick yogurt |
| ¼ cup French dressing or | generous sprinkling of paprika |

Insert meat thermometer in center of thickest portion; bake in moderate oven at 350° F. for 30 minutes, or until internal temperature is 150 to 160° F.

Serve with steamed onions (p. 389), spinach (p. 380), cabbage and carrot salad (p. 277).

## LIVER WITH APPLES

Mix together well:

| | |
|---|---|
| 3 chopped unpeeled cooking apples | ¾ teaspoon salt |
| 1 chopped large onion | freshly ground black peppercorns |

Place in oiled baking dish:

1 pound sliced baby beef, pork, or veal liver

Cover liver slices with apple-onion mixture; top with:

| | |
|---|---|
| 4 slices bacon cut in half | generous sprinkling paprika |

Add:
¼ cup hot water

Cook in moderate oven at 350° F. for 20 minutes.

Serve with eggplant casserole (p. 353), fresh lima beans (p. 413), pear and cottage cheese salad.

*Variations:*

Instead of apples use 1½ cups shredded carrots; add ¼ crushed bay leaf, pinch of thyme, 3 tablespoons chopped parsley.

**Liver with tomatoes:** Omit apples; slice onions thin; cover liver with slices of beefsteak tomatoes; top with onion slices and bacon.

## LIVER CASSEROLE WITH RICE

Cut ¾ pound of baby beef, lamb, or veal liver into 1-inch cubes and shake in paper bag with:

3 tablespoons whole-wheat flour          1 tablespoon powdered milk

Brown in heat-resistant casserole in:

2 tablespoons bacon drippings

Sauté as liver is browning:

6 to 8 green onions with tops or          1 or 2 chopped onions or leeks

Beat or shake until smooth and pour over liver:

2 tablespoons whole-wheat pastry         ½ cup powdered milk
flour                                     1½ cups fresh milk

Add and mix together:

1½ to 2 cups cooked brown or all-        ¼ to ½ teaspoon crushed black
vitamin rice                             peppercorns
1 teaspoon salt                          pinch of savory, orégano, thyme

Simmer 10 to 12 minutes. Serve with steamed collards (p. 384), salad of carrot, pineapple, and raisins (p. 277).

*Variations:*

Omit herbs and add ½ teaspoon or more curry powder.

Omit fresh and powdered milk, add 1 cup tomato purée or any tomato sauce (p. 166).

Use diced kidneys or brain instead of liver; brown kidneys no longer than 5 minutes.

Sauté with onions and liver 1 chopped stalk celery, red bell pepper, fresh pimento, or paprika, or green chili pepper.

Instead of rice use steamed whole-wheat spaghetti, macaroni, or noodles; cooked unground wheat, unpolished whole barley, or whole buckwheat; add after milk is hot.

When liver is to be ground, it should first be dredged in whole-wheat flour and sautéed to solidify the proteins; otherwise valuable juices may be lost when it is being passed through the meat grinder.

## LIVER LOAF

Dredge 1 pound of sliced lamb or baby beef liver in **whole-wheat pastry flour** and sauté quickly on both sides in **bacon drippings**; put liver aside on paper.

Pass through meat grinder into utensil used for sautéing liver:

| | |
|---|---|
| 1 or 2 onions or leeks | 1 clove garlic |
| 1 large handful parsley | 1 chilled bell pepper or pimento |
| 1 stalk celery with leaves | |

Cover utensil and sauté vegetables slowly for 8 minutes.

Meanwhile grind liver and add to vegetables with:

| | |
|---|---|
| pinch each of marjoram, basil, savory | 2½ teaspoons salt |
| 1 or 2 tablespoons brewers' yeast (optional) | ¼ teaspoon crushed black pepper-corns |
| ½ cup each wheat germ and powdered milk | 1 egg |
| | ¼ cup tomato catsup |

Mix thoroughly; put into a loaf pan brushed with oil; bake in a moderate oven at 350° F. for about 40 minutes; insert meat thermometer when nearly done; cook to internal temperature of 185° F.

Serve with sautéed onions, steamed rhubarb chard (p. 379), mixed-fruit salad.

*Variations:*

Use ground liver instead of beef in any meat loaf (p. 134).

Omit part of liver and use brain, pork sausage, ground heart, leftover meats, or hamburger.

**Liver paste:** See page 232.

**Liver patties:** Prepare as in basic recipe, omitting catsup; form into patties, roll in flour, and sauté until brown on both sides. Serve with baked yams (p. 394), artichokes with Hollandaise sauce (p. 164), carrot sticks, celery.

**Stuffed peppers:** Use half the basic recipe for stuffing bell peppers, pimentos, paprikas, or green chili peppers; bake at 350° F. for 15 to 20 minutes; pour **1 or 2 cups tomato sauce** (p. 166) over peppers when nearly done. Vary by using canned peppers, stuff, flatten, dip in beaten egg, and sauté until light brown.

## LIVER STEW

Cut 1 pound unsliced baby beef, lamb, or pork liver into 1-inch cubes; dredge by shaking in paper bag with **whole-wheat pastry flour;** brown in **hot bacon drippings** and set aside on paper; sauté lightly in same utensil:

| | |
|---|---|
| 1 chopped onion | 3 diced stalks celery or |
| 1 minced clove garlic | 1 diced chilled celery root |
| 2 each turnips and carrots, cut into | 2 teaspoons salt |
| fingers | ¼ teaspoon crushed black pepper- |
| 1 quartered unpeeled potato | corns |

When vegetables start to become tender, add:

| | |
|---|---|
| 1 cup soup stock | ½ cup soup stock |
| 3 tablespoons whole-wheat pastry | pinch each of savory, rosemary, |
| flour shaken with | orégano |

Simmer 10 minutes, or until vegetables are tender; add and reheat liver. Serve surrounded by brown or all-vitamin rice with tossed salad (p. 298).

*Variations:*

Instead of soup stock add tomato juice or purée; if sour, sweeten with 1 to 3 teaspoons black molasses.

Add other vegetables, such as peas, corn, zucchini, or string beans.

## MILT, OR SPLEEN

Milt, or spleen, like other glandular meats, contains excellent protein and is outstandingly rich in the B vitamins and in iron. It should be eaten far more frequently than it is, especially when the budget is limited. I often recommend it to mothers of small children who find liver too expensive to serve frequently. A butcher can order it for you. Like liver, it is covered with a membrane of connective tissue.

The membrane can be removed before it is cooked by cutting it along the sides with knife or scissors, then slipping a large knife along each flat surface between membrane and meat. A somewhat easier method is to steam or broil the milt and remove the membrane after it has chilled. The milt can then be diced or cut into steaks and broiled, sautéed, creamed, served with any meat sauce, made into patties or meat loaf, or added to salads or appetizers. Use milt instead of brains, kidneys, or liver in any recipe.

## HEART

Since heart is a muscle meat, its flavor is similar to that of meats used for steaks and roasts. Persons usually enjoy it the first time they eat it. Uncooked heart can be used instead of beef in any recipe in which the meat is sliced, diced, or ground.

## CHICKEN-FRIED HEART

Use 1 to 1½ pounds of young beef, pork, or veal heart; wash under running water, drain, and cut across the fibers into ¾-inch slices; dredge with **salted whole-wheat flour,** pound well with tenderer, and dredge again; form into compact serving sizes and hold together with toothpicks.

Brown well on both sides in **bacon drippings;** reduce heat and sauté slowly about 5 minutes. *Do not cover.* Insert meat thermometer diagonally and take up when internal temperature reaches 140 to 160° F.

Put heart on serving platter; make country gravy seasoned with pinch each of savory and marjoram.

Serve with steamed kohlrabi (p. 360), shredded beets (p. 342), watercress and green onions with French dressing.

*Variations:*

If gravy is not desired, mix ¼ teaspoon each savory and marjoram with the flour used for dredging.

If lamb or veal heart is used, cut into ½-inch slices and dredge without pounding; season gravy with minced clove garlic, ½ teaspoon dill seeds.

**Broiled heart:** Pound slices of pork or beef heart; sprinkle with **minced garlic and lemon juice;** wrap in wax paper and refrigerate overnight; place on baking sheet, brush with **oil,** and broil (p. 64) slowly 10 minutes on each side. If lamb or veal heart is used, broil without pounding.

## HEART MEAT LOAF

Use 1 to 1½ pounds beef, pork, veal, or lamb heart; wash quickly, drain, and snip off tough membranes.

Put through the meat grinder:

| | |
|---|---|
| 1 onion, 2 leeks, or 6 green onions and tops | several sprigs parsley |
| 1 clove garlic | 1 small bunch spinach |

Heat vegetables 5 minutes in **2 tablespoons bacon drippings;** also heat juices extracted by grinding.

Meanwhile pass heart through meat grinder; add to vegetables:

| | |
|---|---|
| ground heart | 1 or 2 tablespoons debittered brew- |
| 3 teaspoons salt | ers' yeast (optional) |
| ¼ to ½ teaspoon crushed black | ½ cup wheat germ |
| peppercorns | ⅓ cup powdered milk |
| pinch each of marjoram and savory | ½ cup fresh milk or tomato purée |
| 1 egg | |

Mix ingredients thoroughly, preferably with fingertips; place in flat baking dish brushed with oil, form into a loaf, and bake in a moderate oven at 350° F. for 30 minutes; cover top with any **tomato sauce** (p. 166) or **condensed canned tomato or mushroom soup;** insert meat thermometer; bake 10 minutes longer, or until internal temperature is 185° F. This is a delicious meat loaf.

Serve with broiled eggplant (p. 354), steamed carrots (p. 346), Bibb lettuce with Roquefort-cheese dressing (p. 293).

*Variations:*

Spread one-third of meat-loaf ingredients ¾ inch thick on baking dish; cover with mound of crumb dressing (p. 155) or leftover mashed potatoes; spread remainder of meat mixture over top.

Use 1 pound ground heart, ½ pound ground round steak, pork sausage, leftover ham, or sautéed liver.

Add ¼ cup soy grits or soy, peanut, or cottonseed flour.

Use ground heart instead of beef in any meat loaf (p. 134), patties (p. 136), or puffs (p. 138).

**Heart with chili:** Substitute ground heart for beef in making chili (p. 200) or use half heart, half kidney.

**Heartburgers:** Grind with heart 1 onion, 1 clove garlic; make into patties and sauté or broil. If lamb hearts are used, mix 1 teaspoon dill seeds with meat.

**Heart cutlets:** Prepare half the basic recipe, using 1 egg; mold into cakes; roll in sifted whole-wheat bread crumbs and sauté until golden brown. Serve with tomato gravy (p. 150), steamed cauliflower (p. 387), tossed salad (p. 298), hot wheat-germ rolls (p. 425).

**Stuffed peppers:** Combine ingredients of basic recipe, using ¾ pound of heart and half the amounts of other ingredients; fill peppers and bake 35 minutes at 350° F.

## HEART IN CASSEROLE

Purchase 1 veal or 4 lamb hearts; slice across the fibers; dredge with whole-wheat pastry flour; brown in bacon drippings in heat-resistant casserole; when slices are well browned, add:

| | |
|---|---|
| 1½ cups soup stock or tomato juice | 2½ teaspoons salt |
| 2 tablespoons vinegar | ½ teaspoon crushed black pepper- |
| 2 teaspoons blackstrap molasses | corns |

Cover casserole and simmer until heart is almost tender, or about 1¼ hours; add:

| | |
|---|---|
| 1 chopped onion | pinch each of basil and savory |
| 1 minced clove garlic | 4 tablespoons whole-wheat pastry |
| 1 chilled diced bell pepper or | flour shaken with |
| pimento | ½ cup soup stock or tomato juice |
| ¼ crushed bay leaf | |

Stir well; cover casserole and simmer 15 minutes.

Serve with steamed parsley and spinach (p. 380), broiled tomatoes (p. 369), cabbage salad (p. 277).

*Variations:*

If oven is in use, combine all ingredients, cover casserole, and steam heart until tender, or about 1½ hours at 350° F.

Add any diced fresh vegetables in time to become tender when heart is done or add leftover vegetables in time to reheat.

**Heart pot roast:** See page 100.

**Heart stew:** See page 106.

**Heart with fruit:** Prepare heart as directed, using soup stock or vege-table-cooking water; omit herbs; add in time to become tender ¼ pound dried apricots or prunes or thick rings of unpeeled apple.

One of the easiest ways to include heart in your menus is to cook it in soup or soup stock each time you make either. To me soup bones and heart are as boon companions as are bacon and eggs. Although some of the flavor of the meat is lost, the soup gains in flavor. Unless part of the heart is to be eaten in the soup, it should be cooked until it is barely tender and the cooking completed as it is reheated. The following recipes are designed to suggest ways of serving heart cooked in soup stock.

## SAUTÉED HEART

Cut cooked heart across the fibers into ½-inch slices; form into compact serving sizes and hold together with toothpicks; dip in **egg** stirred with **½ teaspoon salt, 2 tablespoons milk**, then in sifted **whole-wheat-bread crumbs.**

Meanwhile sauté lightly in **bacon drippings:**

| | |
|---|---|
| 2 chopped onions | dash of freshly ground peppercorns |
| 1 minced clove garlic | pinch each of thyme and basil |

Push onions to one side; brown heart well on both sides.

Serve with steamed shredded carrots (p. 346), creamed chard (p. 373), apricot and cottage cheese salad.

*Variations:*

Omit onions and garlic; sprinkle sautéed heart lightly with dry mustard, curry powder, or ginger.

Cut heart into fingers ½ inch thick; moisten with milk, shake with flour, and brown; add salt, paprika, ½ to 1 cup sour cream.

Use or omit egg and crumbs; heat 1 or 2 cups any tomato sauce (p. 166) or cream sauce (p. 160); slice or dice heart and reheat in sauce or serve with sauce over meat.

**Broiled heart:** Cut cooked heart into ½-inch slices; hold in serving sizes with toothpicks; broil on oiled baking sheet until heated through. Vary by refrigerating overnight with **minced garlic** and **mixed herbs** or by sprinkling with **dry mustard** or **chopped chives** before serving.

**Creamed heart:** Prepare 2 cups of any **cream sauce or brown sauce** (p. 162); dice cooked heart or cut into fingers and add to sauce in time to reheat before serving.

**Heart pie:** Follow directions for kidney pie (p. 106), substituting cooked heart for kidneys.

**Heart salad:** See page 236.

**Heart with apples and prunes:** Sauté in bacon drippings 2 finely diced unpeeled apples; add 12 diced prunes, ½ teaspoon grated lemon rind. Slice cooked heart ¼ inch thick and reheat over fruit. Serve with fruit sandwiched between heart slices. Pork heart is especially delicious prepared in this way.

**Heart with raisin sauce:** Stir 1½ tablespoons whole-wheat pastry flour into 1 tablespoon melted margarine or butter; add 1 cup steamed raisins and juice, 1 tablespoon black molasses, 3 tablespoons lemon juice; reheat heart in sauce; serve sauce between and over heart slices.

**Stuffed heart:** See page 87.

## WAYS OF MAKING INEXPENSIVE MEATS INTERESTING

For value purchased, the least expensive meats are the glandular ones. Meats discussed in this group are inexpensive because little or no waste need be purchased. Luncheon meats and wieners usually contain soy flour as a binder, which offers two to three times more protein than does meat itself. Dried meat is economical by virtue of its protein concentration.

Contrary to popular belief, luncheon meats and wieners are not made from poor quality meats. Although the more flavorful and less tender cuts are used, the meat is as carefully inspected as are the prime cuts of highest quality.

Since sealed dried beef keeps indefinitely, it should be kept on the emergency shelf and used when dinners must be quickly prepared, when there has been no time to market, or when leftover gravies need to be used up.

### DRIED-BEEF CURRY

Heat to simmering:

**2 cups leftover country gravy or medium cream sauce**

Add and stir well:

**4 ounces dried beef**      **2 tablespoons or more crushed pine-**
**½ to 2 teaspoons curry powder**      **apple**

Serve with tossed salad (p. 298) and broiled bananas (p. 406) or steamed all-vitamin rice (p. 204).

*Variations:*

Omit gravy or cream sauce and add dried beef to diluted canned tomato or mushroom soup or to any tomato sauce (p. 166).

Use lamb, chicken, veal, or any leftover meat instead of dried beef or with dried beef.

Heat dried beef in dill, caraway, celery, horseradish, or other seasoned cream sauce (p. 162).

If luncheon meats are to be held for some time, they should be purchased unsliced. These meats are excellent to keep on hand for box lunches and spur-of-the-moment dinners. Of such meats available, liver sausage offers the greatest nutritive value.

## LIVER-SAUSAGE CRISPS

Slice ¾ pound of liver sausage into ½-inch slices; dip in:

| | |
|---|---|
| **1 salted egg stirred with**<br>**2 tablespoons fresh milk** | **whole-wheat-bread crumbs** |

Sauté quickly in **bacon drippings** until brown on both sides.

Put a slice of **raw leek or sweet onion and 1 ring of red bell pepper** on each slice of sausage; sprinkle with **salt.**

After fish appetizer serve with steamed Chinese cabbage (p. 384), corn on the cob (p. 408), salad of watercress and grapefruit with cream dressing (p. 293).

*Variations:*

Broil sliced liver sausage on a baking sheet; use low heat and do not brown. Sprinkle with pickle relish or serve with barbecue sauce (p. 166).

Instead of liver sausage, use bologna, luncheon loaf, or other luncheon meat.

Wieners are cooked before being sold and need no further cooking; yet they are almost invariably cooked too long and at a high temperature. They should be reheated only at low temperature and usually not longer than 5 minutes. Unless they are dipped in batter, attempts to brown them cause them to curl, shrivel, toughen, and lose flavor. When they are to be served alone, heat them by steaming in 2 tablespoons water or, if the oven is in use, save dishwashing by heating them in a paper bag. Wieners are far more nutritious than they have been given credit for; serve them frequently in interesting ways.

## SPANISH WIENERS

Prepare **2 cups Spanish sauce** (p. 167); let simmer 10 minutes.

Meanwhile hold 1 pound wieners together and slice all at one time into ½-inch pieces; drop wieners into hot sauce, stir well, cover utensil, and let heat 5 minutes.

Serve at once with steamed shredded carrots (p. 346), steamed New Zealand spinach (p. 380), assorted finger salads (p. 273).

*Variations:*

Instead of Spanish sauce use any tomato sauce (p. 166).

**French-fried wieners:** Prepare **batter** (p. 183); dip whole or sliced wieners in batter and fry in deep fat at 360° F. for 1 to 3 minutes, or until golden brown. Don't miss this recipe; it's a good one. Serve with quick-cooked shredded beets (p. 342), tossed salad (p. 298).

**Paprika wieners:** Prepare **2 cups medium cream sauce** (p. 161); add 1 pound wieners cut into ½-inch pieces, **2 tablespoons ground parsley and/or chopped chives, ½ to 1 teaspoon paprika;** stir well, cover utensil, and let stand 5 minutes. Vary by adding wieners to any meat sauce with cream-sauce or brown-sauce base (p. 162).

**Stuffed wieners:** Split wieners lengthwise, leaving skin attached; fill with preheated moist bread stuffing (p. 155); wrap each wiener with bacon and fasten with toothpicks; bake until bacon is well browned.

**Wieners with barbecue sauce:** Use long slender wieners, 2 for each person; cut slit lengthwise in each wiener, open slightly, and arrange in low, rectangular baking dish; pour **1 cup barbecue sauce** (p. 166) into slits; heat in moderate oven 10 minutes. Vary by serving with any tomato sauce (p. 166).

**Wieners in blankets:** Follow recipe for beef in blankets (p. 133); serve with sauce made of **2 teaspoons dry mustard** mixed with **2 tablespoons each yogurt and freshly ground horseradish**

**Wieners with eggs:** Buy short, thick wieners, allowing 2 for each serving; pan-broil on grill 1 minute on each side, using high heat to make wieners curl into semicircles. Lower heat, arrange 2 wieners to form a circle, and drop **1 egg** into each; add **1 tablespoon water;** cover utensil and steam slowly 12 minutes; sprinkle with **freshly ground black peppercorns, salt and chives or Chinese garlic.** Serve with quick-steamed rutabagas (p. 391), tossed green salad (p. 298), rye bread (p. 424).

**Wieners with cabbage:** Follow any recipe for cooking green or purple cabbage (p. 384); heat wieners over cabbage 5 minutes before serving.

**Wieners with omelet or scrambled eggs:** Slice ½ pound of wieners into ½-inch pieces; add to omelet (p. 247) or scrambled eggs (p. 240).

**Wieners with sauerkraut:** Mix **2 to 4 teaspoons caraway seeds** with **1 quart sauerkraut;** put wieners on top and cook without added moisture 8 minutes.

**Wieners with sour cream:** Heat **1½ cups sour cream** over direct heat in serving casserole; add **1 tablespoon ground horseradish, ¼ teaspoon salt,** 1 pound wieners cut into ½-inch pieces. Serve as soon as wieners are heated through. Vary by adding seasonings suggested for sour-cream sauces (p. 168).

Ground meats spoil readily, because of the large amount of surface exposed to bacteria. They should not be kept longer than a day unless at a temperature of 40° F. or lower; small quantities to be held should be frozen in an ice tray.

Ground meat in blankets is an adaptation of piroshki, a Russian meat pie so popular as to be served at breakfast, lunch, tea, and dinner. It takes only a few minutes to make and is sufficiently like our pigs in blankets to be enjoyed readily by Americans. If a high-protein dough is used (p. 424), these meat pies are nutritionally excellent, especially for children whose calorie needs are high.

## GROUND BEEF IN BLANKETS

Render drippings from small piece of suet; grate directly into hot fat.

| | |
|---|---|
| 1 or 2 onions | 1 clove garlic |

Cook slowly until onions are transparent; remove from heat and add:

| | |
|---|---|
| ½ pound (1 cup tightly packed) ground lean beef<br>1 teaspoon salt | generous sprinkling ground black peppercorns |

Meanwhile roll any yeast dough (p. 423) ⅛ inch thick; cut into 4-inch squares or circles 5 inches across; put 2 tablespoons ground meat in center of each piece of dough.

Moisten edges of dough with back of wet spoon and pinch together like an apple turnover. Let dough rise a few minutes.

Brush utensil used for heating onions lightly with butter-flavored fat or oil; sauté meat pies slowly, turn, and brown the other side, cooking about 10 minutes; serve piping hot; eat with fingers or cover with gravy or meat sauce. Don't miss this recipe; it's a good one.

After glandular-meat appetizer (p. 265), serve with creamed peas (p. 365), tomato and cucumber salad.

*Variations:*

Season ground meat with a pinch of basil, savory, marjoram, or orégano or with other herbs or seeds.

Instead of ground beef use any leftover meat, supplemented with chopped hard-cooked eggs if needed.

Instead of beef use ground lamb or veal; season veal with basil and lamb with 2 tablespoons capers or 1 teaspoon dill seeds.

Set meat in blankets on oiled baking sheet; let rise a short time; bake about 10 minutes at 400° F., or until brown; serve with gravy or any cream sauce (p. 162).

**Chicken in blankets:** Instead of beef use finely chopped or creamed chicken; serve with chicken gravy.

Vegetables to be used in meat loaves should be quickly heated to prevent loss of vitamin C during the baking. The secret of having a meat loaf hold together and slice well is to cook it to the internal temperature at which egg, the binder, becomes tough. Insert the meat thermometer into the center of the thickest portion when the loaf is nearly done.

## BEEF LOAF

Sauté lightly:

| | |
|---|---|
| 1 chopped onion | 1 minced clove garlic |
| 1 chopped green pepper or pimento | |

Remove from heat and add:

| | |
|---|---|
| 1 pound ground beef | ¼ to ½ teaspoon freshly ground |
| 1 egg | black peppercorns |
| ½ cup wheat germ | 3 teaspoons salt |
| ⅓ cup powdered milk | ½ cup fresh milk |
| 3 tablespoons ground parsley | pinch each of thyme and basil |

Mix thoroughly, preferably with fingertips; mold into a loaf in a shallow baking dish or pack into an oiled loaf pan; sprinkle generously with **paprika**; bake in moderate oven at 350° F. about 40 minutes, or until temperature in center is 185° F.; insert thermometer when loaf is nearly done.

Serve with sautéed parsnips (p. 363), New Zealand spinach (p. 375), cole slaw with yogurt dressing (p. 295).

*Variations:*

Bake in oiled ring mold dusted with sifted crumbs; turn onto platter and fill center with creamed peas, carrots, or onions.

Add 2 slices or more of quickly sautéed and ground liver; ground leftover chicken, ham, beef, turkey, or other meat; or use half beef and half ground lamb, veal, or pork sausage.

Season with savory, tarragon, marjoram, rosemary, or tops of green onions.

Add one or more of the following: ½ cup chopped celery, shredded raw carrot, fresh or frozen peas; 2 tablespoons catsup or chili sauce; 1 tablespoon Worcestershire or dry mustard; ¼ cup soy, peanut, or cottonseed flour, rice polish, or soy grits; add 2 tablespoons brewers' yeast if catsup or chili sauce is used.

Add not more than 1 cup leftover peas, string beans, diced carrots, or other leftover vegetables.

Place one-third of meat-loaf ingredients in baking dish; pat ¾ inch thick; cover with mound of 2 cups of any crumb, cereal, vegetable, or fruit stuffing (p. 155) or leftover macaroni, noodles, rice, or mashed potatoes; cover with remaining meat-loaf ingredients.

Pour over meat loaf 15 minutes before removing from oven 1 or 2 cups tomato sauce (p. 166), leftover gravy, thick cream soup, or can of condensed mushroom or tomato soup.

Double recipe and serve part of the loaf chilled with caper, dill, or other sauce with sour-cream or yogurt base (p. 168).

Instead of fresh milk add ½ cup tomato sauce, drained canned tomatoes, leftover gravy, sour cream, catsup, or chili sauce.

**Chicken loaf:** See page 230.

**Corned-beef loaf:** Grind uncooked corned beef and use instead of fresh beef; add pinch each of savory, marjoram, dash of cloves, 2 tablespoons chili sauce; increase the onions to ½ cup. Serve with broiled eggplant (p. 354), stewed tomatoes (p. 368), watercress-grapefruit salad.

**Duck or goose loaf:** Instead of beef use leftover ground goose or duck; add ½ cup each of tart diced raw apples and chopped celery, dash of nutmeg. Serve with steamed brown rice (p. 204) or buckwheat (p. 407), broccoli (p. 383), cottage cheese and apricot salad (p. 290).

**Fish loaf:** See page 191.

**Ham loaf:** Use equal parts of beef and ground ham or cured shoulder, either leftover or fresh; decrease salt to 1½ teaspoons; season with savory or 2 teaspoons caraway seeds; when almost baked, pour ½ cup spiced peach juice or other sweet pickle juice over top. After tomato-juice appetizer, serve with cauliflower cooked in milk (p. 387), spiced applesauce (p. 460), carrot-raisin salad (p. 277).

**Italian meat loaf:** Add ¼ cup chopped or ground celery and leaves, ⅛ teaspoon celery salt, dash of nutmeg, ½ cup Parmesan cheese. My favorite meat loaf. Serve with baked banana squash (p. 414), tossed salad.

**Lamb loaf:** Use ground lamb breast instead of beef; season as in basic recipe and add one of the following: **3 tablespoons chopped pimentos; 1 teaspoon dill seeds or 1 tablespoon commercial dill sauce; 2 to 4 tablespoons capers.** Serve with baked potatoes, string beans, citrus-fruit salad.

**Meat loaf of big game:** Instead of beef use ground venison, bear, moose, or buffalo meat; if meat is gamy, use **catsup, chili sauce, tomatoes, or sour cream** instead of milk; proceed as in basic recipe. Serve with fried rice (p. 205), pickled crab apples, steamed broccoli (p. 383), finger salads (p. 273).

**Meat loaf of heart:** Use ground beef, veal, pork, or lamb heart; prepare and season as in basic recipe or as directed on page 126. Serve with corn pudding (p. 410), sautéed carrots, tossed salad.

**Mutton loaf:** Choose lean mutton and grind with a small amount of suet, bacon, or salt pork; add **2 tablespoons capers and ¼ teaspoon each marjoram and savory.** Serve with baked banana squash (p. 414), spiced prunes (p. 464), watercress salad (p. 298).

**Pork loaf:** Substitute ground lean pork for beef; omit the garlic and onions; sauté and add **½ cup each diced apples and celery, pinch of thyme, dash of nutmeg;** proceed as in basic recipe. Serve with broiled sweet potatoes (p. 396), apple and carrot salad (p. 275).

**Rabbit loaf:** Use leftover ground rabbit; add **½ cup chopped celery;** use **½ cup tomato purée** instead of fresh milk. Serve with stewed tomatoes and eggplant (p. 353), molded cabbage salad (p. 287).


## GROUND-BEEF PATTIES

Pinch to bits:

### 2 slices whole-wheat bread

Soak in:

### ½ cup milk

Grate into milk and crumbs:

### 1 onion

Add and stir well:

| | |
|---|---|
| **1 pound (2 cups tightly packed) ground beef** | **freshly ground black peppercorns** |
| **⅓ cup powdered milk** | **pinch of sage, basil, savory, or marjoram (optional)** |
| **1 teaspoon salt** | **⅓ cup wheat germ** |

Make into patties 1 inch thick, roll in sifted **whole-wheat-bread crumbs,** and brown both sides in **bacon drippings;** do not cover utensil. When nearly done, pierce with meat thermometer; serve at internal temperature of 155 to 170° F.

Serve with new potatoes (p. 394), zucchini with cheese (p. 366), salad of watercress and shredded raw cauliflower marinated in French dressing.

*Variations:*

Instead of bread crumbs use ½ cup cooked rice; use tomato juice or purée instead of milk with either rice or crumbs; add a pinch of basil with tomatoes.

Make country gravy (p. 150) and pour over meat before serving.

Add ¼ cup rice polish, soy grits, or soy, peanut, or cottonseed flour.

Instead of ground beef use ground leftover stewing chicken or rabbit; ground pork, lamb, or veal; lean mutton ground with a little beef suet or bacon, seasoned with marjoram, savory, rosemary; or use any ground wild game seasoned with mixed herbs.

Sauté onion until transparent before adding to meat; vary by sautéing with onion 2 tablespoons chopped bell pepper and/or celery.

**Ground beef broiled on toast:** Prepare basic recipe or omit crumbs, milk, salt; spread ground meat ½ inch thick on hot toasted whole-wheat or rye bread; broil with slow heat until well browned, or about 10 minutes. Salt and serve topped with a thin slice of raw **leek** or mild-flavored onion. Excellent for quick lunches.

**Ground beef in pepper rings:** Cut **bell peppers, fresh pimentos, chilis, or paprikas** into rings ¾ inch thick; dip in oil and place on baking sheet; combine ingredients for meat patties, pack firmly into pepper rings, sprinkle with **paprika,** or roll in **crumbs;** broil under moderate heat 6 minutes on each side. Vary by using onion rings instead of peppers; pepper or onion should be still crisp when served.

**Ground-ham patties:** Use ground leftover ham instead of beef; prepare as in basic recipe or substitute **rice and tomato purée** for crumbs and milk; serve with mustard and horseradish sauce (p. 169).

**Ground-lamb or veal patties:** Substitute lamb or veal for beef in basic recipe; add **1 teaspoon dill seeds;** serve tomato gravy (p. 150) or tomato sauce (p. 166) over meat.

**Heart patties:** Use ground beef, veal, pork, or lamb heart; prepare as in basic recipe.

**Meat balls:** Make into round balls instead of patties; brown well, cover utensil, and let steam 8 to 12 minutes. Serve with whole-wheat macaroni, noodles, or spaghetti and Italian sauce (p. 166), or red beans and Spanish sauce (p. 167), tossed green salad (p. 298).

Meat puffs, which are easier to make than might be assumed from reading the recipe, are a delightful variation of meat patties.

### BEEF PUFFS

Combine and mix thoroughly, preferably with the finger tips:

| | |
|---|---|
| 1 grated onion | ½ cup powdered milk |
| 1 minced clove garlic | 2 tablespoons catsup or chili sauce |
| 2 tablespoons ground parsley | 2 teaspoons salt |
| 1 chopped pimento (optional) | ¼ teaspoon freshly ground black |
| 1 pound (2 cups tightly packed) |     peppercorns |
|     ground beef | pinch of thyme, savory, or marjoram |
| ½ cup wheat germ | 1 egg yolk |

If more convenient, combine all ingredients except egg yolk and let stand in refrigerator 2 hours or more; just before cooking add egg yolk and fold in carefully:

**2 stiffly beaten egg whites**

Press into balls 1 to 2 inches in diameter, the smaller size if more "browned" taste is desired; roll in egg yolk stirred with 1 tablespoon milk, then in sifted whole-wheat-bread crumbs; brown in hot fat at 280° F. for 7 to 10 minutes; pierce with meat thermometer and take up when internal temperature reaches 175° F. If fat becomes too hot and puffs brown before well done, finish cooking in warming oven.

Serve with baked banana squash (p. 414), artichokes (p. 339), carrot sticks.

*Variations:*

Cook in shallow fat or bake in moderate oven at 350° F. for 15 to 20 minutes.

Add ¼ cup soy, peanut, or cottonseed flour or ¼ cup soy grits. Use any meat or combination of meats, leftovers, seasonings, and liquids suggested under meat loaves (p. 134) or patties (p. 136).

With little effort, pork sausage can be changed from a prosaic to an ever-varied and interesting dish. After making or buying sausage, add one or two seasonings; fry a small amount and taste it. Try different combinations, using any fresh or dried herbs, any member of the onion family, any sauces such as Tabasco or Worcestershire, or cumin, caraway, mustard, or celery seeds. Use seasoned pork sausage for lunches or dinners.

## SEASONED PORK SAUSAGE

Mix together thoroughly:

| | |
|---|---|
| 1½ pounds pork sausage | 1 tablespoon chopped pimento or |
| 1 or 2 teaspoons caraway seeds | green pepper |
| 2 tablespoons ground parsley | 1 grated onion |

Mold into cakes ½ inch thick; pan-broil slowly over low heat; insert meat thermometer momentarily in center of each cake; take up when internal temperature of 165° F. is reached. After lentil soup (p. 326), serve with steamed cabbage (p. 384), stuffed tomato salad (p. 281) with cottage cheese on bed of watercress.

*Variations:*

Omit onions and add 2 tablespoons chives or Chinese garlic; or use dill, cumin, or mustard seeds instead of caraway seeds; or season with basil and serve with tomato gravy (p. 150).

**Pigs in blankets:** Pierce casings of link sausages and pan-broil for 6 to 8 minutes; or season sausage as in basic recipe or any variation and make cakes the size and shape of large wieners; brown over slow heat for 10 minutes; prepare like beef in blankets (p. 133); sauté or bake.

**Sausage with apples and sauerkraut:** Brown seasoned sausage in heat-resistant casserole; remove and drain on paper; brown **apple rings** cut ½ inch thick; pour off all but **1 tablespoon fat**; place **2 to 4 cups sauerkraut** over apples; put sausage on top of sauerkraut; cover and steam until sauerkraut is heated through, or about 8 minutes; wipe edges of casserole and serve. Vary by preparing sausage with apples and finely shredded red cabbage; cook 15 minutes.

**Sausage with green cabbage and yams:** Prepare as above, using slices of yam instead of apples, shredded green cabbage instead of sauerkraut.

Tongue can be cooked most easily in soup stock as it is being prepared. During the winter months, however, when soup is frequently on the menu, cold tongue may be unappetizing. Following are recipes for reheating tongue cooked in soup stock.

## BROWNED BEEF TONGUE

Cut beef tongue diagonally into ½-inch slices; dip in a mixture of:

**1 egg, slightly beaten, mixed with 2 tablespoons fresh milk**

Dredge with:

**sifted whole-wheat-bread crumbs**

Sauté with high heat until brown on each side; sprinkle with salt.

Serve with raw creole sauce (p. 167), asparagus simmered in milk (p. 341), salad of fresh pepper rings stuffed with cheese (p. 275), rye bread (p. 424).

*Variations:*

Use pork or veal tongue; serve with any meat sauce (p. 162).

**Creamed lamb or mutton tongues:** See page 88.

**Pork tongue with apple rings:** Cut tart red apples into rings ⅓ inch thick and brown in bacon drippings; put slices of pork tongue over apples, cover utensil, and cook until apples are tender; serve tongue topped with apple slices. Vary by spreading thick applesauce sprinkled with nutmeg between thin slices or over thick slices of pork tongue; reheat in oven. After cream of avocado soup (p. 321), serve with steamed turnips (p. 392) and celery stuffed with cheese.

**Rolled pork or beef tongue with bacon:** Slice tongue diagonally ⅛ inch thick; mix together **2 teaspoons dry mustard and 2 tablespoons ground horseradish;** spread on tongue, roll tightly, wrap a strip of bacon around each, and hold with toothpicks; bake until bacon is crisp. Vary by filling with leftover creamed vegetables or well-seasoned mashed potatoes. Serve with shredded beets (p. 342), cooked celery with cheese (p. 347), carrot-cabbage salad (p. 277).

Next to milt, tripe is usually the cheapest meat available. It contains little adequate protein and should be served with eggs, cheese, or other proteins on the menu with it. In cooking tripe, include a small amount of bone for flavor and calcium.

## CREAMED TRIPE

Use 1 pound of veal, beef, lamb, or pork tripe and 2 small pieces of bone. Put tripe and bones in utensil with:

**1 cup vegetable-cooking water          2 tablespoons vinegar**

Simmer 2 hours for pickled or precooked tripe, 3½ hours for uncooked tripe, or until tender and cut edge has a clear appearance; add a small amount more liquid if needed; remove from utensil and cool.

Prepare in same utensil, using moisture left from steaming:

### 2 cups cream sauce (p. 161)

After sauce has simmered 10 minutes, cut tripe into small strips or squares with scissors, dropping it directly into sauce; salt to taste; serve as soon as tripe has reheated. Tripe is especially good with dill, caraway, cheese, celery, pimento, or onion sauce.

Serve with baked sweet potatoes, steamed rhubarb chard (p. 380), pineapple and cottage cheese salad.

*Variations:*

Instead of cream sauce use any brown sauce (p. 162), any tomato sauce (p. 166), leftover gravy, or any heated sour-cream sauce (p. 169); if sour-cream sauce is used, heat only to simmering; do not boil.

**Broiled tripe:** Steam tripe as directed in basic recipe; cut into serving sizes, place on oiled baking sheet, sprinkle with **paprika**, and cover with **bacon slices** cut into thirds; broil slowly until bacon is crisp. After meat-vegetable soup (p. 313), serve with steamed turnips, tomato and cottage cheese salad.

**Pepper-pot stew:** Cut raw tripe into 1-inch squares and cook as directed in basic recipe; add at the beginning of cooking **1 cup canned or diced tomatoes, 2 teaspoons salt, 1 tablespoon black molasses;** when tripe is nearly tender, discard bone, add ½ **teaspoon crushed black peppercorns, 1 each diced onion, unpeeled potato, carrot, turnip, pinch each of thyme and savory;** thicken with **4 tablespoons whole-wheat pastry flour** mixed with ½ **cup water;** cook until vegetables are just tender. Serve with salad of apricots and cottage cheese.

**Sautéed tripe:** Cook as in basic recipe; cut into serving sizes, dip in **salted egg diluted with milk,** then in sifted **whole-wheat-bread crumbs;** sauté until golden. After cream of asparagus soup (p. 320), serve with steamed kohlrabi (p. 359), tossed salad.

**Stuffed tripe:** Simmer whole tripe until almost tender; cool slightly and cut into two matching sections, dicing scraps; fill with onion stuffing (p. 157) to which scraps are added; brush surface with bacon drippings and bake in moderate oven at 350° F. for 30 minutes.

**Tripe creole:** Prepare as in basic recipe, using 2 cups creole sauce (p.166) instead of cream sauce.

## MAKE THE BONY MEATS RICH SOURCES OF CALCIUM

Such meats as spareribs, backbones, and pigs' feet supply only about a fifth as much protein as do lean meats such as liver, steaks, or roasts. Since they contain much fat, they are satisfying. Unless the meat is removed from the bones after cooking, as it is in head cheese, additional protein foods should be served at the same meal with bony meats.

If soaked and cooked in vinegar or other acid, these meats can become outstanding sources of calcium, sometimes supplying as much in a single serving as can be obtained from 3 quarts or more of milk. When they are cooked without acid, almost no calcium dissolves out. The amount of calcium dissolved in the gravy or sauce is in proportion to the amount of acid used, the length of time the meat is soaked and cooked with acid, and the amount of bone exposed. Use as much acid in preparing these meats as you can without making them unpalatable. Whenever time permits, soak the bones before cooking. Larger amounts of calcium dissolve out when these meats are stewed than when they are steamed, although stewing causes loss of flavor.

Serve bony meats frequently, especially when you have growing children in the family, or at any time when the calcium requirements are high. Make sure every drop of liquid used for soaking and cooking is eaten with the meat.

### PICKLED PIGS' FEET

Select 8 pigs' feet; clean thoroughly, put into cooking utensil, and add:

3 cups water                              1 cup vinegar

Simmer about 3 hours, or until tender; do not allow meat to fall from bones; put pigs' feet in a glass baking dish; skim fat from broth, and add:

1/4 teaspoon mixed pickling spices        1/4 teaspoon crushed black pepper-
1/2 cup vinegar, or enough to make            corns
    quite tart                            1 tablespoon gelatin soaked in
2 teaspoons salt                              1/2 cup cold water

Add more liquid if needed to bring total to about 3 cups; pour broth over pigs' feet; cover lightly and keep in refrigerator 3 to 5 days before serving. Under no circumstances seal pickled pigs' feet; the protein can neutralize the acid in the vinegar, and botulinus can thrive in the absence of air and acid.

Serve pigs' feet chilled with baked beans, salad of sliced cucumbers, tomatoes, and sweet onions.

*Variations:*

Instead of pigs' feet use 2 pounds or more of spareribs, backbones, or smaller bony sections of oxtail; simmer spareribs and oxtail about 2 hours, backbones 2½ hours. If only 2 pounds of meat are pickled, use half the amounts of other ingredients.

## BRAISED PIGS' FEET

Select 4 pigs' feet; ask butcher to cut in half lengthwise; pack into refrigerator dish and add:

| | |
|---|---|
| ½ cup white vinegar | 1 to 2 cups tomato juice or canned tomatoes |

After soaking 24 to 48 hours, drain well, roll in **whole-wheat pastry flour**, and brown all surfaces in **bacon drippings**; add liquid used for soaking and simmer 3 hours, or until tender; add:

| | |
|---|---|
| ¼ teaspoon crushed black peppercorns | 1 to 2 tablespoons black molasses |
| 1 minced clove garlic | 2 teaspoons salt |
| 1 chopped or grated onion | 4 tablespoons whole-wheat pastry |
| 1 diced stalk celery | flour shaken with |
| 2 diced pimentos or bell peppers | ½ cup tomato juice |

Stir well and simmer 10 minutes.

Serve with potato pancakes (p. 404), carrots with cheese (p. 346), sliced cucumbers with green-pepper rings.

*Variations:*

Add a pinch each of basil and orégano, 1 or 2 teaspoons cumin seeds. Use spareribs instead of pigs' feet. Simmer 1½ to 2 hours.

**Pigs' feet fried in batter:** Soak pigs' feet and cook as in basic recipe without browning, using water instead of tomatoes; omit seasonings; dip in **batter** (p. 183) and fry in deep fat at 360° F. for 3 minutes, or until golden brown. If your butcher is good-natured, ask him to cut the pigs' feet into 2-inch lengths. Serve with corn on the cob (p. 408), eggplant with cheese (p. 353), tossed green salad (p. 298).

**Pigs' feet with ginger:** If possible, have pigs' feet cut into 2-inch lengths; soak, brown, and cook as in basic recipe, using water instead of tomatoes; omit onion, celery, pimento; add with other seasonings **2 or 3 tablespoons chopped preserved ginger or 1 or 2 teaspoons ground ginger.** This is my favorite recipe for pigs' feet. Serve with steamed brown rice (p. 204), broccoli (p. 383), pineapple and cottage cheese salad.

**Stewed pigs' feet:** Prepare like backbones (p. 145). Simmer 3 to 4 hours.

## BARBECUED SPARERIBS

Select 2 pounds or more of meaty, uncut spareribs; put in flat baking dish and pour over meat:

| | |
|---|---|
| 2 tablespoons vinegar | 1 tablespoon blackstrap molasses |
| 2 cups tomato purée or drained and chopped canned tomatoes | |

Let soak 24 to 48 hours; pour off liquid, removing purée with dish scraper; put spareribs on meat rack, insert meat thermometer between bones, and set in broiler compartment; place an upright oven thermometer at same level with meat and adjust temperature to 300° F.; when surface dries, brush with **oil,** then with **black molasses;** barbecue (p. 83) to an internal temperature of 170° F., or about 2 hours.

Meanwhile prepare barbecue sauce (p. 166), using ingredients left from soaking; 20 minutes before time to serve, pour sauce over meat; baste with the sauce once or twice.

Serve with sautéed parsnips (p. 363), rhubarb chard, salad of celery and hard-cooked eggs.

*Variations:*

Select matching sections of spareribs; barbecue as in basic recipe; when well browned and nearly done, spread one section with sauerkraut, put other section on top, cover with sauce.

**Braised spareribs:** Prepare as braised pigs' feet (p. 143).

**Pickled spareribs:** Prepare as pickled pigs' feet (p. 142).

**Spareribs with apples:** Omit tomatoes or purée; brush spareribs well with vinegar; barbecue; 30 minutes before serving cover spareribs with ½-inch rings of tart, cored but unpeeled apples; brush apples with drippings and black molasses; cook until well browned.

**Stewed spareribs:** Prepare as stewed backbones (p. 145).

**Stuffed spareribs:** See page 79.

## STEWED BACKBONES

Select 2 pounds or more of pork backbones cut at each joint. If meat is not to be cooked immediately, pack solidly into a refrigerator dish; pour over meat:

¼ to ½ cup white vinegar
1 or 2 tablespoons black molasses

½ to 1 cup vegetable-cooking water, or enough to cover

After soaking for 24 to 48 hours, simmer in the same liquid 2½ hours, or until meat is tender; put backbones on serving platter, skim fat from broth, and add:

1 minced clove garlic
¼ teaspoon crushed black peppercorns
1 whole cayenne or chili tepine
¼ crushed bay leaf

2 teaspoons salt
½ cup vegetable-cooking water shaken with
3 tablespoons whole-wheat pastry flour

Add more water if needed; stir well, cover utensil, and simmer 10 minutes.

After fruit appetizer, serve with stewed lima beans (p. 413), salad of cottage cheese and spinach (p. 282).

*Variations:*

Soak backbones in vinegar with tomato juice or canned tomatoes instead of water; or omit vinegar and add with water ¼ to ½ cup dry white or red wine.

Shake ⅓ cup powdered milk with thickening; add 2 or 3 drops brown coloring to gravy.

Instead of backbones use pigs' feet or spareribs; simmer pigs' feet 3 to 4 hours, spareribs 1½ to 2 hours.

I would probably never have prepared head cheese or scrapple had it not been necessary to test the following recipes. To my surprise, I found them unusually delicious. Head cheese is quite similar to pressed chicken in taste, and scrapple is a flavorful variation of old-fashioned fried mush. I was even more surprised at the tremendous amount of food one could obtain at little cost. Surely few other cuts of meat can offer so much satiety value for money spent as can hog's head. The heads are carefully cleaned at the slaughterhouses; hence the work of preparing these dishes is slight.

## HEAD CHEESE

Select hog's head, wash thoroughly, put into large utensil, and add:

½ cup white vinegar            4 cups vegetable-cooking water

Simmer about 4 hours, or until meat starts to fall from bones; set head in colander, let head and broth chill overnight; it is much easier to work with and far less greasy if chilled.

Remove meat from bones; dice fine or pass through meat grinder, using large knife, tongue, brain, skin, all lean meat; keep larger amount of fat meat for seasoning. Skim all fat from broth, heat to boiling, and add:

3 teaspoons salt                   ⅛ teaspoon each savory, sage,
½ teaspoon crushed black pepper-     marjoram, basil
  corns                              ½ crushed bay leaf

Mix together:

half of the diced or ground meat   1½ cups hot broth, or enough to
½ cup powdered milk                  moisten

Pack into oiled mold or cardboard milk cartons; chill until firm; slice and serve cold. Use remainder of broth and meat in making scrapple.

Serve head cheese with horseradish sauce (p. 169), sauerkraut, applesauce, carrot salad (p. 277).

*Variations:*

Grind or dice fine and add to head cheese one or more of the following: sweet onion or leek; green pepper, pimento, or green chili pepper; celery; or add 1 or 2 teaspoons caraway seeds.

Dice fat meat taken from hog's head into ½-inch cubes; pan-broil until crisp and well browned; use for seasoning baked or string beans or green leafy vegetables; or add to scrambled eggs or to any food customarily seasoned with crisp bacon.

**Scrapple:** Add enough water to remaining broth to make 1 quart; bring to a rolling boil and stir in slowly 1¼ cups yellow corn meal; stir constantly until mixture thickens, or about 5 minutes; add ½ cup wheat germ and remaining diced or ground meat, salt to taste; cool, pour into loaf pans or milk cartons, and chill. Slice and serve cold or dredge in whole-wheat flour or crumbs and sauté. Vary by using entire hog's head, cooking it in 2 quarts water and stirring 2½ cups corn meal into broth; or use equal parts corn meal and buckwheat flour. Serve with fresh lima beans, broccoli with cheese sauce (p. 163), salad of assorted fruits.

# CHAPTER 8

## MAKE DELICIOUS GRAVIES OR NONE AT ALL

Tender, juicy, and delightfully cooked meat can be almost ruined by having gray, lumpy gravy served over it. There are only two ways of making gravies: by cooking flour in fat and then adding liquid; by adding thickening to meat juices. The causes of failure are the same in both varieties.

All kinds of gravy should have an appetizing color. Brown gravies may be achieved in three ways: by heating fat until a small amount of it changes to carbon; by browning bits of lean meat until some of the protein breaks down chemically; or by heating flour until some of the starch changes to dextrin, a semi-sugar, which is partly caramelized. Browned fat, bits of meat, and flour each give a characteristic flavor which is usually enjoyed. If one or all three are browned, the flavor and the color desired can be obtained. Kitchen bouquet, always the convenient admission of failure, may be used. Tomato gravy and gravy to be served with stewed chicken can be enhanced by a few drops of red or yellow coloring.

The taste of undercooked flour can be avoided if 2 cups or more of flour for gravy are heated in the oven. Spread the flour out on a flat pan and heat it slowly as if you were making Melba toast; stir it occasionally; when it is a light brown, store it in a jar or paper bag for future use. When starch changes to dextrin, or when the flour is highly browned, some of its thickening power has been lost and larger amounts must be used. Gravies made of uncooked flour should be simmered at least 10 minutes to prevent the taste of undercooked flour.

The trick of mixing thickenings in a second is to put the liquid into a jar, add the flour, fasten the lid securely, and then shake it. The liquid must be put in first; otherwise the flour sticks to the bottom. This same procedure is excellent for mixing powdered milk or yeast with liquids. It is surprisingly easy and quick.

What housewife does not have the memory of some guest dinner which she hoped would be particularly good, but the gravy became as full of lumps as a gravel path? Lumps can be avoided by a moment's consideration of why lumps lump. If flour and liquid are not shaken or stirred to a smooth batter, the lumps in the thickening are cooked into small dumplings; this type of lump can be prevented by shaking the thickening a moment. Lumps of a cornstarch-pudding texture are made by pouring smooth thickening drop by drop into boiling liquid; each drop in all its lumpy roundness is cooked immediately and preserved. Such lumps may be prevented if you are careful to keep the liquid to be thickened below the boiling point until the thickening is added and the mixture is thoroughly stirred.

Gravies made by adding flour to fat cannot lump if stirred sufficiently to coat each particle of flour with fat. As little as 1 tablespoon of fat can prevent the particles in 3 tablespoons of flour from sticking together if the two are well mixed. The liquid should be added slowly and the heat kept low until liquid, fat, and flour are blended. If these precautions are taken, there is no need for gravies to be beaten or stirred rapidly. If too large a proportion of fat is used, gravies separate; hence excess fat should be removed before the flour is added.

In my opinion the most delicious gravy has a proportion of 1 or 2 tablespoons of fat to 2 tablespoons of flour. If you use more than 2 tablespoons of fat for each tablespoon of flour, you can expect the fat to separate out. An easy way to ruin gravy is to allow it to be greasy.

The problem of making gravy too thick or too thin can be met by memorizing once and for all the proportions of flour to liquid: 1 level tabelspoon of flour is used to each ½ cup of liquid, including the liquid used in mixing the thickening. If the flour is to be highly browned, allow an extra tablespoon.

The habit of making gravy immediately before the meat is served is frequently inconvenient, has social disadvantages, and often causes the meat to get cold and the housewife to arrive at the table dripping with perspiration. Most gravies can be made in advance and be ready to serve by the time the meat is done. If thickening is to be added to liquid, as in making gravy for stew, part of the meat can be put on the serving platter while thickening is added and the meat returned to the gravy to finish cooking. When meat is to be steamed to tenderness after being browned, as are fried chicken, veal cutlets, and many sautéed meats, the browned meat can be put on a wire rack over the serving platter while the gravy is quickly made; the rack of the meat can then be set over the gravy. Even though the utensil is uncovered, the meat can be steamed to tenderness as the gravy cooks. If the heat is kept low, there is no danger of the gravy's sticking or burning. When more gravy is desired than can be made without coming up over the meat, additional liquid can be added later. Gravy to be served with braised meats which are cooked on a rack can be prepared by this procedure.

When meats are broiled or roasted at extremely low temperature, no fat or meat juices are charred and not more than 1 tablespoon of juice may collect in the dripping pan. In this case gravy can be made of trimmings cut from meat before cooking. A tablespoon or two of lean meat for each cup of gravy desired should be minced and browned in fat. The fat may be rendered from the trimmings of broiled meat or dipped from the dripping pan under a roast. The quantity of liquid in the dripping pan should be estimated. A thick gravy may be prepared with milk, stock, or tomato juice and diluted by the juices in the dripping pan when the meat is taken up and undesired fat is skimmed off. A brown country gravy to serve with meats which are fried in deep fat or braised without searing, such as croquettes, can also be made of bits of meat browned in fat. The juices left from braising may be added immediately before the gravy is served. If gravy is desired with leftover meat after all drippings have been used, bits of cooked meat may be browned in freshly rendered fat or in any bland-flavored fat.

Because of the great nutritive value of milk, prepare country gravy whenever possible. Delicious gravy can be prepared by adding canned mushroom or tomato soup diluted with milk or meat juices to browned fat and bits of meat. When a liquid other than milk is to be added to gravies, tomato and other vegetable juices, vegetable-cooking water, or soup stock should be used instead of water. Gravies can be made creamier in texture, superior in flavor, and richer in protein, vitamin $B_2$, and calcium if powdered milk is beaten with part of the liquid to be used and added a few minutes before the gravy is served. Since meat juices contain much nutritive value, no more gravy should be prepared than is likely to be eaten. Any leftover gravy should be used as cream or brown sauce, added to fresh gravy, meat loaf, or dressing, or reheated with fresh seasonings.

The earmark of good gravy lies in the seasoning. When a person becomes accustomed to well-seasoned gravy, chicken gravy without a pinch of sage or thyme, tomato gravy without orégano or basil, and beef gravy without savory, marjoram, or rosemary seem as flat as if the salt were omitted. The use of crushed peppercorns instead of stale ground pepper makes a striking improvement. Endless variations and delightful flavors can be achieved by adding seasonings. Chopped onions, celery, any variety of fresh peppers, and garlic may be slightly cooked in the fat to be used for making gravy. All gravy should be well salted and tasted for salt before being served.

### GRAVY MADE WITH FLOUR ADDED TO FAT

Measure into a bowl the liquid to be used and keep in a warm place. Brown slightly:

**2 to 4 tablespoons fat**

Add and stir thoroughly:

**4 level tablespoons whole-wheat pastry flour, uncooked or slightly browned**

Brown to the color desired over moderate heat; reduce heat and add slowly while stirring:

| | |
|---|---|
| 2 cups milk, tomato or other vegetable juice, vegetable-cooking water, or soup stock | 1 teaspoon salt |
| | ¼ teaspoon minced fresh herbs or pinch of dried herbs |
| ¼ teaspoon crushed black peppercorns | |

Taste for salt. Simmer for 10 minutes; garnish with **paprika.**

## GRAVY MADE WITH THICKENING ADDED TO LIQUID

Shake to a smooth paste in a small sealed jar, adding liquid first:

½ cup cold milk or vegetable-     4 level tablespoons whole-wheat
cooking water                     pastry flour, uncooked or slightly
                                  browned
Heat:

1½ cups meat juices, meat juices and milk, tomato juice, vegetable-
cooking water, or soup stock

Remove momentarily from heat; stir constantly, and add thickening
slowly; when gravy is well blended, add:

1 teaspoon salt                   ½ teaspoon minced fresh or a
¼ teaspoon crushed white or black     pinch of dried herbs
peppercorns

Simmer 10 minutes. Taste for salt. Garnish with **paprika.**

*Variations:*

If meat is to be steamed until tender, put it on wire rack over serving
platter; prepare gravy, and steam meat while gravy simmers; *do not cover
utensil* unless meat is braised or stewed.

Shake ½ cup powdered milk with 1 cup of the liquid to be used for
gravy; add 5 minutes before serving.

Render the fat for gravy from meat trimmings or dip from dripping
pan; brown in the fat 1 or 2 tablespoons fresh or leftover lean meat until
almost charred; prepare gravy by either method, using any available meat
juice.

For highly seasoned gravies, see brown sauces (p. 162).

To prepare browned flour: Spread 2 cups whole-wheat pastry flour on
a flat baking pan and heat in a moderate oven at 300° F. for 10 to 15
minutes, or until slightly browned; store in a glass jar; a small amount of
flour may be well browned and used for coloring and sweetening.

Omit flour and use canned tomato or mushroom soup diluted to desired consistency with milk; season the tomato soup with a pinch of orégano or basil.

Beef gravy: Vary the seasonings by adding one or two of the following:
marjoram, rosemary, savory, basil, orégano, chives, onions, leeks, parsley,
garlic, mustard, celery, caraway, or cardamom seeds; chili tepine, chili
sauce, Worcestershire, catsup; chopped celery, fresh pepper, or pimento.

**Chicken gravy:** Season with sage or combine with sage one or more of the following: savory, basil, thyme, marjoram, chives, leeks, or a generous amount of ground paprika; chopped canned or fresh pimento, bell pepper, or paprika; add 1 or 2 drops yellow coloring to clear chicken gravy.

**Duck, goose, or small game gravy:** Season like chicken gravy.

**Gravy with big game:** Season like beef gravy, combining 2 or more seasonings if the meat is gamy.

**Lamb gravy:** Season like chicken gravy or combine chervil, rosemary, savory, and marjoram; or omit herbs and add 1 teaspoon dill seeds or fresh dill, or 1 or more tablespoons capers.

**Mutton gravy:** Season like lamb or beef gravy, or combine several herbs or herbs and seeds; add a small amount of Worcestershire and Tabasco.

**Pork or ham gravy:** Season with any one of the following: sage, savory, basil, thyme, chives, parsley, Chinese garlic, minced leeks; celery or mustard seeds. Season ham gravy with mustard or caraway seeds.

**Tomato gravy:** Use tomato juice or canned tomatoes instead of milk or other liquid; add basil, orégano, chili powder, or Worcestershire. If the tomatoes are sour, sweeten with 1 or 2 teaspoons black molasses.

**Turkey gravy:** Season with basil, sage, and thyme; add a mere sprinkle of grated lemon peel and nutmeg or mace.

**Veal gravy:** Season like beef or chicken gravy.

# CHAPTER 9

## DRESS UP YOUR MEATS WITH DRESSINGS

Aside from stuffing turkeys and chickens, few housewives use dressings as frequently as they should. Fish, rabbit, and any number of cuts of meat can be made more interesting and festive by delicious stuffing. Make them frequently.

Since only low heat reaches the stuffing and since aromatic oils cannot escape through the meat, seasonings may be used without sacrificing much of their freshness. Vegetables added to stuffing should first be heated to destroy enzymes and thus retard the destruction of vitamin C during cooking.

Keep crumbs on hand for dressings. As stale bread accumulates, separate the slices, allow them to dry thoroughly, and store them in a paper bag. Whenever you are using the meat grinder, pass the bread through it. Sift out the finer crumbs to use in sautéing meats, and save the coarse crumbs for dressings. Such crumbs keep almost indefinitely, certainly as well as do crackers.

If you wish to stuff chops or steaks—delicious with onion, celery, or fruit dressing—have them cut double thickness; cut a pocket by inserting a knife in one side and rotating it without cutting the edge of the meat. Make a pocket between the bones and meat in such cuts as brisket, plate, shoulder, and breast of lamb or veal, or a standing rump roast. You can select matching sections of spareribs, round steaks, ham slices, flank, or plate, put the dressing between them, and tie them around the edges. Any roast having a bone in the center, such as a ham, a leg of lamb, an arm roast cut from the chuck, or a fresh pork shoulder, can be boned and the resulting space filled with dressing. The cut should be made along the underside of the roast, where it will not show, and the bones removed by following them with a sharp knife. If you especially enjoy dressing and are preparing a cut in which a pocket cannot easily be made, as in many pot roasts, make a

153

dressing rich with drippings, bake it separately, and serve in mounds around the meat. And do not overlook stuffed meat loaves (p. 135).

Underestimate the amount of dressing which a pocket will hold. Since stuffing swells as steam is formed, be sure to pack it lightly into the available space. This point I'm afraid I shall never learn. I invariably think of how delicious the dressing will be, pack it in tightly, and then feel distressed when it bursts forth from its pocket and ruins the appearance of the meat.

One of the cutest culinary tricks I know is lacing up a roast (it isn't original). Close the pocket by slipping large trussing pins or hardwood toothpicks—the fat variety sold for spearing cherries and olives in cocktails—through either side of the opening about 1 inch apart. I have even used thin nails, for lack of something better. Then lace around both ends of the pins or toothpicks or nails with a string, as hiking boots are laced. After the roast is put on a serving platter, the toothpicks or pins or nails can be removed and the string falls away. If the meat or skin is thin, the "spikes" should be set farther back from the opening.

Achieve variety in your menus by stuffing any of the following cuts of meat and by using many different types of dressings. The page references give the method of cooking each cut.

**Beef:** brisket (p. 99); chuck, including 4 or more ribs (p. 99); flank, rolled or matching sections (p. 99); heel of round, rolled or with pocket cut in center (p. 77); heart (p. 87); liver, unsliced (p. 78); plate, pocket, or matching sections (p. 98); rump, rolled or standing roast with pocket (p. 77); steaks, thick (p. 64); meat loaf (p. 135).

**Lamb or mutton:** breast, boned and rolled or with pocket between ribs and meat (p. 100); chops, thick (p. 66); heart (p. 87); leg, boned (p. 78); liver, unsliced (p. 122); shoulder, pocket between bones and meat (p. 78); steaks, thick (p. 66); lamb loaf (p. 136).

**Pork, fresh or cured:** chops, thick (p. 66); whole or half ham, boned (p. 78); ham or shoulder slices, matched (p. 70); heart (p. 87); leg, fresh, boned (p. 79); liver, unsliced (p. 78); shoulder or picnic ham, boned (p. 79); spareribs, matching sections (p. 144).

**Veal:** breast, boned and rolled or with pocket between ribs and meat (p. 79); chops, thick (p. 71); heart (p. 87); leg roast, boned or with pocket (p. 79); leg steaks, matched (p. 71); rump, boned and rolled or with pocket (p. 100); shoulder, pocket between bones and meat (p. 100); veal loaf (p. 134).

Since one person enjoys dressing made largely of crumbs and few vegetables, and another wants vegetables with little bread, and still another hates sage while someone else loves it, recipes for dressings should not give exact measurements. Juggle the ingredients around to suit yourself. By all means do not waste time to measure ingredients except by eye. The throw-it-together method usually produces the best stuffing; tasting it as you make it is the best guide.

## CRUMB DRESSING

Heat in a utensil large enough to hold a quart:

**4 to 6 tablespoons bacon drippings, butter-flavored fat, or drippings rendered from the meat to be stuffed**

Vary the amount of drippings with fatness of meat; chop fine or run through the meat grinder directly into fat:

| | |
|---|---|
| 1 or 2 onions | 1 handful parsley |
| 1 clove garlic | 1 chilled bell pepper or pimento |
| 1 to 4 stalks celery with leaves | (optional) |

Cover utensil and sauté vegetables 5 to 8 minutes; remove from heat and add:

| | |
|---|---|
| 2 or 3 cups dry whole-wheat-bread crumbs | ¼ teaspoon crushed black peppercorns |
| ½ cup wheat germ | 1 teaspoon salt |
| ⅓ cup powdered milk | pinch to ½ teaspoon sage, thyme, marjoram, or savory |

If a moist dressing is desired, add:

**1 to 2 cups meat juices from dripping pan, from braising meat, or from stewing giblets; or milk or leftover gravy**

Mix thoroughly; taste for seasonings; stuff into the meat.

This recipe, or approximately 4 cups of dressing, is enough for stuffing a chicken, a rabbit, a large beef roast, or 2 matching flank steaks.

*Variations:*

Add leftover vegetables, such as peas, diced carrots, or celery root; or substitute leftover potatoes or rice for part of the crumbs.

*Variations:*

If for fowl, proceed as directed on page 156; use broth from stewing giblets for cooking buckwheat.

Steam the buckwheat; when nearly done, add the fat and diced vegetables.

**Rice stuffing:** Prepare as in basic recipe or as directed on page 157.

**Whole-wheat stuffing:** Prepare as in basic recipe, using cooked unground wheat. Use for stuffing meat loaf (p. 134), beef, lamb, or pork.

**Wild-rice stuffing:** Prepare as in basic recipe, using wild rice instead of buckwheat; cook like brown rice (p. 204). Use for stuffing wild duck or other wild or tame fowl.

Fruit stuffings can be delightful additions to meat. Unfortunately, they are little used, possibly because of some of the recipes which exist. For example, the mixture of dried apricots with onions and sage, which I find in several recipe books, is my idea of a horrible concoction. Yet what could be more delicious than a richly browned broiled pork chop stuffed with crushed pineapple, perhaps slightly caramelized, or diced crabapple pickles? You may, of course, add crumbs to fruit dressings or vice versa, but I do not recommend it.

## APPLE DRESSING

Estimate the cups of dressing needed. Select **tart apples,** such as Jonathans, which will not cook to a mush; chill thoroughly, core, and dice without peeling.

Brown the apples in **hot bacon drippings or fat** rendered from the meat to be stuffed, allowing **2 tablespoons fat** for each cup of apples; add:

| | |
|---|---|
| pinch of salt | ¼ cup walnuts, pecans, almonds, |
| dash each of nutmeg and cinnamon | or other nuts for each cup of apples (optional) |

Stir well; use for stuffing ham, pork, goose, duck, wild fowl, lamb, or beef.

*Variations:*

Add ¼ cup seedless raisins for each cup of apples; steam with the apples until soft and plump; or use half apples and half diced and well-drained cling peaches, crushed pineapple, cooked dried apricots, or cooked prunes.

**Apricot stuffing:** Steam dried apricots in a small amount of water until they are just soft and all water is absorbed; dice and prepare as in basic recipe. Use 1 or 2 cups for stuffing lamb, beef, pork, or small wild game.

**Peach stuffing:** Use canned cling peaches; drain well and prepare as in the basic recipe. Use 2 cups for stuffing beef heart or flank steak; 1 cup for veal, pork, or lamb chops.

**Pineapple stuffing:** Drain crushed pineapple well in a strainer or use finely diced sliced pineapple; sear in very hot bacon or pork drippings until slightly brown; omit spices and nuts. Vary by adding bits of crisp bacon. Use 2 cups for stuffing boned ham or shoulder or fresh pork roasts; 1 cup for pork chops or matching ham steaks.

**Prune stuffing:** Pit cooked prunes; dice or leave whole; prepare as in basic recipe, keeping heat high until moisture has evaporated; add grated rind of ¼ lemon or orange. Use 2 cups for stuffing flank steak or beef heart or breast of veal; 1 cup for pork chops.

**Spiced-fruit stuffing:** Dice any spiced or sweet-pickled fruit, such as figs, crab apples, cling peaches, or prunes; you need not heat; use or omit nuts. Use 1 cup for stuffing small cuts such as pork chops, matching ham steaks, veal or lamb chops, or flank steak to be broiled.

# CHAPTER 10

## WHEN IN DOUBT, SERVE SAUCES WITH MEATS, FISH, OR VEGETABLES

One of the easiest ways to make food interesting is to serve it in or with a sauce. If you don't know how to serve a meat, fish, or vegetable, dice it and serve it in a sauce. If you are thinking, "We'll have the same vegetables again today," steam them and serve a sauce over them. If a conglomeration of leftovers has accumulated and you don't know what to do with them, prepare a sauce and throw them into it. If you want to make friends think you are an excellent cook, make a sauce and give it a French name. Sauces make further seasoning unnecessary; they banish monotony; and few take as long as 10 minutes to prepare.

Sauces have not gained the popularity in America which they deserve. The reason, I hold, is their names: sauce Bercy, which is essentially clear chicken gravy; poulette sauce, or chicken stock thickened with egg yolks; sauce allemande, Béarnaise sauce, and so on. One of my cookbooks offers a little masterpiece of a recipe for making soubise sauce: you are to add 2 cups of velouté sauce. It took considerable scrambling around to discover that velouté sauce was thickened chicken or veal gravy, and that soubise, which means smothered, refers to smothered onions added to it. So what? Since we have an excellent language of our own, why not use it? Surely a rose by any other name would smell as sweet. You may recognize recipes for foreign sauces in the following pages, but their names are missing.

Cook cream sauces over the direct heat. Making them in a double boiler usually leaves a raw-flour taste and wastes time and fuel. Compared with the usual variety of cream sauces, which taste strikingly like wallpaper paste, sauces made with flavorful whole-wheat flour have a delightful taste. The richness contributed by

160

the powdered milk makes the addition of cream superfluous. Use cream sauces frequently as a means of working milk into your menus. Whenever you prepare cream sauce, make 1 or 2 cups more than you need and keep it stored in the refrigerator. Instead of mixing a dab of thickening each time you prepare creamed vegetables—a ridiculous procedure—cook the vegetables in milk and thicken it to the consistency desired with previously prepared sauce. Although thick cream sauce requires less storage space than medium sauce, when chilled it is difficult to dilute quickly.

I use butter-flavored shortening in making cream sauces. As far as I know, no one has yet discovered that they are not made with butter.

## MEDIUM CREAM SAUCE

Melt in a saucepan, preferably with a rounded base:

**4 tablespoons butter-flavored shortening, margarine, or butter**

Add and mix thoroughly without browning:

**¼ cup whole-wheat pastry flour**

Add gradually, stirring rapidly:

**1 cup fresh milk**

When milk and flour are well blended, add:

| | |
|---|---|
| ¼ to ½ teaspoon crushed white or black peppercorns | ½ teaspoon Worcestershire (optional) |
| 1 teaspoon salt | 2 or 3 drops yellow coloring |
| ¼ teaspoon paprika | |

Simmer 5 to 8 minutes; meanwhile shake or beat until smooth:

| | |
|---|---|
| 1 cup fresh milk | ½ cup powdered milk |

Stir in the milk; simmer 3 minutes, being careful that sauce does not boil.

Double the recipe; store amount not needed for immediate use in a covered jar in refrigerator.

*Variations:*

For thin cream sauce, use 2 tablespoons each flour and fat, keeping other ingredients the same; for thick cream sauce, use ½ cup each flour and fat.

**Brown sauce:** Brown fat lightly, using fat from soup stock or meat broth when available; add and brown the flour; use soup stock, meat broth, or fresh milk; add brown coloring; salt to taste if the stock or broth has not been salted. Since brown sauce is essentially brown gravy, use leftover gravy when available.

**Tomato-cream sauce:** Heat 1 can condensed cream of tomato soup (1⅛ cups); add ⅓ cup powdered milk blended with ¾ cup fresh milk; salt to taste; omit the other ingredients of basic recipe. This is an excellent sauce to prepare when time is limited.

Probably I would never in my lifetime have made all the following sauces if I had not had to test them. For three days, from early morning until evening, an assistant and I did nothing but make sauces, hundreds of them. I was amazed at how easily they can be prepared, how many problems in menu planning they solve, and how delicious they are. I take no credit for their deliciousness; they are largely standard recipes found in every cookbook.

I would heartily recommend that you do as we did—start at the beginning and systematically prepare every sauce, using each basic sauce. After you have once prepared them, you have them at your fingertips and will probably use them, as I have, again and again. Let us suppose you have steamed lamb hearts or tongues on hand; not an especially exciting entree, certainly, but diced and dropped into a delicious sauce or sliced and served attractively with an appetizing sauce over them—that's something else again. Almost any meat, fish, fowl, or vegetable may be similarly improved with a well-seasoned sauce.

Unless otherwise stated, use as a base for any of the following sauces:

2 cups medium cream sauce or          2 cups medium brown sauce or
2 cups tomato-cream sauce or          leftover brown gravy

*Merely add the following ingredients to the basic sauce. Heat and serve the food in the sauce, serve the sauce over the food, or serve the sauce separately. When meat, fish, fowl, or vegetables are served in the sauce, salt to taste.*

**Caper sauce:** 4 to 6 tablespoons capers, 2 tablespoons ground parsley. Serve with fish, lamb, brains, or sweetbreads.

**Caraway sauce:** Simmer 5 minutes in basic sauce 1 or 2 tablespoons caraway seeds; add 3 tablespoons ground parsley. Serve over steamed cabbage or sauerkraut, with spareribs, fresh or leftover pork or ham.

**Celery sauce:** Simmer 5 minutes in basic sauce 1½ cups finely chopped celery or 1 teaspoon celery seeds; add 4 tablespoons ground parsley. Serve with baked or broiled fish, hard-cooked eggs, baked or steamed unsliced liver or heart.

**Cheese sauce:** Remove basic sauce from heat and add 1½ cups diced nippy cheese 3 minutes before serving. Serve over broccoli, cauliflower, spinach, or other vegetables; or add ½ to 1 teaspoon anise or dill seeds and serve over steamed or broiled fish.

*Cheese-pimento sauce:* Use pimento cheese or add 4 tablespoons diced pimentos.

**Curry sauce:** 1 minced clove garlic, 3 tablespoons grated onion, ½ to 4 teaspoons curry powder. Serve with shrimp, fish, chicken, lamb, rice, or potatoes. This is a delicious sauce.

**Dill sauce:** 2 tablespoons or more minced fresh dill or commercial dill sauce; or cook in the sauce 1 to 3 teaspoons crushed dill seeds. This is my pet sauce. Serve with fish, lamb, veal, eggs, or potatoes.

**Egg sauce:** Just before serving add 1½ teaspoons Worcestershire, ¼ cup lemon juice or tarragon vinegar, 2 to 4 diced or sliced hard-cooked eggs. Serve over steamed spinach, broccoli, or any green leafy vegetable; decorate baked fish with sliced eggs and pour the sauce over it.

**Horseradish sauce:** Just before serving add ¼ cup freshly grated horseradish and 1 or 2 teaspoons dry or prepared mustard. Serve with fresh or leftover ham, pork, beef, heart, tongue, liver, or kidney.

**Hot tartar sauce:** Heat ⅔ cup medium cream sauce; add ⅓ cup mayonnaise, 2 tablespoons each ground parsley and tarragon vinegar, ½ cup chopped pickles, 1 grated onion, 1 teaspoon dry or prepared mustard. Serve with fish or sea food; use for low-calorie diets instead of the usual variety of tartar sauce.

**Mock Hollandaise sauce:** Heat 1 cup medium cream sauce; just before serving beat in 2 egg yolks, 2 tablespoons margarine or butter, ¼ cup lemon juice. Serve with asparagus, broccoli, artichokes, steamed spinach or other greens, fish, lean fowl, or hard-cooked or poached eggs.

**Mushroom sauce:** Sauté 5 minutes in butter-flavored fat 1 or 2 cups sliced mushrooms; proceed with basic sauce, using the same utensil; or use canned mushrooms and liquid; or dilute 1 can condensed mushroom soup with ¾ cup fresh milk mixed with ½ cup powdered milk. Serve with hard-cooked eggs, fish, ham, croquettes, veal patties, noodles, or steamed rice.

**Mustard sauce:** Just before serving add 2 to 4 tablespoons dry or prepared mustard. Serve with tongue, heart, baked liver, corned beef, ham, or pork.

**Olive sauce:** ½ cup chopped ripe or sliced stuffed olives; salt the sauce to taste after olives are added. Serve with fish, eggs, broccoli, asparagus, spinach, or other green vegetables, broiled tomatoes or eggplant; leftover veal, lamb, or ham.

**Onion sauce:** 2 cups ground onions, a generous dash of cayenne; cook the onions in sauce only 5 minutes. Serve over steamed sliced heart or tongue, unsliced baked liver, hard-cooked eggs, leftover lamb, veal, or pork.

**Pimento sauce:** ½ cup chopped canned or sautéed fresh pimentos; 2 tablespoons ground parsley. Serve with fish, eggs, lamb, liver, or leftover pork.

**Piquant sauce:** Sauté **3 chopped onions, 1 minced clove garlic, 2 finely diced carrots;** make basic sauce, using same utensil; add **pinch of thyme, a dash of nutmeg;** just before serving add **4 tablespoons ground parsley, ¼ cup lemon juice or tarragon vinegar.** This is a delicious sauce. Serve with fish, lamb, heart, liver, tongue, veal, rice, spinach, or any greens.

**Sauce delicious:** 1 grated onion; just before serving, beat in 2 egg yolks, 2 tablespoons lemon juice or sherry, 4 tablespoons Parmesan cheese. Serve with tongue, heart, sliced beef, fish, broccoli, spinach, or other steamed green vegetable.

One of the most overrated misconceptions is the belief that Hollandaise sauce is difficult to make. Egg protein starts to thicken at 130° F. In the presence of an acid, such as lemon juice or vinegar, it thickens, or curdles, very quickly. If you heat Hollandaise sauce above 135° F. you can expect it to curdle. Even if you do not use a thermometer, you can make beautiful Hollandaise in about 5 minutes if you keep the heat low and take the sauce from the heat as soon as it thickens.

### EASY HOLLANDAISE SAUCE

Combine in a saucepan, preferably with a rounded base:

**2 egg yolks**
**2 tablespoons lemon juice or vinegar**
**½ teaspoon salt**

**¼ teaspoon freshly ground white peppercorns**
**dash of cayenne**

Fasten the cooking thermometer to edge of saucepan so that bulb of the mercury reaches top of sauce; put saucepan over low direct heat and beat constantly with a wire whisk or 6-pronged fork, or if the pan has rounded base, with a rotary eggbeater. Add in 4 portions:

¼ pound (½ cup) soft margarine or butter

As soon as 1 portion of margarine or butter is beaten in, or melted, add another portion. Remove from heat as soon as it is thick. Do not allow sauce to heat beyond 135° F. at any time.

Serve at once with broccoli, asparagus, artichokes, baked or broiled fish, veal, or broiled chicken.

*Variations:*

If heat cannot be controlled, cook in top of double boiler, over but not touching boiling water.

Use 1 tablespoon lemon juice and 1 tablespoon sherry or dry white wine; or make with tarragon or wine vinegar.

Add any of the following: 1 teaspoon or more grated onion; dash of nutmeg; ½ teaspoon dry or prepared mustard; 1 tablespoon ground parsley or minced tarragon leaves.

If to be served with fish, add ½ teaspoon or more grated lemon rind, dill sauce, or dill or anise seeds.

## VINEGAR SAUCE

Combine and heat over simmer burner:

| | |
|---|---|
| ¾ cup brown soup stock | ⅛ teaspoon freshly ground pepper- |
| 1 tablespoon grated onion | corns |
| | 1 teaspoon salt |

When hot, beat in:

| | |
|---|---|
| 2 egg yolks | 3 tablespoons margarine or butter |

Simmer 2 or 3 minutes, or until thick; *do not boil.* Remove from heat and add:

2 tablespoons tarragon or wine vinegar

Serve at once over baked or broiled fish, steaks, broccoli, steamed spinach, or other cooked greens. This is a delicious sauce.

*Variations:*

Add any of the following: 2 teaspoons horseradish or dry or prepared mustard; 2 drops Tabasco and 1 finely diced cucumber; 2 tablespoons chopped fresh dill or 1 teaspoon dill seeds or commercial dill sauce; 3 tablespoons chopped chives or ground parsley.

## TOMATO SAUCE

Sauté lightly in bacon drippings:

| | |
|---|---|
| 1 or 2 chopped onions | 1 green pepper |
| 1 minced clove garlic | 1 finely diced carrot |
| 1 chopped stalk celery with leaves | |

Stir well and add:

| | |
|---|---|
| 2 cups tomato purée or drained and chopped canned tomatoes | 1 or 2 tablespoons brewers' yeast (optional) |
| 1 teaspoon salt | ¼ to ½ teaspoon crushed black |
| pinch of basil and/or orégano | peppercorns |
| 1 teaspoon blackstrap molasses | |

Cook slowly 10 minutes, stirring occasionally. Before serving add **2 tablespoons ground parsley.** Serve with macaroni, spaghetti, noodles, rice, lamb, pork, fish, beef, or broiled eggplant.

*Variations:*

Season with one or more of the following: ¼ crushed bay leaf; 3 or 4 whole cloves; 1 teaspoon Worcestershire or dry mustard; bits of crisp bacon; a pinch of thyme, marjoram, rosemary, or savory; ¼ teaspoon mustard or celery seeds.

**Barbecue sauce:** A dash each of Tabasco, allspice, and nutmeg; 2 tablespoons vinegar, 1 tablespoon blackstrap molasses.

**Chili sauce:** Use 2 each large onions and green chili peppers; add ¼ teaspoon mustard seeds, 1 tablespoon each blackstrap molasses and vinegar, a generous dash of nutmeg.

**Creole sauce:** Omit carrots and celery; sauté ½ cup mushrooms with onions and peppers; use 1 cup each tomato purée and brown sauce or leftover brown gravy; add 8 or 10 sliced stuffed olives.

**Italian sauce:** Add a pinch each of savory, basil, and orégano; when available, use 1 cup Italian paste diluted with 1 cup water.

**Mexican sauce:** Use 2 fresh chili peppers or add 1 to 3 teaspoons chili powder; add ¼ teaspoon cumin seeds and orégano.

**Spanish sauce:** Before salting add 1 teaspoon beef extract or 1 bouillon cube; or use 1 cup brown sauce instead of 1 cup tomatoes; season with ¼ crushed bay leaf, and a pinch of basil.

Uncooked sauces are usually served with chilled foods. If they are served with hot foods, their charm lies in having the sauce thoroughly chilled and the food piping hot. The following creole sauce is a delicious one; don't miss it.

## UNCOOKED CREOLE SAUCE

Pare 2 raw tomatoes and squeeze out as much juice as possible; use the pulp for the sauce, or use chilled tomato purée. Combine:

| | |
|---|---|
| 1 chopped onion | ¾ cup chilled tomato purée |
| 1 diced bell pepper, pimento, or paprika | ½ teaspoon salt |
| 2 finely diced raw tomatoes without juice or | ⅛ teaspoon freshly ground peppercorns |
| | pinch each of orégano and basil |

Let stand in refrigerator 20 minutes or longer. Serve over kidneys, chops, steaks, jellied fish, sliced tongue or heart, broiled or sautéed liver, or cold baked liver.

*Variations:*

Add any of the following: finely diced celery; chopped chili pepper; minced clove garlic; 2 tablespoons or more French dressing; or omit herbs and add minced fresh dill, commercial dill sauce, or 1 teaspoon dill seeds.

Fresh herbs and other seasonings may be added to butter, margarine, or cooking fat, which may then be used for seasoning meats, fish, and vegetables. Herb butter makes a delicious sandwich spread. The freshness of the herbs is retained. Such fats may be kept for many weeks in a tightly sealed jar in the refrigerator.

## HERB BUTTER

Combine:

| | |
|---|---|
| ¼ pound (½ cup) soft butter, margarine, or butter-flavored cooking fat | ½ teaspoon each minced fresh or pinch of pulverized dried savory, marjoram, basil, tarragon |
| 1 tablespoon ground parsley | 1 minced clove garlic |
| 1 tablespoon minced chives | ¼ teaspoon paprika |

Blend well, pack into a small jar, and cover; keep in refrigerator. Serve on fish, steak, chops, baked or steamed potatoes, or other vegetables; add to fat-free bouillon; use for sandwiches.

*Variations:*

Add any of the following: 1 tablespoon minced canned pimento, anchovy paste, or grated onion; any single minced fresh herb or any two or more herbs, omitting herbs in basic recipe.

**Garlic butter:** Melt butter with 1 or 2 mashed garlic cloves; let stand 20 minutes or longer; discard the garlic. Use on toasted rye bread, steaks, or serve melted with mussels.

**Lemon butter:** Melt fat; omit other ingredients; add 3 tablespoons lemon juice, grated rind of 1 lemon. Serve with fish or green vegetables.

**Spiced sauce:** Heat 2 tablespoons fat prepared as in basic recipe; add 1 tablespoon each catsup, Worcestershire, wine vinegar or lemon juice, ½ teaspoon dry mustard. This sauce is delicious over broiled or sautéed kidneys, brains, liver, steamed heart, or any barbecued meat. Don't miss it.

An almost endless variety of delicious sauces can be made by adding seasonings to sour cream or to thick commercial yogurt. The sauces made with yogurt and whipped evaporated milk are lower in calories than those prepared with cream, and should be used by persons wishing to reduce. Serve these sauces with meat and fish aspics, cold sliced meat, chilled fish fillets, or chilled steamed vegetables. They add much to hot-weather dinners and buffets.

## SOUR-CREAM OR YOGURT SAUCE

Combine and stir well:

| | |
|---|---|
| 1 cup sour cream or thick yogurt | ½ teaspoon dry mustard |
| 2 tablespoons lemon juice or vinegar | 2 to 4 tablespoons grated onion (optional) |
| 1 teaspoon salt | 2 tablespoons ground parsley |
| 1 teaspoon Worcestershire | dash of cayenne |

Serve with cold meats, fish, aspics, or chilled vegetables.

*Variations:*

Instead of sour cream or yogurt whip ½ cup sweet cream no earlier than ½ hour before serving; add the seasonings of basic recipe; or whip

⅓ cup chilled evaporated milk, add seasonings and 3 tablespoons mayonnaise. For reducing diets use evaporated-milk sauce, which is quite delicious.

Add any one or more of the following: 1 minced clove garlic; 1 tablespoon minced fresh or pinch of any dry herb; ¼ cup or more chili sauce, catsup, Parmesan or other nippy grated cheese, ground mixed pickles, or sliced stuffed or diced olives; 1 chopped green chili pepper; 2 to 4 tablespoons chives, capers, or minced fresh dill; 1 diced cucumber or 2 diced hard-cooked eggs with 3 tablespoons chili sauce; 1 or 2 teaspoons dry mustard, dill sauce, or dill or anise seeds. If anise is used, serve with fish; add 2 teaspoons caraway seeds if to be served with cold pork. The sauce is customarily given the name of the principal seasoning.

**Almond sauce:** Omit seasonings except salt and lemon juice; add ¼ cup chopped toasted almonds, ½ cup finely diced unpeeled red apple, dash of nutmeg. Serve with cold fowl or lamb.

**Citron-cherry sauce:** Omit seasonings; add ¼ cup each finely diced citron and maraschino cherries. Serve with beef, lamb, or pork.

**Lemon sauce:** Use lemon juice; add grated rind of 1 lemon. Serve with fish.

**Mint sauce:** Omit seasonings; add 4 tablespoons minced leaves of fresh mint; let stand 30 minutes. Serve with lamb, mutton, or fruit aspic.

**Mustard-horseradish sauce:** Use 2 teaspoons dry mustard; add 2 tablespoons freshly ground horseradish. Serve with tongue, heart, liver, kidney, cold meats, ham, or pork.

**Onion sauce:** Add 2 shredded onions or finely diced leeks. Serve with fish, mutton, pork, or cold baked liver.

**Pineapple-curry sauce:** Omit seasonings; add ½ cup well-drained crushed pineapple, 1 to 3 teaspoons curry powder, 2 tablespoons shredded coconut. Serve with cold lamb, chilled rice, or leftover chicken.

**Tartar sauce:** Add to ½ cup mayonnaise or to basic recipe ½ cup ground mixed pickles, dash of Tabasco, pinch of chervil, basil, ½ teaspoon dill or anise seeds; if mayonnaise is used, dilute with 2 tablespoons tarragon vinegar. Serve with fried shrimp or other sea food.

# CHAPTER 11

## GET ACQUAINTED WITH FISH

The consumption of fish in America has increased rapidly. It is to be hoped that the nation will eventually become a fish-eating people. In years past, about a third of the fish caught were discarded as trash fish, many of which fishermen considered delicious. One such fish, the monkfish, when served recently to a group of dietitians was judged to be ham. It behooves each housewife to become acquainted with every kind of fish available and to learn how to prepare it so that it will be consistently delicious.

Fish contains approximately the same amount of protein as does meat and has a comparable content of essential amino acids, or health-building qualities. All fish are rich sources of phosphorus, and ocean fish and sea foods are excellent sources of iodine, although fresh-water fish often have goiters because of lack of iodine. Since fish are very active and the B vitamins are necessary for energy production, their flesh is a rich source of these vitamins provided the juices are not lost before or during cooking. Unfortunately, vitamins A and D are stored almost entirely in fish liver, which is rarely eaten.

Serve fish not only in the place of meat but in addition to it, especially when your protein requirements are high or when you serve meats or meat substitutes low in protein. Steamed fish or other sea food may be prepared in advance, kept frozen in an ice compartment until needed, and served in salad or an appetizer on the same menu with meat. Well-prepared fish can do much to overcome the widespread iodine and protein deficiencies which exist in America.

Since the muscles of fish are tender and delicate, juices are easily lost after fish is cut or the skin removed. Much flavor is lost even during a short period of soaking. Shrimps, scallops, oysters, and other shellfish contain a sweet substance known as glycogen, which is lost readily if these foods are washed slowly, soaked, or cooked in water. Fish should be washed thoroughly but rapidly, and dried immediately; it should not be touched unnecessarily with any liquid which is not to be eaten. I do not recommend any salted fish if it must be soaked to be edible.

Fish cookery differs markedly from that of meat. Fish, except for roe, contains little fat. Whereas well-marbled beef averages 33 per cent fat and ham 50 per cent, many fish contain only 1 per cent or less. The so-called fat fish, such as shad, mackerel, herring, and lake trout, average 7 to 10 per cent fat, and salmon alone sometimes reaches 14 per cent. Since fat is a poor conductor of heat, the lack of fat allows heat to penetrate fish more rapidly than it does meat. Furthermore, fish is usually flat in shape, with a large amount of surface through which heat can pass quickly. The cooking time of fish, therefore, is based not on pounds of weight, as it is in meat, but upon thickness.

With the exception of abalone, the connective tissue between the muscle fibers of fish is in extremely thin sheets. When submitted to heat, these thin sheets break down almost as soon as they are warm. The problem of cooking fish, therefore, is exactly opposite to that of cooking meat. If meats are to be delicious, the connective tissue must be softened without the meat proteins becoming tough. In fish cookery the problem is to cook the proteins of the muscle fiber without allowing the connective tissue to break down. If the connective tissue of fish does break down in cooking, juices carrying vitamins, minerals, sweet glycogen, and delicious flavors are quickly lost. The fish is left dry and unappetizing.

Older recipe books often mention moist fish, meaning fish which contain some fat, and dry fish, meaning lean fish, which were habitually overcooked. It should be clearly understood that such a thing as a dry fresh fish does not exist. The flesh of all fresh fish contains from 65 to 80 per cent moisture, which was essential to the life processes of the fish. If the fish is properly cooked, these juices are retained. The flavor and deliciousness of any fish are in proportion to the amount of juices retained during cooking.

The juices of ocean fish and sea food contain the same amount of salt as does ocean water. Steamed shrimps, for example, which have not been overcooked or soaked before cooking, taste not only quite sweet but well salted. Fresh-water fish likewise must have salt to live. Since added salt draws out juices, flavor, and nutritive value, most fish should be salted only when it is served. When fish tastes flat without added salt, juices have been lost during cooking. Since gravy is not prepared with fish, nutritive value and flavor drawn out are usually wasted. If fish is rolled in flour or crumbs or dipped in batter which needs salt and which catches juices as they are drawn out, it may be salted before being cooked. If the fish is stuffed, the salt in the dressing pulls juices into it. In each case, however, the fish itself is left drier and less salty. Since the cooking time is short, seasonings other than salt should be added at the beginning of cooking so that the aromatic oils may be extracted.

To have a basis for preparing fish consistently juicy, you should know the temperatures at which fish proteins are cooked and the connective tissue is broken down. Fish takes on the flavor of being cooked as soon as the fiber proteins become firm, or are coagulated. Coagulation starts when the internal temperature of the fish reaches 130° F.; if held at this temperature, fish will become well cooked. Coagulation is usually complete by the time the internal temperature reaches 140° F. The proteins become progressively more firm as the heat increases.

Since the sheets of connective tissue in fish are extremely thin, they start breaking down around 150° F. If the fish is cooked beyond this internal temperature, the connective tissue breaks down rapidly. As in meat, the contracting proteins act as a hand squeezing water from a sponge, and the juices, flavor, and much nutritive value are squeezed through the broken connective tissue. The fish or sea food is robbed of flavor and left dry. To cook fish perfectly so that no juices are lost and yet all proteins are well cooked, the internal temperature should be checked with a meat thermometer whenever possible; the fish should be taken up as soon as the internal temperature reaches 140° to 145° F. Fish is most enjoyed at this degree of doneness.

There are many so-called tests for doneness: The fish is supposedly done when it curls, flakes, pulls from the bones, or comes to the surface during French frying. These are actually tests for overcooked fish after connective tissue has already broken down and juices have been lost. Since fish cooks when little more than warm, it continues to cook after it has been put on the serving platter. For this reason you should err on the side of cooking it too little rather than too much. Except when using up leftovers, do not precook fish which is to be creamed, added to casseroles, or French fried.

To boil fish is nothing less than criminal treatment of good food. Not only do flavor and nutritive value quickly soak out, but the temperature is 62° F. above that at which juices are lost. For example, shrimps when boiled lose more than half of their moisture content and shrink to half their original size. Stewing likewise soaks out flavor, and is not recommended unless the fish is stewed in sauce with which it is to be served. Even in this case, the fish is usually far more delicious if steamed above the sauce. Since moist heat penetrates about twice as quickly as does the dry heat of broiling and roasting, it is extremely difficult to steam or stew fish without overcooking it. Because fish is habitually so overcooked that it is dried out, many recipe books recommend that lean fish be stewed. After the connective tissue is broken down, however, the tiny dried-out muscles again absorb moisture, but lost flavor cannot be recaptured.

No attempt should be made to brown fish without the aid of paprika, flour, crumbs, batter, or some cereal. When fats which burn easily, such as margarine and butter, are used to coat fish before roasting or broiling, a delicate suggestion of a golden color may be attained without overcooking. Further browning causes marked deterioration of flavor. Beauty should be achieved through garnishes. A rich brown can be most easily obtained by sprinkling the fish generously with paprika before cooking it, although the aromatic oils are sacrificed.

Frozen fish should be thawed slowly at room temperature and cooked immediately. If heated while still frozen, the outside becomes overcooked while the center is still chilled; the expansion of steam is so great that the fish usually falls to pieces. If time permits, fish should be allowed to reach room temperature before being put on to cook.

If the thousands upon thousands of recipes for preparing fish were stripped of their seasonings, they would be reduced to three or four basic recipes. The seasonings are no more than sauces cooked with the fish. Time and effort can be saved by learning the basic ways of cooking fish, using the method which appeals to you, and serving the sauce you happen to enjoy. Since most fish are lean, fish sauces are usually rich in fat.

The principles and methods of cooking fish remain identical regardless of the type of fish; the same is true of shellfish. Bass and mackerel are baked the same way; trout and squid are fried alike. A fish having approximately the same size or cut in the same manner as another can be substituted in any recipe. To feel that you must have a separate recipe for each variety of fish limits your horizon. Many excellent fish have recently appeared on the market for which no recipes exist. They are not needed. If you are buying fillets, buy one from a kind of fish which is new to you. If you are making salad or creamed fish, add a small, unfamiliar fish to the familiar ones you plan to use. Prepare recipes using a combination of two or more varieties of fish. The ones you have not yet discovered may be far more delicious than your favorites. By such an approach, by careful cooking, and by the use of a wide variety of sauces and seasonings, monotony can be avoided indefinitely.

When you plan to serve fish, decide first whether you wish to bake, fry, broil, or cream it. Then glance through the sauces, and decide how you would like it seasoned. Prepare the sauce and cook the fish in it; or pour the sauce over the cooked fish; or serve them separately. By following such a procedure you will need no recipes except basic ones. In general, large fish are usually baked, small ones are fried, and fillets and steaks are broiled or sautéed. Any fish, however, may be broiled, baked, creamed, or fried.

In buying fish, allow ⅓ pound per person if it contains no bones and ½ pound if it is not trimmed.

Since the kinds of fish available in different parts of the country vary widely, I have purposely not suggested specific types of fish with each recipe but rather the size and type of cut. Try every variety of fish available to you and each new variety as it appears in your market. Each of the following fish can be delicious when well cooked and interestingly seasoned:

*Fish*

| | | |
|---|---|---|
| anchovies | flounder | shad |
| barracuda | haddock | shad roe |
| bass, black | hake | shark |
| striped | halibut | skate |
| bloater | mackerel | smelt |
| bluefish | monkfish | squid |
| bonita | mullet | sturgeon |
| bream | muskellunge | sturgeon roe, |
| bullhead | perch | or caviar |
| butterhead | pickerel | sucker |
| carp | pike | swordfish |
| catfish | pompano | terrapin |
| cod, black | red snapper | trout, fresh-water |
| ling cod | salmon | sea trout |
| rock cod | salmon roe | tuna |
| yellow cod | sand dabs or sole | turbot |
| eel | sardine | whitefish |

*Shellfish*

| | | |
|---|---|---|
| clams | lobster | prawns, or giant shrimp |
| crabs | mussels | scallops |
| crawfish | oysters | shrimp |

## HOW TO CLEAN FISH

Clean fish on several layers of newspapers. If it is slimy, rinse quickly with hot water. Using the blunt edge of a knife or a fish scaler, remove the scales by forcing under them from tail toward head. If the fish is to be cooked whole, leave head and fins on and do not cut skin unnecessarily.

A fillet is a slice from which the bones have been removed. To prepare fillets, skin the fish before cutting it open. Cut off head, tail, and fins with kitchen shears. Use small scissors and slit skin down the backbone and lengthwise along center of abdomen. Start at gills and gently remove skin from head toward tail, cutting with scissors when necessary. Cut through abdominal wall and remove vital organs. Wash inside of fish quickly and dry immediately. Remove bones by cutting along both sides of the backbone from the inside of the fish; loosen flesh from bones by pushing it back with dull edge of a knife. If fish is large, cut in half along backbone before removing ribs.

The ribs from any small fish to be cooked whole may be taken out by cutting them from inside the body cavity along either side of the backbone. A knife can be slipped under the ribs, cutting them free. The backbone should be left, to retain the shape of the fish.

To prepare fish steaks, clean the fish, remove organs, and slice across the grain without skinning or removing bones.

To clean shrimp to be used in any way except for salad and appetizers, wash quickly and remove shells before cooking. Cut along sand vein to depth of $\frac{1}{16}$ inch. Wash out sand vein by holding your thumb over part of the water faucet to increase water pressure. Dry shrimp immediately.

Clean lobster and crab by washing thoroughly. Unless they are to be steamed whole and eaten chilled, cut open lengthwise and crack shells with hammer or nutcracker. Remove meat from crab claws and body; from the claws, tail, and body of the lobster. Discard intestinal vein; remove stomach and liver by holding under running water.

To remove odor of fish from hands, wash with soda or vinegar.

### FISH CAN BE COOKED WITHOUT ODOR

How many hundreds of times have you heard housewives remark, "I don't cook fish because I don't like the odor in the house"? The fact is that when fish is properly cooked, there is no odor. The substances which cause the unpleasant odor volatilize, or evaporate, at temperatures of 150° F. and above; fish should not be allowed to reach this temperature. Whenever you smell fish cooking, you may be sure it is being overcooked.

On one occasion, two assistants and I prepared dozens of fish recipes in a small apartment, cooking practically every variety of fish and sea food sold on the market. During the course of the day, nine friends dropped in, and each was greeted at the door with the question, "Do you know what we are cooking?" To our delight each friend answered with a puzzled expression, "No. Why?"

If for no other reason than to prevent the escape of unpleasant odors, a meat thermometer should be used in cooking fish. To attempt to cook fish without a thermometer is to invite olfactory disaster.

For other ways of serving fish, see the following recipes:

Fish appetizers (p. 265)                    Fish omelet (p. 248)
Fish salads (p. 235)                        Fish soufflé (p. 210)
Fish chowders and bisques (p. 324)          Fish to be served cold (p. 226)

To bake fish means to cook it on a rack with dry heat surrounding all surfaces. If it is put on a pan, moisture quickly collects, steams the lower part of the fish, and invariably overcooks it. To facilitate handling and lifting the fish out intact in case it overcooks, it may be laid on a thin cloth, such as a sugar sack. A piece of heavy paper may be placed a few inches below it to catch juices which may escape; thus unnecessary dishwashing is avoided.

Hundreds of recipes for "baked" fish recommend that the fish be cooked in an oven and covered with a sauce. In this case, the lower part of the fish is stewed, the upper part steamed. Juices from the fish pass into the already well-seasoned sauce, robbing the fish of flavor not needed by the sauce. Since moist heat penetrates quickly, such fish is almost invariably overcooked unless a thermometer is used and the temperature is carefully watched.

When baking fish, achieve variety by using different kinds of stuffing (p. 155) and by serving it with different sauces (p. 162). Since the skin prevents evaporation, small whole fish may be stuffed and baked as well as large ones. If you wish to "bake" fish in a sauce, prepare any type of sauce and pour it over the fish before it is put in the oven.

## BAKED, STUFFED FISH

Select any whole fish weighing 2 to 3 pounds, such as salmon, trout, shad, mackerel, fresh tuna, or herring; or use several small fish.

Clean the whole fish without removing tail, fins, and head. Let the fish reach room temperature. Stuff with **rice, mushroom, eggplant, celery, or onion dressing** (p. 157), preferably still hot.

Place fish on a cloth and put on a wire rack from oven; set fish with its back up rather than on its side. Insert a meat thermometer into thick flesh behind gills; brush with soft **bacon drippings, oil, margarine, or butter.** *Do not salt.*

Set in preheated, slow oven at 300° F.; place an upright oven thermometer on level with fish. Put cardboard or paper on wire rack 3 inches or more below fish. After a few minutes, check oven thermometer and take reading of meat thermometer.

Allow approximately 20 minutes for heat to penetrate 1 inch, 30 minutes for 2 inches, 35 minutes for 3 inches; take fish from oven when the internal thermometer reading is 140° F.

Lift fish to serving platter by rolling from cloth; garnish with **sprigs of parsley** and **lemon sections,** surround with steamed carrots.

Serve with herb butter, caper sauce, or other sauce (p. 162), salad of endive and cucumbers.

*Variations:*

If the stuffing is cold when fish is put into the oven, insert a meat thermometer in the stuffing and cook to 135° F.; allow 10 to 15 minutes longer for cooking time. Serve with piping-hot sauce.

Tie a string from head to tail to hold the fish in a semicircle, or fasten with skewers in the shape of an S.

**Baked fillets of fish:** Select fillets from halibut, red snapper, trout, or other fish. Insert a thermometer into one fillet. Brush or spread with **herb-seasoned butter or fat;** lay on a wire rack, not on a pan; sprinkle generously with **paprika.** Bake as in basic recipe. Serve with olive sauce (p. 164), steamed purple cabbage (p. 385), tossed salad.

**Browned fillets:** Dip the fillets in **milk and sifted whole-wheat-bread crumbs** seasoned with **4 teaspoons minced dill;** or add **dill sauce** to milk. Insert thermometer, lay fish on rack, sprinkle with **paprika,** and dot with **bacon drippings;** bake as in basic recipe. After tomato-juice appetizer, serve with Hollandaise sauce (p. 164), steamed carrots, rhubarb chard, lettuce salad with Roquefort-cheese dressing.

**Fillets baked with barbecue sauce:** Dip the fillets in any **tomato sauce,** such as barbecue, Spanish, or Italian sauce, or in catsup; roll in **sifted crumbs** and lay on heavy paper; insert the meat thermometer, dot generously with **bacon fat,** and bake as in basic recipe. Serve with tartar sauce (p. 169), hash-browned potatoes (p. 403), salad of tomatoes, cucumbers, and green peppers.

**Stuffed fillets:** Select 2 matching fillets weighing about 2 pounds each; spread one with **celery, onion, or crumb stuffing** (p. 157), lay the other fillet on top. Insert thermometer into either fillet, brush with oil, and bake as in basic recipe. After citrus-fruit appetizer, serve with **cheese sauce** (p. 163), string beans, avocado and tomato salad.

## FISH "BAKED" IN SAUCE

Clean 2 or 3 pounds of fish, using 1 large fish, several small ones, or fish fillets or steaks; stuff whole fish if desired.

Prepare in a heat-resistant baking dish **2 cups medium cream sauce** seasoned with **capers, cheese, dill, mushrooms, or other seasoning** (p. 162).

Insert meat thermometer in the center of a steak or fillet or into thick muscles behind gills of whole fish; place fish in a baking dish with thermometer near the edge of utensil; dip the sauce over fish.

Sprinkle over the top of fish:

¼ cup toasted whole-wheat-bread       ground paprika
crumbs

Put into a preheated slow oven at 300° F. Allow approximately 10 minutes for heat to penetrate fish or fillets 1 inch thick, 15 minutes for fish 2 inches thick, 20 minutes for fish 3 inches thick. Check thermometer reading frequently. Remove from oven as soon as internal temperature reaches 140° F.

After citrus-fruit appetizer, serve fish with spiced red onions (p. 389), vegetable salad set in lemon gelatin (p. 290).

*Variations:*

Instead of cream sauce use any sauce with a base of sour cream or yogurt (p. 168).

If the sauce is cold when fish is put into the oven, double the baking time given in basic recipe.

Instead of cream sauce use any tomato sauce, such as barbecue, chili, Spanish, or Italian sauce (p. 166).

**Baked fillets with pickles and onions:** Brush a shallow baking dish with oil and put in layer of thinly sliced **onions or leeks,** a layer of sliced **dill pickles,** then the fish fillets; omit sauce; put slices of **lemon** on top, sprinkle with **paprika;** bake as in basic recipe, allowing 20 minutes for fillets 1 inch thick. Vary by sprinkling fish with dill or anise seeds. Serve with sautéed parsnips (p. 363), steamed spinach (p. 380), apple and carrot salad (p. 275).

**Baked fish with mushrooms:** In the utensil to be used for baking, sauté **1 cup chopped mushrooms and 2 tablespoons onions;** add the fish and **½ cup sauterne or sherry.** Bake as in basic recipe. Serve with broiled tomatoes (p. 369), mashed banana squash (p. 415), grapefruit and avocado salad.

**Baked fish with oysters:** Put a layer of uncooked fish fillets in bottom of a baking dish; add layer of **fresh oysters, grated onion, ground parsley, salt, and paprika;** repeat until dish is filled; dot the top with **bacon drippings** and sprinkle with **browned crumbs and paprika;** insert a meat thermometer in the center of dish; bake in moderate oven at 350° F. for about 40 minutes, or until internal temperature is 140° F. Serve with fresh peas, creamed new potatoes, mixed-fruit salad.

**Baked roe:** Select shad or other roe; wash and dry, being careful not to break membrane. Dip in **milk,** roll in **toasted and sifted whole-wheat-bread crumbs,** place on a flat baking dish, insert a meat thermometer, and bake to 150° F., or about 30 minutes. Cover with the sauce a few minutes before taking from oven; sprinkle with **parsley.** After glandular-meat appetizer (p. 266), serve with zucchini with cheese (p. 366), shredded beets (p. 342), assorted finger salads (p. 273).

**Fish with fried rice:** Prepare **fried rice** (p. 205) in a heat-resistant baking dish; when rice is almost tender, cover the top with **fillets** about 1 inch thick; insert a meat thermometer; dot the fish with **bacon drippings,** sprinkle with **paprika,** and bake as in basic recipe. Serve with tossed salad (p. 298).

Broiling is one of the easiest and most successful methods of cooking fish. As a rule, the fish should not be more than 1½ inches thick; as long as this qualification is met, any fish can be broiled. Small fish, such as fresh-water trout, may be stuffed and broiled whole. Larger fish should be cut in half along the backbone or sliced into steaks or fillets of serving sizes.

Fish to be broiled successfully should be set on a wire rack. If it is put on a baking sheet or pan, the utensil becomes hot; juices collect and change to steam which penetrates quickly; overcooking can scarcely be prevented. If you wish to cook the fish in a low baking dish, broil only the top surface; do not turn it.

## BROILED FISH

Select steaks or fillets not more than 1½ inches thick; unless the steaks are to be rolled in crumbs, do not remove skin. Leave small fish whole.

Carefully punch a hole for the meat thermometer in thickest part of the flesh. If whole fish are being broiled, insert thermometer into flesh behind gills. Move thermometer about to make sure it does not touch bone. Set fish on broiler rack.

Brush fish with **bacon drippings or oil;** *do not salt;* sprinkle generously with **paprika.**

If using gas heat, set broiler pan on top ledge so that fish is about 1 inch from heat; keep the flames very small. If using electricity, set about 5 inches from heating unit. Leave the broiler door open.

Use pancake turner and turn fish after 8 to 10 minutes, or when half the thickness has become opaque. Read the thermometer frequently and take up the fish as soon as 140° F. is reached. Allow 15 minutes for cooking fish 1 inch thick, 18 minutes if 1½ inches thick.

Garnish with **ground parsley.** Serve with herb butter seasoned with fresh dill, tarragon, and chives (p. 167), or with lemon butter (p. 168), or sauce of sour cream (p. 168).

After fruit appetizer (p. 261), serve with creamed leeks (p. 388), steamed radish tops (p. 380), finger salads (p. 273).

*Variations:*

If a browned crust is desired, dip in milk or 1 egg stirred with 2 tablespoons fresh milk and then in sifted whole-wheat-bread crumbs, cereal crumbs, whole-wheat flour, or yellow cornmeal; sprinkle with paprika.

If egg or milk is used, season with freshly ground peppercorns and a pinch of sage, tarragon, fennel, thyme, or basil; or add 1 teaspoon dill sauce, dry mustard, paprika, minced fresh herbs, or crushed anise.

**Broiled lobster:** Cut a live lobster in half and broil as in the basic recipe or drop the whole lobster into rapidly boiling water; boil 2 minutes, allow to simmer 10 minutes longer. Remove from water, split, clean (p. 175); crack claws. Dot with **margarine or butter,** sprinkle with **browned crumbs and paprika.** Broil under low heat 8 to 10 minutes. Vary by filling cavity before broiling with creamed lobster (p. 189) prepared from the claws, or after broiling with cole slaw garnished with paprika; or place a lettuce leaf in cavity and top with sliced lemon. Serve with baked yams, mixed-fruit salad.

**Broiled roe:** Choose shad, bass, barracuda, or other roe with membrane unbroken; roll in **oil and sifted and toasted crumbs.** Broil on a baking sheet about 20 minutes on one side, or to an internal temperature of 150° F. *Do not turn.* Serve with melted butter to which lemon juice, chives, and ground parsley are added, steamed carrots, cauliflower with cheese sauce (p. 163), head lettuce salad.

**Broiled scallops:** Place 4 to 7 scallops on each of 4 skewers; brush with **oil or bacon drippings,** sprinkle with **paprika;** broil 3 to 4 minutes on each side. Serve with dill sauce (p. 163), string beans, beet pickles, tomato and cottage cheese salad.

**Fish with herbs:** If fish steaks or fillets are to be held several hours before cooking, brush surfaces with oil and sprinkle with minced fresh dill or tarragon or crushed anise or dill seeds; pile steaks or fillets on top of each other so that seasonings can penetrate from both surfaces. Broil as in basic recipe. Serve with fresh lima beans (p. 413), Brussels sprouts (p. 383), cucumber salad (p. 278).

**Seasoned broiled fish steaks or fillets:** Spread surfaces of uncooked fish with **mayonnaise.** Broil with or without rolling in crumbs or flour. Vary by sprinkling with shredded nippy cheese or Parmesan cheese just before taking from broiler. Serve with French-fried potatoes (p. 398), steamed kale, tossed salad.

Frying in deep fat is an excellent method of cooking small fish or sea food, particularly if the surface is irregular. Unfortunately fish cooked by this method are almost invariably dried out. Until you have used a meat thermometer when French-frying fish, you can hardly believe that it cooks as quickly as it does. For example, in testing recipes, we found that jumbo shrimps required only 1 minute in fat at 360° F. to reach the internal temperature of 140° F., and that before they cooled sufficiently to be eaten, they had reached 160° F. Shrimps that were fried 2 minutes were only half the size of those cooked 1 minute, and not nearly as delicious. After the fish is removed from the fat, the piping-hot crust causes cooking to continue until the crust has cooled. The cooking time of fried fish, therefore, must not be thought of as the time it is immersed in fat; instead, count from the time it is put on to cook until it is actually cooled or eaten. The browning itself should be done so quickly that the inside can little more than become warm.

Even when fat used for frying is heated until extremely hot, the cold fish usually cools it from 100° to 200° F. In order not to cool the fat so much that the fish becomes overcooked before the crust becomes delightfully brown, only a small amount of fish or sea food should be browned at one time. Bacon drippings are especially satisfactory for cooking fish because they do not burn easily.

The problem of crust flaking off during the cooking can be met by dipping the fish or sea food in crumbs and letting it dry before browning. Restaurants which specialize in sea foods often dip their fish several hours before time to fry them. Too, the crust will have less tendency to flake off if powdered milk is used in the batter.

## BATTER FOR FRENCH-FRIED FOODS

Sift together:

| | |
|---|---|
| ⅓ cup whole-wheat pastry flour | 1 tablespoon mustard (optional) |
| 3 tablespoons powdered milk | 1 teaspoon salt |

Add and stir well:

| | |
|---|---|
| ¼ cup fresh milk | 1 egg |

Dip fish or other food in batter one piece at a time; place in wire basket and fry immediately in deep fat.

*Variations:*

If especially light batter is desired, beat egg white until stiff and fold in last.

Vary batter by omitting mustard and adding any of the following seasonings: 1 teaspoon crushed dill, anise, or celery seeds or minced fresh basil, fennel, or dill.

## FRENCH-FRIED FISH

Use cod, flounder, lake haddock, barracuda, red snapper, halibut, or other fish.

Clean and trim fish, removing skin and bones; pat dry with paper towels and cut into serving sizes not more than 1 inch thick, or into pieces allowing two or more per serving.

Dip in **batter** or shake in a paper bag containing:

| | |
|---|---|
| ½ cup whole-wheat flour or | 1 tablespoon powdered milk |
| ¾ cup sifted whole-wheat-bread crumbs | 1 teaspoon salt |

If flour or crumbs are used, let dry 10 minutes.

Heat **bacon drippings or vegetable oil** 2 inches or more deep in a pan used for French frying. Place 3 or 4 pieces of fish in wire basket; when heated fat reaches 360° F., set basket in fat and brown fish as quickly as possible, not longer than 2 minutes. Pierce the servings with meat thermometer and take up at 130° to 135° F. Drain the browned fish on absorbent paper and keep in a warm place.

Reheat fat to 360° F. and continue frying until the remainder of fish is browned.

Fry a few slices of raw potato in fat to clear it; strain. This fat may be used for frying doughnuts, potatoes, etc., or for general cooking.

Garnish the platter with **parsley** and **pickled beets.** Serve fish with caper or horseradish sauce with sour-cream or yogurt base (p. 168) or with uncooked creole sauce (p. 167); steamed celery root (p. 348), lettuce and cucumber salad.

*Variations:*

Dip fish in 1 egg stirred with 2 tablespoons fresh milk, 1 tablespoon powdered milk, 1 teaspoon salt: roll in whole-wheat flour or sifted bread crumbs.

**Shrimp:** If fresh shrimp are used, do not precook before frying; remove the shells and sand veins (p. 176); dry quickly, dip in batter seasoned with **1 teaspoon dill or anise seeds.** Fry as in basic recipe; allow them to be in fat only 1 minute. Serve with steamed shredded beets (p. 342), roasted corn on the cob (p. 408), citrus-fruit salad with French dressing.

**Mock scallops:** Use halibut fillets or fillets of other white-fleshed fish; cut into 1¼-inch cubes; dip in batter seasoned with **dill,** adding ½ **teaspoon sugar.** Fry 1 minute, as in basic recipe. Serve with fresh peas (p. 364), tossed green salad (p. 298).

**Scallops:** Dip in batter seasoned with **basil;** fry 1 minute, as in basic recipe (p. 183) or in shallow fat (p. 185). Serve with creamed corn (p. 409), steamed chard (p. 374), sliced tomatoes and cucumbers.

**Fish croquettes:** Add **2 cups of any steamed and flaked or leftover fish** to ½ **cup thick cream sauce** (p. 161) seasoned with **1 or 2 tablespoons capers or dill sauce or 1 teaspoon dill or anise seeds;** add ½ **teaspoon each salt, Worcestershire, and paprika, 1 tablespoon grated onion, 1 egg.** Stir well, mold into croquettes, dip in **sifted crumbs,** and fry as in basic recipe, 1 to 2 minutes. Vary by adding ½ cup shredded American cheese. Do not miss this recipe; these are delicious croquettes. Serve with creamed kohlrabi (p. 359), New Zealand spinach, apple, celery, and walnut salad (p. 275).

*Potato-fish croquettes:* Use ½ to 1 cup leftover mashed potatoes instead of cream sauce. Vary by adding 2 tablespoons chili sauce as well as the seasonings in fish croquettes.

Only small fish which are to be cooked whole, such as mackerel, smelt, squid, and fresh-water bass or trout, should be fried rather than sautéed. In order that all contours of the fish may be evenly browned, the fat used should be the depth of half the thickness of the fish. Although butter browns easily, it is not recommended for frying; it usually causes fish to stick. As in deep-fat frying, cooking continues as long as the fish is warm. The fat should be very hot before the fish is put into it, and the fish should be taken up the minute it is delicately golden.

## FRIED FISH

Clean 2 pounds or more of small whole fish. Mix well and use for dredging fish:

| | |
|---|---|
| ¼ cup whole-wheat flour or yellow corn meal or | 1 teaspoon salt |
| ½ cup sifted whole-wheat-bread crumbs | 1 teaspoon pulverized thyme or grated lemon rind |

Heat until very hot:

**½ cup or more of bacon drippings or butter-flavored fat**

Lay fish in hot fat; turn as soon as golden, or in 2 to 5 minutes; brown the other side; *do not cover utensil;* take up immediately after both sides are browned.

Serve with chilled creole sauce (p. 167) or caper sauce (p. 162), baked yams, steamed cabbage (p. 384), tossed salad (p. 298).

*Variations:*

Season the crumbs with basil, fennel, crushed dill, or dill or anise seeds.

**Fried skate and roe:** Fry fish as in basic recipe; fry roe more slowly, cooking 10 to 12 minutes, or to 160° F. Serve with vinegar sauce (p. 165) or lemon butter (p. 168) poured over fish, steamed parsley and spinach (p. 376), mixed-vegetable salad set in lemon aspic (p. 286).

**Stuffed squid:** Choose small squid 5 to 6 inches long; remove tentacles and bone, or shell, from inside of back; stuff with **crumb dressing** (p. 155) and fry as in basic recipe. Serve with Spanish sauce (p. 167), quick-steamed carrots (p. 346), beet pickles, finger salads (p. 273).

Fish which has a flat surface, such as fish steaks and fillets, should be sautéed, or cooked by easily controlled direct heat, rather than fried. When the slices are sufficiently thick, use a thermometer and take up the fish when the internal temperature is 140° F.

## SAUTÉED FISH

Select 4 fish steaks or fillets, such as bonita, cod, halibut, barracuda, shark; dip in **batter** (p. 183) or shake in a paper bag containing:

| | |
|---|---|
| ¼ cup whole-wheat flour or yellow corn meal or ½ cup sifted whole-wheat-bread crumbs | 1 tablespoon powdered milk freshly ground white peppercorns |
| **1 teaspoon salt** | 1 teaspoon fresh basil, tarragon, or dill |

Insert the meat thermometer in the center of one serving parallel to surface.

Heat grill and brush with **bacon drippings, cooking fat, or oil;** set fish on grill; *do not cover at any time.*

Turn fish as soon as the undersurface is golden brown; take it up when the thermometer reading is 140° F. or when fish has cooked 5 to 8 minutes.

Serve with celery sauce (p. 163), steamed turnips (p. 392), fresh peas cooked in milk (p. 364), salad of tomatoes and cottage cheese (p. 280).

*Variations:*

As soon as fish is taken up, heat in same utensil 3 tablespoons each lemon juice or vinegar, water, and chives; pour over fish.

**Fish patties:** Dice **2 cups leftover fish or 1 pound fresh fish fillets;** add **1 finely chopped onion, ½ stalk celery, 1 fresh or canned pimento, 1 teaspoon each salt and anise or dill seeds, 1 egg, ¼ cup each wheat germ and powdered milk;** mix well, make into patties, roll in crumbs, and sauté as in basic recipe. Vary by adding leftover mashed or chopped potatoes. Serve with buttered beets (p. 343), zucchini with cheese (p. 366), shredded carrot and pineapple salad (p. 277).

Although there is much danger of overcooking when fish is steamed, the method is preferable to baking if time is limited. Steamed fish should be cooked with the utmost care and the time be closely checked. To prevent loss of flavor and sweetness, the fish should be set on a rack so that water cannot soak out the juices. Since the penetration of moist heat is extremely rapid, the internal temperature should be checked with a meat thermometer.

If the oven is in use, fish may be steamed in an ordinary paper bag in the oven; thus dishwashing is eliminated. The thermometer should be inserted and the bag closed with string or paper clips in such a way that thermometer readings may be taken. The dead-air space inside the bag acts as an insulator and causes the temperature inside to be from 50° to 75° F. below that of the oven; the fish is steamed slowly and stays delightfully moist and juicy.

## STEAMED FISH

If the fish is more than 2 inches thick, cut in half along the backbone or into slices of uniform thickness.
Put into a utensil below rack:

**½ cup water**

Insert a meat thermometer in a piece of fish; as soon as water boils, put fish on rack, cover utensil, and note the time.

If fish is 1 inch thick, steam no longer than 3 to 4 minutes; if 2 inches thick, steam 6 to 8 minutes. Add 2 to 3 minutes if fish is chilled.

Check internal temperature near end of cooking time; remove from steam immediately when internal temperature reaches 140° F. Sprinkle with **paprika and chopped parsley.**

Serve with olive sauce (p. 164) or tartar sauce (p. 169), hash-browned potatoes (p. 403), sautéed carrots, tossed salad.

*Variations:*

If fish is to be used for appetizers (p. 265) and salads (p. 235), remove skin and bones after steaming, and separate into flakes.

**Fish steamed in a paper bag:** Put fish fillets, steaks, or whole fish on 2 or more paper towels. Season fish with **fresh basil, fennel, dill, or thin slices of lemon, onion, or dill pickle.** *Do not salt.* Insert a meat thermometer; slip the fish into an ordinary paper bag, fold over the opening and fasten with paper clips so that the thermometer extends and may be read easily. Put in a preheated oven. Remove when internal temperature reaches 140° F. Serve with any sauce or lemon butter (p. 168). Whole fish for salads and appetizers may be steamed in this manner.

**Steamed fillets:** Cut fillets into serving sizes and steam as in basic recipe. Serve with Hollandaise sauce, tartar sauce, or any sauce having a cream-sauce base. Any cream sauce can be prepared in same utensil to be used for steaming fish; set rack over the sauce, cover utensil, and steam the fish as in basic recipe. Serve cream sauce over the fish.

**Steamed lobster, crabs, or crawfish:** Wash thoroughly and steam as in basic recipe; cook crawfish 5 to 6 minutes, crabs 8 to 10 minutes, and lobster 10 to 12 minutes. Shellfish will continue cooking as they cool. Split in half, clean, and serve with lemon butter (p. 168) or tartar sauce (p. 169).

**Steamed shrimp, clams, and mussels:** Wash thoroughly, but do not remove shells; put on a rack over boiling water, cover utensil, and steam no longer than 2 minutes; remove from heat and take off lid of utensil to let steam escape; cover utensil again and let stand 3 to 4 minutes to cook from heat inside shells. Use steamed shrimp for salads or appetizers; serve clams and mussels hot with lemon butter or garlic butter (p. 168).

Although creamed dishes and casseroles may be prepared with leftover or canned fish or sea food, a far more delightful flavor can be gained by making these dishes with uncooked fish or sea food. When the uncooked fish or sea food is diced, it should be added to the hot cream sauce or casserole dish only 3 minutes before serving. Since fish should not be heated above 150° F., the simmering liquid can quickly overcook it. Any cream sauces or brown sauces may be used in preparing creamed fish and fish casseroles.

A friend who attempted to prepare the following recipe felt sure that the uncooked diced fish would be raw if not heated longer than 3 minutes; therefore she allowed the cream sauce to boil a minute or two after the fish was added. The diced fish contracted into tiny tough lumps and the fish juices diluted the sauce into a thin soup. If you are skeptical about the cooking time, pierce a small cube of fillet with a meat thermometer, making sure the mercury is in the exact center. Serve the creamed fish when the temperature reaches 130° F. The temperature will continue to rise to 140° F. after it is served. It is hard to realize how quickly fish can overcook until you have checked the temperature with a cooking thermometer.

## CREAMED FISH WITH DILL

Prepare 2 cups dill sauce (p. 163), using thick cream sauce as the base. No more than 3 minutes before serving, add to the simmering sauce:

2½ cups diced uncooked fish fillets        1½ teaspoon salt

Reheat sauce to simmering; *do not boil.*
Garnish lightly with **ground parsley.**
After citrus-fruit appetizer, serve with Brussels sprouts, sautéed shredded carrots (p. 346), salad of cottage cheese and tomato.

*Variations:*

Instead of fresh fish use flaked leftover or canned fish. Salt to taste.

Take from their shells uncooked shrimp, crab, lobster, clams, mussels, or oysters; add to dill sauce, dicing crab or lobster into 1-inch cubes. If canned shellfish is used, substitute the liquid for part of the milk in the sauce.

Omit dill from the sauce and add 1 or 2 teaspoons anise seeds. To my way of thinking, this dish is food for the gods.

Instead of cream sauce, heat 2 cups sour cream or yogurt; season with dill, anise, paprika, or other seasonings suggested for sour-cream sauces (p. 168). Proceed as in basic recipe.

Instead of dill sauce, add fish or shellfish to any cream sauce or brown sauce (p. 162) such as caper, celery, cheese, curry, mock Hollandaise, hot tartar sauce.

Prepare the sauce in a heat-resistant casserole; add fish, wipe edges, and sprinkle the top with grated cheese and toasted whole-wheat-bread crumbs.

**Casserole with potato chips:** Prepare sauce in a heat-resistant casserole; add diced fillets or canned tuna and small package of potato chips; sprinkle with paprika and brown surface under the broiler. Vary by combining 1 can condensed mushroom soup, potato chips, and diced fillets or flaked tuna; omit salt; heat in a moderate oven 30 minutes.

**Curried shrimp:** Prepare 2 cups curry sauce (p. 163); add 1 teaspoon salt, 2 cups diced raw or canned shrimp. Garnish with strips of canned pimento and ground parsley. Serve in a bed of steamed brown or all-vitamin rice (p. 204) with cooked carrots (p. 344) and endive-cucumber salad.

**Lobster Newburg:** Sauté lightly in margarine or butter 3 or 4 cups diced uncooked lobster or 2 cups flaked steamed or canned lobster; add 2 tablespoons sherry, ¾ teaspoon salt, 2 cups simmering cream sauce. As soon as heated, serve with steamed celery root, tossed salad. Prepare crab, shrimp, or any diced white fish fillets in the same manner.

In making fish casseroles, vegetables may be quickly cooked, a sauce prepared in the same utensil, and the fish or sea food added. By varying the kinds of fish, sea foods, sauces, and vegetables used, an unlimited number of casserole dishes can be prepared. Follow this procedure and create your own recipes.

## FISH IN CASSEROLE

Heat in a heat-resistant casserole or baking dish:

**3 tablespoons bacon drippings or butter-flavored fat**

Sauté lightly in fat:

**1 cup finely diced carrots**          **1 tablespoon chopped onion**
**1 chopped green pepper**

Add and mix well:

**3 tablespoons whole-wheat flour**     **1½ teaspoons salt**
**¼ teaspoon crushed white pepper-**
**corns**

Stir in slowly:

**1½ cups canned or diced fresh to-**   **½ cup chili sauce**
**matoes**

Cook until slightly thick and add:

**2 tablespoons ground parsley**

Lay across the top:

**1½ pounds fresh fillets, fish steaks, or small whole fish**

Insert a meat thermometer in the center of steak or fillet or in the flesh behind gills of whole fish.

Sprinkle top with **browned whole-wheat-bread crumbs, paprika, and** dots of **bacon drippings or other fat.**

Put in the oven at 325° F. and bake about 12 minutes, or until the internal temperature of fish reaches 140° F.

Serve with steamed summer squash (p. 367), French-fried potatoes (p. 398), finger salads (p. 273).

*Variations:*

Cook the vegetables until tender on top of the range; 3 minutes before serving add 2 cups diced uncooked fish fillets or flaked steamed or left-over fish; wipe edges of casserole, sprinkle top with buttered and toasted crumbs, and serve without baking. Vary by using fresh or canned shellfish.

Blend fat and flour and add 2 cups of any tomato sauce (p. 166).

Sauté with other vegetables ½ cup fresh or canned mushrooms or chopped celery.

Add a pinch of basil, tarragon, dill, or fennel, or 1 teaspoon dill or anise seeds.

Sauté vegetables and prepare 2 cups of any cream sauce, brown sauce (p. 162), or tomato sauce (p. 166); add diced fish or shellfish, or cover with fresh fish, and bake as in basic recipe. Vary by adding peas, string beans, cauliflower, potatoes, leeks, or other vegetables.

Add any diced leftover vegetables to casserole before adding fish.

**Fish or sea food in rice casserole:** Prepare fried rice (p. 205) in a heat-resistant casserole, using 1 cup uncooked rice; when rice is tender, stir in 1 teaspoon salt, 2 cups uncooked diced fish fillets or diced fresh or canned crabmeat, lobster, clams, oysters, or shrimp. Sprinkle with whole-wheat-bread crumbs and brown under broiler. Serve with tossed salad.

**Fish or sea food with eggplant:** Prepare eggplant creole (p. 353) in a heat-resistant casserole; 3 or 4 minutes before serving stir in 2 tablespoons ground parsley, 1 teaspoon salt, 2 cups diced uncooked or canned shrimp, clams, oysters, lobster, or crab, diced uncooked fillets, or flaked steamed or leftover fish. Cover top with buttered and toasted crumbs. Serve with egg and celery salad (p. 235).

**Fish or sea food in corn and tomato casserole:** Prepare as in basic recipe, omitting carrots; when sauce is thick, add a **No. 2 can of corn**, 1 teaspoon salt, 2 or 3 cups diced uncooked or canned shrimp, crab, lobster, or other shellfish, diced fish fillets, or flaked leftover fish; heat to simmering, sprinkle top with buttered and toasted crumbs, and serve immediately with tossed salad.

**Fish or sea food with mixed-vegetable casserole:** Combine and simmer 8 minutes in a casserole with 2 tablespoons margarine or butter, 2 cups each shredded unpeeled carrots and potatoes, 1 grated onion, 1 finely chopped pimento, 2 tablespoons ground parsley; 3 minutes before serving add 2 teaspoons salt and 2 cups diced uncooked or canned shrimp or other sea food, fish fillets, or flaked, canned or leftover fish. After mixed-fruit appetizer, serve with vegetable-gelatin salad (p. 285).

## FISH LOAF

Mix together:

| | |
|---|---|
| 2 cups diced uncooked fish or sea food | 1 chopped pimento |
| ½ cup wheat germ | 1½ teaspoons salt |
| ½ cup powdered milk | dash of cayenne |
| 2 tablespoons ground parsley | freshly ground white peppercorns |
| 1 grated onion | 2 eggs |
| | ½ cup fresh milk |

Pack in a shallow baking dish brushed with oil and sprinkle with toasted whole-wheat-bread crumbs; dot with bacon drippings, margarine, or butter-flavored fat.

Bake in a moderate oven at 350° F. for 35 to 40 minutes; test the center with meat thermometer; serve when internal temperature reaches 150° F.

Serve with creamed peas (p. 365), spiced beets (p. 343), assorted finger salads (p. 273).

*Variations:*

Prepare any soufflé (p. 209) and add 2 cups uncooked fish or flaked leftover fish.

Add any leftover vegetables, such as peas or diced carrots, potatoes, string beans, or shredded uncooked carrots.

Add 1 teaspoon dill or anise seeds or 2 tablespoons minced fresh dill or fennel.

Use canned or flaked leftover fish instead of uncooked fish.

# CHAPTER 12

## MEAT SUBSTITUTES AND EXTENDERS

Most of the so-called meat substitutes, such as dry beans, peas, rice, and macaroni, are not true substitutes for meat. They supply only about 4 to 6 grams of protein per serving, compared with an average of 18 to 20 grams in a serving of meat and fish. The proteins they contain lack several of the essential amino acids and hence do not have the health-building value of meats, fish, eggs, or milk. Generous amounts of meats, cheese, or other adequate proteins should be added to meat substitutes whenever possible. It is difficult, however, to add sufficient protein to make them nutritionally equivalent to meat. When you serve these foods, plan your menus to include other sources of protein, such as fish or glandular-meat appetizers; meat, fish, cheese, or eggs added to the salad; high-protein bread, and perhaps a dessert made of milk and eggs.

There is one exception among legumes which is a true meat substitute—soybeans. They cannot be made to taste identical with the usual variety of beans, but can be equally delicious when well prepared. Soybeans differ from other beans in that they contain about three times more protein, a small amount of sugar, and no starch. They supply essential amino acids, calcium, and B vitamins. They should be served frequently, especially when the budget is limited.

By far the easiest way to prepare soybeans is to freeze them after they have soaked and before they are cooked. This procedure decreases the cooking time about 2 hours and causes them to taste more like navy beans. Since soybeans are relatively new to Americans, seasonings should be heavily relied upon to make them palatable.

The most satisfactory means of working soybeans into your menus is by using soy grits, in which each raw bean is broken into

8 or 10 pieces. Although I have used soy grits in dozens of recipes, not once have I considered a recipe containing them a failure. They are inexpensive and bland in flavor, cook in a few minutes, and can be added to any number of foods without altering the taste. They can be substituted for cooked soybeans; thus the long cooking is avoided and the seasonings are more evenly distributed. Precooked soy grits are available, but those quickly cooked at home probably retain greater nutritive value.

## COOKED SOYBEANS

Soak in an ice tray 2 hours or longer in **2 cups water:**

### 1½ cups dry soybeans

Place in freezing compartment and freeze until solid, preferably overnight. Remove from refrigerator and drop into:

### 1 cup hot soup stock or vegetable-cooking water

Cover utensil and simmer about 2½ hours; do not allow the beans to boil at any time; add more soup stock if needed. When nearly tender, add:

| ½ teaspoon crushed black pepper-corns | 1 or 2 minced cloves garlic |
|---|---|
| 2 teaspoons salt | seasonings suggested in variations as desired |
| 3 to 5 tablespoons bacon drippings | |

Continue cooking until tender, or about 15 minutes; remove lid of utensil, allowing excess liquid to evaporate; add:

### 2 to 4 tablespoons chopped parsley

Serve with steamed broccoli, sautéed carrots, salad of spinach and cottage cheese (p. 282).

*Variations:*

Soak beans overnight without freezing; simmer 4 to 5 hours in water used for soaking.

Pass cooked soybeans through meat grinder and substitute for meat in making meat loaf (p. 134) or patties (p. 136); add 2 teaspoons meat extract before salting; use tomato purée or catsup for liquid in loaf; omit liquid from patties. Soybean loaf and patties are surprisingly good.

Instead of soybeans use 1½ cups or less uncooked soy grits; add 1½ cups boiling stock or vegetable-cooking water and the seasonings of basic recipe or any variation; simmer 10 to 15 minutes.

*Add any of the following groups of seasonings to cooked soybeans about 15 minutes before serving or to uncooked soy grits; prepare soy grits as directed above.*

**"Baked" soybeans:** 2 to 4 tablespoons blackstrap molasses; evaporate moisture until consistency is that of baked beans. Add 1 tablespoon dry mustard and 2 sliced onions 5 minutes before serving.

**Chinese soybeans:** ¼ cup blackstrap molasses, 2 chopped onions, 1 teaspoon powdered ginger or 3 tablespoons diced preserved or candied ginger, 1 diced apple, 1 to 2 tablespoons soy sauce; salt to taste after soy sauce is added; serve while apple is still crisp.

**Creamed soybeans:** 2 diced pimentos, 2 finely diced carrots, 3 tablespoons chopped parsley, pinch of basil, 1 cup or more undiluted evaporated milk; evaporate moisture before adding milk; sprinkle generously with Parmesan cheese.

**Savory soybeans:** 2 finely diced carrots, 2 chopped onions, 1 diced stalk celery; pinch each of rosemary, savory, marjoram.

**Spanish-style soybeans:** 2 chopped chili peppers or bell peppers with 1 or 2 teaspoons chili powder, ¼ cup tomato catsup, 1 or 2 chopped onions; add ½ cup shredded American, Jack, or Parmesan cheese just before serving.

**Soybean chili:** Instead of kidney beans use cooked soybeans in preparing chili (p. 200).

**Soybeans with bacon:** 2 or 3 diced and pan-broiled strips of bacon or salt pork, 2 chopped onions, a pinch of savory, a dash of smoke-flavoring.

**Soybeans with beef:** 3 or 4 drops Tabasco, 1 cup leftover diced beef or beef heart, tongue, or liver, 2 diced leeks or onions, pinch of marjoram.

**Soybeans with chicken:** Diced leftover chicken; a pinch of thyme, sage, or basil; season with chicken fat if available.

**Soybeans with green onions:** ½ to 1 cup each green onions with tops and chopped celery; a pinch each of savory, basil, marjoram; 1 tablespoon Worcestershire.

**Soybeans with ham:** 1 or 2 teaspoons caraway seeds, ½ to 1 cup each chopped onions and diced leftover ham or smoked tongue.

**Soybeans with tomatoes:** 2 to 4 tablespoons blackstrap molasses, 1 cup canned or fresh tomatoes, or ½ cup tomato catsup, 1 each chopped onion, bell pepper, stalk celery; a pinch of basil; 5 minutes before serving add 1 tablespoon dry mustard.

**Soybeans with wieners:** ½ cup tomato catsup, chili sauce, or other tomato sauce, 1 diced onion, 4 or 5 sliced wieners.

**Soybeans with vegetables:** 1 cup canned tomatoes, 1 each diced carrot, onion, green pepper; ¼ teaspoon celery seeds, 1 tablespoon black molasses.

You will use soy grits more frequently as a meat extender if you keep soaked or partially cooked soy grits on hand at all times. The uncooked grits can be added to soups, cereals, or any moist food. When the moisture in a recipe is limited, however, the grits should be soaked or precooked unless it is desirable to have a nut-like texture, as it may be in cookies.

## SOFTENED SOY GRITS

Combine:

**1 cup boiling vegetable-cooking water**          **1 cup uncooked soy grits**

Soak until all moisture is absorbed; if a softer texture is desired, simmer 5 minutes. Cool and store in a covered jar in the refrigerator.

Add ¼ cup of the cooked soy grits to omelet, scrambled eggs, or any soufflé (p. 209); ½ cup to meat loaf or meat patties, to any casserole, croquettes, cooked beans, corn pudding, chili, creamed meats, stuffing for peppers, or other meat substitutes.

Use either uncooked or softened soy grits in desserts, depending upon texture desired.

The cooking time of dry beans, peas, and lentils varies widely, depending on the age of the legumes and the locality in which they were grown. When these legumes are soaked before cooking, vitamins and minerals pass into the water; therefore they should be cooked in the water used for soaking. Under no circumstances should they be parboiled and the liquid drained.

Soaking legumes is unnecessary if the dry legume is quickly washed and dropped into boiling water so slowly that boiling does not stop. As in popping corn, the starch grains burst and break the outside covering of the legume. After the covering and starch grains have burst, water is absorbed rapidly and the cooking time is shortened. When all the beans, lentils, or split peas have been put into the water, the heat should be lowered immediately to prevent the protein from becoming tough. A simmering temperature should then be maintained until the beans are tender. Soda, which appears to harm a number of B vitamins, should not be used in cooking legumes.

The cooking time of legumes can be decreased almost half by soaking them and then freezing them before putting them on to cook. Use the method which is most convenient for you.

If salt, fat, or molasses is added at the beginning of cooking, the cooking time is prolonged. Fat coats the outside covering and prevents moisture from passing readily into the legume. The acid in molasses toughens the outside covering. Salt attracts water away from the legume rather than into it. Add these seasonings and others only after the legume is starting to become tender.

So-called baked beans are not actually baked but are cooked by the heat of simmering liquid. They can be "baked" over a simmer burner far more quickly and with less fuel cost than in an oven. The difference in taste between boiled and baked beans lies in the seasonings and the amount of liquid evaporated. Any dried beans may be prepared in a heat-resistant casserole and the top browned slightly under the broiler to give the appearance of baked beans.

## DRIED BEANS

Bring to a rolling boil:

### 1 quart water

Put in a wire strainer and wash rapidly under running water:

### 2 cups dry navy beans, lima beans, kidney beans, or other dry beans

Add beans slowly to boiling water so that boiling does not stop; reduce heat immediately after all beans are in the water.

Simmer until beans are almost tender, or 1½ to 2½ hours; add and stir well:

| | |
|---|---|
| ½ teaspoon crushed black peppercorns | ½ to 3 teaspoons salt |
| 4 to 6 tablespoons bacon drippings or 3 slices of salt pork, diced | seasonings suggested under variations if desired |

Add more water if needed; if more moisture is left than is desired, finish cooking without covering utensil. Allow 2½ to 3 hours as total cooking time for dry navy beans, 2 to 2½ hours for lima or kidney beans. Taste for seasonings.

After sea-food appetizer (p. 265), serve with creamed spinach (p. 373), cottage cheese and pear salad.

*Variations:*

Soak beans overnight and bring slowly to boiling in water used for soaking, or soak in ice tray for 2 hours, using 2 cups water; freeze 2 hours and cook 1½ to 2 hours; add 1 cup vegetable-cooking water or soup stock during cooking.

If recipe is doubled, use 4 cups beans to 6 cups water.

*Prepare beans as in basic recipe; when they start to become tender, add the following seasonings:*

**Black-eyed beans:** 1 minced clove garlic, 2 chopped onions, and 2 chili tepines or small whole cayenne pepper; discard the pepper before serving.

*With ham:* 1 chopped pimento, a pinch of basil, diced leftover ham; or cook with a ham bone or ham stock; or add smoke flavoring to taste.

*With onions:* 2 sliced onions, 2 teaspoons Worcestershire; add 1 tablespoon dry mustard 5 minutes before serving.

*With sausage:* ½ cup tomato juice, ½ pound pork sausage made into small balls, 2 or 3 chopped stalks celery with leaves, 2 chopped onions, 1 minced clove of garlic; omit fat; just before serving add 2 tablespoons sherry. Vary by including fat and using sliced wieners instead of sausage; add 5 minutes before serving.

**Fresh kidney beans, Mexican style:** Omit fat; mash half the beans; heat ¼ cup vegetable oil or bacon fat until it starts to brown; add beans, 2 minced cloves garlic, a pinch of orégano and/or cumin seeds; simmer 10 minutes; before serving add 1 cup grated or shredded Jack, American, or Swiss cheese. These beans are delicious; don't miss them.

**Kidney beans:** 1 each finely chopped onion and green pepper; 1 minced clove garlic; instead of 1 cup water use 1 cup tomatoes.

**Kidney beans with chives:** Add 5 minutes before serving 3 tablespoons chives, 2 tablespoons parsley, 2 teaspoons Worcestershire.

**Lima beans, "baked":** 2 chopped onions, 1 to 3 tablespoons blackstrap or dark molasses, 1 tablespoon dry mustard, leftover ham scraps or smoke-flavoring to taste; prepare in a heat-resistant casserole; remove lid and let excess moisture evaporate; brown slightly under broiler. Vary by seasoning with part of the fat rendered from 4 slices bacon; put bacon strips on top before browning.

**Lima beans, creamed:** Use margarine or butter; add a pinch of basil, 2 diced pimentos, 3 tablespoons chopped parsley; 1 cup top milk or evaporated milk shaken with ½ cup powdered milk; cook in 3 cups water and evaporate excess moisture before adding milk.

**Lima beans with lentils:** Cook together 1 cup each lima beans and lentils; add 1 diced carrot, 1 each chopped onion, green pepper, pimento, 1 minced clove garlic, ½ cup catsup or chili sauce.

**Lima beans with vegetables:** 2 finely diced carrots, 1 chopped onion or leek, 2 tablespoons parsley, 1 tablespoon Worcestershire.

**Navy beans, "baked":** 2 to 6 tablespoons blackstrap molasses added to taste; cook in a heat-resistant casserole, evaporate excess moisture; use salt pork instead of bacon drippings; brown surface under broiler; add 4 teaspoons dry mustard immediately before browning.

**Navy beans "baked" with tomatoes:** 2 cups tomatoes, 3 tablespoons blackstrap molasses, 1 or 2 finely chopped onions, 1 minced clove garlic; cook in a heat-resistant casserole; evaporate the excess moisture; brown surface under broiler.

**Navy beans with bacon:** Pan-broil slowly 4 slices bacon without browning and use part of the drippings to season beans; finish cooking the beans until tender; put into a shallow baking dish, cover with thin slices of fresh tomatoes, sweet onion or leeks, strips of bacon; set under a slow broiler until tomatoes are cooked; serve when onions are hot but still crisp.

**Navy beans with ham:** Cook with a ham bone, with the skin from cured ham or bacon, or in ham stock; just before serving add scraps of leftover ham, 2 teaspoons each Worcestershire and dry mustard; if no ham is available, add smoke-flavoring to taste.

**Savory navy beans:** a pinch each of basil, savory, and thyme; 1 each chopped onion, stalk celery with leaves; minced clove garlic; 1 pimento or ripe bell pepper or green chili pepper.

Split beans and lentils are not served often enough. If cheese, meat, or other adequate protein is added to them, they become excellent meat substitutes, particularly for use when the budget is limited.

## LENTILS AND SPLIT PEAS

Prepare lentils and split peas in the same way as dry beans (p. 197,) using 2 or 3 cups water for 2 cups lentils or split peas; simmer lentils 2 hours, split peas ¾ to 1 hour.

When they are almost tender, add **salt, white peppercorns, 4 to 6 tablespoons fat,** and any of the following seasonings:

**Creamed lentils or split peas:** 1 cup top milk or evaporated milk shaken with ½ cup powdered milk; 2 diced pimentos, 2 tablespoons ground parsley, ¼ teaspoon thyme; use margarine or butter.

**Lentils or split peas with chicken:** 1 diced carrot, 2 chopped pimentos, a pinch each of sage and basil; chicken fat, margarine, or butter; leftover diced chicken if available.

**Lentils or split peas with vegetables:** 1 diced carrot, 1 chopped onion or leek, 2 stalks celery with leaves, 1 green pepper, 2 tablespoons ground parsley, ½ cup tomatoes or tomato sauce; just before serving add ¼ cup grated Parmesan or other cheese. Vary by adding 3 or 4 sliced wieners or smoked pork sausages, 1 cup diced ham, or bits of crisp bacon.

*With caraway seeds:* 3 to 4 teaspoons caraway seeds in addition to vegetables; use or omit cheese; add smoke-flavoring to taste. Don't miss this recipe.


## CHILI WITH MEAT AND BEANS

Heat in large utensil:

### ¼ cup vegetable oil or bacon drippings

Add and fry until well brown, to develop a pronounced meat flavor:

### 4 tablespoons ground lean meat

Add and sauté lightly:

¾ cup chopped onions                    2 minced cloves garlic
½ cup chopped green pepper

When onions are transparent, add:

2 cups cooked red kidney beans          1 cup soup stock, tomato purée, or
   (p. 197)                                liquid from beans
1 pound ground meat                     2 teaspoons salt
1 to 3 teaspoons chili powder           2 teaspoons minced fresh or ½ tea-
                                           spoon dried orégano

Mash about half the beans; stir well, and serve as soon as they are heated through.

Serve with tossed green salad (p. 298) and cucumber pickles.

*Variations:*

Use canned kidney beans; omit liquid from recipe and use juice from beans.

Add ½ to 1 teaspoon cumin seeds with the onions and garlic.

If available, use 3 diced fresh chili peppers or 1 dried chili instead of ground chili powder; discard the dried chili before serving.

Use cooked soybeans instead of kidney beans or add ½ cup or more soy grits to basic recipe.

Macaroni, spaghetti, and noodles are available prepared from whole-wheat flour and from whole-wheat flour combined with soy flour. Brown rice is well known. All-vitamin rice is prepared by treating unmilled rice with steam under pressure. As the steam penetrates the rice, the B vitamins dissolve in it and are carried into the heart of the rice. The rice is then milled. It cooks quickly and does not differ in taste or appearance from devitalized white rice. All of these products are far superior nutritionally to refined ones. If you sincerely wish your family to maintain excellent health, use these products from which the minerals and vitamins have not been removed. Keep them covered in a dry, cool place; discard them if they smell rancid.

It has been found that as much as 20 per cent of the B vitamins are lost when rice is washed by being dipped from one pan of water to another. Wash rice quickly under running water. Since most of the minerals and the B vitamins may pass into the cooking liquid, water in which rice, macaroni, or spaghetti is cooked should not be drained off. The liquid should be carefully measured and no more used than is actually needed. If these foods are to be served in a sauce made of milk, cook them in milk; if to be served with a tomato sauce, cook them in soup stock or vegetable-cooking water.

The trick of cooking rice, macaroni, and other starchy food so that each grain or particle is separate is to drop the food so slowly into hot liquid that boiling or simmering does not stop. When the starch in the food is cooked immediately, it does not have time to soak out to thicken the cooking liquid or hold the particles together. The reverse of this procedure can be used when thickening is needed. Instead of making cream sauce when preparing macaroni and cheese, for example, and thus adding starch to starch, add cold milk when the macaroni is almost tender; some of the starch from the macaroni soaks into the milk and when heated thickens the sauce. To prevent rice or macaroni from boiling over, add a small amount of fat.

Rice, macaroni, noodles, and spaghetti can be cooked more quickly and economically over a simmer burner than in an oven. Since the shorter the cooking time, the greater the retention of B vitamins, the longer oven cooking is not recommended.

## MACARONI, SPAGHETTI, NOODLES, OR RICE COOKED IN MILK

Heat to simmering in a heat-resistant casserole:

1½ cups fresh milk

Add so slowly that simmering does not stop:

| | |
|---|---|
| 1 cup brown or all-vitamin rice or | 2 tablespoons butter-flavored fat, |
| 1½ cups whole-wheat macaroni or | margarine, or butter |
| spaghetti or | ¼ to ½ teaspoon crushed white |
| 2 cups whole-wheat or soy noodles | peppercorns |

Cover and simmer until tender; allow 15 to 20 minutes for cooking noodles, macaroni, spaghetti, or all-vitamin rice, 40 to 45 for brown rice. Add:

| | |
|---|---|
| 1 teaspoon each salt and Worcestershire | ½ cup or more cold fresh milk shaken with |
| 1 cup diced American cheese or ingredients suggested in variations | ½ cup powdered milk |

Do not boil after powdered milk or cheese is added; wipe edges of casserole; sprinkle over top:

| | |
|---|---|
| ½ cup toasted whole-wheat-bread crumbs | ½ cup shredded American cheese generous amount of paprika |

Cover casserole until cheese is melted, or heat lightly under broiler.

Serve with Chinese mustard (p. 377), salad of carrot, cottage cheese, pineapple.

*Variations:*

If utensil does not hold steam, use 2 cups milk at the beginning of cooking and add more as needed.

Cook with creamed rice or noodles 1 tablespoon or more poppy seeds.

*Follow the basic recipe, merely adding the ingredients suggested below. When fresh vegetables are used, cook them with the rice, macaroni, or noodles, adding them only in time to become tender; stir sea food, cheese, or leftover meat into the sauce just before adding crumbs.*

**With chicken:** 2 diced pimentos, 2 tablespoons ground parsley, 1 cup diced leftover chicken, 2 tablespoons chicken fat or margarine, a pinch each of sage and basil. Vary by adding 1 cup peas.

**With clams:** 1 to 2 cups chopped fresh or canned clams with broth, ¼ cup ground parsley, a few sliced stuffed olives.

**With ham:** 1 cup diced leftover ham, 1 tablespoon dry mustard; use ham drippings instead of other fat. Vary by adding 1 or 2 teaspoons caraway seeds instead of mustard.

**With liver:** 2 tablespoons chopped celery, 1 chopped onion, 1 chopped bell pepper, a pinch each of savory and marjoram; 1 cup diced sautéed liver.

**With meat balls:** Add 8 small uncooked meat balls (p. 137); simmer 5 to 7 minutes.

**With mushrooms:** Sauté ½ cup fresh or canned mushrooms in the same utensil before adding milk.

**With oysters:** 1 pint fresh or canned oysters, 2 tablespoons ground parsley, 2 tablespoons chili sauce. Vary by omitting chili and adding 1 teaspoon dill or anise seeds; or by using shrimp, lamb, or veal instead of oysters.

**With peas:** 1 cup fresh or frozen peas, 1 chopped leek or sweet onion, 1 diced pimento; stir 1 cup cheese into sauce.

**With salmon or other fish:** 1 each finely chopped onion and pimento or green pepper, 1 stalk chopped celery and leaves, 2 tablespoons ground parsley, 2 cups canned salmon, diced fresh fillet, or flaked steamed fish.

**With seeds:** Add 2 to 4 teaspoons poppy seeds 15 minutes before serving; include or omit cheese. Poppy seeds are particularly delicious with rice or noodles. Or add 1 to 3 teaspoons crushed dill seeds with any recipe in which cheese is used.

**With shrimp:** 1 cup or more of uncooked fresh or canned shrimp and the broth, 2 diced hard-cooked eggs, 2 teaspoons minced onion, a dash each of cayenne, nutmeg, and celery salt.

**With vegetables:** ½ cup each diced carrots, finely chopped celery and onion, 2 or 3 strips crisp bacon broken to bits; sauté vegetables lightly in bacon drippings before adding to the noodles, rice, or macaroni; add bacon just before serving.

## MACARONI, SPAGHETTI, RICE, OR NOODLES
## TO BE SERVED WITH SAUCES

Bring to a rolling boil:

   1½ cups soup stock, tomato juice, or vegetable-cooking water

Add so slowly that boiling does not stop:

| | |
|---|---|
| 1 cup brown or all-vitamin rice or | ¼ to ½ teaspoon crushed black |
| 1½ cups whole-wheat macaroni or | peppercorns |
| spaghetti or | 1 teaspoon salt |
| 2 cups whole-wheat or soy noodles | |

Cover the utensil and simmer until the food is tender, or about 15 to
20 minutes for all-vitamin rice, macaroni, spaghetti, or noodles, 40 to 45
minutes for brown rice.

Pour over macaroni or spaghetti, or stir rice or noodles into:

   2 cups Italian sauce (p. 166)

Sprinkle over top:

   ½ cup Parmesan or other nippy cheese

After fruit appetizer (p. 261), serve with tossed salad (p. 298).

*Variations:*

Instead of Italian sauce prepare 2 cups tomato, creole, Mexican, or
Spanish sauce (p. 166). Add to sauce any of the following: 6 slices crisp
pan-broiled bacon broken to bits; meat balls (p. 137) or ½ pound ground
lean beef, preferably heart; leftover diced chicken, ham, liver, tongue,
veal, or lamb. Add tuna, diced fresh fish fillets, or leftover flaked fish to
tomato sauce and noodles or rice.

Use macaroni or spaghetti made of soy flour mixed with whole-wheat
flour.

If utensil does not hold steam, cook in 2 or more cups soup stock or
vegetable-cooking water; use any remaining cooking liquid in making
sauce; add 1 teaspoon beef extract or 1 bouillon cube when using vegetable-cooking water.

If the cooking time is not more than 20 minutes and sauce is to be
mixed with macaroni, etc., prepare sauce, add liquid, and proceed with
basic recipe, using only one utensil.

# FRIED RICE

Place in a wire strainer and wash quickly under running water:

1½ cups brown rice

Shake dry and fry in:

3 tablespoons oil or bacon drippings

Keep heat high, stir frequently, and cook until rice is well browned; add slowly:

2 cups soup stock or vegetable-cooking water

Simmer 30 minutes and add:

¼ to ½ teaspoon crushed black peppercorns
1 minced clove garlic
1 chopped onion

1 cup canned tomatoes or 2 diced fresh tomatoes
1½ teaspoons salt
pinch each of basil and orégano

Cook until tender; allow about 45 minutes for the total cooking time. Just before serving add:

2 tablespoons ground parsley

1 cup diced American, Swiss, or Jack cheese

After sea-food appetizer (p. 265), serve with creamed cabbage (p. 384), tossed green salad (p. 298).

*Variations:*

Before browning rice pan-broil 3 or 4 strips bacon; remove when crisp, break into bits, and add just before serving.

When rice begins to be tender, stir in 2 beaten eggs and the cheese; turn into a ring mold; bake at 325° F. for 15 minutes, or to the internal temperature of 185° F.

If all-vitamin rice is used, brown the rice, reduce heat, and sauté vegetables; add 1 cup each tomatoes and soup stock; cook 15 to 20 minutes.

Omit or decrease cheese and add 1 cup of any of the following just before serving: diced leftover beef, chicken, heart, tongue, lamb, or veal; fresh or canned shrimps, oysters, or other shellfish and juice; diced uncooked fish fillets or flaked steamed fish; omit orégano if sea food is used and add 1 teaspoon dill or anise seeds.

Use noodles instead of rice; add seasonings of basic recipe or any variation and ½ cup whole ripe olives.

## CHEESE LOAF

Simmer over low heat for 3 minutes:

| | |
|---|---|
| 1 diced green pepper | ½ cup fresh milk |

Remove from heat and add:

| | |
|---|---|
| 2 cups (1 pound) diced American cheese | 1 cup whole-wheat-bread crumbs |

When the cheese has melted, add:

1 small can diced pimentos and juice
1 teaspoon salt
¼ teaspoon freshly ground white peppercorns
2 tablespoons ground parsley

1 cup cooked whole-wheat macaroni, spaghetti, noodles, brown rice, or all-vitamin rice
¼ cup powdered milk
3 eggs slightly beaten

Mix well, pour into a loaf pan brushed with oil, and bake in slow oven at 300° F. for 25 minutes.

Serve with mushroom sauce (p. 163), string beans (p. 356), tossed green salad with strips of leftover ham or other meat.

*Variations:*

Add 1 cup shredded raw carrot or diced leftover carrots or other vegetables; or 1 cup finely shredded fresh spinach, mustard, or other greens. Heat the raw vegetables with green pepper. Use 1¾ cups bland cheese and ¼ cup Parmesan or other strong-flavored cheese.

Select firm and thick-meated peppers for stuffing. Since fresh peppers are among the richest known sources of vitamin C, which can easily dissolve in cooking water, they should not be parboiled. When it is desirable to precook them, steam them over a small amount of water, but try not to touch them with water except to wash them. Pimentos, green chili peppers, and fresh paprikas have more flavor than bell peppers have and should be used for stuffing when available. Since the vitamin C content doubles with ripening, red bell peppers are preferable to green ones. To preserve vitamin C, peppers should be kept chilled, heated rapidly, and cooked the shortest time possible. When they are to be baked, fill them with preheated stuffing without precooking them and serve while they are still slightly crisp.

## PIMENTOS STUFFED WITH CHEESE

Shred:

### 2 cups Jack or American cheese

Stuff firmly into:

### 8 canned pimentos

Beat until fluffy:

### 2 whole eggs

Add and beat slightly:

**1 tablespoon whole-wheat flour**          **2 tablespoons powdered milk**

Flatten the pimentos and dip in **egg**; fry 3 or 4 at a time in:

### ¼ cup oil or bacon drippings

Be extremely careful to keep heat low; brown lightly on both sides; set on hot serving platter and keep in a warm place; heat **2 cups Spanish sauce** (p. 167) and pour over pimentos. Do not miss this recipe; these peppers are a choice delicacy.

Serve with fried rice (p. 205) or fried kidney beans (p. 406), tossed salad (p. 298).

*Variations:*

Add to shredded cheese 3 tablespoons chopped ripe olives.

**Baked peppers with cheese and eggs:** Remove stem end and seeds from 4 large bell peppers or fresh pimentos trimmed to stand straight; stuff half full of shredded cheese; drop **1 egg** on top of each pepper, season with **salt and dash of cayenne;** use 8 pimentos if they are small; stir **4 eggs** together, add **1 teaspoon salt,** and pour over cheese in peppers. Bake in a moderate oven at 350° F. for 12 to 15 minutes.

**Chili relleno, or stuffed chili peppers:** Select fresh green chili peppers with thick meat; do not remove stems or seeds; put peppers under broiler and sear with high heat on all sides; wrap quickly in a damp towel and steam until skin is loose; remove skin, make a slit on one side, fill, and prepare as in basic recipe. Use canned chili peppers when no fresh ones are available. This is my favorite of all Mexican dishes. If fresh bell peppers are used, mix **1 or 2 teaspoons ground chili powder** with the cheese used for stuffing.

**Peppers filled with creamed meat or vegetables:** Fill fresh peppers with creamed leftover chicken, ham, shrimp, oysters, macaroni and cheese, or creamed peas or asparagus mixed with cheese. Add to creamed food **3 tablespoons each powdered milk and ground parsley; pinch of basil;** heat to simmering and put into peppers; sprinkle with **grated cheese, browned crumbs and paprika;** bake in moderate oven at 350° F. for 10 minutes.

**Peppers stuffed with meat:** Prepare half the recipe for any meat loaf (pp. 124, 126, 134), using 1 whole egg; stuff into peppers and bake in moderate oven at 350° F. about 35 minutes, or to internal temperature of 175° F. Vary by stuffing with ingredients of any recipe for croquettes (p. 220); sprinkle with **crumbs, grated cheese, paprika,** and bake 30 to 35 minutes.

**Stuffed peppers with omelet:** Steam 4 whole peppers until soft, or about 3 minutes; cut a gash in one side, remove seeds, and stuff with cheese. Prepare fluffy omelet (p. 247), add **1 or 2 teaspoons chili powder,** and pour over peppers. Bake in a slow oven at 300° F. for 30 minutes. Cut omelet so that each serving contains a pepper. Serve with Spanish sauce (p. 167), string beans, assorted finger salads.

Well-made soufflés are the most nutritious of all meat substitutes and are superior to muscle meats in that they supply larger amounts of the essential amino acids. The temperature inside a soufflé when ready to serve is usually not high enough to harm the proteins and B vitamins.

Few recipes offer such an opportunity to work eggs, cheese, milk, and other nutritious foods into the menu as do soufflés. Powdered milk, wheat germ, soy or peanut flour, and soy grits may be added to improve the nutritive value without harming the flavor. Since cheese blends well with other foods, it may be added to almost every variety of soufflé. Serve soufflés frequently, especially when cooking for one whose health is below par.

A soufflé should be baked in much the same way as an angelfood cake, or at 300° F. If the oven becomes too hot, the soufflé, being largely protein, toughens and shrivels. Since raw eggs are not firm until cooked, an undercooked soufflé naturally falls. If the soufflé is allowed to cool before it is served, the steam inside it contracts and causes it to shrink. The soufflé will be a success if you control the baking temperature, give it time to cook, and keep it warm until it is served.

## CHEESE SOUFFLÉ

Heat to simmering: **1 cup whole milk**

Meanwhile beat together, and add to the hot milk:

| | |
|---|---|
| ½ cup cold milk | 1½ teaspoons salt |
| ½ cup powdered milk | ⅛ teaspoon freshly ground white |
| 3 tablespoons whole-wheat flour | peppercorns |

Simmer 5 minutes, stirring constantly; remove from heat, cool slightly; add and stir well:

| | |
|---|---|
| 4 egg yolks | 1 to 2 cups diced American cheese |
| ¼ teaspoon dried basil or celery | 2 or 3 tablespoons ground parsley |
| salt (optional) | 1 or 2 teaspoons Worcestershire |

Beat stiffly and fold in:

**4 egg whites**

Pour into casserole brushed with oil and place in a slow preheated oven at 300° F.; set an upright oven thermometer on same level with soufflé and check temperature carefully; bake 45 to 50 minutes.

After fruit appetizer, serve with mustard greens, beet aspic (p. 291).

*Variations:*

Instead of cheese add 1 to 2 cups finely diced cooked tongue, heart, leftover beef, pork, or veal, 1 grated onion, a pinch each of savory and marjoram.

Add one or more of the following: ½ cup fresh or canned mushrooms; ¼ cup diced fresh or canned pimentos, chopped ripe olives, or sliced stuffed olives; 1 each finely chopped onion, celery stalk, or bell pepper. If fresh vegetables are added, simmer 5 minutes in milk before adding other ingredients.

Add any leftover vegetable, such as peas, diced carrots, artichoke heart, chopped kale, broccoli, spinach, asparagus, celery, or string beans.

Omit flour; instead of fresh milk use 1½ cups leftover gravy, medium cream sauce (p. 161), brown sauce (p. 161), or condensed tomato or mushroom soup. Or use tomato juice or purée instead of fresh milk, adding flour and powdered milk.

Add ½ cup wheat germ or ¼ cup precooked soy grits or soy or peanut flour. If tomatoes are used instead of fresh milk, mix 1 to 3 teaspoons debittered brewers' yeast with powdered milk.

*Follow the basic recipe, merely adding the ingredients suggested below; decrease the amount of cheese as desired, but omit it only when 1½ cups or more of meat or fish are added. Simmer the fresh vegetables in the hot cream sauce until heated through.*

**Carrot soufflé:** 2 cups raw shredded carrots, 1 each chopped onion and green pepper or pimento.

**Chicken soufflé:** 1½ cups diced steamed chicken (p. 86), 1 cup uncooked fresh or frozen peas, 2 diced pimentos; a pinch of sage; use liquid left from steaming chicken instead of fresh milk. Make soufflés of duck, turkey, other fowl, or rabbit in the same manner.

**Corn soufflé:** 1 to 1½ cups fresh, frozen, or canned corn; heat in milk only if corn is fresh; reduce cheese to 1 cup.

**Crab, lobster, or shrimp soufflé:** 1½ to 2 cups diced or flaked crab, shrimp, or lobster; 1 teaspoon anise or dill seeds or ¼ teaspoon Chinese allspice; use liquid from canned sea food instead of part of the milk.

**Fish soufflé:** 1 to 2 cups diced uncooked fish fillets or flaked leftover fish, 1 tablespoon minced fresh dill or 1 teaspoon dill or anise seeds, 1 or 2 diced pimentos. Vary by using smoked salmon, cod, or other fish.

**Ham soufflé:** 1 cup or more diced leftover ham, 2 tablespoons green-onion tops or chives, a pinch each of basil and savory; vary by adding 1 or 2 teaspoons caraway seeds.

**Liver soufflé:** Use leftover liver or dredge ¾ pound lamb, beef, or veal liver in whole-wheat flour and sauté quickly; remove the liver and heat milk in same utensil; grind liver or dice fine; add with ½ cup chopped onions or leeks, a pinch each of savory, marjoram and rosemary. Vary by adding 1 or 2 teaspoons dill or caraway seeds. This is really a delicious soufflé.

**Mushroom soufflé:** ½ to 1 cup sliced fresh or canned mushrooms; use the liquid from canned mushrooms instead of part of the milk; omit cheese or use mild-flavored cheese. Vary by adding 1 cup diced artichoke hearts.

**Pea soufflé:** Use 2 cups chilled fresh peas or thawed frozen peas; put through the meat grinder without cooking; add chopped pimentos if desired; use mild-flavored cheese or omit cheese. This is a wonderful soufflé. Vary by using cooked split peas (p. 199).

**Potato soufflé:** 1 cup or more diced or mashed leftover potatoes, 1 grated onion, 1 or 2 teaspoons dill or caraway seeds.

**Spinach or broccoli soufflé:** 2 to 3 cups finely shredded or chopped raw spinach or ground uncooked broccoli, 1 grated or chopped onion; use 1 cup cheese. This is the best soufflé yet; it has the freshness of a spring garden. Vary by using kale, chard, New Zealand spinach, or other greens.

**Soufflé of sweetbreads or veal brains:** 1 cup or more finely diced brains or sweetbreads, 3 drops Tabasco, 2 tablespoons pimento or chopped celery.

**Spanish soufflé:** Use tomato purée, canned tomatoes, or diced fresh tomatoes instead of fresh milk; add 1 each chopped onion, green chili pepper, or bell pepper; 1 teaspoon chili powder, 1 minced clove garlic, 1 to 3 teaspoons brewers' yeast, a pinch each of orégano, basil and cumin seeds. Vary by adding diced ham, beef heart, liver, brains, chicken, or fish instead of cheese.

Whole, unground wheat is excellent to use as a meat extender. If hard wheat is purchased, the protein content is similar to that of rice, macaroni, and other meat extenders. The cooked wheat may be served with any cream sauce (p. 162), mixed with fresh meat, fish, or cheese, and made into patties, croquettes, or casserole dishes. Its flavor soon comes to be enjoyed; it should be served frequently, especially if the budget is limited.

## COOKED WHOLE WHEAT

Place in a wire strainer and wash quickly under running water:

**1½ cups whole, unground wheat**

Add slowly to:

**3 cups boiling soup stock or vegetable-cooking water**

Reduce heat and simmer until tender, or about 3 to 4 hours; add **1 teaspoon salt**

Add seasonings suggested in any recipe for soybeans (p. 195), split peas, or lentils; substitute an equal amount of cooked wheat for rice, macaroni, or noodles in any recipe given on page 203; use instead of rice in any casserole dish (p. 219), croquettes (p. 220), meat patties (p. 136), or cheese loaf (p. 206); add to omelets or scrambled eggs.

Serve with cooked mustard greens and tossed salad containing meat or sliced hard-cooked eggs.

*Variations:*

Soak wheat overnight; cook in same liquid used for soaking.

Cook wheat in a pressure cooker 30 minutes.

Although the recipe for tamale pie seems complicated, it can be prepared in about 15 minutes. Unfortunately, several utensils must be used in making it, but if you happen to enjoy Mexican food, the dishwashing is justified.

## TAMALE PIE

Brown thoroughly in **bacon drippings** to develop a pronounced meat flavor:

### 4 tablespoons ground lean beef

Add and sauté lightly:

1 chopped onion                          1 chopped green pepper, preferably
                                         fresh chili pepper

Add:

1 cup canned or diced fresh toma-        1 to 3 teaspoons chili powder
toes                                     pinch of orégano and basil
8 to 12 ripe olives (optional)          ½ to 1 teaspoon cumin seeds (op-
1¼ teaspoons salt                        tional)

Simmer 10 minutes, remove from heat, and stir in:

½ pound ground lean beef, prefer-        1 cup fresh, frozen, or canned corn
ably heart                               (optional)

Set filling aside. Prepare corn meal mush by mixing together thoroughly:

1 cup yellow corn meal                   1 teaspoon salt
½ cup powdered milk

Add and mix:

### 1 cup cold milk

Stir constantly while adding corn meal mixture to:

### 2 cups simmering milk

Stir until mixture thickens, or about 5 minutes, being extremely care-ful to use low heat after thickening starts. Immediately pour half the mush into a flat oiled baking dish, spreading evenly; add and spread the filling and cover with remaining mush; sprinkle generously with **paprika**. Bake in moderate oven at 350° F. for 10 minutes; brown top slightly under broiler.

Serve hot with steamed New Zealand spinach, tossed green salad.

*Variations:*

Instead of ground fresh meat use 1 or 2 cups diced or ground leftover ham, chicken, veal, lamb, heart, tongue, or liver; or use finely diced wieners.

Add ½ cup softened soy grits (p. 196) to corn meal mush, to filling, or to both.

**Corn meal mush:** Prepare as in basic recipe; serve as a cereal or pour into a square mold, chill, slice, dredge in flour, and sauté until golden brown on both sides. This is delicious mush which browns much more easily than the ordinary variety. The protein content can be still further increased by adding ½ cup soy grits.

**Rice or spaghetti pie:** Instead of corn meal mush use **fried rice** (p. 205) seasoned only with salt; prepare as in basic recipe; or use **spaghetti or rice** cooked in **milk** (p. 202); add sautéed onion, bell pepper or pimento, and ground meat to **1 can condensed tomato soup,** omitting other ingredients of basic recipe; proceed and bake as in basic recipe. Use leftover rice or spaghetti when available. After melon appetizer (p. 261), serve with steamed beet tops (p. 380), shredded carrot salad (p. 277).

**Tamale loaf:** Brown meat, sauté vegetables; add tomatoes and seasonings, and **1½ cups soup stock;** mix corn meal and powdered milk with soup stock and add to heated moist ingredients; when thick, add corn and remaining meat. If tomatoes are sour, add **1 to 3 teaspoons black molasses.** Bake as in basic recipe. Serve with steamed parsley and radish tops (p. 380), apple and celery salad (p. 276).

## FILLED THIN PANCAKES

Beat stiff:

> 2 egg whites

Add and beat enough to blend:

| | |
|---|---|
| 2 egg yolks | 1 teaspoon black molasses (op- |
| ⅓ cup whole-wheat flour | tional) |
| 1 teaspoon salt | 1 cup fresh milk |
| ¼ cup powdered milk | |

Bake on a moderately hot grill; use 3 tablespoons of batter for each pancake, making it about 5 inches in diameter; stack and keep in a warm place.

Meanwhile prepare filling by cooking in 2 tablespoons oil or bacon drippings:

1 chopped onion                             1 clove garlic

When onion is transparent, discard garlic and add:

1 bunch finely shredded spinach      ½ bunch finely shredded parsley

Keep heat high, turn frequently, and cook only until greens are wilted; add:

**1 cup diced leftover ham, veal, lamb, or chicken**

Put 1 tablespoon of filling on each pancake, fold sides of pancake over filling, and set folded side down in a casserole; sprinkle over top:

**1 cup shredded yellow cheese**

Set in a moderate oven until cheese melts. Serve hot with heated Spanish sauce (p. 167).

After sea-food appetizer (p. 265), serve with summer squash, apricot salad (p. 290).

*Variations:*

Add 1 cup shredded American cheese, such as a nippy Cheddar, to spinach if no leftover meat is available.

Make a filling of any chopped, quickly cooked greens, such as broccoli, chard, kale, New Zealand spinach, or equal parts of mustard or radish tops and spinach.

Bake the pancakes in advance, fill with hot filling, and reheat in the oven.

**Blinee, or blintzes:** Make filling for pancakes by passing through a wire strainer or food mill 1 pound, or 2 cups, dry cottage cheese, or hoop cheese; stir into cheese 1 egg, 1 teaspoon salt, and 2 tablespoons each sugar, powdered milk, and whole-wheat flour; stir well. Bake pancakes until golden on one side; turn and put 2 tablespoons in each pancake; fold over and sauté until pancake is golden brown and filling is heated through. Serve piping hot with chilled sour cream or thick yogurt. After meat-vegetable soup (p. 313), serve with steamed turnip tops (p. 380), celery with avocado filling (p. 274). The trouble with this recipe is that your family will probably not let you stop making blinee once you learn how.

Pancakes filled with shredded cheese: Shred 2 cups American, Jack, or Swiss cheese; add 4 tablespoons each chopped ripe or stuffed olives and minced chives. Fold into pancakes and heat in a hot serving dish for about 5 minutes; pour heated Spanish sauce (p. 167) over pancakes, and sprinkle with grated cheese. Serve with broiled eggplant (p. 354), salad of egg, parsley, celery (p. 235).

## CHOW MEIN

Fry in 1½ cups fat at 360° F. until light brown:

½ pound Chinese noodles

Remove to hot platter and arrange in form of nest.

Drain fat, leaving 3 to 4 tablespoons; use the same utensil and sauté lightly:

| ½ pound lean raw pork, diced in ½-inch cubes | 1 chopped onion<br>4 stalks chopped celery |

Cook 8 minutes and add:

| 1 pound fresh or a No. 2 can bean sprouts and juice | 1 can sliced mushrooms and juice<br>1 tablespoon or more soy sauce |

Stir well; salt to taste after soy sauce is added; cook for 5 minutes; put in center of noodles.

Serve with fried shrimp (p. 184), head lettuce with French dressing.

*Variations:*

If available, add 2 or more peeled and sliced water chestnuts.

Use leftover pork or chicken cut in thin strips; add after sautéing vegetables.

**Chicken chow mein:** Omit pork; sauté onions and celery in margarine or butter; add with bean sprouts and mushrooms 1 or more cups diced leftover chicken, ½ cup diced fresh pineapple or well-drained and diced canned pineapple. Serve with noodles or steamed rice (p. 204), whole tomatoes stuffed with cottage cheese.

**Pork chop suey:** Omit noodles and mushrooms; use 1 pound pork cut into strips 2 inches long, 1 cup each chopped onions and celery; proceed as in basic recipe; add bean sprouts and soy sauce. After fish appetizer (p. 265), serve with tomato, green pepper, cucumber, and cottage cheese salad.

## EGG FOO YUNG, OR EGG AND VEGETABLE PATTIES

Chop or cut fine or pass through the meat grinder:

| | |
|---|---|
| 2 onions | 4 strips uncooked bacon |
| 3 green peppers | |

Add:

| | |
|---|---|
| 1 pound fresh or a No. 2 can bean sprouts | ½ teaspoon salt |
| | 4 whole eggs |

Beat together thoroughly. Drop from a tablespoon onto a hot **oiled** grill and sauté until light brown on both sides.

Serve with soy sauce, rice (p. 204), parsley and spinach (p. 373), finger salads.

*Variations:*

Substitute 1½ cups slightly cooked chopped celery for bean sprouts. Add 1 can sliced mushrooms or 1 cup diced cooked beef, chicken, shrimp, or fish.

If available, add ¼ cup peeled and sliced water chestnuts.

The following meat extenders are built around using leftover meats, of which the creamed meats are perhaps the most delicious. Before I gave much thought to cooking, I often prepared creamed chicken, combined all ingredients, let the chicken overcook, and then wondered brainlessly why the amount of chicken seemed to disappear and the sauce needed more thickening. If meats have been properly cooked, leftover meats still contain 50 per cent or more water. In case cream sauce is allowed to boil after meat has been added, you can expect the meat to shrivel, meat juices to be squeezed out, and the sauce to become too thin.

### CREAMED CHICKEN

Prepare **2** cups medium cream sauce (p. 161), using chicken stock instead of part of the milk when available; cook in sauce:

| | |
|---|---|
| 1 cup fresh or frozen peas | pinch of sage or thyme |
| 2 diced fresh or canned pimentos | 1 diced carrot, or add leftover carrot later |
| 1 or 2 drops yellow coloring | |

Simmer 10 minutes, or until peas are barely tender. Add no earlier than 5 minutes before serving:

**2 or 3 cups diced leftover chicken**

Serve over hot wheat-germ biscuits cut with doughnut cutter (p. 432), with steamed banana squash (p. 415), assorted finger salads (p. 273).

*Variations:*

Instead of 2 cups chicken use 1 cup chicken and 1 cup or more diced hard-cooked eggs, roasted fresh pork, veal, or lamb, or use drained canned tuna quickly washed under running hot water; or add 1 cup diced uncooked sweetbreads or brains 10 minutes before adding chicken.

Use leftover turkey, duck, goose, or other fowl instead of chicken.

If preparing creamed chicken for a large group, steam 1 mature rabbit with every 1 or 2 chickens; if nothing is said about it, no one will know the difference.

Add 1 small can mushrooms; use juice from mushrooms in preparing the sauce; if desired, omit sage and add 2 tablespoons sherry just before serving.

**Creamed beef:** Prepare 2 cups celery, curry, horseradish, mustard, olive, or onion sauce (p. 162); proceed as in basic recipe, using diced leftover beef; use or omit vegetables; make a sauce of leftover gravy when available. Supplement beef with diced wieners if needed.

**Creamed ham or pork:** Prepare 2 cups caraway, curry, dill, olive, mustard, pimento, piquant, or horseradish sauce (p. 161); omit vegetables; proceed as in basic recipe, using diced leftover ham or pork. Supplement with diced wieners or hard-cooked eggs if needed.

**Creamed lamb or veal:** Prepare 2 cups caper, celery, curry, dill, mushroom, olive, pimento, or piquant sauce (p. 161); omit vegetables; prepare as in basic recipe, using diced lamb or veal.

Dozens of out-of-date recipes for casserole dishes which need to be cooked no longer than 15 minutes specify cooking times ranging from 1 to 3 hours. Casserole dishes are made almost without exception of leftover meats or meats which need only to be heated through, such as clams, shrimp, oysters, and sweetbreads. The vegetables are customarily diced and hence will cook in 10 to 12 minutes; often only leftover or canned vegetables are used. Besides being a waste of fuel, the long cooking indicated in many recipes cause unnecessary destruction of proteins and B vitamins, and probably the complete destruction of vitamin C.

Nutritive value, time, and dishwashing can be saved if such dishes are prepared over a surface burner in a heat-resistant casserole. Attractive casseroles made of thick but lightweight aluminum alloys and of certain types of pottery have proved satisfactory for cooking over direct heat. The busy mother who wants to put the meal in the oven and forget it may prepare the casserole earlier. It is better to reheat it quickly than to cook it slowly.

If toasted crumbs are desired, they may be prepared in advance, toasted in the oven or under the broiler, and sprinkled over the casserole after the edges have been wiped clean.

Increase the nutritive value of casserole dishes by adding powdered milk and/or generous amounts of cheese. Merely covering the utensil permits the cheese to melt. It supplies sufficient fat so that the crumbs need not be buttered. If you follow this procedure, a casserole dish can be prepared with almost no bother.

Since casserole dishes must depend upon the ingredients you have on hand, you should originate your own recipes for them. Prepare any cream sauce, brown sauce, or tomato sauce (p. 162), add vegetables and leftover meat, and sprinkle with crumbs and cheese.

## LAMB AND PEAS IN CASSEROLE

Prepare **2 cups medium cream sauce** (p. 162); add and cook in the sauce:

| | |
|---|---|
| 1½ cups fresh peas | 1 diced stalk celery with leaves |
| 1 finely chopped onion or leek | pinch each of sage and basil |

When peas are tender, add:

| | |
|---|---|
| 2 diced canned pimentos (optional) | 1 to 2 cups or more diced lamb |
| 1 teaspoon each salt and Worcestershire | |

Stir well and simmer 10 minutes; turn off heat; stir in **2 tablespoons ground parsley**; wipe edges of casserole and if desired, sprinkle top with:

| | |
|---|---|
| ¼ cup toasted whole-wheat-bread crumbs | ½ to 1 cup shredded American cheese |
| | generous amount of paprika |

Cover until cheese melts, or heat slightly under broiler, as desired.
After jellied consommé, serve with beet tops, cottage cheese and apricot salad with French dressing.

*Variations:*

Prepare any cream sauce (p. 162), vinegar sauce (p. 165), tomato sauce (p. 166), or brown sauce (p. 161); add vegetables, leftover meats, cheese, and crumbs.

Instead of peas use 2 cups diced zucchini, carrots, corn, cauliflower broken into flowerlets, leeks, or other vegetables; cook each vegetable only long enough for it to become tender.

Omit lamb and add 1½ cups diced leftover beef, veal, chicken, sliced kidney, canned or diced fresh tuna, quickly sautéed and diced liver, or diced cooked heart or tongue.

Supplement leftover meat with any canned or quick-cooking fresh meat; combine canned tuna or diced sweetbreads with leftover chicken; fresh sliced kidneys with leftover beef; sliced wieners with leftover pork; lamb liver with leftover lamb.

*Use the basic recipe in preparing any casserole dish; substitute the same amounts of the following vegetables, seasonings, and meat for peas, herbs, lamb; cook vegetables only long enough to become tender.*

Diced carrots, 1 chopped green pepper, diced cooked heart, chicken, tongue, or beef with dash of nutmeg, a pinch each of thyme and basil, or diced leftover veal, mutton, flaked fish, canned tuna, or shrimps with chopped fresh dill, dill sauce, or 1 teaspoon dill seeds.

Diced leftover ham, 2 or 3 diced sweet potatoes or 3 cups shredded cabbage.

Leftover diced pork or pork heart or tongue, 2 diced raw potatoes, 1 teaspoon caraway or dill seeds.

Diced cooked heart, 2 cups fresh string beans, a pinch each of basil and thyme.

A few fresh string beans, 1 diced carrot, ½ cup peas, leftover veal, chicken, or lamb, a pinch each of thyme, savory, and marjoram.

Cook 1 each diced potato, carrot, and turnip in tomato sauce (p. 166); add leftover diced tongue, Worcestershire, a pinch each of savory, basil, and marjoram. Also delicious with either brown sauce (p. 161) or cream sauce.

Use diced carrots, 1 cup leftover brown or all-vitamin rice, meat or fish; the herbs of basic recipe.

Canned or fresh corn, a pinch of basil, flaked fish, diced leftover ham, veal, beef, heart, or sliced wieners; use tomato sauce instead of cream sauce.

Although croquettes are customarily cooked in deep fat, they can be prepared much more easily by sautéing with equally good flavor and fewer calories.

## HAM CROQUETTES

Mix together:

| | |
|---|---|
| 2 cups chopped ham | 2 tablespoons each ground parsley |
| 1 cup cold thick cream sauce | and grated onion |
| (p. 161) or leftover gravy | freshly ground black peppercorns |
| 1 egg | salt to taste |

Form into oblong patties, roll in crumbs, and sauté in **butter-flavored cooking fat or bacon drippings;** or fry in deep fat at 350° F. for 5 minutes, or until brown.

Serve with horseradish sauce (p. 163), Brussels sprouts with cheese (p. 383), tossed green salad.

*Variations:*

If oven is being used, bake at 350° F. for 20 minutes.

Omit cream sauce and add any one of the following: 1 cup rice, mashed or finely diced leftover white or sweet potatoes, or shredded and quickly sautéed raw white or sweet potatoes.

Add to basic recipe any one or more of the following: a pinch each of basil and savory; 1 tablespoon caraway seeds, catsup, dill sauce, or chili sauce; ¼ cup powdered milk, wheat germ, or precooked soy grits; ½ cup cooked soybeans or cooked whole wheat.

Make 2 cups thick cream sauce; use 1 cup in croquettes; dilute the remainder and prepare horseradish sauce. Use this same procedure in making sauces to serve with croquettes suggested below.

*Follow the basic recipe, merely omitting ham and adding ingredients suggested.*

**Beef, veal, or lamb croquettes:** Diced leftover beef, veal, or lamb; 1 teaspoon Worcestershire, 1 tablespoon chili sauce.

**Cheese and rice croquettes:** Omit cream sauce and use 1 cup cooked rice, ½ cup shredded American or pimento cheese.

**Cheese and vegetable croquettes:** 1 cup shredded American cheese and 1 cup or more leftover vegetables, such as peas, corn, diced carrots, broccoli, or potatoes; or combine several leftover vegetables.

**Chicken croquettes:** Diced or ground chicken, ½ teaspoon paprika, a pinch of sage, 2 diced pimentos.

**Crab, lobster, or oyster croquettes:** 2 cups flaked crab, lobster, or chopped raw or canned oysters; add 1 tablespoon dill sauce, capers, or lemon juice.

**Fish croquettes:** Use finely diced uncooked or flaked leftover salmon, halibut, or other cooked or canned fish. Add 1 teaspoon dill sauce or anise or dill seeds.

## HASH OF LEFTOVER MEAT

Heat in frying pan:

### 4 tablespoons bacon drippings

Shred quickly into fat:

### 2 chilled unpeeled potatoes

Keep heat high, turn frequently, and brown well; add:

**1 finely shredded carrot (optional)**    **1 cup or more ground leftover beef,**
**1 small shredded onion**    **veal, lamb, or chicken**
    **freshly ground black peppercorns**

Mix well, reduce heat; cover utensil and steam until heated through; add:

**1 teaspoon salt**    **¼ teaspoon celery salt**

Serve with applesauce, mustard-spinach, salad of carrot and green pepper.

*Variations:*

Sauté onion and shredded carrot lightly; add ground meat and leftover mashed potatoes; make into patties, roll in whole-wheat flour or wheat germ, brown on both sides; serve with leftover gravy seasoned with savory.

Use finely chopped leftover steamed or baked potatoes; add 2 tablespoons chives, 1 teaspoon Worcestershire or caraway seeds.

Add 1 or 2 cups uncooked ground beef or corned beef 3 to 5 minutes before serving; do not cover utensil after meat is added. Corned-beef hash prepared in this way is particularly delicious.

# CHAPTER 13

## MEATS AND MEAT SUBSTITUTES
## FOR HOT-WEATHER DINNERS AND BUFFETS

The diet of most people during hot weather is often appallingly inadequate in many respects. The days are sometimes so hot that you do not enjoy cooking, and the family does not relish eating unless foods are particularly attractive and appetizing. The intake of meats, cereals, and breads may be so decreased that protein, salt, and the B vitamins become dangerously deficient. At the same time much salt and large amounts of the vitamins which dissolve in water are lost through perspiration. Cokes and iced tea sweetened with refined sugar frequently satisfy hunger pangs. The mother who keeps her family adequately fed during hot weather must be alert to their nutritional needs.

Why not serve your summer dinners in the delightful buffet, or smörgåsbord, style? Have your entire dinner of chilled foods, or perhaps serve one hot dish and the other foods chilled. The variety of foods which may be served cold is almost endless: appetizers and juices, jellied bouillons, sliced meats, fish, meat or fish aspics, plates of assorted sliced cheese or a bowl of cottage cheese, chilled vegetables marinated in French dressing or other tart sauce, frozen purées, salads, and the old stand-bys, sliced tomatoes and stuffed eggs. Such foods can be prepared in the cool of the morning and kept in the refrigerator until dinnertime.

If hot-weather fatigue is to be prevented, the salt, vitamin C, and B vitamins lost in perspiration must be replaced. Add a larger amount of salt to foods than you would at other times and serve salted potato chips, perhaps spread with cheese, salty fish, ham, salted nuts, and other well-salted food at each lunch and dinner. Vitamin C may easily be obtained from fresh fruits, tomatoes, and salads. See that the B vitamins are supplied by serving only dark breads, by emphasizing glandular meats in appetizers, salads,

222

and cold cuts, and by serving yogurt with chilled fruits and salads, and as a beverage.

There is a prevalent idea that only a small amount of meat should be eaten during hot weather. This belief is largely a hangover from the times when refrigeration was unknown and meats spoiled too easily to be safe. It is true that meat causes the activity of the body cells to be speeded up for a few minutes after it is digested, but the mere act of drinking cold water has a greater stimulating effect on the cells; energy is produced to maintain body temperature, momentarily reduced by cold drinks. This stimulating effect is no argument against eating either meats or cold foods. Even during the winter, chilled foods are equally as nourishing as are hot foods, although they may be less appetizing.

If adequate protein is obtained from milk, cheese, eggs, yeast, wheat germ, and other foods, meats may be avoided without loss of health. It is difficult, however, to obtain sufficient protein from these foods without careful planning, especially during the summer when the appetite may be jaded. If you sincerely want your family to have the best health possible, you should learn the approximate protein content of foods and estimate the amount each member of your family eats daily. These figures should be so familiar that you can count protein grams as easily as the change in your purse. Unless you do such counting, it is much safer to serve meats during the summer. The quantities of food eaten need not be large or the calorie intake high.

## HOT-WEATHER DINNERS WITH COLD MEATS

The cold meats which are customarily served are so excellent that there is little to add about them. By varying the kinds of meat sauces served with cold cuts, monotony can be avoided indefinitely. The sauces of whipped evaporated milk and yogurt, both of which are low in calories, are especially suitable during hot weather. If the meat does not slice well, the entire platter of meat may be covered with sauce and attractively garnished with parsley, radishes, and sliced eggs or stuffed olives. Many meat stuffings are delicious when cold, especially those of vegetables, grains, or fruits; do not overlook them during the summer months. Aspics of tart fruit juices and frozen purées hit the spot on hot summer evenings when served with meat; try purple-plum purée with roast beef and see if you do not find it delicious.

Almost any vegetable can be delicious when served cold if it is first steamed, chilled, and marinated in French dressing or mayonnaise. Several vegetables of contrasting colors can be arranged on a bed of lettuce or on the same platter with the meat. The sauces made of yogurt, sour cream, or whipped evaporated milk mixed with mayonnaise can also be served with chilled vegetables.

In restaurant windows or on Swedish smörgåsbords one sometimes sees beautiful glazed meats which appear bafflingly professional. The glazing is achieved merely by brushing the chilled meat with any aspic base or jellied consommé just before it congeals. The gelatin may be dissolved in the juice left from canned fruit or peach or watermelon pickles. The glazing takes about two minutes to make and brush on, and is well worth the effort.

Following are suggestions for hot-weather menus in which cold meat serves as the entree:

See **aspic recipe** (p. 234) or **jellied consommé** (p. 312) for glazes; **meat sauces** (p. 162).

**Cold corned beef:** Serve with horseradish sauce made with yogurt or whipped evaporated milk, marinated string beans, potato salad, watercress in tomato aspic.

**Chilled liver:** Steam uncut lamb or baby beef liver; chill, slice, and cover with raw creole sauce. Serve with marinated cauliflower, cottage cheese, tossed green salad, chilled raspberries with yogurt.

**Chilled brains:** Steam, dice, marinate in a little French dressing; serve covered with ground pickle or cucumber sauce of mayonnaise and whipped evaporated milk; garnish with parsley. After fruit appetizer, serve with marinated broccoli, egg-celery salad, sliced tomatoes, sweet onions.

**Barbecued veal:** Slice cold fillet of veal and put the slices together as if uncut; cover with a glaze of jellied consommé and serve surrounded with diced cubes of consommé; garnish with parsley or capers. After tomato-juice appetizer, serve with three-layer salad (p. 288), marinated parsnips, sliced cucumbers, green peppers.

**Ham or shoulder:** Braise or roast. After jellied bouillon, serve with horseradish sauce of sour cream or yogurt, marinated turnips, sliced tomatoes, tossed salad.

**Dried-beef rolls:** Mix cream cheese generously with horseradish and parsley; roll inside slices of dried beef; surround with assorted sliced cheeses. After shrimp cocktail, serve with marinated celery root, carrot-parsley salad.

**Cold roast beef:** Serve with aspic of purple plums, marinated celery and carrots, cole slaw of green cabbage, yogurt dressing.

**Glazed ham:** Decorate the surface with thin half slices of orange and maraschino cherries; hold in place with a glaze of ham stock left from steaming; chill the remaining glaze, dice, and arrange around the meat. Serve with mustard sauce, marinated potatoes, applesauce with toasted wheat germ (p. 460), tossed salad.

**Cold lamb:** Serve with caper sauce; if the slices are unattractive, cover with caper sauce. Serve with apricot aspic (p. 290), marinated broccoli, assorted finger salads.

**Roast lamb or mutton:** Make a glaze of mint aspic (p. 235) and serve with aspic cubes, marinated rutabagas, sliced tomatoes and cucumbers on a bed of watercress.

**Roast chicken:** Stuff with rice or buckwheat stuffing (p. 157); make a glaze of stock seasoned with sage and thyme. Serve with marinated string beans, fruit salad.

**Roast or barbecued brisket of beef:** Slice and serve with a strip of thick plum purée across each slice, marinated cauliflower, sliced tomatoes with green pepper rings, tossed salad.

**Cold roast pork:** Serve with frozen applesauce seasoned with cassia buds, marinated onions and turnips, beet aspic (p. 291).

**Baked fish:** Stuff with onion dressing; chill, glaze with aspic seasoned with dill or anise seeds. After frozen tomato juice (p. 262), serve with cold sweet potato chips, green cabbage and cucumber salad.

**Cold sliced heart:** After citrus-juice appetizer, serve with mustard-horseradish sauce, marinated broccoli, carrot sticks, tomato and cottage cheese salad.

**Braised shoulder of lamb:** Slice and serve with pineapple-curry sauce, marinated carrots, celery stuffed with avocado, tomato-watercress salad.

**Diced cold meat:** Dice scraps of leftover veal, lamb, pork, or beef; fold into citron-cherry sauce. After frozen tomato-juice appetizer, serve with marinated asparagus, spiced beets, tossed salad of endive, grapefruit, and watercress.

**Pork tongue:** Chill and slice; drop into cold aspic seasoned with caraway seeds; put together again as if uncut; glaze and set in a bed of aspic; decorate the aspic with slices of hard-cooked egg. Serve with horseradish sauce, marinated zucchini, sliced tomatoes and leeks, mixed-fruit salad.

**Wieners or luncheon meat:** Dice into ½-inch cubes 1 pound wieners, bologna, or other luncheon meat; combine with 2 cups mustard sauce with a base of whipped evaporated milk and mayonnaise (p. 169). After fruit appetizer, serve with stuffed eggs (p. 246), marinated parsnips, tossed salad of avocado, watercress, radishes.

### FISH TO BE SERVED CHILLED

Although fish salads and appetizers have become popular in America, other forms of chilled fish are used far too little. Steamed fish (p. 187), chilled, well seasoned, attractively arranged and garnished, is excellent for luncheons and hot-weather dinners. Any of the cold sauces, whether with a base of sour cream, yogurt, whipped cream, or whipped evaporated milk and mayonnaise, can be served with them. Every kind of fish available may be used. In preparing nutritious lunches, summer-evening dinners, and buffets, serve chilled fish frequently.

Following are suggestions for serving fish as the entree or on buffet dinners.

See **baked fish** (p. 177), **steamed fish** (p. 187), **chilled sauces** (p. 169).

**Baked fish ring:** Buy 2 whole fish or more; clean and stuff with **onion stuffing** to which is added a **generous amount of pimentos** (p. 157); tie a string from heads to tails to form a curve and prop mouths open with toothpicks; bake with back of fish up; chill and arrange around platter with the tail of one fish in the mouth of the other, making a complete circle; fill center with **potato salad**, garnish with **tomato sections, capers, and paprika.** Serve with any chilled sauce.

**Fish with beet pickles:** Steam 2 pounds fillets ½ inch thick; chill and arrange slices of **beet pickle** between layers of fillets; pour **2 to 3 tablespoons French dressing** over top and garnish with **lemon sections dipped in ground parsley and/or thin slices of onion or leek.** Bony fish may be flaked and mixed with chopped beet pickles or diced tart apple and chilled sauce.

**Fish with sour cream and capers:** Steam 2 pounds fillets, chill; pour over the fillets **2 cups caper sauce** with a sour-cream base; garnish with **sliced tomatoes, lemon sections dipped in ground parsley, and paprika.** Vary by flaking steamed fish; stir with 1 cup sauce and pour the other cup over the top; use any variety of fish and any uncooked sauce. Garnish with sliced radishes and stuffed olives.

**Fish with pickles, parsley, eggs:** Steam small whole fish, fillets, or steaks; chill; arrange on platter, flaking bony or whole fish if used; cover with finely chopped beet or dill pickles, generous layer of ground parsley, 2 or 3 hard-cooked eggs forced through a sieve. Garnish with onion rings and slices of beet pickles and eggs.

**Fish flakes with radishes:** Steam and flake 2 pounds whole fish or 1½ pounds fillets; chill; slice thin 1 bunch radishes, add to the flaked fish, and mix with basic yogurt or sour-cream sauce. Put on platter and surround with lettuce or endive; garnish with tomato sections.

**Fish flakes with mushrooms:** Steam and flake 2 pounds fish, or use shrimps or other sea food; add 1 can sliced mushrooms with liquid and 3 tablespoons tart French dressing. Chill and garnish with strips or rings of pimento; or serve with any sauce with base of sour cream.

**Fish platter:** Steam 2 pounds fillets cut into serving sizes; steam 2 unpeeled potatoes, chill, peel, and slice; place fish on serving platter, cover with sliced potatoes, 1 or 2 each sliced cucumbers and sweet onions or leeks; pour over all 1 cup French dressing; let stand 2 hours or more. Surround with celery sticks and tomato sections; garnish with parsley.

**Fish with cucumber sauce:** Steam 2 pounds or more fillets; put on platter and chill; pour over fish 1 cup cucumber sauce; garnish with slices of hard-cooked egg and 2 tablespoons capers.

**Fish with hard-cooked eggs:** Steam thin fillets; put half the fillets on a platter and cover with slices of hard-cooked eggs and leeks; add another layer of fillets; cover with sauce of sour cream to which chopped mixed pickles are added; garnish with a few slices of hard-cooked eggs and ground parsley. Vary by covering with sliced eggs and tartar sauce diluted with vinegar and seasoned with dill sauce or fresh dill and ground parsley.

**Fish with leeks:** Steam 2 pounds thin fish fillets and chill; alternate in a bowl layers of fish with thin slices of fresh leeks or sweet onions; pour over the fish ½ cup French dressing, let stand in refrigerator 2 hours or more. Garnish with sprigs of parsley and lemon slices. Or use bony fish; flake and mix with chopped leeks and French dressing.

**Glazed fish with aspic cubes:** Stuff a whole fish with onion dressing (p. 157) and bake; use dill-seasoned aspic as a glaze (p. 228). Turn remaining aspic into flat pan and let congeal. Dice aspic into tiny cubes and serve around glazed fish. Garnish with parsley, sliced stuffed olives, and tomato sections.

**Roe with capers and olives:** Steam ½ pound herring, shad, or other roe; remove the membranes and mash, mixing with 2 tablespoons each grated onion, ground parsley, capers, and sliced stuffed olives. Chill, and garnish with paprika.

**Roe with egg sauce:** Mix 1 cup (½ pound) raw or steamed roe with a sauce of yogurt or sour-cream base and 2 or 3 diced hard-cooked eggs; garnish with slices of hard-cooked eggs, chopped chives, and ground parsley.

**Roe with onion sauce:** Mix 1 cup (½ pound) caviar or uncooked salmon roe with **1 cup onion sauce;** add **4 to 6 minced radishes.** Serve with wheat-germ crackers.

**Rolled fish fillets with pimentos:** Select small fillets or cut large fillets into thin strips 2 inches wide; cut **canned pimentos** in half and spread over each fillet; roll and hold with toothpicks; steam quickly; chill and pyramid on platter, cover with **caper or other sauce** having base of whipped evaporated milk, sour cream, or yogurt; garnish with **ground parsley and tomato sections.** Vary by preparing rolls and setting in aspic (p. 228) or by spreading chopped pimentos between steamed fillets in layers in loaf pan and covering with aspic.

**Spiced fish flakes:** Buy 2 pounds or more of any small bony fish, such as smelt, sardines, fresh herring, sand dabs. Steam quickly, using ¼ cup water. Flake fish, add bones to water used for steaming with ¼ cup vinegar, 4 each of cloves and cassia buds, ¼ crumbled bay leaf, ¼ teaspoon each celery and dill seeds, crushed white peppercorns; boil slowly 10 minutes and cool. Strain through fine-mesh strainer and pour over flaked fish; add **3 tablespoons each chives and ground parsley, 1 tablespoon oil;** chill; garnish with **slices of dill pickles.**

Fish for aspics has customarily been boiled in order to season the liquid. The fish, however, should not be robbed of flavor. If the aspic is made of fillets prepared at home, the trimmings and bones may be used to flavor the stock; otherwise, a small bony fish should be purchased for making the aspic.

## FISH ASPIC

Select or prepare 2 pounds or more fillets.

Chop bones left from preparing fillets or chop a small whole fish into ½-inch pieces; put bones or chopped fish into utensil to be used for steaming and add:

| | |
|---|---|
| 1¼ cups vegetable-cooking water | ¼ crushed bay leaf |
| ¼ cup vinegar | 1 teaspoon dill or anise seeds (op- |
| 1 sliced clove garlic | tional) |
| ¼ teaspoon crushed white pepper-corns | 1 teaspoon salt |

Simmer 10 minutes; set rack over water and add:

**2 pounds or more of fillets**

Steam as directed on page 187; remove fillets to large platter as soon as internal temperature of 140° F. is reached.

Meanwhile soften:

**1 tablespoon gelatin in**                    **½ cup vegetable-cooking water**

Strain water used for steaming into softened gelatin; stir well, pour onto platter around the fish, chill.

When gelatin is chilled but not congealed, set in aspic around fish:

**thin slices of leeks or onion and     slices of stuffed olives
lemon**

Let stand, and garnish platter with **sprigs of parsley.**

*Variations:*

If small or bony fish are to be used, steam them above 1 cup vegetable-cooking water; flake the fish and put bones, trimmings, vinegar, and seasonings into the water; simmer 10 minutes, strain into softened gelatin, cool, and add the flaked fish, 3 tablespoons sliced stuffed olives, 2 tablespoons grated onion, and ¼ cup mayonnaise; chill in an oiled ring mold or a loaf pan.

**Flaked fish loaf:** Steam over **1 cup vegetable-cooking water** enough fish or shrimp, crab, or lobster to make 2 cups when flaked; soften **1 tablespoon gelatin** in ½ cup vegetable-cooking water; stir gelatin and **2 tablespoons vinegar** into hot liquid used for steaming fish; cool, and add **½ cup chopped celery, 1 chopped green pepper, 2 tablespoons sliced stuffed olives, ½ cup mayonnaise, 1 teaspoon salt, ¼ teaspoon paprika;** chill in loaf pan or a fish mold; serve on bed of **watercress with sliced cucumbers.** Canned salmon or shrimp may be used.

**Whole fish in aspic:** Stuff whole fish weighing 2 pounds or more with **onion or celery stuffing** (p. 157); bake (p. 177). Double the basic recipe for fish aspic, using small bony fish and adding **2 tablespoons each chopped onion and celery leaves.** Before straining add **3 crushed eggshells** to clarify the liquid. Pour 3 cups of the aspic into large loaf pan brushed with oil; when it starts to congeal, place whole fish in center of aspic with back down; chill; when gelatin has set, mix **3 tablespoons each chopped parsley and pimento** with the remaining cup of aspic and pour over fish; chill until set. Unmold on large platter and garnish with **tomato and lemon** sections. Fish prepared in this manner is strikingly beautiful.

## CHICKEN LOAF

Select stewing chicken and steam (p. 86) until tender; skin and chop feet and cook with neck and wing tips in water and vinegar under a rack.

Remove meat from bones and put through meat grinder with:

1 slice sweet onion or leek          1 small stalk celery with leaves
1 fresh or canned pimento            few sprigs of parsley

Evaporate the broth left from steaming to 1 cup and strain into the chicken; mix well and add:

salt to taste                        freshly ground white peppercorns

Mold in quart cardboard milk carton or garnish top of oiled mold with **slices of hard-cooked eggs and ground parsley;** press chicken firmly into the container. Chill thoroughly, unmold, slice.

Serve with marinated cauliflower (p. 224), cottage cheese or assorted sliced cheeses, tossed salad.

*Variations:*

If bones are not used in preparing broth, soak 2 teaspoons gelatin in ¼ cup water and dissolve in hot broth; season broth with pinch of sage, basil, or tarragon.

Grind with chicken 1 small can mushrooms; add liquid from mushrooms to broth.

**Chicken loaf with rice or noodles:** Remove bones from broth and add enough water to make 2 cups; cook in broth ½ cup brown or all-vitamin rice or 1 cup whole-wheat or soy noodles; proceed as in basic recipe. Serve with marinated parsnips (p. 364), assorted sliced cheese, tomato aspic (p. 287) on bed of watercress.

**Pressed tongue:** Use 1 veal or pork tongue, either fresh or smoked, or 1½ pounds lamb tongues. Steam with 2 tablespoons vinegar, 2 cups water, and 1 pound beef soup bones sawed into small pieces; when tender, skin tongues while hot, discard bones. Soak 2 teaspoons gelatin in ½ cup cold water and dissolve in hot broth. Proceed as in basic recipe, increasing onion or leek or adding garlic as desired. If lamb tongues are used, vary by adding dill sauce to taste or by cooking 1 teaspoon dill seeds in broth. Serve with baked navy beans (p. 199), tossed salad (p. 298).

**Veal loaf:** Use 1 pound lean veal and veal knuckle sawed into ¾-inch pieces; add 2 tablespoons white vinegar, 2 cups vegetable-cooking water, and steam until the veal is tender. Proceed as in basic recipe. Serve with potato salad (p. 402), sliced tomatoes, spiced beet pickles (p. 343), watercress with Roquefort dressing.

## HAM LOAF

Soak 1 tablespoon gelatin in:

> ½ cup tomato juice, water, or ham stock

Dissolve in:

> 1 cup hot tomato juice, vegetable-cooking water, or ham stock

Cool; add after liquid has cooled:

| | |
|---|---|
| ¼ teaspoon paprika | 1 chopped or ground bell pepper |
| 1 teaspoon Worcestershire | 2 tablespoons ground parsley |
| 2 cups ground ham | 1 small ground onion or 2 table- |
| ¼ cup mayonnaise | spoons onion juice |

Pour into cardboard milk carton or oiled loaf pan. Chill; invert on platter and garnish with tomato sections, parsley, lettuce leaves.

Serve with potato salad seasoned with dill, sliced tomatoes, tossed salad.

*Variations:*

Use 1 cup ham and any one of the following: 3 diced hard-cooked eggs; 1 cup shredded American cheese; ½ cup each shredded American and Swiss cheese, 1 tablespoon fresh dill or dill sauce; 1 cup shredded Swiss cheese; 1 or 2 teaspoons caraway seeds added to hot liquid; 1 cup pimento cheese or American cheese with 3 diced pimentos.

Instead of ham, use leftover veal, tongue, heart, lamb; or 1 cup meat with 3 diced eggs or 1 cup shredded cheese; add ½ cup mayonnaise.

**Cottage-cheese loaf:** Soak 1 tablespoon gelatin in ½ cup pineapple juice and heat over simmer burner to dissolve; add 1 cup crushed pineapple; chill well; add 2 cups cottage cheese; mold. This is a delicious loaf.

**Cheese loaf:** Instead of ham in basic recipe, use 2 cups shredded American or Swiss cheese; heat 2 tablespoons chopped dill or 1 to 2 teaspoons dill seeds in vegetable-cooking water or tomato juice.

**Fish loaf:** Use fish stock or vegetable-cooking water; instead of ham, add 2 cups flaked fish, crab, or lobster, ½ cup mayonnaise, the other seasonings of basic recipe, ¼ teaspoon celery seeds, 2 tablespoons capers.

Mock liverwurst is one of my favorite recipes, and I hope you will also like it. Use it not only during hot weather but also for box lunches, between-meal snacks, sandwiches, and buffets throughout the year. Few foods can compare with it nutritionally. It is excellent to serve to persons who are anemic, deficient in calcium or B vitamins, or who are reducing.

## MOCK LIVERWURST, OR LIVER PASTE

Sauté lightly in **bacon drippings** without browning:

| | |
|---|---|
| **1 sliced carrot** | **1 sliced onion** |

When onion is transparent, add and steam above vegetables:

| | |
|---|---|
| **1 pound sliced lamb, veal, or baby beef liver** | **¼ teaspoon crushed black peppercorns** |

Steam liver 8 minutes. Pass liver, vegetables, and 1 clove garlic through meat grinder 2 or 3 times, using smallest knife; add and mix well:

| | |
|---|---|
| **2½ teaspoons salt** | **1 to 3 teaspoons brewers' yeast** |
| any juices left from sautéing or grinding | (optional) |
| pinch of sage or thyme | **1 to 4 tablespoons wheat germ** (optional) |
| **hickory sauce or smoke-flavoring** to taste (optional) | **½ to 1 cup powdered milk,** or enough to make firm |

Turn liver paste onto wax paper; form into a roll the size of commercial liverwurst. Chill thoroughly; cut in diagonal slices.

Serve with celery root marinated with French dressing (p. 348), pineapple-cucumber aspic with cream cheese (p. 288), tossed green salad.

*Variations:*

Use pork liver; omit sage and add 1 or 2 teaspoons crushed caraway seeds. Or season lamb liver with dill seeds.

Omit powdered milk, sage, garlic, smoke-flavoring; add 2 to 4 tablespoons soft margarine or butter; serve on crackers. This paste is similar to pâté de foie gras.

Aside from hot-weather dinners, salads which contain meat, eggs, fish, or cheese are excellent for lunches throughout the year with nothing more than milk or yogurt, whole-grain bread, and butter. Serve this kind of salad in addition to the entree whenever the protein requirements are high, especially if you have adolescent youngsters. Meat, eggs, cheese, or fish may be added to any tossed salad (p. 298).

Although the amateur at cooking likes to have amounts of each ingredient specified, the quantities of meat and vegetables used in a salad should vary, depending on the needs of your family and the other foods you are serving at the same meal. If a salad or an aspic is the principal protein dish, add only 1 or 2 tablespoons of each of the vegetables mentioned. If the salad is to be served with an entree, increase the amount of vegetables used. In making aspics, use well-seasoned soup stock rich in flavor made from seared bones or vegetable-cooking water which fairly bulges with vitamins and minerals. Have fun making attractive designs by setting slices of hard-cooked egg, avocado, stuffed olives, and other ingredients at the sides and bottom of the mold before pouring the gelatin into it.

The average housewife has two or three salads which she serves as entrees in hot weather: usually tuna, chicken, and egg and celery salad. Often she makes little attempt to increase the variety. Actually the number of excellent meat or fish salads is almost unlimited. Such salads are splendid for using up leftovers or for introducing the nutritionally superior meats which, if not enjoyed, can be well disguised by the clever use of seasonings.

There are only two ways to prepare salads to be served as entrees. Since the ingredients are essentially the same whether the meat, fish, egg, or cheese salad is combined with mayonnaise and served on greens or added to an aspic, I have listed the ingredients for each type of salad following the two basic recipes. Serve them in either manner you desire.

## MEAT, FISH, EGG, OR CHEESE SALADS

Use the ingredients specified on pages 235 to 237.

Dice or flake:

### 1 to 2 cups meat or fish

Unless flavor alone is especially enjoyed, marinate with:

### 1 to 3 tablespoons French dressing for each cup of meat or fish

Wash the vegetables; prepare the eggs; chill all ingredients; shortly before serving combine the vegetables, meat or fish and/or cheese or eggs, seasonings, mayonnaise, boiled dressing, or other salad dressing. Add onions and/or garlic as desired.

Arrange on a bed of **watercress, endive, romaine, or lettuce;** garnish with **pimento, red or green pepper rings, tomato sections, olives, or radishes.**

## MEAT OR FISH ASPIC SALADS

Soak **1 tablespoon gelatin** in:

>   ½ cup vegetable-cooking water or tomato juice

Dissolve it in:

**1 cup boiling soup stock, vegetable-cooking water, or tomato juice**

Add and stir well:

| | |
|---|---|
| 2 tablespoons vinegar or lemon juice | 3 tablespoons finely chopped onion |
| 1 teaspoon salt | 1 teaspoon Worcestershire |
| ⅛ teaspoon each celery salt and paprika | 2 or 3 drops Tabasco |

Chill, and when the gelatin starts to congeal, add:

**1½ to 2 cups solid ingredients, or chopped vegetables and meat, fish, eggs, or cheese specified on pages 235 to 237**
Pour into a mold brushed with oil; chill until firm.
Unmold on a bed of watercress, romaine, endive, or lettuce.
Serve with mayonnaise or other salad dressing.

*Variations:*

Use 1 package lemon or lime gelatin; dissolve in 1¾ cups boiling vegetable-cooking water; omit unflavored gelatin and seasonings; use as a base for fish or cottage cheese salad.

Decrease the amount of gelatin to 1 or 2 teaspoons if firmly jelled soup stock is used in making aspic.

Omit vinegar or lemon juice if tart tomato juice is used.

Clear soup stock or vegetable-cooking water with eggshells (p. 310); remove all fat from the stock.

When available, use ¼ cup rose-hip extract (p. 489) instead of stock or water.

**Fruit-juice aspics:** Omit the seasonings; instead of stock or vegetable-cooking water, use apple or pineapple juice for aspics containing ham or pork, tart plum juice for aspics of beef, grapefruit juice for lamb or mutton. Omit vegetables and use 2 cups diced meat.

**Glaze for meat or fish:** Prepare the basic aspic, using cleared soup stock or vegetable-cooking water; omit onion; when aspic starts to congeal, brush over meat or fish, applying 2 coats or more; pour any remaining aspic into shallow pan so that it is no more than ½ inch thick; chill, dice, serve around cold meat. Glazed meats and fish are extremely attractive and well worth the effort of preparing them.

**Mint aspic for lamb or mutton:** Steep **1 cup crushed mint leaves** in **1 cup boiling unsweetened pineapple or grapefruit juice;** cool; strain out the leaves; reheat the juice and dissolve in it **1 tablespoon gelatin** soaked in **½ cup juice;** add **2 tablespoons each sugar and lemon juice and 1 drop green coloring.** Mold and serve with roast lamb or mutton; or add diced cold lamb before molding. Mint flavoring may be used instead of fresh leaves.

*Add the ingredients listed below to aspic recipe; or combine with mayonnaise or other dressing and serve as a salad on a bed of greens. If an aspic is to be served as the entree, use a small amount of vegetables for coloring and seasonings, and 1½ to 2 cups eggs, meat, or fish. If an aspic or salad is to be served in addition to the entree, use larger proportion of vegetables. Add a generous amount of salt if weather is hot.*

Diced roast beef, set in aspic of purple-plum juice or combined with diced fresh purple plums and mayonnaise.

Steamed brains (p. 115), parsley, American cheese, diced pickle.

Steamed brains, chopped ripe olives, pimentos, shredded carrot.

Steamed brains, chopped celery, parsley, set in tomato aspic or served on whole tomato cut petal fashion.

Cottage cheese, 1 cup or more, 2 diced hard-cooked eggs, parsley, celery, chives; serve with tomatoes or add to tomato aspic; vary aspic by adding ¼ cup mayonnaise or ½ cup sour cream.

Cottage cheese, 1 cup or more, sliced hard-cooked eggs, shrimps or flaked fish, chives, parsley; use eggs to decorate aspic mold; for a salad, arrange eggs and shrimps over tomato slices, put cheese at one side.

Sliced hard-cooked eggs, diced American cheese, chopped pimentos, celery, parsley; set in tomato aspic or add tomato wedges; use 4 or more eggs.

Chicken or turkey, celery, diced pimento, dash of nutmeg.

Chicken or turkey, parsley, fresh or canned asparagus; supplement the chicken with lean diced veal or pork.

Chicken or turkey, diced broccoli stalk, shredded carrot.

Flaked fish, such as halibut or cod, chopped cucumber, green pepper, fresh dill or dill sauce.

Flaked fish, parsley, diced celery; set in tomato aspic seasoned with basil, or add tomatoes and fresh basil.

Flaked salmon or other fish, hard-cooked eggs, sliced stuffed olives, green pepper or pimento.

Flaked fish, parsley, shredded raw carrot; season boiling liquid used in aspic with 1 teaspoon anise seeds or marinate the fish in French dressing to which anise seeds are added.

Flaked fish, diced beet pickle, parsley, diced American cheese.

Flaked fish, celery, diced hard-cooked eggs or wedges of unpeeled red apple, parsley.

Flaked crab or lobster, celery, cucumbers, parsley, avocado; add ½ cup mayonnaise to aspic.

Steamed or canned shrimp, parsley, sliced stuffed olives, chopped celery; leave shrimps whole; set in tomato aspic or add sliced tomatoes.

Diced steamed shrimp, chopped celery, diced unpeeled cucumbers, pimento, chips of Roquefort cheese. This is a delicious salad.

Flaked white fish, chopped mixed pickles, celery set in lime gelatin.

Flaked kippered fish, such as herring or salmon, diced beet pickles, wedges of tart raw apple, parsley.

Flaked fish, parsley, celery stalk and leaves; use thin slices of cucumber, carrot, and lemon to decorate the mold.

Diced ham, celery, green peppers, sliced hard-cooked eggs, fresh dill or dill sauce.

Diced ham, parsley, green peppers; set in tomato aspic or add tomatoes to salad; season with basil or 1 teaspoon caraway seeds.

Diced lean corned beef, parsley, green peppers, 1 tablespoon each prepared mustard and ground horseradish; add tomato or celery to salad; set in well-seasoned soup stock.

Diced heart, diced cucumbers, shredded carrot; or add 2 cups diced heart to an aspic of plum juice, omitting vegetables.

Diced heart, shredded raw cauliflower, parsley, green peppers; add ¼ cup mayonnaise to aspic.

Diced steamed liver, parsley, celery, leeks; set in tomato aspic or add tomato sections to salad.

Diced steamed liver, green pepper, parsley, chopped green onions with tops.

Diced steamed lamb liver, 2 teaspoons fresh dill or dill seeds, celery, parsley, chives.

Diced roast pork, celery; set in an aspic of apple juice or add diced red apples to salad.

Diced steamed sweetbreads (p. 117), pimentos, celery, sliced hard-cooked eggs, parsley.

Diced sweetbreads, asparagus, shredded carrot.

Diced sweetbreads, avocado wedges, chopped pimento, celery; set in a gelatin of bland vegetable-cooking water to which 2 tablespoons lemon juice are added.

Diced sweetbreads, diced cucumbers, sliced stuffed olives, chips of Roquefort cheese.

Diced sweetbreads, sliced canned mushrooms, pimento, celery, parsley, 2 tablespoons capers.

Steamed kidney, chopped green onions with tops, shredded raw carrot, parsley; dice kidney and marinate in tart French dressing; set in tomato aspic or add tomato sections to salad.

Diced lamb, a small amount of celery; set in mint aspic or add minced mint leaves to salad.

Diced lamb, celery, shredded raw cauliflower, pimento, fresh dill or dill sauce.

Diced lamb, chopped dill pickle, green peppers, minced raw broccoli bud and chopped stalk; set in tomato aspic or add tomato to salad.

Diced tongue, green peppers, parsley, shredded carrot; set in an aspic of stock or tomato juice, or add tomatoes to salad.

Diced tongue, diced cucumbers, green onions with tops, sliced radishes, hard-cooked eggs.

Diced tongue, shredded raw cauliflower, parsley, pimento.

Diced veal, celery, parsley, chives, pickle relish.

Diced veal, shredded carrots, chopped cucumber, pimento.

Diced veal, grated Parmesan cheese, parsley, finely shredded mustard leaves or watercress.

# CHAPTER 14

## SERVE EGGS AND CHEESE DAILY

Eggs and cheese supply adequate protein which has an abundance of amino acids essential to health. Aside from other vitamins and minerals, cheese furnishes calcium and vitamin $B_2$; eggs supply iron and vitamins A and $B_2$. Ideally an egg and a serving of cheese should be eaten daily, either alone or added to other foods. Although emphasis has often been put on the 1-egg cake and other ways of "economizing" on eggs, the liberal use of eggs and cheese should be looked upon as an economy which aids in preventing illnesses and saves money from medical bills, drugs, and lost working hours. In 1940, the annual consumption of cheese per person was only 8 pounds, and of sugar 92 pounds; the improvement in health would be startling if these amounts could be reversed.

Contrary to popular opinion, cheese is neither "hard to digest" nor constipating; soft-cooked and raw eggs are not "easy to digest." These beliefs are based on early studies of the length of time foods stayed in the stomach; if a food left the stomach quickly, the assumption was that it was easily digested and vice versa. Later studies showed that foods pass through the stomach much as liquids pass through a funnel. Protein foods of firm texture, such as cheese and hard-cooked eggs, are held in the stomach until their proteins are digested to liquid. Extremely soft-cooked or raw eggs leave the stomach so rapidly that almost no digestion can take place; hence few nutrients from such eggs can reach the blood.

Aside from the fact that the nutrients are poorly absorbed, there are two reasons why undercooked eggs should not be eaten. Avidin, a substance in raw egg white, combines with biotin, one of the B vitamins, and prevents it from reaching the blood. Persons deficient in biotin become ill and mentally depressed, and suffer from eczema. The protein of egg white, albumen, dissolves in water or

238

digestive juices and may pass into the blood undigested. When undigested protein reaches the blood, allergies may result. There is evidence that well-meaning mothers have produced allergies and eczemas in their children because of the belief that soft-cooked eggs are "easy to digest." Eggs should be cooked until the white is no longer a semiliquid and the yolk is at least slightly firm. Hundreds of recipes which call for raw egg white, as in ice cream, mayonnaise, Bavarian cream, gelatin sponges, and eggnogs, have probably done much harm. If the egg is beaten and stirred into hot liquid, it cooks quickly and is safe to use.

If you submit either eggs or cheese to high temperatures, the protein quickly becomes tough and some of its health-promoting value is destroyed. Cook both cheese and eggs gently with low heat at all times. Except when the temperature is low, as in a soufflé, cheese should be added to hot foods a few minutes before serving. Melt cheese under the broiler if you like, but avoid browning it.

Except in hot weather, eggs for beating should be kept in a cool place rather than in a refrigerator.

Since a generous calcium intake is advantageous and calcium deficiencies are widespread, eggshells should be used as a source of calcium. Sterilized shells from hard-cooked eggs can be crushed and added to a little lemon juice or diluted vinegar; as the acid combines with calcium, it loses its sourness; the strained liquid can then be added to fruit drinks, gelatins, or almost any cooked food. The continuous use of such liquid can do much to relax nerves and prevent tooth decay and fragility of bones. Since many people drink lemon juice before breakfast and eat an egg for breakfast, a wise procedure is to allow the lemon juice to stand overnight with the washed egg in it.

Since vitamin $B_2$ is destroyed by light, cheese should be kept covered. Purchase cottage cheese in a carton instead of that kept in open pans at a delicatessen counter. Keep other cheeses covered with wax paper in the refrigerator; use cream cheese soon after unwrapping. During cooking, vitamin $B_2$ is destroyed by light so quickly that foods should be kept covered every minute possible. When eggs are fried or scrambled in an open pan, as much as 48 per cent of the vitamin is lost whereas no loss occurs when the utensil is covered. Casserole dishes containing cheese should be kept carefully covered even when on the table.

In order to use eggs frequently in salads, sandwiches, and other foods, hard-cook a dozen at a time and keep them in the refrigerator ready to be used. Keep on hand several kinds of cheese, including grated cheese. Add generous amounts of cheese to soups, salads, egg dishes, and meat substitutes. Almost any cooked vegetable is delicious when cheese is added to it; serve such vegetables frequently. Make it a rule to serve both eggs and cheese daily.

I have given methods of cooking eggs for breakfast in the basic recipes. Eggs prepared with more elaborate seasoning and served with vegetables, cheese, and other foods are intended for lunches and dinners.

## SCRAMBLED EGGS

Brush grill or frying pan with **butter-flavored fat or bacon** drippings; heat to moderate temperature.

Break directly into pan:

### 4 to 6 eggs

Heat until white starts to set; stir in:

**¼ to ½ cup evaporated or top milk    1 teaspoon salt**
**⅛ teaspoon ground peppercorns**

Cook over extremely low heat for 10 to 12 minutes, stirring 2 or 3 times. *Keep the utensil covered as much as possible.* Serve with crisp bacon.

*Variations:*

Add any one of the following to scrambled eggs a few minutes before serving: 1 to 2 tablespoons minced chives, leeks, fresh dill, Chinese garlic, diced pimento, or ground parsley; ½ cup thinly diced sautéed kidneys, steamed brain, or shredded or cubed American cheese; ¼ cup Parmesan cheese or shredded dried beef; 1 cup diced leftover chicken, rabbit, ham, sautéed liver, or other meat; sautéed fresh or canned mushrooms; or ¾ cup flaked leftover or smoked fish.

Use tomato purée or sauce instead of milk, or add 2 tablespoons catsup or chili sauce.

Before cooking eggs cut ¼ to ½ pound link sausages into 1-inch pieces and pan-broil until nearly done; drain fat, add eggs, and cook as in basic recipe; or cut 3 or 4 wieners into ½-inch pieces and add with milk. Vary by using any of the highly seasoned sausages.

Surround scrambled eggs with steamed or fried rice, French-fried potatoes, or steamed kale, spinach, or other greens; top with grated cheese or cheese sauce (p. 163).

Sauté lightly before adding eggs 1 chopped or grated onion, chopped celery, and/or chopped green or red bell pepper.

**Spanish-style eggs:** Sauté lightly before adding eggs **1 chopped green or red bell pepper or fresh chili pepper;** or when eggs are almost done, add **1 diced pimento and 2 tablespoons chili sauce.** Stir in ½ **cup shredded or diced cheese.**

In order to poach eggs satisfactorily, use only fresh eggs, one to five days old. The whites of older eggs will run when dropped into water. To prevent the white from breaking apart or being uneven, the water should not be boiling or moving in any way when the egg is dropped into it; however, it should be as hot as possible without boiling. Vinegar may be added to the water to make the egg white coagulate more quickly, but the acid causes the white to have a curdled, rough appearance.

When you have purchased eggs of unknown age, break one into a cup and observe the texture of the white and the contour of the membrane covering the yolk. If the white seems quite jelly-like and the yolk tends to be spherical, the egg is fresh. The white of an older egg is more liquid and the yolk is somewhat flat on top.

If you wish to poach eggs which are not strictly fresh, the only method which can assure a symmetrical form is to cook them in an egg poacher, in muffin tins partly filled with hot water, or in rings, which are the easiest to use and wash. Poaching rings can be made out of large biscuit cutters slightly bent into oblong shapes and with the handles removed.

My pet method of cooking breakfast eggs, which can substitute for poaching, frying, or baking, is to steam them. If the utensil used holds heat, you can cover the eggs, turn off the heat, and forget about them while you have your fruit or juice; you return to find them perfectly and evenly cooked on both top and bottom. I heartily recommend this method to you.

## POACHED EGGS

Select strictly fresh eggs; use a shallow utensil filled to the depth of 1 inch with water; add:

### 1½ teaspoons salt

Bring water to boiling; turn down heat until the water is quiet; crack an egg, hold it just above the surface of the water, and slip it in gently; drop in other eggs, cover utensil, and simmer slowly until whites are firm, or 8 to 10 minutes; or remove from heat and let stand 15 minutes.

Lift from liquid with pancake turner and place on **buttered whole-wheat toast.** Sprinkle with freshly **ground black peppercorns.**

*Variations:*

Cover poached eggs with any cream sauce (p. 162) or creamed fish, lobster, crab, or shrimp (p. 189).

Garnish with rings of green or red bell pepper, fresh pimento, or paprika; or place pepper rings on moist grill, drop an egg inside each, add ¼ cup water, cover, and steam eggs.

Serve covered with sautéed pimentos, onions, and/or mushrooms.

Poach eggs in 2 cups medium cream sauce, such as dill, pimento, or cheese sauce; serve sauce over eggs.

Serve poached eggs on nest of buttered spinach, chard, or beet tops.

**Eggs with tomato sauce:** Prepare 1 or 2 cups tomato sauce (p. 166); poach eggs in sauce; serve sauce over eggs. Vary by using creole, Spanish, or other tomato sauce.

**Mock poached eggs, or steamed eggs:** Put ½ cup water in heated pan or grill; set poaching rings in water, drop in eggs, sprinkle with salt and freshly ground peppercorns, cover and steam over extremely low heat; if utensil and lid hold heat, turn off heat. If oven is in use, steam there.

No egg should be so mistreated as to be fried, or actually cooked by the heat of hot fat. Almost invariably fat reaches such a high temperature that the egg white touching it becomes brown and tough; the white next to the yolk is often left uncooked. Only enough fat should be used to prevent the eggs from sticking to the grill or frying pan. The heat should be kept low at all times. Again I would recommend that a little water or milk be added to produce steam, that the utensil be covered, and that the egg be allowed to cook gently so that no part of it is tough. Eggs cooked with butter-flavored fat are particularly delicious.

## "FRIED" EGGS

Heat grill or shallow frying pan until moderately hot; brush lightly with **butter-flavored fat or oil**; break and drop gently into it:

**4 to 8 whole eggs**

Add:

**2 tablespoons top milk or water**

Cover utensil and cook over extremely low heat until white is firm, or about 12 to 15 minutes; sprinkle with **salt and freshly ground black peppercorns.**

*Variations:*

Sauté breaded slices of eggplant (p. 354) and tomatoes; place tomatoes over eggplant and an egg on top of each serving.

Serve eggs on buttered toast and sautéed tomatoes; place crisp bacon on top.

Sprinkle ¼ cup shredded or grated cheese over top of eggs 4 minutes before serving.

Baking eggs is one of the easiest methods of cooking them. The dry heat penetrates slowly, and the eggs cook evenly from both top and bottom; almost no attention need be given them. It is usually recommended that eggs be baked in custard cups, which are a nuisance to oil, handle, and wash. Bake them directly on a hot grill or in a frying pan, or a baking dish, or in poaching rings.

## BAKED EGGS

Heat grill, frying pan, or baking dish to moderate temperature; brush lightly with **oil or fat** and break into it:

**4 to 8 eggs**

Sprinkle with **salt and freshly ground peppercorns**; place in a preheated slow oven at 325° F. and bake for 15 to 18 minutes.

*Variations:*

If oven is in use, add 2 or 3 tablespoons water or milk, cover utensil, and let eggs steam in the oven; substitute for frying or poaching eggs.

After egg white has set, lay slices of bacon across the top, or cover the eggs with ½ cup grated cheese and/or ¾ cup barbecue or Spanish sauce (p. 167).

Sprinkle grated American cheese over eggs and serve in indentations made in mounds of cooked spinach.

**Eggs in bacon rings:** Fasten bacon into rings with toothpicks; drop an egg into each ring; bake as in basic recipe.

**Eggs in meat cups:** Pan-broil for 1 minute at high temperature **thin slices of bologna or any luncheon meat,** making them curl into cups; drop an egg into each cup, bake, and serve with cheese sauce or mustard sauce (p. 164). Vary by baking eggs on slices of ham; or serve ham slices on toast, broiled tomato slices on ham, and baked egg on top of tomato; cover with any cream sauce (p. 163), preferably Hollandaise or mock Hollandaise.

**Eggs with leftover meat:** Combine **1½ cups ground leftover meat, ½ cup whole-wheat-bread crumbs, 1 teaspoon salt, freshly ground pepper-corns, ¾ cup gravy or milk;** put meat in flat baking dish, make indentations to hold eggs, and bake as in basic recipe.

**Eggs with rice or noodles:** Put **leftover rice or noodles** into oiled casserole; make depressions with tablespoon, place egg in each depression, season, and bake. Cover with **shredded cheese** or serve with cheese sauce (p. 163).

**Eggs with sausage:** Shape large sausage cakes with a hollow in the top side; bake cakes slowly 10 to 12 minutes; drop eggs into hollows and bake. Or arrange link sausages in circles, drop an egg into each circle, season, and bake.

**Eggs with sauce:** Break the eggs into baking dish; bake; prepare any cooked sauce (p. 163) and pour over eggs before taking from oven.

The old expression, "She can't even boil an egg," implies that it is easy. Actually, to boil eggs perfectly at all times is extremely difficult. If you let the heat become too high for too long a period, the egg becomes tough and the sulfur compounds in the yolk break down, leaving an unappetizing green ring. If the heat is not high enough to toughen the outside, the egg white pulls apart when you remove the shell. You may enjoy a soft-cooked egg with a certain texture which you want in every egg served you. The texture of either a hard-cooked or a soft-cooked egg depends on the initial temperature of the water and the eggs, the number

of eggs cooked, the amount of water used, the degree to which
the utensil holds heat, the temperature to which the water is
heated, and the length of time the eggs are left in it. If that is
easy, I give up. The more water used, the more slowly it will heat
or cool, and the longer the eggs will cook before they reach boiling
and/or after the water is removed from the heat. The only way
perfection can be obtained is to measure the water and to use a
stop watch and a thermometer, none of which I expect a housewife to do.

## BOILED EGGS

*Method I:* Use a deep utensil and bring to boiling approximately:

**1 quart water**

Use eggs which have been left at room temperature; slip carefully into
water:

**4 to 8 eggs**

Cover utensil; reheat water to boiling, but let boil no longer than 5
seconds; move the utensil from heat and let stand 8 minutes for soft-
cooked eggs; 25 minutes for hard-cooked ones, or until water has cooled.

*Method II:* Put cold eggs into cold water; heat to boiling, but boil no
longer than 5 seconds; move utensil from heat and let stand 5 minutes
for soft-cooked eggs; 20 minutes for hard-cooked ones, or until water is
cold.

*Method III:* If the oven is in use, set eggs on rack in oven at 350° F.;
let cook 15 to 18 minutes for "soft-boiled" eggs, 35 to 40 minutes for
"hard-boiled" eggs; decrease or lengthen the cooking time depending on
oven temperature. This is a very satisfactory way to cook eggs and it
saves dishwashing.

Creamed eggs are an excellent meat substitute or extender and
should be served frequently for lunches, dinners, or even late
breakfasts. If the sauces used are varied, creamed eggs need never
be monotonous. These dishes are especially valuable to use when
one must prepare food for an invalid, a convalescent, or a small
child who requires a smooth but high-protein diet. Even more
powdered milk could be used in making the cream sauce than I
have specified on page 161, and cheese may be added to any sauce.

## CREAMED EGGS

Prepare **2 cups pimento, caper, cheese, caraway, dill, curry, mushroom, olive, onion, or piquant sauce** (p. 162), using a base of cream sauce, brown sauce, leftover gravy, or tomato-cream sauce.

Stir into hot sauce:

> **4 to 6 hard-cooked eggs, sliced or cut in half lengthwise**

As soon as eggs have heated through, or in about 5 minutes, serve over **whole-wheat toast** or **wheat-germ biscuits** cut with a doughnut cutter; garnish with **parsley** and **paprika**. Serve with cooked asparagus, lettuce salad with Roquefort-cheese dressing.

*Variations:*

Slice eggs in half lengthwise while hot and place on hot serving platter; pour sauce over them, garnish, and serve.

Prepare dill, mushroom, olive, onion, pimento, or cheese sauce; slice eggs over hot cooked asparagus, spinach, kale, chard, broccoli, or other green vegetable; cover with sauce.

Before adding eggs, cook in sauce 1 cup peas, diced carrots, celery, diced broccoli, or asparagus; or add leftover vegetables.

Use 4 eggs; add 1 cup diced ham or other leftover meat or ¼ pound chipped dried beef; or use dill sauce and add 1 cup diced uncooked or flaked leftover fish, shrimps, lobster, or crab; or add 1 or 2 teaspoons anise seeds to medium cream sauce, and add eggs and fish or sea food.

Instead of cream sauce prepare Spanish, Mexican, creole, or other tomato sauce (p. 166); add eggs as in basic recipe. Vary by using stuffed eggs; reheat in tomato sauce and serve with sauce over them; sprinkle with grated cheese.

## STUFFED HARD-COOKED EGGS

Cut **4 hard-cooked eggs** lengthwise and remove yolks; mash yolks with fork and add:

| | |
|---|---|
| 2 tablespoons mayonnaise | dash of paprika, cayenne, or freshly |
| 1 teaspoon salt | ground black peppercorns |
| ½ teaspoon each mustard and | |
|    Worcestershire | |

Fill egg whites with yolk mixture.

*Variations:*

Add about 2 tablespoons of any one of the following: caviar with lemon juice; minced celery, pimento, green pepper, or fresh cucumbers; nippy cheese; diced ripe or stuffed olives; chopped nuts; chives with chopped pimento, 1 or 2 drops Tabasco sauce; finely chopped chicken or other leftover meat; ground parsley and 2 or 3 minced anchovies or 2 teaspoons anchovy paste; sour or dill pickles; steamed shrimp diced with 1 teaspoon chili sauce; or add fresh dill, commercial dill sauce, or dill or caraway seeds.

If a fluffy omelet is not to be tough and is to hold its shape after it is taken from the oven, it must be cooked at low temperature until the egg white is firm. A quickly cooked omelet will invariably fall and/or shrink.

### FLUFFY OMELET

Use eggs which are at room temperature. Beat until smooth:

½ cup fresh milk                    ½ cup powdered milk

Add and beat slightly:

4 to 6 egg yolks                    ¼ teaspoon freshly ground black
1 teaspoon salt                        peppercorns

Beat until stiff and fold in:

4 to 6 egg whites                   ½ teaspoon salt

Turn into baking dish brushed with **bacon drippings;** sprinkle with **paprika;** bake in preheated slow oven at 325° F. for 30 minutes.

Serve from baking dish.

*Variations:*

Use ¾ cup fresh milk; add and beat with yolks ½ cup toasted wheat germ or 4 tablespoons soy or peanut flour.

Add to egg yolks leftover peas, diced carrots, asparagus, broccoli, other cooked vegetables, canned mushrooms, or pimentos.

At the table serve over omelet any cream sauce or tomato sauce (p. 166), creamed ham, chicken livers, or sweetbreads; or creamed vegetables, such as asparagus or peas.

**Artichoke omelet:** Remove edible part from leaves of **2 or 3 artichokes** and mix with chopped artichoke hearts; add the artichokes, **1 minced clove garlic, and 1 finely chopped onion** to egg yolks.

Bacon and bean sprouts with omelet: Add 1 cup raw or canned bean sprouts and 2 slices crisp bacon, broken to bits.

Cheese omelet: Mix with egg yolks 1 cup shredded or grated cheese; sprinkle top of omelet with cheese.

Corn omelet: Add to egg yolks 1 cup raw, canned, or leftover corn, ½ teaspoon more salt.

Creole omelet: Sauté lightly in the utensil in which omelet is to be baked 1 chopped onion, 1 diced tomato, 1 chopped green pepper; add ¼ teaspoon each salt and paprika; mix with egg yolks before folding in whites. Vary by adding link sausage or wieners cut into ½-inch pieces.

Fish omelet: Add 1 cup any diced raw or flaked steamed fish to egg yolks before folding in whites.

Mushroom omelet: Add to egg yolks before folding in whites ½ to 1 cup sautéed fresh or canned mushrooms; use liquid from canned mushrooms instead of part of the milk.

Parsley-anchovy omelet: Decrease salt in basic recipe to ½ teaspoon; add 2 teaspoons or more of anchovy paste, 4 tablespoons ground parsley.

Rice omelet: Add ½ to 1 cup leftover rice and 1 tablespoon each catsup and Worcestershire to egg yolks before folding in whites.

Tomato omelet: Add ¾ cup of any tomato sauce (p. 166) to omelet instead of fresh milk; or roll slices of tomato in toasted whole-wheat-bread crumbs, sprinkle with salt, cayenne, and grated cheese, and place on bottom of baking dish; pour omelet over tomatoes.


## QUICK EGG OMELET

Beat until smooth:

½ cup fresh milk                    ½ cup powdered milk

Add and beat slightly:

4 to 6 eggs                         ¼ teaspoon freshly ground black
1½ teaspoons salt                      peppercorns

Pour into heated omelet pan or frying pan brushed with butter-flavored fat or bacon drippings; cover and heat slowly 6 to 10 minutes; loosen the edges with spatula and fold toward center, letting any uncooked egg run to sides of pan. Again cover utensil, and heat slowly 5 to 8 minutes. Fold edges toward center and sprinkle with:

2 to 4 tablespoons chopped chives, parsley, or Chinese garlic

Garnish with paprika.

*Variations:*

Mix with eggs before cooking 2 teaspoons minced fresh dill or dill sauce; or season with ¼ teaspoon celery seeds or salt or 1 teaspoon caraway or dill seeds.

Add diced leftover meat or ham to eggs before cooking.

**Crab or lobster omelet:** Fold omelet over 1 cup minced crab or lobster mixed with 2 tablespoons chili sauce; cover and serve as soon as heated.

**Kidney omelet:** Add thinly sliced raw kidney; fold omelet over kidney, cover the utensil, and heat 5 minutes before serving; or sauté the kidney 5 minutes, drain on paper, bake the omelet, add the kidney, and reheat.

**Oyster omelet:** Before folding omelet over add 1 cup chopped raw oysters or mix oysters with ½ cup thick cream sauce (p. 161), dash of cayenne, and ½ teaspoon salt; fold into omelet and heat for 5 to 8 minutes.

**Spanish omelet:** Sauté lightly 1 each chopped onion and green or red bell pepper or fresh chili pepper; add eggs; cook as in basic recipe. Vary by heating 1 cup of any tomato sauce (p. 166) and serving over omelet.

## THIN OMELETS, OR PFANNKUCHEN

Sift together or mix thoroughly:

¼ cup whole-wheat pastry flour      1 teaspoon salt
⅓ cup powdered milk

Add and beat well:

1 cup fresh milk      4 eggs

Heat grill or 8-inch frying pan and brush with a generous amount of butter-flavored fat; sauté a fourth of the batter until light brown on both sides; keep hot while cooking 3 more thin omelets.

Transfer to hot serving plates; add to each 4 tablespoons grated cheese, creamed shrimp or chicken, applesauce, or fresh sweetened berries; roll, and serve while piping hot.

*Variations:*

Separate eggs, beat whites until stiff, and fold into other ingredients; cover utensil until time to turn.

Cut bacon strips into 2-inch lengths and pan-broil until crisp; drop into each omelet. Vary by adding diced ham or thin slices of fresh ham.

**Swedish pancakes:** Add to basic recipe 2 tablespoons melted butter-flavored fat; use ½ cup whole-wheat flour; bake and serve as in basic recipe.

## FRENCH TOAST

Beat until smooth:

½ cup fresh milk                    ½ cup powdered milk

Add and beat slightly:

2 to 4 eggs                         1 tablespoon blackstrap molasses
1 teaspoon salt

Soak in mixture until soft:

6 or 8 slices stale whole-wheat, soy, wheat-germ, or rye bread

Sauté slowly in **butter-flavored fat** until browned on both sides.

Serve with applesauce, apricot purée, or other fruit sauce, or with fresh crushed and sweetened berries.

*Variations:*

Instead of fresh milk use tomato juice or tomato purée or any tomato sauce (p. 166). Serve with ham or bacon.

Increase black molasses to 3 or 4 tablespoons; add to batter ½ teaspoon cinnamon, ¼ teaspoon nutmeg.

Separate eggs, beat whites stiff, and fold in after other ingredients are combined.

Cheese dishes have been so scattered throughout the book that only a few are given here. I hope that you will scatter cheese throughout your menus in the same manner. As is shown in the vegetable recipes, shredded cheese may be added to almost any vegetable in the place of butter. It may be sprinkled on the surface of many soups. Its uses are unlimited. Keep cheese on hand at all times and serve it daily.

See **cheese soufflés** (p. 209), **peppers stuffed with cheese** (p. 207), and **cheese-filled pancakes** (p. 214).

When cottage cheese is made at home from milk which has been allowed to sour, the lactic acid causes calcium to dissolve into the whey, which is discarded. Calcium is well retained in cheese made with rennet, or junket. For this reason I do not recommend that cheese be made with sour milk. The cheese should not be washed to remove whey; too many vitamins and minerals are unnecessarily lost.

## COTTAGE CHEESE MADE WITH RENNET

Heat to lukewarm, or 110° F.

### 1 quart skimmed milk

Soak in 1 tablespoon water:

### 1 rennet, or junket, tablet

Add tablet to milk, stir well, and let stand until set.

Place in a large pan of hot water or over extremely low heat; fasten a cooking thermometer to edge of utensil or let dairy thermometer float on surface; stir frequently until desired temperature is reached; heat to 110° F. for soft-curd cheese, 120° F. for farmer-style cheese.

Pour into a strainer lined with a clean cloth; gather corners of cloth around curds and squeeze out whey; put cheese into a dish and add:

| | |
|---|---|
| 1 teaspoon salt | ½ cup sour cream or commercial yogurt |

Garnish lightly with **paprika.**

*Variations:*

Season occasionally with any of the following: 1 tablespoon chives, Chinese garlic, or minced fresh dill, basil, burnet, or parsley; 1 teaspoon crushed caraway, dill, celery, or mustard seeds. Let cheese stand ½ hour before serving.

## CHEESE CUTLETS

Use approximately **3 cups dry cottage cheese** before cream is added; or purchase **1 pound hoop cheese, or dry cottage cheese.** Press cheese through coarse strainer or food mill; add and mix well:

| | |
|---|---|
| 1 egg if cheese is moist; 2 if it is dry | 2 tablespoons sugar |
| 1 tablespoon whole-wheat flour | 1 teaspoon salt |

Mold into patties, roll in **whole-wheat flour,** and sauté slowly in **butter-flavored oil or fat;** cook until golden brown on both sides.

After vegetable soup (p. 317), serve with chilled sour cream or yogurt, green asparagus, fruit salad.

## WELSH RAREBIT

Combine and beat in utensil which holds heat or in top of double boiler:

¾ cup top milk or evaporated milk     1 teaspoon dry or prepared mustard
½ cup powdered milk               few grains cayenne
¼ teaspoon salt

Heat milk to simmering, stirring frequently; *keep covered as much as possible;* remove from heat and add:

### ½ pound or 2 cups diced mild cheese

Stir well, and cover utensil; let stand 6 to 8 minutes, or until cheese is melted; stir again.

After shrimp cocktail (p. 265), serve over buttered toast or slices of broiled tomato (p. 369) or eggplant (p. 354) with string beans, salad of Bibb lettuce with French dressing.

*Variations:*

Use 1 cup fresh milk and add 1 egg or 1 cup soft whole-wheat-bread cubes; add other ingredients and proceed as in basic recipe.

Use 1 cup mild American cheese combined with 1 cup Swiss, Jack, or pimento cheese or 1½ cups American and ½ cup Roquefort cheese; add Roquefort immediately before serving.

Instead of milk use tomato purée or any tomato sauce (p. 166).

**Baked rarebit:** Cut **2 or 3 slices stale whole-wheat bread** into fingers 1 inch wide; place sticks over bottom and along sides of flat baking dish brushed with oil; combine ingredients of basic recipe and add **2 egg yolks;** beat stiff and fold in **2 egg whites;** pour into the oiled baking dish, garnish with **paprika,** and bake in a slow oven at 325° F. for 30 minutes.

**Cheese fondue I:** Combine **1 cup soft whole-wheat-bread cubes** with **1 cup fresh milk;** add ingredients of basic recipe without heating, and **2 eggs beaten separately;** bake in slow oven at 325° F. for 25 minutes.

**Cheese fondue II:** Put **4 slices whole-wheat bread** into oiled baking dish; sprinkle **diced cheese** over it; mix **2 eggs** with other ingredients of basic recipe, using 2½ cups milk; bake at 350° F. for 30 minutes.

**Mushroom or tomato rarebit:** Use **1 can condensed mushroom or to-mato soup** and ¼ cup each **fresh milk and powdered milk;** omit salt; heat, and stir in cheese.

**Oyster rarebit:** Heat in milk 1 minute before adding cheese **1 cup raw oysters;** proceed as in basic recipe; omit mustard and add **1 teaspoon dill sauce or seeds or minced fresh dill.**

**Spanish rarebit:** Omit milk; sauté lightly 1 each chopped green pepper and onion; add ¾ cup tomato purée or diced pulp and cook 5 minutes; salt, remove from heat, and add cheese.

Few foods discussed in this book can compare in nutritive value or deliciousness with cheese snacks. The recipe was originated by Mrs. Mabel Garvey. If you have teeth instead of dentures, I think you will agree with me that she was inspired. Cheese snacks have a strange cycle of being tender when first baked, then becoming tough for a few days, then becoming extremely crisp. If the best flavor is to be attained, the cheese must be nippy. Mrs. Garvey recommends that Cheddar be used.

## CHEESE SNACKS

Combine:

| | |
|---|---|
| ½ cup hot water, preferably boiling | ¾ teaspoon salt |
| ½ cup soy grits | generous dash of cayenne |
| 1 cup grated nippy cheese, preferably Cheddar | |

Stir well, or until cheese is partially melted; add:

½ cup powdered milk

Drop on an oiled baking sheet and mash wafer-thin with prongs of a fork; or put cheese mixture in a shallow 11- by 16-inch baking pan; cover with wax paper and roll with rolling pin to ⅛ inch thick; sprinkle top generously with **paprika**, pierce with a fork at 1-inch intervals; bake at 325° F. for 12 to 15 minutes. While hot, cut into fingers or squares the size of soda crackers.

Serve with soups, salads, between meals, or in box lunches. Store in a dry place; reheat slightly to freshen.

*Variations:*

Omit cayenne and add 1 to 3 teaspoons dill, caraway, poppy, or cumin seeds or ½ teaspoon celery seeds; or sprinkle seeds over top before baking. Don't miss dill seeds; cheese snacks with dill are delicious.

If soft texture is desired, cook soy grits in ¾ cup water for 5 minutes; remove from heat, add cheese and other ingredients. Add any of the following (all are delicious): 2 tablespoons grated onion, ground parsley, or finely diced pimento; pinch of thyme, sage, marjoram, basil, or other herbs or combination of herbs.

Use ½ cup heated tomato catsup or chili sauce instead of hot water.

Instead of soy grits use ½ cup unrefined barley grits, steel-cut oats, buckwheat grits, or cracked wheat.

If soft texture is enjoyed, instead of soy grits use ½ cup wheat germ and middlings, quick-cooking rolled oats, or ¾ cup wheat germ or coarsely ground yellow corn meal.

A friend of mine set out to make butter but could find neither a recipe for making it nor an acquaintance who knew how. She tells me that two persons informed her in dead earnest that it was made from buttermilk. To anyone who has lived on a farm and has spent hours churning, such lack of information seems incredible. Even when she learned how to make butter, it developed a peculiar flavor a few days later; she had failed to sour the cream rapidly and to pasteurize it to destroy foreign bacteria and wild yeasts.

Although butter can be made of sweet cream, most dairymen will tell you that it has about as much flavor as does lard. The delightful flavor of butter, which is principally butyric acid, develops during the souring of the cream. So-called sweet butter is made of sour cream, but is not salted.

## HOMEMADE BUTTER

Collect sweet cream, keeping it in the refrigerator; when 1½ quarts or more have accumulated, pour into a cooking utensil such as the top of a large double boiler; fasten cooking thermometer to utensil or float dairy thermometer on surface; heat to 160° F. and hold at this temperature for 15 minutes; cool to 125° F. and add:

2 tablespoons commercial yogurt or yogurt culture

Stir well and set in pan of warm water or in oven; keep between 90° and 115° F. until it becomes quite sour and thick, or from 3 to 4 hours.

Or instead of adding yogurt, cool to 75° F. and add:

**4 tablespoons fresh commercial sour cream**

Keep between 70° and 80° F. until it sours and thickens, or about 24 hours.

Chill thoroughly, letting cream drop to temperature of 60° F. if possible; the more sour and chilled the cream is, the easier it is to churn.

Churn, shake in a 2-quart jar, or beat with electric mixer or rotary eggbeater until bits of butter separate; then churn, shake, or beat slowly until butter forms into large particles. Press particles together with wooden spoon or butter paddle; drain off buttermilk; wash butter 3 times in ice-cold water; drain well; fold butter over and over, squeezing with spoon or paddle until no more liquid can be pressed out.

Unless sweet butter is desired, add for each cup of butter:

**1 teaspoon salt**                     **2 drops butter coloring**

Press into mold and chill.

*Variation:*

If the taste is not delightful, add 3 to 5 drops butter-flavoring for each cup of butter.

# CHAPTER 15

## APPETIZERS CONTRIBUTE TO HEALTH

If full health for your entire family is to be your goal, appetizers should appear frequently on your menus. Appetizers play a triple role in contributing to health. They add the esthetic values of beauty and leisure to a meal. Their tartness stimulates the flow of digestive juices. They satisfy the appetite only sufficiently to decrease a desire to overeat; thus weight is kept within bounds.

An appetizer may be a glass of chilled vegetable juice or unsweetened fruit juice; fresh fruit or fresh fruits mixed with canned fruits; or almost any type of fish in catsup or chili sauce. Many delicious juices may be prepared at home by anyone who has a garden and fruit trees; a generous supply should be canned for winter use. The small amount of water left when vegetables are steamed, the vitamin C content of which is often greater than that of orange juice, can be added to vegetable-juice cocktails.

Appetizers of fruit and vegetable juices supply minerals and vitamins A, C, and P; fish cocktails provide protein and iodine. Family needs should determine which type of appetizer is to be served. Since foods rich in sugar or fat readily satisfy the appetite, the purpose of an appetizer should not be defeated by serving such foods as heavily sweetened fruits or juices, avocados, or Thousand Island dressing. Cracked ice should not be added to juices, as it dilutes their nutrients. All appetizers, however, should be served chilled.

People who own liquefiers, or blenders, have unlimited possibilities for preparing appetizers of outstanding health value. A liquefier reduces foods of the texture of carrots and apples to bits readily suspended in liquids; thus solid food can be drunk. All ingredients should first be chilled to prevent the air which is whipped into them from destroying part of the vitamins A and C. After being prepared, such appetizers should stand in the refrigerator until the air bubbles have escaped. If these juices are drunk immediately, the air quickly heats to body temperature and expands. In case they are gulped rather than sipped, still more air is swallowed; this air also expands and pushes against the stomach walls. The conclusion is usually reached that the ingredients have caused "heartburn," or indigestion. Such difficulties are avoided if the drink is sipped.

Special care should be taken to make drinks prepared in a liquefier delicious. The health enthusiast often defeats his own purpose by combining unpalatable concoctions containing an overabundance of mustard greens, watercress, spinach, and alfalfa. All these greens have outstanding nutritive value, but when large amounts are liquefied, they taste like newly mowed grass. Soon the liquefier is left unused.

If properly used, a liquefier can contribute much to health, especially in feeding babies, invalids, and elderly persons who have difficulty in chewing. A combination of any juice and fruit or vegetable may be used provided one finds it delicious. Since this choice is a personal one, no recipes for making these appetizers have been included.

Commercially prepared fresh juices are often of little value as appetizers. By the time they are brought home, vitamins C, A, and probably $B_2$ are largely destroyed; notice the color of most carrot juice, for example. The bacterial content of such juices is high, and the price even higher for value received. If juices cannot be drunk immediately after being prepared, frozen or canned juices should be used.

Appetizers of all varieties can serve as vehicles by which many nutritional deficiencies may be prevented or overcome. Calcium can be made palatable by soaking eggshells in lemon juice (p. 239); the juice may then be added to any appetizer. A few tablespoons of bland rose-hip extract make appetizers rich in vitamin C without altering their flavor. Whenever guavas and fresh peppers, both outstanding sources of vitamin C, are available, they should be used in all appetizers in which their taste blends with the other ingredients. Mild, debittered brewers' yeast can be stirred into appetizers of grapefruit or tomato juice without its presence being discovered. If no other source of vitamin D is obtained, 3 or 4 drops of this vitamin in the form of viosterol in propylene glycol may easily be added. In this form it mixes readily with water, is tasteless, and is sold inexpensively at drugstores.

The contribution which appetizers enriched with calcium, vitamins C, D, and the ten or more B vitamins can make in maintaining health cannot be overemphasized; if they are not served before dinner, they should be served at breakfast, lunch, or between meals. The ingredients and the amounts of each ingredient used in appetizers must depend, however, upon the food likes and dislikes of your family, the extent of your desire to build and maintain health, the degree of health you strive for, and the foods you have on hand. The ingredients and amounts in the following recipes, therefore, are only suggestions.

Form the habit of serving appetizers several times each week, either in the living room or at the table. They contribute much toward making each dinner a guest meal.

### TOMATO-JUICE APPETIZER

About ½ hour before serving combine in each of 4 serving glasses:

1 cup, or 8 ounces, tomato juice
1 tablespoon lemon juice
1 teaspoon or more mild-flavored brewers' yeast (optional)
1 to 3 drops Tabasco
¼ teaspoon Worcestershire

1 teaspoon chives (optional)
¼ teaspoon minced fresh basil or pinch of dried basil
red coloring if needed
¼ teaspoon salt

Give juice a swirl with fork and set in refrigerator. Stir again just before serving; taste for salt. Garnish with sprig of **watercress or parsley.**

*Variations:*

Instead of basil use orégano, marjoram, savory, or rosemary. Gradually increase yeast to 1 tablespoon as the taste becomes enjoyed.

Omit other seasonings and use ½ teaspoon freshly ground horseradish; add crushed seeds of mustard, celery, dill, or caraway.

Instead of ¼ cup tomato juice use ¼ cup vegetable-cooking water.

**Tomato-grapefruit appetizer:** Omit half the tomato juice and use fresh or canned grapefruit juice; omit Worcestershire, chives, basil, Tabasco. Serve immediately if ingredients are chilled.

**Tomato-sauerkraut appetizer:** Use equal amounts of sauerkraut juice and tomato juice; season as in basic recipe. Taste before adding salt.

Any fruits or juices whose colors and flavors blend may be combined in preparing appetizers. Since few fruits supply vitamin C in generous amounts, citrus fruits or citrus juices should be served more frequently than other fruits unless rose-hip extract or guavas are used. Sea food has long been served with lemon juice, but is even more delicious with tart grapefruit juice.

## GRAPEFRUIT HALVES WITH OYSTERS

Cut into halves:

**2 grapefruits**

Remove cores and cut sections loose from fibers; put in each center:

**3 raw or canned oysters or shrimps**     **dash each of salt and paprika**
**1 teaspoon freshly ground horse-**     **2 drops Tabasco**
**radish**

Set in refrigerator until served.

*Variations:*

Instead of oysters or shrimps use small amount of flaked steamed fish; add 1 teaspoon lemon juice.

Omit oysters and seasoning; garnish grapefruit with a maraschino cherry, or a sprig of mint, or unstemmed strawberry.

## ORANGE-APRICOT APPETIZER

Combine directly in each of 4 serving glasses:

**⅔ cup orange juice**        **⅓ cup apricot juice or thin purée**

Stir; set in refrigerator until time to serve; garnish with a sprig of **mint.**

*Variations:*

Instead of apricot juice use unsweetened pineapple juice, grapefruit juice, loganberry, strawberry, or other berry juices, a mild-flavored grape juice, or any juices light in color. Garnish with thin slices of fresh apricot or orange or grated orange rind.

Omit apricot juice and add grapefruit, pineapple, or apple juice, or pear and lime juice.

## ORANGE APPETIZER WITH MARASCHINO CHERRIES

Peel, dice, and remove seeds from:

### 2 large oranges

Put into each of 4 serving glasses:

½ diced orange                    2 teaspoons sliced green or red
2 tablespoons cut pineapple slices    maraschino cherries

Stir, and set in refrigerator until time to serve.

*Variations:*

Use sliced strawberries or seeded purple grapes instead of maraschino cherries.

Add 1 tablespoon lime juice and slices of papaya, guava, or diced sapote or kumquat.

Instead of pineapple use sliced fresh apricots, peaches, plums, or California persimmons; diced cantaloupe or Persian melon; seeded or seedless grapes; seeded black cherries and/or white cherries; grapefruit sections or wedges of unpeeled yellow pear or plum.

**Orange-pear appetizer:** Instead of pineapple use sliced unpeeled pear or white seedless grapes soaked in grapefruit or apple juice to which are added a few drops of green coloring; let stand 15 minutes and drain before combining with the other ingredients. Vary by adding diced loquats or fresh guavas.

**Persimmon-grapefruit appetizer:** Omit cherries and pineapple; prepare orange and small grapefruit sections and alternate in serving glasses with wedges of large California persimmons.

Melon to be used for appetizers may be cut into balls or cubes. Any melon with firm pulp may be used and served with fruit juice or mixed with assorted fruits.

## CANTALOUPE-RASPBERRY APPETIZER

Mix directly in each of 4 serving glasses:

⅓ cup cantaloupe cubes or balls    ¼ cup fresh orange juice
⅓ cup fresh red raspberries

Garnish with single **fresh mint leaf.** Set in refrigerator until time to serve.

*Variations:*

Instead of raspberries, combine melon with diced unpeeled red apple or yellow pears; diced orange, grapefruit, or tangerine sections; diced fresh or canned pineapple; fresh whole or sliced boysenberries, youngberries, or strawberries; sliced peaches, plums, or apricots; diced fresh guavas, sapote, or papayas; seeded and halved Concord or other purple grapes. Cantaloupe with purple plum is especially attractive and delicious.

Omit the cantaloupe and use cubes or balls of watermelon, muskmelon, Persian melon, or honeydew.

**Cantaloupe baskets:** Cut two small cantaloupes in half and remove seeds; fill the centers with chilled unstemmed strawberries or unstemmed black or white cherries.

**Mixed-melon appetizers:** Use equal parts of cantaloupe, honeydew, and watermelon or papaya cubes or balls; add the juice if desired.

Any fresh fruits whose colors and flavors blend and enhance each other may be used in preparing a fruit appetizer.

### BLACK RASPBERRY-PEACH APPETIZER

Mix directly in each of 4 serving glasses:

⅓ cup black raspberries                    ⅓ cup unsweetened pineapple juice
⅓ cup diced yellow peaches

Set in refrigerator until time to serve.

*Variations:*

Instead of raspberries use strawberries or other berries; unpeeled red apple or yellow pear; seeded and halved purple or Concord grapes; or slices of purple plum.

Substitute for peaches any fresh light-colored fruit and for pineapple juice any light-colored unsweetened juice.

**Apricot-grape appetizers:** Combine ⅓ cup each wedges of fresh apricots and seeded halves of purple grapes, seeded black cherries, or wedges of purple plums; sweeten to taste.

**Guava appetizers:** Add 1 to 3 diced strawberry or pineapple guavas to any mixed-fruit cocktail; as the taste becomes familiar, cut guava into thin slices; serve sliced or diced guavas alone with orange, grapefruit, pineapple, or apple juice; add 1 tablespoon lime or lemon juice.

**Loquat or papaya appetizers:** Slice or dice loquats or papayas; add to any appetizers of mixed fruits; serve alone with fruit juice if the flavor is enjoyed.

**Persimmon-pear appetizers:** Dice fresh unpeeled pear and let soak ½ hour in 1⅓ cups apple, pineapple, or grapefruit juice to which green coloring is added. Meanwhile freeze 2 large unpeeled California persimmons until solid. Just before serving, cut persimmons into ⅓-inch cubes, combine with pears and other ingredients, and pour ⅓ cup colored juice over each appetizer.

Surely no more delightful appetizers could be served on a sweltering hot evening than a frozen fruit sauce or a juice chilled with frozen cubes of sauce. Frozen sauces may be served as the first course or with the entree. One of the most beautiful appetizers is made of yellow tomatoes. I make a point of canning them each year just for appetizers.

## FROZEN YELLOW-TOMATO APPETIZER

Mix in freezing tray an hour or more before time to serve:

| | |
|---|---|
| 3 cups yellow-tomato purée | 1 teaspoon Worcestershire or dill |
| ¼ cup lemon juice | sauce |
| | salt to taste |

Set in freezing compartment; in ½ hour stir thoroughly to prevent crystals from becoming large; freeze to a firm mush. Immediately before serving stir in:

½ cup finely chopped fresh paprika, red bell pepper, or pimento

Put into chilled serving glasses. Garnish with a single leaf of watercress or parsley.

*Variations:*

Substitute yellow-tomato juice for purée.

Vary seasonings by adding crushed celery or mustard seeds, Tabasco, dry mustard, minced fresh basil or dill, or freshly ground horseradish.

Use red-tomato juice or purée instead of yellow; just before serving add ½ cup finely chopped green pepper.

Instead of yellow-tomato purée use vegetables prepared in the liquefier, such as carrot, celery, and mixed fresh vegetables blended with liquid from canned asparagus or peas, red-tomato juice, apple juice, or vegetable-cooking water. Season like tomato-juice appetizer (p. 258).

**Frozen applesauce:** Use applesauce cooked with 1 teaspoon cassia buds; add a few drops of red coloring; if sauce is not tart, add lime or fresh lemon juice.

**Frozen apricot purée:** Substitute apricot purée for tomato purée. Garnish with bits of purple plum or a light sprinkling of finely chopped mint or a green maraschino cherry.

**Frozen nectarine purée:** Use nectarine juice or purée instead of tomato purée; add green coloring, garnish with halves of a red maraschino cherry.

**Frozen pear or peach purée:** Increase tartness by adding 2 to 4 tablespoons fresh lemon or lime juice; add a few drops of yellow, green, or red coloring.

**Frozen persimmons:** Freeze well-ripened California persimmons in ice tray. Immediately before serving, shred quickly without peeling. Garnish with mint leaves. Serve with lemon sections.

**Frozen strawberry or youngberry purée:** Instead of tomato purée use strawberry or youngberry purée; add red coloring to strawberries if needed, and garnish with mint leaves or halves of green maraschino cherry.

Cubes of firmly frozen sauce are easily broken apart with a spoon; hence juices chilled with cubes of frozen sauce may be served at the table. After the juice is drunk, the sauce may be eaten with a long-handled ice-tea spoon.

## PINEAPPLE JUICE WITH FRUIT-PURÉE CUBES

Hold a tray of ice cubes carefully under running water and remove 4 cubes from each end; set remaining cubes back in tray and fill empty spaces at one end with:

### 1 cup apricot purée

Fill the empty spaces at the other end with:

### 1 cup purple-plum purée

Freeze until solid enough to hold shape.
Put into each of 4 chilled serving glasses:

### ⅔ cup clear pineapple juice

Set in refrigerator until the family is seated at the table; just before serving put into each glass:

**1 cube frozen apricot purée**      **1 cube frozen purple-plum purée**

*Variations:*

Omit pineapple juice; freeze purée cubes only enough to hold shape; serve 3 cubes of contrasting color from large sherbet glasses; serve at the table from a glass ice bucket if desired.

Instead of pineapple juice use apple juice or strained grapefruit juice.

Use any purée darker in color than the clear juice, or two or more purées of contrasting colors.

When fresh juices are squeezed or canned juices opened in advance of using, loss of vitamin C occurs even if they are covered and kept in the refrigerator. The vitamin is preserved over a longer period when the juices are frozen until needed.

Cubes of frozen juices may become extremely hard and should be used only with other juices when the appetizer is to be served in the living room before dinner. Frozen cubes should be made of light-colored juices. Decorative cubes are fun to make, need take only a few minutes to prepare, and are enjoyed by old and young alike.

## APPLE JUICE WITH DECORATIVE JUICE CUBES

Pour into ice tray:

### 2½ cups clear light-colored apple juice

Set in freezing compartment until ice crystals form over the top.

Quickly make flower arrangements in center of each cube by using fresh raspberries and tiny strawberries; bits of orange and lemon peel; halves or wedges of red or green maraschino cherries; small mint, parsley, or watercress leaves.

Freeze until solid; add enough apple juice to fill tray; complete freezing.

When the family has gathered, serve an ice bucket of decorative cubes in the living room, using 2 cubes for each glass; fill glasses with chilled clear apple, grapefruit, or pineapple juice.

*Variations:*

Make decorative cubes of any strained, light-colored juice.

Make frozen cubes of any contrasting color, but of light-colored juice, such as orange, apricot, strawberry, or white grape, and serve in any clear juice. If dark-colored juices are used for frozen cubes, the entire drink becomes muddy and takes on the color of the cubes as they melt.

Any mild-flavored and properly cooked fish may be used for appetizers instead of crab, oysters, and lobster which are customarily used. Shellfish are available to few and prohibitive in price to many. When well seasoned, fish appetizers are often thought to be made of shellfish and taste as delicious.

## FISH APPETIZER

Steam ½ **pound fillets** of any white-fleshed fish (p. 187). Flake the fish and add:

| | |
|---|---|
| ½ teaspoon salt | freshly ground white peppercorns |
| 2 tablespoons lemon juice or tarragon vinegar | dash of celery salt |
| 2 or more tablespoons capers | ½ cup catsup |

Stir, taste for seasoning, and chill.

Put into cocktail glasses and garnish with **ground parsley** or a small sprig of **parsley or watercress.**

*Variations:*

Use barbecue or chili sauce instead of catsup.

Add 1 tablespoon or more of any one or a combination of the following: chopped, grated, or minced fresh pimento, paprika, or red or green bell pepper; chopped onions or leeks; green-onion tops, chives, or Chinese garlic cut with scissors; chopped parsley or celery.

Omit capers and season with 1 or 2 teaspoons dill sauce or fresh horseradish, 1 to 3 teaspoons minced fresh fennel, dill, marjoram, or thyme; or add ½ teaspoon anise, dill, or celery seeds; let stand ½ hour after seasonings are added.

Instead of fish use steamed shrimp, flaked crab, lobster, or chilled uncooked or canned oysters or clams; or serve oysters or clams in half shells with sauce.

Sweetbreads and chicken livers are customarily served as canapé appetizers. You will probably agree, however, that canapés are a nuisance to make and become soggy quickly. An easier way of serving these meats as appetizers is to steam, chill, and combine them with a delightfully seasoned barbecue sauce or catsup.

## SWEETBREAD APPETIZER

Steam ½ **pound lamb or veal sweetbreads** (p. 117); chill, remove all membranes, and cut into small cubes.

Combine with sweetbreads and stir thoroughly:

¼ to ½ cup chili sauce
2 tablespoons chopped leeks, raw onion, chives, or Chinese garlic
2 tablespoons chopped pimento, fresh paprika, or bell pepper

2 tablespoons diced celery
salt to taste
sprinkling of ground black pepper-corns

Let stand in refrigerator ½ hour before serving.

*Variations:*

Add 1 teaspoon minced fresh basil, savory, tarragon, marjoram, or dill.

**Appetizers of brain:** Use ¼ pound lamb, veal, or beef brain; steam the brain with **vinegar** (p. 115); if flavor is disliked, add a **generous amount of parsley, 1 or 2 diced hard-cooked eggs, 1 teaspoon chopped tarragon, dill, or other fresh herbs.**

**Appetizers of kidney:** Use 2 lamb or 1 veal kidney; cut in half lengthwise and cut out all white tissue; dice, mix with **1 tablespoon vinegar,** and steam 5 minutes; chill and proceed as in basic recipe.

**Appetizers of liver:** Rabbit, lamb, veal, and baby beef liver may be used as well as livers of chicken, duck, and goose. Broil gently (p. 166), cut into ⅓-inch cubes, and combine with ingredients of basic recipe; rub with **garlic** the bowl used for mixing.

# CHAPTER 16

## SERVE YOUR SALADS FIRST

A raw vegetable or a salad largely of raw fruits or vegetables should be served at each lunch and dinner throughout the entire year. Raw foods contribute vitamins, minerals, and bulk, and are particularly important as sources of vitamin C. Leftover cooked vegetables may be added to salads in order to avoid further nutritive losses caused by reheating, but "salads" of canned beans, boiled potatoes, or macaroni (curses on the person who invented such a dish!) do not count. If you like such foods chilled, serve them with fresh salads, but not as a substitute for salads.

Salads need not be elaborate or take much time to prepare. A single raw vegetable will suffice: radishes, green onions, celery, carrot sticks, or strips of fresh pimento, paprika, or bell pepper. These raw vegetables may be served with an appetizer, a soup, or the entree.

Salad dressings add more nutritive value than mere calories. Most vegetable oils are excellent sources of vitamins $B_6$, E, and K, and of unsaturated fatty acids. Corn, peanut, cottonseed, and soybean oils appear to be nutritionally superior to olive oil. It is wise to vary the kinds of oil used or to mix two or more varieties, thereby allowing one oil to supply nutrients which another lacks.

Make it a rule to serve a salad as the first course. Larger amounts are eaten when persons are most hungry. Salads satisfy the appetite sufficiently to decrease the danger of overeating; thus they help to maintain or reduce weight and to break the habit of wanting an oversweet dessert.

The salads most superior nutritionally are those made of green leaves. Although fruit salads are excellent, fruits are generally eaten in other ways. Unless raw green leaves are eaten in salad, they are not eaten at all. The concentration of vitamins and minerals in deep-green leaves is greater than in any other type of

267

fresh food. Not only is vitamin A, or carotene, many times richer than in the bleached leaves, but also much richer are vitamins C, E, K, P, $B_2$, folic acid, some eight or more other B vitamins, iron, copper, magnesium, calcium, and other minerals. When leaves are bleached, they can no longer function normally as active parts of the plant; their need for vitamins and minerals is so reduced that these substances are largely removed from them. The salads of intensely green vegetable leaves should therefore be served most frequently. Few food habits could be of more value to health than that of taking a tossed green salad with each dinner, as do the Italians and French.

Many people avoid salads which contain onions, garlic, and green peppers, believing these excellent foods do not digest, because an aftertaste is sometimes noticeable. "Burping" indicates only that a person is so malnourished as to be highly nervous or that he has eaten so rapidly that he has gulped air; similarly, an overly hungry baby swallows so eagerly that its back must be patted to bring up air bubbles. The air enclosed in the stomach absorbs volatile oils from foods and when heated to body temperature, expands and forces its way upward, carrying odors with it. If the person having such difficulty eats slowly, chews his food thoroughly, sips all liquids, and builds up his general health, his trouble disappears. Then he can enjoy all of the ingredients of fresh salads.

Parsley has such outstanding nutritive value that large amounts should be added not only to most salads but to every food possible. Since parsley has a rough texture, it should be ground so that large amounts can be eaten and the nutrients be well absorbed. The nutrients in the firmer leaves are enclosed in cells surrounded by a substance known as cellulose which human beings lack enzymes to digest. The entire contents of such cells can reach the blood only when the cell walls are broken open by cutting, chopping, or chewing. Although from all cells the vitamins and minerals which dissolve in water can pass into the digestive juices, vitamins A, K, and other nutrients which cannot dissolve in water are largely lost. Grinding parsley has other advantages: a bale is reduced to a thimbleful; so many aromatic oils escape that the flavor becomes bland; thus it can be used as a food rather than a garnish, and ½ cup or more may be added to salads without the taste predominating. If parsley is chilled before being ground, and is kept covered in a refrigerator with no moisture except its own juices, no nutritive loss need occur. It will keep many days.

Use every variety of vegetable in salads. Examples which are particularly delicious, but are not customarily eaten raw, are: tiny uncooked or frozen peas; raw Jerusalem artichokes; raw broccoli buds, stalk, or shredded leaves; raw shredded cauliflower and Brussels sprouts; raw turnip, kohlrabi, rutabaga, and asparagus tips; bits of celery-root leaves and stalk. Among the green leaves which should be eaten raw are tampala, mustard-spinach, young radish tops, endive, chard, kale, wild greens, and New Zealand spinach. Make a point of adding all of these uncooked vegetables to your salads.

There is no reason why invalids, elderly persons who have difficulty in chewing, babies taking their first solid food, and people suffering from such conditions as ulcers or colitis should be denied delicious and appetizing salads. In such cases, salad vegetables are well tolerated if they are shredded, grated, or ground, mixed with cottage cheese, set in gelatin, or combined with soft foods, such as sliced eggs, avocado, or peeled tomatoes.

The nutritive value of salads depends on the method of handling and preparing the ingredients. In buying vegetables, purchase those which have been trimmed the least. If the roots and outside leaves or tops have been left on, the vitamin content is increased after the vegetable is gathered until wilting sets in. Except for foods which have a heavy peeling, such as oranges, bananas, pears, and apples, buy only the amount of salad fruits and vegetables which can be stored in the refrigerator. If you have a garden, gather the food just before time to chill and prepare it for the table.

Except for fruits or vegetables which bruise easily, such as berries or watercress, the following rules must be observed in preparing salad ingredients if nutritive losses are to be prevented:

Wash the vegetable or fruit carefully but quickly, using cold water; rinse and drain.
Dry thoroughly.

Unless you have a moisture-controlled refrigerator, keep all vegetables in a covered refrigerator pan, preferably on a rack above ⅛ inch of water.

Chill as quickly as possible.

These recommendations have often been made, but housewives rarely follow them, largely because the reasons behind them have not been given.

Vitamin A and particularly vitamin C are destroyed by combining with oxygen. The combination of oxygen and vitamins is brought about largely by the action of enzymes. The best-known enzymes are those in the stomach and intestines which aid in the digestion of foods. Enzymes exist in all plants. During the growth period and until a fruit is ripe, these enzymes help to synthesize, or make, vitamins. When the food is overripe or after it is gathered, these same enzymes bring about the destruction of the vitamins. The saving of vitamins, therefore, means preventing enzyme action and keeping oxygen away from the food.

Since the rules for handling, preparing, and cooking foods are based on preventing enzyme action, the housewife should know certain facts about enzymes. Their action is inhibited by cold, or refrigeration. They are particularly active at room temperature. Their activity decreases as the temperature approaches boiling, or 212° F., and they are destroyed by boiling. The action of the enzyme which destroys vitamin C is inhibited by acid; the enzymes which affect $B_2$ are active only in the light. Leafy vegetables kept in the light and at room temperature can lose half of their vitamins $B_2$ and C in a day. The skin on such foods as apples, oranges, and pears largely prevents contact with oxygen; hence the vitamins they contain are not readily destroyed at room temperature.

If fruits and vegetables are to retain their delightful flavor, they must be washed quickly, dried immediately, and not soaked even to freshen them. Quick washing, however, does not imply careless washing. The sweetness of most vegetables is due to three sugars: sucrose, or table sugar; glucose, or grape sugar; and fructose, or fruit sugar. Just as sugar dissolves quickly in coffee, so do these sugars speedily dissolve out during slow washing or soaking. Since vegetables contain less sugar than do fruits, their flavor is more quickly harmed. Soaking also causes loss of many aromatic oils, of minerals which give a salty tang, and of acids which give piquancy to the taste. When foods are washed slowly or soaked, serious nutritive losses occur. Vitamins C, P, and all the B vitamins readily dissolve in water. For example, peas soaked for 10 minutes have been found to lose 20 to 40 per cent of the vitamin $B_1$ and 35 per cent of the vitamin C in the water. These vitamins and some ten or more others and all minerals except calcium dissolve out in approximately the same proportion when any vegetable is soaked. The cumulative loss of nutrients in a year's time through slow washing is tremendous.

Except for fruits and vegetables which have soft textures, such as berries and watercress, or heavy peelings, such as oranges, potatoes, and dry onions, all should be washed as soon as they are brought into the house, then quickly chilled, and stored in a dark place. To prevent enzyme action, only cold water should be used in washing them, and they should be washed so thoroughly that they will not need to be touched by water again. Since drying is essential to delicious salads and prevents nutrients and flavors from passing into the water clinging to the surface, vegetables should be dried with considerable care. A soft Turkish towel should be kept for drying smooth vegetables. Leafy vegetables are most easily and quickly dried in a whirling bag, a cheesecloth bag about 18 inches square. When vegetables are whirled in such a bag—in the back yard, out a window, or over the bathtub—the water is thrown from them by centrifugal force, and they are dried in a minute. The fruits and vegetables should then be immediately stored in a refrigerator pan.

Unless you have a moisture-controlled refrigerator, the type of refrigerator pan, or hydrator, used is important. Ideally it should be fitted with a rack under which is kept ⅛ inch of water to supply continuous moisture, yet which would prevent the vegetables from touching the water. A rack sold with a roaster may be used. The lid of the pan should fit tightly to prevent the escape of moisture. A towel laid over the vegetables in such a utensil will become wringing wet in a short time. Similarly, wilted or shriveled vegetables soon become crisp without water touching them.

To stop enzyme action, fresh foods should be chilled as quickly as possible and be kept chilled continuously, whether they are to be used for salads or for cooking. The food should not be left unnecessarily long at room temperature because the destruction of vitamins is rapidly resumed as the vegetables become warm.

Losses may occur during the preparation of salads. Contact with any equipment which contains copper brings about instant destruction of vitamin C, causing the surfaces to turn brown. When fruits or vegetables are cut, chopped, peeled, grated, or sliced, a large amount of surface is exposed to air and light, and vitamins are rapidly destroyed unless the food is so chilled that enzyme action cannot take place. Little or no loss occurs if the salad ingredients are thoroughly chilled, quickly cut or shredded with stainless-steel or well-tinned equipment, and immediately served or returned to the refrigerator without dressing.

When such foods as shredded lettuce, sliced avocado, and diced apples become brown along a cut surface, a chemical action occurs involving the destruction of vitamin C. If no copper-containing metal is allowed to touch the food, and if enzyme action is inhibited by thorough chilling and by immediately adding an acid such as lemon juice, vinegar, or French dressing, discoloration can be prevented, and nutritive value and attractiveness saved.

Plates used for individual servings of salad should be set in the refrigerator and chilled. Since housewives are aware that salad ingredients should be chilled, I have not stressed chilling ingredients in the recipes, assuming that it will be done. Because sweets readily satisfy the appetite, salads should not be sweet, particularly those served at dinner. Unsweetened gelatin is preferable for molded salads, and dressing should be sweetened little if at all.

I recently discussed American salads with a charming woman from Holland. "They are beautiful ornaments without taste," she remarked. I was forced to agree with her. Although the rules for preparing delicious salads are indeed simple ones, no salad can be worthy of its name until Americans learn not to soak salad vegetables.

When you serve a properly prepared salad, you serve health in the making.

## FINGER SALADS

The following raw vegetables may be served alone or combined:

Large broccoli stalk, peeled and cut into sticks.
Sticks of unpeeled carrot.
Celery stalks or curls.
Cucumber fingers, peeled or unpeeled.
Peeled kohlrabi slices, sticks, or wedges.
Green onions with 4 to 5 inches of the tops.
Thin slices of large onion.
Green or red bell pepper sticks or rings.
Pimento or fresh paprika sticks or rings.
Cabbage or cauliflower stalk cut into sticks.
Unpeeled turnip slices, sticks, or wedges.
Radishes, preferably not made into "roses."
Whole cherry tomatoes with stems; the bottom half may be dipped in French dressing, then into ground parsley or chopped chives.
Young rutabaga sticks, peeled or unpeeled.
Potato fingers; these should be used for winter salads when sources of vitamin C are inadequate.

## FINGER SALADS WITH FRENCH DRESSING

The following raw vegetables may be soaked, or marinated, in French dressing and served by toothpick. If several are served at one time, vary the seasonings used.

Cauliflowerlets no more than ½ inch in diameter; add ¼ cup ground parsley or 1 tablespoon grated orange peel for each cup of flowerlets.
Tiny clusters of broccoli buds garnished with paprika.
Raw unpeeled beets, cut into fingers slightly larger than shoestring potatoes; for each cup of beets add 3 tablespoons chives cut fine with scissors, or minced fresh thyme.
Stalk of chard or tampala 2 to 3 inches long; for each cup add 1 tablespoon chopped fresh basil, burnet, chives, or parsley.
Brussels sprouts, no more than ¾ inch in diameter.
Rings of raw zucchini or small wedges of young summer squash; add to each cup 2 teaspoons minced mixed herbs or 1 tablespoon Chinese garlic.
Unpeeled eggplant, cut into sticks ½ inch square and 2 to 3 inches long; for each cup add 2 tablespoons chives and 1 tablespoon fresh horseradish or 1 teaspoon dill seeds.

Raw potato sticks; for each cup add 1 teaspoon caraway seeds or 2 tablespoons chives cut fine with scissors; serve for winter salads when vitamin C is inadequate.

Tomato quarters; to 2 cups tomato quarters add ¼ cup ground parsley and 1 tablespoon chopped fresh basil or 2 tablespoons chives.

Red apple wedges; cut each apple into 8 to 10 wedges; add to each cup ½ teaspoon cumin, caraway, or dill seeds.

## FINGER SALADS COMBINED WITH OTHER FOODS

**Stuffed celery stalks:** Cut the stalks into 3- to 5-inch lengths and stuff with any of the following fillings, combined with mayonnaise:

Chopped hard-cooked egg, chives, pimento.

Equal parts of peanut butter, shredded carrot, and ground parsley.

Mashed avocado mixed with lemon juice, Chinese garlic, Worcestershire, freshly ground white peppercorns.

Cottage cheese mixed with chopped chervil, burnet, or parsley.

Liver paste (p. 232) or mashed liverwurst with shredded carrot, a few drops of Tabasco.

Salmon, sardine, or anchovy, finely flaked or mashed and combined with grated onion.

Cottage, cream, pimento, shredded American, Swiss, or Roquefort cheese, mixed with chives, parsley, fresh basil, dill, or caraway seeds; add enough milk or mayonnaise to moisten.

**Stuffed celery-stalk rings:** Use the stalks of an entire head of celery; pull apart, wash, and dry thoroughly; save the heart for other uses; spread the inside of stalks with any filling suggested above; when stalks are filled, start with center stalks and press firmly together, working from the heart outward and reconstructing the entire head; tie stalks together, chill for ½ hour or more; cut into slices ½ inch thick.

**Cream-cheese balls:** Combine cream cheese with vegetables and herbs, such as shredded carrots, raw beets; tiny fresh or frozen raw peas; finely chopped purple cabbage or celery; ground parsley, chervil, or celery leaves; chives; chopped fresh sage, rosemary, burnet, or other fresh herbs; or add dill, caraway, anise, celery, or mustard seeds; make into balls.

**Rainbow-cheese balls:** Season cream cheese with cumin, caraway, dill, or celery seeds; make into balls of different colors by rolling them in ground nuts; ground parsley or celery leaves combined with fresh herbs; shredded American cheese or finely grated carrots; paprika or minced canned or fresh pimento.

**Cream-cheese scrolls:** Mix cream cheese with ground or grated carrots, raw beets, parsley, spinach, mustard greens, or other vegetables; season with 1 tablespoon fresh horseradish and roll into scrolls in chipped beef; cut into 1-inch lengths.

**Stuffed cucumbers:** Cut the ends of cucumbers, scoop out seeds with an apple corer; fill centers with pimento cheese, chicken salad, or any filling suggested for celery; slice crosswise and serve.

**Stuffed green pepper or pimento rings:** Choose 3 or 4 bell peppers or pimentos of different sizes, or use one or more of both peppers and pimentos; dry thoroughly; remove stem end, seeds, and center tissues; cover inside surface of largest pepper with any firm cheese filling; press next largest pepper firmly inside largest one and line with the filling; repeat process; leave smallest pepper empty; chill and slice in ½-inch slices. A different filling may be used inside each pepper. Interesting combinations for pimentos are cream cheese mixed with ground parsley; liver paste; grated Swiss cheese seasoned with dill sauce. For green peppers, use pimento cream cheese, liver paste, and any yellow filling. Don't miss these rings; they are both attractive and delicious.

**Stuffed whole baby peppers or pimentos:** Select peppers or pimentos not more than 2 inches in diameter; leave stem end intact, cutting across top; fill with any cream cheese or cottage cheese combined with vegetables; chicken or shrimp salad, gelatin salad; or an aspic topped with cheese spread; put stem end in place and serve whole.

**Stuffed raw onion or leek:** If onions are used, make sure this recipe is to be served to onion-lovers. Cut base and top from leeks or round sweet onions no more than 1 inch in diameter; separate the onion into layers by holding under running water; dry by whirling; stuff with any firm, bland filling, such as cottage, grated American, or cream cheese, combined with minced or ground greens, grated carrot, or shredded pimento.

## APPLE SALADS

Generally choose red apples for salads and do not peel. Quarter, core, dice, and mix immediately with lemon juice, French dressing, or mayonnaise to prevent discoloration. Unless other dressings are mentioned, serve the following salads with mayonnaise on a bed of watercress, endive, chopped mixed greens, romaine, or other lettuce. Combine a large proportion of diced raw apples with the following ingredients:

Shredded carrot, orange sections; sprinkle with coconut meal; serve with fruit dressing (p. 292).

Shredded pineapple, carrot, grated orange peel, a few raisins.

Celery, carrot, ½ teaspoon dill or caraway seeds.

Diced or sliced banana, a few maraschino cherries, 2 to 4 minced mint leaves.

Green pepper, kohlrabi, diced ham, 1 teaspoon caraway seeds.

Shredded purple cabbage, celery, raisins.

Celery, cubes of American cheese, 1 teaspoon cumin seeds, French dressing.

Celery stalk and leaves, chopped walnuts.

Fresh pimento, celery, ground parsley, multiplying-onion tops.

Seedless grapes, diced cantaloupe; serve with yogurt dressing.


## AVOCADO SALADS

As soon as an avocado is cut, sprinkle or brush with vinegar, lemon or tomato juice, or French dressing to prevent discoloration. Use a large proportion of avocado combined with the following ingredients, sprinkle with salt, and serve on a bed of greens with French dressing:

Fill halves with chicken, crab, shrimp, or fish salad.

Fill halves with grapefruit and orange sections; garnish with diced fresh or canned pimento.

Pile in alternate layers sliced tomato, paper-thin slices of leek or sweet onion, rings of avocado sliced crosswise; if salad is main luncheon dish, put stuffed egg in center of top avocado slice or serve with cottage cheese.

Arrange in a circle on a flat plate orange or grapefruit slices alternating with avocado rings, thin slices of leek or sweet onion; in the center place cheese balls rolled in ground nuts.

On a bed of greens, alternate rings of avocado and unpeeled California persimmon; or cut both in wedges; if persimmons are extremely soft, freeze whole in freezing tray, slice, and serve frozen. This is a beautiful and delicious salad.

Combine grapefruit sections, wedges of avocado, and persimmon.

Alternate rings of avocado with slices of oranges; have an orange slice on top and garnish with mint leaves.

Add diced or sliced avocado to any tossed salad (p. 298).

Mix large dices of avocado with pineapple cubes and chopped ripe olives.

Slice tomatoes and avocado on a bed of endive; add ⅓ cup cottage cheese seasoned with chives to each serving; garnish with chives.

## CABBAGE SALADS

Shred very thin or chop fine all cabbage to be used for salads. Use Chinese cabbage and savoy cabbage when available. Combine following ingredients, using a large proportion of cabbage; salt to taste:

Equal amounts of green and purple cabbage; season with onions, celery, dill or caraway seeds, chives, or Chinese garlic; serve with yogurt dressing.

Green cabbage, chopped onion, tomato wedges, sliced cucumber, minced clove garlic; toss with oil and tarragon vinegar or mix with yogurt dressing or mayonnaise.

Shredded carrots, savoy cabbage, fresh or canned pimento, chopped onion, ground parsley; stir with mayonnaise or Thousand Island dressing.

Shredded cabbage, diced apricots, orange sections, celery salt; serve with French dressing.

Shredded purple cabbage, diced celery stalks and leaves, young rutabaga fingers, fresh marjoram leaves; toss with oil and vinegar. (Oil should always come first.)

Shredded cabbage, quartered tomatoes, chopped green peppers, sliced cucumbers, minced fresh basil; mix with yogurt or sour cream.

Shredded green cabbage, diced pineapple, apple, and/or banana, a few peanuts, 5 or 6 fresh mint leaves; stir with mayonnaise.

Shredded cabbage, chopped green pepper, grated onion or chopped chives, chopped dill pickle; stir with mayonnaise.

## CARROT SALADS

Combine the following ingredients with a large proportion of chilled unpeeled carrots which have been grated or shredded; serve on a bed of greens.

Sliced stuffed olives, diced red apple, a few celery seeds, mayonnaise.

Drained crushed pineapple, a small amount of raisins, French dressing.

Ground parsley, chopped fresh or canned pimento, a few leaves of savory.

Chopped green pepper or diced red apple, 2 or 3 mint leaves, mayonnaise.

Shredded cabbage, chives or onion, ground parsley.

Chopped bell pepper, celery, onion, ground parsley.

Diced raw chayote, avocado, green pepper.

## CUCUMBER SALADS

If cucumbers are tender and thinly sliced, the skins are usually palatable enough to be left on. Cucumbers with skins lacking bitterness are now available and should be raised or purchased when possible. The atrocious habit of soaking cucumbers in vinegar should be avoided; slice them just before they are to be served. Combine the ingredients listed below in any amount desired, using cucumbers as the principal ingredient; season with salt and pepper, and serve on shredded spinach, mustard, watercress, or other greens.

Green pepper and pimento rings, sliced leeks or paper-thin slices of sweet onions; a few minced leaves of marjoram; serve with French dressing.

Shoestring sticks of small cucumbers, kohlrabi, unpeeled carrots, turnips, lettuce, 4 to 6 minced basil leaves; toss with oil, vinegar, a small amount of Worcestershire.

Moisten cucumber slices with tarragon vinegar; sprinkle with salt, paprika, celery salt.

Mix cucumber, radish, and thin carrot slices with sour cream; add a few drops Tabasco; sprinkle with dill seeds.

Mix equal amounts of sliced cucumber and sweet onion; fold into 1 cup sour cream or commercial yogurt.

Slice radishes, cucumbers, raw turnips; add a small amount of chopped fresh dill; serve with yogurt dressing.

Slice green onions and cut the tops with scissors; combine with sliced tomatoes, cucumbers, and a few minced leaves of basil; serve with a tart French dressing.

Sprinkle cucumbers with caraway, cumin, or dill seeds; serve with yogurt dressing mixed generously with chives.

See cucumber aspic (p. 287), cucumber aspic with sour cream (p. 287), cabbage-cucumber aspic (p. 287), pineapple-cucumber-cheese aspic (p. 288), cucumber-pineapple aspic (p. 290).

Bell peppers and fresh pimentos and paprikas are of such outstanding nutritional value that a baby should be allowed to cut his teeth on them, and everyone should eat them like apples. They should be added to all vegetable salads. As soon as the taste for these peppers has been cultivated, they should be served whole in salads in the same way that whole tomatoes are served stuffed or cut in petal fashion.

Since the vitamin C content of bell peppers doubles on ripening, use red ones when available instead of green ones. I frequently find that persons unaccustomed to eating ripe bell peppers imagine them to be hot. Actually they are much sweeter and more mild than green ones. Moreover, their beautiful color is reason enough for adding them generously to salads.

## STUFFED BELL PEPPER SALAD

Remove the tops and centers from:

4 large red or green bell peppers, paprikas, or pimentos

Combine and mix well:

| | |
|---|---|
| 2 cups (1 pound) cottage cheese, sieved hoop cheese, or grated American cheese | 2 tablespoons chives cut with scissors |
| 1 small grated onion or leek or | ¼ cup milk or salad dressing |

Stuff cheese filling into each pepper; chill, serve whole or slice crosswise, and arrange on salad greens, using 1 pepper for each serving.

Garnish centers with **paprika.**

*Variations:*

Instead of cheese fill peppers with any fish, chicken, or meat salad.

Omit the cheese and make a filling by combining 1½ cups shredded carrots or cabbage, ½ cup drained crushed pineapple; add 2 tablespoons mayonnaise.

Fill the peppers with any cabbage salad (p. 277).

**Bell pepper-watercress salad:** Combine 3 diced green or red bell peppers with 1 bunch shredded watercress, 1 grated onion, ½ cup or more yogurt dressing.

**Paprika-cucumber salad:** Combine 1 cup each diced cucumbers and leeks, add fresh paprika; add minced clove garlic, ½ teaspoon salt, ¼ cup tart French dressing. Serve on a bed of endive.

**Pimento-cabbage salad:** Combine 1 cup diced fresh pimentos, 2 cups finely shredded cabbage, 1 minced clove garlic, 1 grated onion, ½ teaspoon salt, ⅓ cup mayonnaise. Serve on a bed of Bibb lettuce.

**Pimento-carrot salad:** Combine 1 cup each shredded fresh pimentos and raw carrots, ½ cup chopped leeks, ¼ cup ground parsley, 1 teaspoon salt, ¾ cup sour cream.

## COMBINATION TOMATO SALAD

Cut in half crosswise:

### 2 large tomatoes

Place tomato halves cut side up over **lettuce leaves** on individual salad plates.

Lay across top of each half **4 or 5 steamed or canned asparagus tips.**

Cut chilled **green or red peppers** into **¼-inch rings** and put over tomatoes and asparagus.

Serve with French dressing or mayonnaise.

*Variations:*

Add slices of 1 hard-cooked egg to each serving.

If salad is main dish for lunch, serve with sliced eggs and cottage cheese.

Instead of asparagus use fingers of carrot, turnip, kohlrabi, or stalks of broccoli, chard, cabbage, cauliflower, or tampala.

Omit asparagus and add marinated tips of broccoli bud or cauliflowerlets.

Cut 4 whole, unpeeled tomatoes toward the stem end into 6 or 8 petals; set tomatoes on a bed of mixed greens, separate the petals slightly, and put into center of each 1 tablespoon mayonnaise. Vary by filling centers of tomatoes with cottage or mashed cream cheese or chopped hard-cooked eggs generously garnished with parsley; any meat or fish salad; or place ½ deviled egg in the center of each tomato.


## SLICED TOMATOES

Border a salad bowl with **lettuce** or **endive** and slice in alternate layers:

**4 large tomatoes**                     **1 large cucumber**
**2 or 3 leeks or 1 large sweet onion**

Pour over salad:

### ¼ cup French dressing

Garnish with **ground parsley,** cover bowl, and let stand in refrigerator 15 minutes before serving.

*Variations:*

Sprinkle over tomatoes 1 teaspoon minced fresh or a pinch of dried basil, tarragon, or orégano.

Put slices of avocado over tomatoes, and/or rings of bell pepper, pimentos, or paprikas over cucumbers.

Add a layer of any of the following vegetables cut into paper-thin slices: raw carrots, turnips, kohlrabi, rutabagas, beets; shredded raw cauliflower; tender buds of broccoli, shredded stalks of cabbage, cauliflower, tampala, chard.

## STUFFED TOMATOES

Cut ½-inch slice from stem end of:

### 4 large unpeeled tomatoes

Remove pulp, chop, and combine with:

| | |
|---|---|
| **1 diced cucumber** | **½ teaspoon salt** |
| **1 small grated onion** | **¼ cup mayonnaise** |

Put filling into salted tomato and serve on **shredded spinach** or **mustard-spinach**.

*Variations:*

Add any chopped leftover vegetables to the filling.

Fill tomatoes with any meat or fish salad (p. 235).

Instead of cucumber use 1 cup shredded carrots, turnips, or kohlrabi; finely diced celery, tart apple, or green pepper; or tender buds and diced stalk of raw broccoli or cauliflower.

Make filling of ½ cup each diced celery and apple, 1 tablespoon grated onion or chopped chives, 2 tablespoons mayonnaise.

All varieties of cheese may be added to any kind of salad. The following salads are particularly advantageous for persons who need a high-protein or a high-calcium diet, as do adolescents, expectant mothers, convalescents, women during menopause, and persons preparing for surgery. Salads of ground vegetables and cheese are excellent for babies, persons who cannot chew well, and persons who must live on smooth diets. When cheese is a principal ingredient of a salad, a mild-flavored cheese should be used.

## COTTAGE CHEESE WITH GREENS

Combine the following ingredients:

| | |
|---|---|
| 2 cups cottage cheese | 2 tablespoons chives |
| ¼ cup ground parsley | 1 chopped pimento (optional) |
| ½ cup ground spinach and/or | 2 drops Tabasco |
| ½ cup shredded carrots | ½ teaspoon each salt and Worcestershire |

Serve on a bed of watercress, shredded young mustard greens, tampala, or Bibb lettuce.

Top with:

mayonnaise, French, or Thousand Island dressing, dash of paprika

*Variations:*

Decrease or increase amount of parsley and spinach used, or add any other ground or finely shredded greens.

Instead of cottage cheese use 3 to 6 ounces mashed cream cheese; 2 cups sieved hoop cheese, or dry cottage cheese; or shredded American, Swiss, or Jack cheese, blended with enough milk, mayonnaise, or dill sauce to hold together.

Instead of parsley and spinach use a combination of leaves such as mustard and spinach; New Zealand spinach and celery stalk and leaves; ground leaves from pea vines and parsley; watercress and tampala; Bibb lettuce and mustard-spinach; tampala and Chinese cabbage; celery stalk and leaves and green-onion tops.

Omit chives; add green onions and tops cut with scissors, and fresh dill.

**Cheese-avocado salad:** Mash 1 avocado, add 1 grated onion, combine with other ingredients.

**Cheese-carrot salad:** Omit spinach and use 1 cup shredded unpeeled carrots; or add crushed pineapple with carrots and omit chives.

**Cheese-fruit salad:** Omit chives and serve salad on 1 banana cut lengthwise, 1 slice of pineapple, 2 apricot halves, or a canned or fresh peach or pear half placed on a bed of watercress.

**Cheese-green pepper salad:** Add ¼ cup or more chopped green pepper to basic recipe, or use instead of spinach or carrot. Vary by using chopped fresh pimento or by combining shredded kohlrabi and any finely chopped fresh peppers with shredded American cheese; add other ingredients and seasonings of basic recipe; or season with 1 teaspoon dill sauce.

**Cheese-pea salad:** Omit parsley or spinach and add ¾ cup ground raw peas or leaves from pea vines. Use Jack, cottage, or cream cheese.

**Cheese-tomato salad:** Omit carrots; use 1 cup spinach, ground with a few leaves of fresh basil; serve with slices of tomato on a bed of watercress.

**Cheese-watercress salad:** Omit carrots and/or spinach; add 1 cup chopped watercress to basic recipe. Vary by using shredded Swiss or pimento cheese.


## FRUIT SALADS

Fruit salads should be served at lunch or at the end of the dinner course except when they are combined with a generous amount of vegetables.

Salads can be made of almost any single fruit or a combination of two or more fruits. When only canned fruit is available for salads, use individual salad plates covered with a generous quantity of shredded greens. If fresh fruits are used, place them attractively between the curved leaves of head lettuce or on a bed of romaine or crisp watercress. Following are suggestions for fruit salads to be served on individual plates.

Fresh or canned peach, apricot, or pear halves; serve with French dressing; vary by adding cottage cheese or cream-cheese balls (p. 274), by sprinkling with walnuts, pecans, or shredded coconut, or by serving with sour cream, yogurt, or peanut-butter dressing (p. 294).

Sliced fresh or canned peaches or sliced bananas, diced celery, ½ cup walnuts; combine with cream dressing.

Cut firm peaches into bite sizes; combine with mayonnaise and any one of the following fruits: seedless grapes, diced honeydew melon, firm plums, fresh or canned apricots, sliced bananas, diced pineapple, orange sections, diced grapefruit sections, white cherries, unpeeled diced apples or pears. Instead of peaches use fresh apricots cut into sixths.

Fresh or canned apricot quarters, seeded black cherries, cream dressing.

Cut California persimmons crosswise into ½-inch slices; arrange on a bed of crisp watercress; serve with tart French dressing. This is the most beautiful salad I know of and one of the most delicious.

Firm purple plums, diced cantaloupe, honeydew, or Persian melon; serve with French dressing or cream dressing.

Cut bananas in half lengthwise; sprinkle with chopped peanuts, walnuts, pecans, or coconut; or omit nuts and serve with cottage cheese or balls of cream cheese; use French or cream dressing; if nuts are not added, serve with peanut-butter dressing.

Cover a whole banana with cream cheese ¼ inch thick; roll in ground nuts; slice and serve with French dressing on a bed of watercress.

Slice bananas ½ inch thick; combine with cream dressing or mayonnaise and seedless grapes, white cherries, apricots, or other fruits suggested under peach salads.

## FRUIT SALAD BOWL

Line a salad bowl attractively with the leaves of:

### 1 head romaine lettuce

Arrange in alternate layers:

**2 cups fresh or canned pineapple, diced or sliced**
**2 cups grapefruit sections**

**1 red apple cut into thin wedges**
**1 cup seeded or seedless grapes**
**2 sliced oranges**

Garnish with **black or maraschino cherries** and serve with mayonnaise or fruit dressing.

*Variations:*

Sprinkle with anise or poppy seeds.

Use equal amounts of each fruit; arrange separately on a platter over lettuce or watercress. Garnish with sprigs of fresh mint.

Omit any one fruit and add slices of chilled banana moistened with lemon juice.

Omit pineapple and grapefruit; combine grapes, apples, orange sections with fresh or canned cherries or sliced bananas, a few leaves of chopped mint or lemon balm.

Combine in layers diced unpeeled pears, red raspberries, sliced bananas.

Substitute one of the following for any fruit suggested: fresh whole strawberries; diced cantaloupe, honeydew, or Persian melon; fresh or canned apricots and/or peaches; seeded tangerine sections; firm or frozen California persimmon; fresh figs; dices of avocado.

**Grapefruit salad:** Combine 2 to 3 cups grapefruit sections, ½ cup chopped almonds, 1 green pepper or pimento cut into strips. Serve on a bed of endive with Roquefort-cheese dressing.

**Orange-green pepper salad:** Cover individual salad plates with romaine lettuce; alternate on lettuce sections of orange or grapefruit, wedges of unpeeled pear, pieces of green pepper. Serve with mayonnaise.

**Pear salad:** Arrange fresh or canned unpeeled pear halves on lettuce; cover with cottage or cream cheese and cherries, strawberries, or youngberries; serve with yogurt or fruit dressing.

**Stuffed-prune salad:** Remove stones from steamed dried prunes or spiced prunes; stuff with cream cheese mixed with nuts, parsley, or pimento; arrange on orange slices on a bed of watercress.

## MELON SALADS

Combine the following ingredients in any amounts desired and serve on individual salad plates or from salad bowl on a bed of lettuce, romaine, watercress, or endive:

Grapefruit sections, diced slices of cantaloupe or honeydew or Persian melon, topped with cottage cheese.

Unstemmed strawberries, cubes or balls of cantaloupe or Persian melon; serve with fruit dressing.

Melon balls or diced slices, white grapes, fresh peach, sliced canned or fresh pineapple; serve with mayonnaise.

Cantaloupe and/or honeydew balls, pineapple cubes, Brazil or hazelnuts or toasted almonds.

## GELATIN SALADS

The liquid used in making gelatin salads should be as rich as possible in vitamins and minerals; hence I have recommended vegetable-cooking water in the basic aspic recipe. When rose-hip extract is available or calcium-rich lemon juice (p. 239) is prepared, either should be used instead of part of the vegetable-cooking water. The gelatin used most frequently should be the unflavored and unsweetened variety. If sweetened gelatin is used, or if much fruit is added, the sugar content becomes so high that such a salad should be served as a substitute for dessert. Raw pineapple and papaya contain enzymes which quickly digest protein; hence they must not be used in a gelatin salad unless they are heated to boiling.

If any of the following salads are to be given to a baby, a person who has difficulty in chewing, or one on a smooth diet, the solid ingredients may be ground.

## ASPIC FOR VEGETABLE SALADS

Combine in aluminum measuring cup:

1 tablespoon unflavored gelatin      ½ cup vegetable-cooking water

Let gelatin soften for 5 minutes and dissolve by heating over simmer burner; pour into mixing bowl and add:

| | |
|---|---|
| 1¼ cups vegetable-cooking water | 1 tablespoon or more grated onion |
| ¼ cup vinegar or fresh lemon juice | 3 tablespoons ground parsley |
| 1 teaspoon salt | 1 diced bell pepper or pimento |
| 1 to 3 teaspoons sugar | ½ teaspoon freshly ground white peppercorns |

Chill until gelatin starts to thicken and add any combination of vegetables and seasonings listed below.

Taste for seasonings; pour into a ring mold brushed lightly with oil. Chill and unmold by turning on edge and tapping lightly to loosen sides.

Serve on a bed of watercress, endive, romaine, lettuce, or mixed chopped greens with a small bowl of dressing in center.

*Variations:*

Instead of ¼ cup vegetable-cooking water substitute ¼ cup rose-hip extract (p. 489) or calcium-rich lemon juice (p. 239).

### Add to the basic recipe any of the following ingredients and seasonings:

**Artichoke jellied ring:** Substitute French dressing for vinegar; remove pulp from leaves of 4 steamed artichokes and combine with chopped artichoke hearts; add 2 diced hard-cooked eggs, ¼ cup sliced stuffed olives. Omit or use less salt if olives are included. Serve with center filled with fish or meat salad.

**Asparagus aspic:** ½ cup young raw asparagus tips cut into ⅛-inch slices, ½ cup celery, ½ teaspoon mustard seed, 2 tablespoons mayonnaise.

**Aspic of Brussels sprouts:** Increase onion and pimento to ¼ cup each; add 1 cup finely shredded raw Brussels sprouts and 1 teaspoon caraway seeds heated as gelatin dissolves.

**Beet aspic:** 1 cup finely shredded raw beets; use green pepper instead of pimento; tarragon or marjoram vinegar.

**Broccoli aspic:** 1 cup shredded tender buds and diced stalk of broccoli; use ½ cup finely diced leeks or increase onion.

**Cabbage aspic:** 1 cup finely shredded green cabbage; increase diced pimento to ¼ cup; add ¼ cup celery, dash of cayenne, fresh dill or 1 teaspoon dill sauce. Vary by using ¾ cup each shredded green and purple cabbage or by steeping 2 teaspoons dill or caraway seeds in warm gelatin.

**Cabbage-cucumber aspic:** ¾ cup each shredded purple cabbage and diced cucumber.

**Carrot aspic:** 1½ cups shredded carrots; or 1 cup shredded carrot and ½ cup drained crushed pineapple; omit onion if pineapple is used.

**Cauliflower aspic:** 1 cup finely shredded cauliflower, ¼ cup each pimento and chopped leeks or sweet onions.

**Chard aspic:** ½ cup each shredded young green chard and rhubarb chard, using leaves and stalks; increase onion and green pepper to ¼ cup each; use wine or tarragon vinegar.

**Cucumber aspic:** 1½ cups diced cucumber, ¼ cup chopped celery; a few drops of green coloring.

**Cucumber aspic with sour cream:** 1½ cups diced cucumber; use ½ cup sour cream or yogurt instead of ½ cup vegetable-cooking water; add 2 tablespoons chives or Chinese garlic cut fine with scissors.

**Dandelion aspic:** ½ cup shredded young dandelion greens, 2 sliced or diced hard-cooked eggs, 3 or more tablespoons Roquefort or Neufchatel cheese; instead of vinegar use ¼ cup French dressing.

**Green-pepper aspic:** Before adding vegetables pour gelatin to depth of ¼ inch in a flat mold; slice 2 eggs into gelatin and let chill; into remaining gelatin stir 2 tablespoons diced ripe olives, 1 cup chopped green peppers, ¼ cup each chopped pimentos, celery and leaves; pour into mold when gelatin holding eggs has congealed.

**Mixed greens in aspic:** Shred spinach, New Zealand spinach, watercress, chard, tampala, and assorted greens, making 1½ cups in all; use ¼ cup chopped onion or leek; a few fresh basil leaves.

**Mustard greens in aspic:** Select tender young mustard greens or use mustard-spinach; shred and add 1 cup with 1 cup cottage cheese.

**Tomato aspic I:** Instead of vegetable-cooking water use tomato juice; add 3 tablespoons chili sauce, 1 to 3 teaspoons horseradish, 1 teaspoon minced fresh basil, a few drops red coloring, and the other ingredients of basic recipe.

**Tomato aspic II:** Use tomato juice instead of vegetable-cooking water; add 1 to 3 teaspoons Worcestershire, 3 drops Tabasco, 1 teaspoon horseradish.

**Turnip aspic:** 1 cup shredded young turnips or turnip tops, ¼ cup each diced onion and pimento; add 1 teaspoon caraway seeds softened with gelatin, or season with fresh dill.

**Watercress aspic:** 1½ cups shredded leaves and diced stalk of watercress; or use ¾ cup each watercress and grapefruit sections.

Gelatin salads are especially attractive when made of two or more layers of contrasting colors. Almost any two recipes may be combined provided the colors and flavors harmonize. The mold used must be large enough to hold a quart or more, and each layer must be thoroughly chilled before the next layer is added. Such salads are easy to make if the gelatin and liquids are accurately measured, and are particularly desirable when serving a large group.

## PINEAPPLE-CUCUMBER-CHEESE ASPIC

Put into aluminum measuring cup:

2½ tablespoons unflavored gelatin      ¾ cup cleared, cold vegetable-cooking water

Soak 10 minutes and heat over the simmer burner until the gelatin is clear; stir thoroughly.

Add exactly ⅓ cup of dissolved gelatin to:

### 2 cups crushed pineapple and juice

Stir and pour into a large mold brushed lightly with oil; chill quickly. Meanwhile combine ⅓ cup of dissolved gelatin with:

1½ cups clear vegetable-cooking      1 teaspoon salt
water                                2 tablespoons mayonnaise
1 cup diced cucumbers                1 to 3 drops green coloring
1 tablespoon grated onion

Chill, but do not allow to congeal.
Add remaining gelatin to:

2 packages mashed cream cheese      1 teaspoon dill sauce (optional)
½ cup milk

Stir well, and add cheese as soon as pineapple has set; when cheese layer has set, add gelatin containing cucumbers; chill thoroughly.

Unmold by turning on edge and tapping to loosen gelatin from the sides of the mold; put large plate over mold, turn upside down; surround with lettuce, romaine, or sprigs of watercress.

*Variations:*

Use combinations of recipes on page 287 for layers containing pineapple and cucumbers; add to the cheese ½ tablespoon gelatin softened in ¼ cup water.

Instead of cream cheese use 2 cups shredded American cheese blended with ¾ cup milk.

**Apricot-grape aspic:** Proceed as in basic recipe and stir ⅓ cup of the dissolved gelatin with 1¾ cups apricot purée and ½ cup orange or grapefruit sections; pour into mold and chill; add ⅓ cup of dissolved gelatin to 1¾ cups Concord grape juice; add the remaining gelatin to cream cheese, omitting dill; add and chill a layer of cheese before chilling grape juice. This salad is both beautiful and delicious.

**Carrot-cabbage aspic:** Soak 2 tablespoons gelatin in ½ cup vegetable-cooking water and heat to dissolve; combine 1½ cups each cold vegetable-cooking water and shredded carrots; add ¼ cup French dressing and ¼ cup of dissolved gelatin; taste for salt, pour into a mold, chill. Combine remaining gelatin with 1½ cups each finely shredded green cabbage and vegetable-cooking water, 1 teaspoon salt, ⅓ cup mayonnaise, 3 tablespoons grated onion. When carrot gelatin is firmly set, add cabbage gelatin and chill. Vary by using gelatin measurements in basic recipe and divide the layers with cream cheese; or substitute any other diced or shredded vegetables for carrots and cabbage.

**Celery-beet aspic:** Dissolve gelatin as in basic recipe; combine ⅓ cup of dissolved gelatin with 1½ cups vegetable-cooking water, 1 cup finely diced celery, 1 each chopped green pepper and leek or sweet onion; add green coloring, ¼ cup tarragon vinegar, 1 teaspoon each sugar and salt; pour into a mold and chill. Combine ⅓ cup of dissolved gelatin with 1½ cups each vegetable-cooking water and shredded raw beets, ¼ cup tart French dressing, 1 teaspoon each salt, sugar, and ground horseradish. Combine remaining gelatin with 2 cups grated Swiss cheese, ¾ cup cold milk, 1 or 2 teaspoons caraway seeds. When celery gelatin has chilled, add and chill layer of cheese; finally add layer of shredded beets.

**Pineapple-avocado aspic:** Follow basic recipe except to omit cucumbers and onion. Arrange slices of chilled avocado attractively in a thin layer of gelatin on oiled mold; chill; add the green gelatin mixed with 1 cup diced avocado; add cheese layer; add pineapple last.

**Tomato-cucumber aspic:** Prepare as in basic recipe except to omit pineapple and combine ⅓ cup of dissolved gelatin with 1¾ cups salted tomato juice or purée, 1 teaspoon Worcestershire, 1 grated onion. Mold cucumber gelatin first; add layer of cheese, and finally tomato aspic.

## ASPIC FOR FRUIT SALADS

Soften for 5 minutes:

1 tablespoon unflavored gelatin in      ½ cup cold pineapple, grapefruit,
                                          or apple juice

Heat slowly over simmer burner until gelatin is dissolved; add:

1¼ cups chilled pineapple, grape-     pinch of salt
fruit, or apple juice                 ¼ cup fresh lemon or lime juice

Stir well, and chill until gelatin starts to congeal; add any group of ingredients listed below.

Pour into a mold brushed lightly with oil. Chill and unmold by turning
on edge and tapping to loosen sides; or mold in shallow pan, cut into
cubes, and serve on individual salad plates on a bed of **lettuce or watercress.**

*Variations:*

Instead of juices suggested use unsweetened apricot, orange, grape, or
berry juice, or sweetened plum juice, or any thin fruit purée.

**Apricot and prune aspic:** Add 1 cup sliced fresh or canned apricots,
½ cup cooked pitted prunes.

**Banana aspic:** Add 2 diced bananas mixed with lemon juice of basic
recipe, ½ cup seedless grapes or sliced cherimoyas or guavas.

**Carrot-pineapple aspic:** Add 1 cup grated carrots, ½ cup crushed
drained pineapple.

**Cheese-apricot aspic:** Add ¾ cup each fresh or canned apricot wedges
and cottage cheese.

**Cherimoya aspic:** Add 1 cup sliced cherimoyas and ½ cup seedless
grapes, sliced peaches, pears, or guavas.

**Cranberry-pineapple aspic:** Add 1 cup ground raw cranberries, ½ cup
crushed pineapple, ¼ cup sugar, 1 teaspoon orange rind; or omit pineapple and use 1½ cups cranberries sweetened to taste.

**Cucumber-pineapple aspic:** Add ½ cup crushed pineapple, 1 cup diced
cucumber, 1 tablespoon chopped pimento, few drops green coloring.

**Mixed fruit aspic:** Dice 1½ cups of any firm fresh fruits and/or well-
drained canned fruits; or use 1 cup diced fruit and ½ cup broken nuts or
shredded watercress or other greens.

**Sapote and melon aspic:** Add ½ cup sliced sapote, 1 cup cantaloupe,
honeydew, or Persian melon cubes or balls.

**Watercress and grapefruit aspic:** Add 1 cup each grapefruit sections
and shredded watercress.

## LIME AND COTTAGE CHEESE SALAD

Dissolve 1 package of lime gelatin in:

¾ cup boiling vegetable-cooking water, unsalted and cleared with egg-shells (p. 310)

Stir well and add:

1¼ cups cold vegetable-cooking water    pinch of salt

Chill until gelatin starts to congeal; add:

2 diced fresh or canned pimentos    1 pound cottage cheese

Pour into ring mold brushed lightly with oil; chill until set; to unmold, set on edge and tap to loosen gelatin from sides; surround with curly endive and serve with a tart French dressing.

*Variations:*

Add 1 cup diced cucumbers, ½ teaspoon salt.

Instead of cottage cheese add 1 cup grated American, Swiss, or Jack cheese, or 1 pound sieved hoop cheese.

Use orange or lemon gelatin instead of lime.

Cranberry aspic: Omit pimentos and cheese; substitute cherry gelatin for lime and add 1 cup ground raw cranberries (½ pound before grinding), 1 small orange ground with ½ cup nuts, ½ to ¾ cup sugar, 1 teaspoon grated lemon rind.

Orange gelatin with avocado: Use orange gelatin instead of lime; before adding cottage cheese pour warm gelatin into a mold with flat base to depth of ¼ inch; chill until it starts to congeal and arrange slices of avocado attractively in gelatin; add the cheese and pimentos to the remaining gelatin and pour into mold.

Raspberry gelatin with beets: Add 1 tablespoon each grated onion and green pepper and 1½ cups grated raw beets to raspberry gelatin; prepare as in the basic recipe; add or omit cheese and pimento.

Raspberries and pineapple in aspic: Omit cottage cheese and pimento of the basic recipe; use raspberry gelatin; add ½ cup each crushed drained pineapple and fresh or frozen raspberries.

Strawberry gelatin with grapefruit: Add 1 cup grapefruit sections to strawberry gelatin; prepare as in basic recipe; add or omit cheese.

Two-tone salads: Prepare orange gelatin to which is added 1 cup grapefruit sections; pour into a mold holding 1½ quarts and chill; when set, pour on it a salad prepared as in basic recipe. Combine any two salads of contrasting colors and blending flavors; prepare both at the same time, but keep at room temperature the color which is to be at the bottom of the mold when served; after the first color has set, add the other.

## COOKED SALAD DRESSING

Mix in a saucepan:

| | |
|---|---|
| 1 tablespoon whole-wheat pastry flour | 2 eggs |
| | 2 tablespoons margarine or butter |
| 1 teaspoon each salt and dry mustard | 1 clove garlic |
| | 1 cup top milk or evaporated milk |
| 1 to 3 teaspoons sugar | |

Stir continually while simmering until it is thick; use cooking thermometer and heat only to 185° F.; *do not boil;* cool, and beat in:

⅓ cup vinegar or lemon juice

Store in covered jar in refrigerator.

*Variations:*

Vary by using tarragon or wine vinegar or any vinegar seasoned with herbs; or use ¼ cup vinegar or lemon juice and add 2 tablespoons sherry.

Add any of the following: 1 chopped cucumber and/or 2 tablespoons chopped onion, ground parsley; green or red bell pepper, or pimento, or ¼ cup chopped celery; ½ cup minced cooked ham or ¼ cup peanut butter.

Cream dressing: Omit garlic; use 1 or 2 tablespoons sugar; add ½ cup whipped evaporated milk or whipped cream. Serve on fruit salads.

Fruit dressing: Use lemon juice; omit garlic; instead of milk use grapefruit, pineapple, or orange juice with 1 teaspoon grated orange or lemon rind.

Sour-cream dressing: When cold, add 1 cup whipped sour cream, few grains of cayenne.

Thousand Island dressing: Add 3 or more tablespoons each chopped sour or dill pickle, ground parsley, chili sauce; 1 chopped hard-cooked egg.

## FRENCH DRESSING

Combine in a pint jar:

¾ cup salad oil
¼ cup vinegar or lemon juice
¼ cup catsup or chili sauce
1 teaspoon honey or sugar
1 clove garlic cut in half

1 teaspoon salt
½ teaspoon paprika
¼ teaspoon freshly ground white
peppercorns

Cover jar and shake until ingredients are well blended; keep in refrigerator or a cool place; shake well each time before using.

*Variations:*

If tart dressing is desired, use ½ cup oil to ¼ cup vinegar or lemon juice.

Add any one or more of the following. 4 to 6 drops Tabasco; 1 finely chopped onion or leek; ⅛ teaspoon curry powder or celery salt; 1 teaspoon dry mustard; 2 or more tablespoons chopped red or green bell pepper or pimento; 1 or 2 tablespoons chopped chives, Chinese garlic, freshly ground horseradish, or chutney; 2 tablespoons each finely chopped celery and onion; 2 tablespoons anchovy paste; 1 tablespoon Worcestershire.

Use tarragon or wine vinegar; or before making dressing add to vinegar 1 or 2 tablespoons minced fresh or ½ teaspoon dry basil, burnet, marjoram, orégano, or other herb or combination of herbs; heat vinegar to simmering, cool, and strain into other ingredients.

**Avocado dressing:** Omit or use catsup; instead of oil add 1 cup mashed avocado.

**Cheese dressing:** Add ¼ cup or more mashed cream cheese or crumbled Roquefort cheese; omit or use catsup.

**Cream dressing:** Omit catsup; combine ⅓ cup each oil and cream or evaporated milk; add 2 tablespoons vinegar or lemon juice and seasonings of basic recipe. Vary by adding 1 package mashed cream cheese.

**Olive dressing:** To ½ cup of basic recipe add 4 tablespoons chopped ripe olives or sliced stuffed olives, 1 tablespoon ground parsley, 1 chopped green pepper.

**Nut dressing:** Omit catsup and garlic; combine the seasonings with ½ cup oil, ¼ cup each lemon juice, and ground walnuts, pecans, other nuts, or peanut butter. Serve on fruit salads.

**Salad-seasoned vinegar:** Omit oil; double the amount of vinegar, combine with other ingredients, add 6 drops Tabasco, 1 teaspoon Worcestershire. Heat vinegar with fresh or dried herbs as directed above if desired. Use for tossed salads.

Tomato-soup dressing: Omit catsup and use ½ cup oil; combine 1 can condensed tomato soup with other ingredients of basic recipe; add 1 tablespoon Worcestershire, 1 teaspoon dry mustard, 1 tablespoon grated onion; increase vinegar or lemon juice if tart dressing is desired. Salt to taste.

## MAYONNAISE

Combine and beat together well:

2 egg yolks
1 teaspoon salt
4 tablespoons vinegar or lemon juice
⅛ teaspoon celery salt (optional)

1 to 3 teaspoons sugar
¼ to 1 teaspoon dry mustard
¼ teaspoon freshly ground white peppercorns

Add slowly, beating constantly:

1½ cups salad oil

Store in a cool place.

*Variations:*

To 1 cup mayonnaise add one of the following: ½ cup whipped evaporated milk or whipped cream; ½ cup chili sauce and 2 tablespoons chopped green or red bell pepper; ¼ cup chopped sour or dill pickle and 2 tablespoons chopped onion; 2 tablespoons each chopped sour pickle, sliced stuffed olives, capers, ground parsley; 1 teaspoon paprika and ¼ cup tomato catsup; ½ cup chopped cucumber; 2 to 4 tablespoons grated horseradish.

Cheese dressing: To 1 cup mayonnaise add ½ teaspoon Worcestershire, ¼ cup grated American or crumbled Roquefort cheese or 1 package mashed cream cheese. Vary by adding ½ cup chilled evaporated milk whipped with 2 tablespoons lemon juice.

Liver-sausage dressing: To ½ cup mayonnaise add ¼ cup mashed liver sausage, 1 tablespoon chopped chives, ¼ cup sliced stuffed olives or chopped pimento.

Peanut butter and banana dressing: To ½ cup mayonnaise add 1 mashed banana, 4 tablespoons peanut butter, ¼ cup cream or evaporated milk. Serve with fruit salads.

Thousand Island dressing: To 1 cup mayonnaise add ¼ cup each chopped mixed pickles and chili sauce, 2 diced hard-cooked eggs, 2 tablespoons each chopped pimentos and onion.

## REDUCING SALAD DRESSING

Chill in ice tray until crystals form around edges:

**½ cup evaporated milk**

Whip until thick, add the following ingredients, and beat slightly:

| | |
|---|---|
| 2 to 4 tablespoons lemon juice or<br>tarragon or wine vinegar<br>¼ to ½ teaspoon dry mustard<br>½ teaspoon salt | ½ to 1 teaspoon paprika<br>1 minced clove garlic<br>1 finely chopped or grated onion |

Let stand in refrigerator 15 minutes before serving.
Serve on head lettuce or any mixed-vegetable salad.

*Variations:*

Add 1 teaspoon minced fresh basil, marjoram, burnet, savory, or dill.
Omit garlic and onion; use 4 tablespoons lemon juice and serve on fruit salads.

Add any seasonings suggested under mayonnaise and French dressing.
Add 1 to 3 tablespoons mayonnaise or salad oil.

Add one or more of the following: 1 teaspoon Worcestershire; 3 drops Tabasco; 1 tablespoon catsup or chili sauce; ½ to 1 teaspoon curry powder; 1 teaspoon caraway, cumin, or dill seeds.

Substitute 1 cup condensed tomato soup for evaporated milk; add seasonings of basic recipe.

**Cheese dressing:** Add to basic recipe 4 tablespoons shredded American cheese or crumbled Roquefort cheese.

**Sour-cream dressing:** Instead of evaporated milk add seasonings of basic recipe to 1 cup sour cream; or use sour cream as a dressing without adding seasonings. Serve on moderately low-calorie diet instead of mayonnaise.

**Yogurt dressing:** Omit evaporated milk; add seasonings to commercial yogurt; omit vinegar or lemon juice if yogurt is tart. For fruit salad use yogurt without adding seasonings. This dressing is much lower in calories than is mayonnaise.

### THE MOST IMPORTANT RECIPE IN THE BOOK

If you learn nothing more from this book than a few pointers on making tossed salads (which were taught to me by a French chef), the years of work required to write it will be justified. Few

foods are so sinned against as are tossed salads. Haven't you seen
them mistreated to the point of disgust—watery, wilted, tasteless, greasy, or with the vegetables so chopped that they seem already to have been chewed? The reason tossed salads are often
abominably made, I believe, is that the "musts" in preparing
them are so simple that they are overlooked as being unimportant.
When you once get the knack of making them well and form the
habit of eating them daily, all other salads seem insipid. No other
salad can compare with them in nutritive value.

If a tossed salad is to be worthy of its name, the ingredients
*must* be free from clinging drops of moisture; whirl them well.
The salad oil *must* be added first. Previously prepared French
dressing *must not* be used. The leaves *must* be so well tossed that
each surface glistens with oil before lemon juice or vinegar and
seasonings are added. There are sound gastronomic and nutritional reasons for each of these rules.

Tossing a salad consists of gently picking up the ingredients between a fork and a spoon, preferably large and wooden, lifting
them 4 to 6 inches above the bowl, and whirling them slightly as
they are dropped. The purpose of tossing is to allow the oil, which
clings tenaciously to dry leaves, to seal the surfaces from oxygen,
which can destroy vitamins, and from moisture, which can soak
out vitamins, minerals, and flavor; to distribute and hold seasonings, which will adhere to the oil and give a delightful taste; and,
most important, to prevent salt from drawing moisture out of the
leaves, which causes them to wilt immediately and allows vitamins
and minerals to be lost in the juices left in the salad bowl.

If the leaves are not well whirled, if a moist ingredient is added
before the salad is tossed, or if French dressing is used so that the
vinegar moistens the ingredients, oil will not adhere to the leaves;
seasonings cannot be well distributed; the leaves wilt quickly; and
juices carrying delicious flavors, sugars, aromatic oils, vitamins,
and minerals are drawn out by the salt. The delightful crispness
and the delicious taste are soon gone and can never be recaptured.

Make your tossed salad a work of art by using contrasting colors
and by letting each ingredient retain its natural beauty as nearly
as possible. Break rather than shred such vegetables as lettuce,
endive, and Brussels sprouts. Leave the tips of watercress, New

Zealand spinach, and other tender greens in attractive sprigs. Cut bell peppers, fresh pimentos, and unpeeled tomatoes into fourths or sixths so that their color and texture can be seen. If foods are difficult to chew, as are carrots, rutabagas, Jerusalem artichokes, or kohlrabi, cut them into narrow strips like shoestring potatoes, which can be easily broken with a fork, yet can add vividness and beauty. If stalks contain stringy fibers, as do celery, chard, and watercress stems, cut them across the fibers into small pieces. Mince or shred only the foods which are disliked or are unfamiliar when eaten raw, such as raw beets, cauliflower, or broccoli.

The amount of oil used and the proportion of oil to vinegar or lemon juice should depend upon your family's taste and calorie needs. A single tablespoon of oil is sufficient to cover all surfaces of the leaves in a salad for a family of four, provided the salad is well tossed. If a high-calorie diet is desired, as much as 3 or 4 tablespoons of oil may be used to 1 tablespoon of vinegar or lemon juice. I personally use 3 tablespoons of oil to 2 of vinegar in making a large salad.

Perhaps it is only imagination, but it seems to me that a wooden salad bowl is essential in making wonderful tossed salads. The argument for such a bowl is that the pores in the wood hold and gradually free into the salad the aromatic oils from garlic and herbs. If you have such a bowl, above all do not wash it and clog the pores with soap; wipe it out with paper. If carefully cleaned without washing, it will keep fresh for years; the germicidal effect of garlic is probably responsible.

The ingredients in a tossed salad should depend on the likes and dislikes of your family; therefore I have avoided giving amounts in the following recipe. When once you have captured the knack of preparing delicious tossed salads, no recipes are needed.

The recipe for tossed salad is given in such detail that it will probably bore many persons. I beg of you to follow it patiently only once; after that you need never glance at it. With each salad you make, however, practice to develop beauty and speed.

Form the habit of serving a tossed salad almost daily throughout the year. Make the tossing of the salad a family ceremony carried out at the table, its design being to whet appetites and to add graciousness to everyday living.

## TOSSED SALAD

Set individual salad plates in refrigerator to chill.

Select, wash, and dry fresh herbs if available; cut a clove of garlic in half; crush well between the fingers or with a hammer; rub wooden salad bowl vigorously and thoroughly with herbs and garlic; mince and leave in bowl, or discard.

Chop or dice onions; cut chives, green-onion tops, and Chinese garlic with scissors; put into salad bowl.

Break lettuce, tips of watercress, or other tender leaves into salad bowl, leaving them in attractive pieces or sprigs.

Lay parallel on the chopping board all leaves, stalks, and stems with stringy fibers, such as spinach, chard, broccoli, celery, or watercress stems; shred all at the same time, cutting across the fibers; push from board into salad bowl.

Cut as shoestring potatoes and drop directly into bowl the raw root vegetables, broccoli stalk, or vegetables of solid texture; shred such vegetables as cauliflower, broccoli bud, and beets; slice cucumbers and radishes.

Add **2 to 5 heaping tablespoons ground parsley and/or other ground leaves,** any leftover vegetables to which no moisture clings, any diced leftover meat, flaked, steamed, or canned fish, or cubed solid cheese.

Add at the table or as early as 30 minutes before serving:

### 1 to 3 tablespoons vegetable oil

Toss 30 times if 1 tablespoon of oil is used, 20 times for 2 tablespoons, 15 times for 3 tablespoons; count tosses carefully and do not stop until all surfaces shine with oil; not earlier than 10 minutes before serving, add:

| | |
|---|---|
| 1 to 3 tablespoons vinegar or lemon juice | mustard, freshly ground horse-radish |
| 1 to 1½ teaspoons salt | cottage cheese or crumbled cream cheese |
| ¼ teaspoon freshly ground pepper-corns | moist ingredients such as tomatoes, grapefruit, canned pineapple, or canned asparagus tips |
| seasonings such as Tabasco, Worcestershire, dill sauce, dry | |

Toss 10 to 12 times; taste for seasonings; add any ingredient to remain on top as a garnish, such as sliced stuffed olives, hard-cooked eggs, or chips of Roquefort cheese; or any ingredient too soft to toss, such as ripe avocado or California persimmon; sprinkle with ground parsley and paprika and, if needed, salt.

Serve immediately or set in refrigerator until time to serve.

*Variations:*

Use tarragon or wine vinegar or any herb vinegar (p. 293); or use fresh lime juice instead of lemon juice.

Add any of the following seasonings with the vinegar or lemon juice: 1 or 2 tablespoons sherry, port, sauterne, or other wine; 2 or more tablespoons catsup, chili sauce, or other tomato sauce; ¼ cup yogurt, sour cream, or whipped sweet cream or evaporated milk; a dash of celery salt, paprika, curry powder, chili powder, or cayenne; chopped mixed pickles, anchovy paste, or chutney; 1 or 2 teaspoons mashed caraway, cumin, dill, or celery seeds; or add the combined seasonings of your favorite French dressing.

*Merely follow the basic recipe, using the raw vegetables suggested below as the principal ingredients:*

Endive, lettuce, fresh pimento, grapefruit sections, a pinch of celery seeds, chips of Roquefort cheese.

Spinach, onion, carrots, finely shredded purple cabbage, Chinese garlic; add freshly ground horseradish and 2 to 4 tablespoons yogurt after tossing; garnish with slices of hard-cooked eggs.

Watercress, tender dandelion greens, carrot sticks; a few nasturtium leaves and buds, fresh thyme, chervil, or burnet.

Bibb lettuce, kohlrabi, watercress, onion, celery, leaf and stalk of rhubarb chard; add 3 drops Tabasco, and 1 cup steamed veal brains (p. 115).

Diced uncooked broccoli stalks and buds, the large stalks peeled; lettuce, shredded beet tops or root, ground parsley, diced fresh pimento, fresh marjoram; add diced leftover ham if available.

Watercress, shredded raw cauliflower, endive, chives, garlic, stalk and leaves of rhubarb chard, shoestring carrots.

Young turnip tops, mustard greens, chicory, head lettuce, green pepper, shoestring sticks of raw rutabaga or turnip, cubes of American cheese.

Celery, romaine, Chinese cabbage or spinach, sliced radishes, turnip fingers, chives, cottage cheese; season with Worcestershire, mustard, celery seeds.

Chicory, mustard greens, romaine, sliced cucumbers, ground parsley, pimento rings, onion slices; add strips of cold tongue if desired.

Spinach, loose-leaf lettuce, Jerusalem artichoke, pimento, green onions, celery, a few leaves of fresh sage or thyme.

Shredded savoy cabbage, uncooked peas, thinly sliced zucchini, mustard-spinach, shoestring kohlrabi, tomato quarters, a few tarragon leaves.

Watercress, lettuce, celery, grapefruit, wedges of California persimmon.

Young dandelion leaves, watercress, sliced radishes, chives, mustard leaves, celery, cucumbers; add a few shrimps and dill sauce.

Kale, endive, broccoli bud and leaves, shredded raw beets, onion, celery; a few leaves each fresh of rosemary, basil, savory.

Watercress, lettuce, avocado, sections of tomato or grapefruit; add ¼ cup whipped evaporated milk with seasonings.

Young radish tops, lettuce, mustard-spinach, tomatoes, avocado, green onions, a few thyme or burnet leaves.

Swiss chard, mustard leaves, green onion, tomato quarters, green pepper, dices of Swiss cheese, a few fresh orégano leaves.

Young dandelions, shoestring carrots, sliced radishes, zucchini, celery and leaves, Bibb lettuce, red bell pepper or fresh paprika, Chinese garlic, chervil.

Chinese mustard, watercress, celery, avocado, shoestring carrots, pimento cheese, thin slices of Jerusalem artichoke.

Endive, spinach, watercress, chives, pimento, shoestring Jerusalem artichoke, carrot sticks, fresh dill.

Lettuce, celery, watercress, diced canned pineapple, cottage cheese.

Young collards, endive, chives, pimento, flaked fish, dill sauce.

Lettuce, Brussels sprouts, avocado, sliced leeks, radishes, tomatoes.

Chicory, watercress, dandelion greens or lamb's-quarters, garlic, bits of crisp bacon.

# CHAPTER 17

## SOUPS ARE FUN TO MAKE

Except for cream soups, little can be said in favor of soups as they are usually made. The flavor of the bones is incompletely extracted, the vegetables are generally watery and overcooked, and the nutritive value is close to nil. Delicious soups rich in vitamins and minerals can be made by improving the methods of preparing them and by imitating the thrifty French, famous for their soups. Before fresh vegetables are added, stock rich in flavor should be prepared. Soup stock may be defined as soup minus the vegetables; it is largely extract of bones and meat scraps. The success of the soup depends on the amount of flavor extracted into the stock. If you want excellent soup, be thrifty and go on a salvage drive. The more vegetables and bones you use in making soup stock, the more delicious the soup will be.

The first trick of making good soup stock is to save vegetable parings: tomato trimmings; pea hulls, washed before hulling; wilted stalks of celery and asparagus, tops of green onions, turnips, radishes, beets, and young carrots not eaten as greens or used in salads; wilted or outer leaves of lettuce, cabbage, spinach, chard, kale, parsley, and other greens; the peelings of squash, carrots, beets, turnips, cucumbers, rutabagas, kohlrabi, and any vegetable so shriveled or tough as to require peeling; unused stalks of cauliflower, cabbage, broccoli, and lettuce; the seeds and stems of peppers. Put nothing into the garbage except bits of vegetables actually decayed or impractical to clean, such as the rough peeling of celery root. Each time you prepare vegetables, keep all the parings and trimmings aside and put them directly into a large utility bag made of strong material sold for shower curtains; keep the bag in the refrigerator until it is bulging.

Second, save bones and meat scraps left on the plates after meals and from trimming meat before cooking it. Since the pasteurization point is 140° F. and the bones will be heated to 212° F. or a higher temperature, they will be as sterile as surgical gauze by the time the soup is made. Collect every variety of bones: pork, veal, lamb, beef, chicken, turkey, rabbit, and game. As the small bones and meat scraps accumulate, put them into another utility bag and keep them next to the freezing unit; whenever you have a large bone, such as a ham bone or a turkey carcass, make soup stock the following day.

Third, collect leftovers which are usually thrown into the garbage: vegetable salad left in the bowl and on the plates; cooked vegetables left on the plates; and any leftovers which cannot be used in other ways. These scraps will also be thoroughly sterilized. Before washing dishes, put these leftovers into a covered refrigerator dish. When parings, bones, meat scraps, and leftover salad and vegetables have accumulated, it is time to make soup, jellied bouillon, aspic, or a glazed meat served with jellied consommé.

The flavor and nutritive value gained from bones is proportional not only to the amount of bones used but also to the amount of bone surface exposed to heat and liquid, or to the size of the pieces into which the bones are sawed or chopped. A hatchet, a hardwood chopping board, and a meat saw are essential in making delicious and nutritious soups. Chop or saw the bones into as small pieces as possible; you will be rewarded by having a soup stock with a better flavor and a rich mineral content.

The minerals in bones are held in a base of connective tissue, like a solid bed of gristle the exact shape of the bones. Contrary to the purpose in cooking meats, the purpose in making soup is to break down the connective tissue from the bones and thereby extract the flavor and the gelatin. When connective tissue is submitted to heat, it combines with water and changes to gelatin, which, although not a complete protein, has food value and a rich flavor when unrefined. Although the customary method of making soup is to simmer it at 185° F., the connective tissue is changed to gelatin slowly and incompletely at low temperatures but quickly and quite completely at high temperature. Since there are no vitamins to be harmed by submitting bones to extreme heat, a higher temperature is preferable. Delicious soup stock can be made in half an hour in the pressure cooker.

An essential step in making delicious soups is to sear the chopped or sawed bones, particularly when fresh bones are used. As the protein in the bits of meat clinging to the bones is broken down by heat, the "browned-meat" flavor so much enjoyed is developed. If care is taken that no meat scraps are charred, the delightful flavor of the soup will be in proportion to the degree to which the bones have been browned.

All well-made soup stock should be rich in calcium, which can be dissolved by adding vinegar. Acid also hastens the breakdown of connective tissue and thus shortens the cooking time. Since salt attracts, or draws out, the juices from the bones and scraps, it is important that salt be added with the water and vinegar. As the stock is boiled, calcium combines with acid and the taste of vinegar disappears. If any odor of it remains, the lid of the utensil may be removed and the vinegar quickly evaporated off by rapid boiling before the vegetable parings are put in.

The vegetable scraps and parings used in making soup stock should be cooked only a short time. Their flavor must be retained; little vitamin C should be destroyed; and the sulfur compounds of the strong-flavored vegetables must not be allowed to break down. Care should be taken that the parings do not contain a large proportion of any vegetable that is unpopular or has too prominent a flavor. Like the bones, the more thoroughly the vegetables are chopped, the more flavor and nutritive value pass into the stock. An understanding of the quantities of nutrients gained from vegetable parings will serve a dual purpose of emphasizing the nutritive value of scraps which are usually thrown away and of showing the tremendous harm done when vegetables are washed slowly, soaked, or boiled.

Of the known vitamins, vitamins $B_1$, $B_2$, $B_6$, C, and P, niacin, pantothenic acid, para-aminobenzoic acid, folic acid, cholin, inositol, and biotin dissolve in water as readily as does sugar. Out of these twelve vitamins, only folic acid and vitamin C are harmed at boiling temperature. Unless submitted to heat for a long period, vitamin $B_1$ is destroyed only by a temperature above boiling. Vitamins A, or carotene, E, and K do not dissolve in water; but when vegetables are chopped or are cooked until the cell walls soften and break down, these vitamins are spilled into the cooking water. When vegetables are thoroughly chopped and quickly cooked in soup stock, therefore, the larger amount of all of these fifteen vitamins passes into the stock.

The minerals lost when vegetables are soaked or boiled are those gained in making soups. Studies have shown that when vegetables are boiled only 4 minutes, even though they are not chopped, an average of 50 per cent of their phosphorus, sodium, magnesium, potassium, iron, and manganese passes into the cooking water. These minerals occur in the form of salts as easily dissolved in water as is table salt. Other studies have shown that when vegetables are boiled until the cell walls are soft and then are allowed to stand for a half hour, as cooked vegetables often do in restaurants, as much as 90 per cent of their total minerals may pass into the water. It is a safe assumption that if vegetable parings and scraps are well chopped and boiled slowly for 15 minutes, the greater part of their minerals is extracted into the stock, although further soaking may be advantageous. Properly prepared soup stock, therefore, can be outstandingly rich in vitamins and minerals.

The stock made of bones which have been chopped should be strained through a cloth or a cloth bag to remove bone splinters. The cloth or bag should also be used to squeeze all the juices and nutrients from the parings. A cloth sugar sack, for example, should be kept especially for making soups.

When bones are not otherwise available, they should be purchased for making stock. Bones of young animals contain more connective tissue than do those of older animals. It is for this reason that veal bones are usually recommended for making jellied bouillons. The meat of veal, however, lacks flavor and makes less delicious soup than ribs, backbones, shoulder blades, and other bones trimmed from mature young beef when rolled roasts are prepared. These bones are excellent for making soups as well as jellied bouillons, consommés, and aspics provided about ⅛ inch of meat is left on them. Since they are not customarily used for soup but are sold for chicken feed and fertilizer, they can be obtained from the butcher at almost no cost. I have made as much as a gallon of delicious and stiffly jellied stock from 10 cents' worth of such bones. When the flavor of the stock is to be obtained largely from meat rather than bones, beef shank and oxtails are best to use.

Soup stock may be used in preparing dozens of dishes other than soup. Rice, macaroni, noodles, gravies, sauces, stews, casserole dishes, and many others are far more delicious when cooked with stock than with water. The stock adds many nutrients which these foods would otherwise lack. A single pint of stock can be made to equal a quart or more of milk in calcium content. Delicious jellied bouillons, aspics, and jellied meats and fish prepared with well-made stock should be served far more often than they customarily are.

Although a large amount of stock may be prepared at one time, the soup itself should usually be prepared for only one meal. Fresh vegetables to be eaten in the soup should be cooked for the shortest time possible. Instead of cooking the vegetables in the soup stock, a far more delightful flavor can be obtained by sautéing them in a little fat taken from the stock; the flavor thus remains in the vegetables and they do not become watery and soggy. The seasoned stock should be added only a few minutes before the soup is served.

Although it is sometimes desirable to cook meat with soup, such meat usually becomes stringy and lacks flavor. The full nutritive value of the meat is retained and freshness of flavor is achieved if the meat is ground and added to the soup just before it is served. Since the pieces of ground meat are small, heat can penetrate and cook them almost instantly. When leftover meat is to be eaten in soup, it should be added only in time to heat through.

The nutritive value of soups can be greatly increased with almost no cost by adding soy or peanut flour to them. These products are almost pure protein and yet are rich in vitamins and minerals; they thicken the soup only slightly, and if used in moderate amounts, do not alter its taste. Cream soups are made creamier and more delicious as well as more nutritious by the addition of powdered milk. It is especially important to use these products when the budget is limited, when the protein requirements are high, or when meat substitutes or meats low in protein are served at the same meal with soup.

Cream soups may be made of the tough ends of asparagus,

broccoli, and celery, and of fresh pea hulls if the leaves from pea
vines are also used. Cream soups which deserve special mention
are those made of avocado and celery root, which are similar in
taste to delicate cream of pea and celery soups, respectively. Delicious soups, such as cream of chicken or turkey soup, can be
prepared with stock and powdered milk.

Since vegetable parings usually accumulate more quickly than
do bones, and since their vitamin and mineral content is far too
great to be wasted, their nutrients should be extracted and the
water used in general cooking. I have given the name vegetable-
cooking water to such extract and have included it in hundreds
of recipes throughout this book. Any water left from steaming
vegetables should also be added to it.

Every housewife who is sincerely interested in her family's
health should make it a habit to throw nothing into the garbage
except inedible parts of food; such a habit can make the difference
between rosy cheeks and pale ones, steady nerves and irritability.
When generous amounts of vegetables are used and little water is
added, a cup or two of vegetable-cooking water or stock can be
the equivalent of a pound or more of vegetables in minerals and
water-soluble vitamins. No family can afford to waste such a po-
tential source of health.

Few dishes prepared by a housewife give her such a thrifty feeling as do good soups. They need cost almost nothing and take
little time to prepare. The nutritive value they save would thrill
any health-minded person. The woman who prepares delicious
soups realizes that persons who use only canned soups miss a
great deal of fun. If friends drop in on a cold evening or your husband gives a poker party, some onions can be quickly sautéed,
seasonings and rich stock added, and the soup served piping hot
generously sprinkled with cheese; in less than 10 minutes you can
have a delicious soup. Neither the soup nor the praise will be forgotten soon.

It is easy to get into a rut by serving two or three kinds of soup
without varying the seasonings or ingredients. Many excellent
vegetables, such as zucchini, savoy cabbage, kohlrabi, and greens,
are rarely used in soups; bouillons and consommés are not served
frequently enough, either hot or chilled; delightful fish bisques are

scarcely known. I hope you will try each recipe before preparing
a particular one the second time. Although measurements of vegetables are given in cups, they are intended to be only approximate;
they should be measured with the eye, and the quantities varied
with your family's food likes and needs. Make it a rule to serve
soup once or twice each week, often having it as the main dish of
the meal. What food could be better to build up blood and relax
tense nerves than properly made soup rich in vitamins and minerals?

## SOUP GARNISHES AND ACCOMPANIMENTS

Soup should be made appealing by the aroma of herbs and other
seasonings, by attractive garnishes, and by interesting accompaniments. Garnishes and accompaniments need take only a few minutes to prepare, and the effect is an added "something" which
makes the cook into an artist. Try each of the following garnishes
and accompaniments.

**Almonds, toasted and chopped:** Sprinkle on bouillons or a bland cream
soup, such as cream of asparagus soup.

**Apple:** Cut unpeeled red apple into tiny wedges, sprinkle on the surface
of any soup where tartness or color is needed; delicious with chicken
bouillon.

**Bread sticks:** Cut stale whole-wheat, wheat-germ, or rye bread into
sticks without removing the crust; serve heated, lightly toasted, fried
with garlic, dipped in fat and melted cheese, or topped with cheese which
is then melted and garnished with paprika or ground parsley.

**Bacon bits:** Pan-broil until crisp; break into bits and sprinkle over
thick soups before serving.

**Caraway, cumin, and dill seeds:** Sprinkle lightly on vegetable and meat
soups; use caraway or dill seeds on cream of potato soup.

**Cheese:** Sprinkle grated Parmesan, Swiss, or shredded American cheese
on any variety of soup; use chips of Roquefort on a bland cream soup,
such as cream of celery or asparagus.

**Cheese puffs:** Make cheese puffs (p. 435) no more than 2 inches in
diameter. Fill with cream cheese or shredded American cheese.

**Chili sauce and catsup:** Put a single teaspoon of sauce or catsup in the
center of each serving if color and seasoning are needed.

**Crackers:** Serve wheat-germ, soy, rye, or whole-wheat crackers. They
may be sprinkled with cheese and reheated.

**Eggs:** Slice or grate hard-cooked eggs and use on any vegetable or cream soup. If protein is needed, a hard-cooked egg may be cut in half lengthwise and used for each serving.

**Eggs stuffed** (p. 246): Use as soup accompaniment.

**Finger salads** (p. 273): When a low-calorie diet is desired, serve instead of crackers or breadstuffs.

**Grated orange or lemon rind:** Add a light sprinkling of orange rind to cream soups; add lemon rind to vegetable soups and fish bisques.

**Lemon slices:** Cut extremely thin and float 1 slice on the surface of bouillons or cream soup; top with a single mint leaf or a tiny sprig of parsley, or dust lightly with paprika.

**Nutmeg, mace, or ground clove:** Add a faint suggestion rather than a sprinkling to any vegetable or cream soup; add nutmeg to cream of spinach or chicken soup.

**Nuts:** Serve with one-dish-meal soups to supply additional protein; reheat roasted peanuts, almonds, soy nuts (p. 549), or other nuts.

**Orange slices:** Use a small orange, slice thin, float on the center of cream soups, such as cream of avocado or pea leaf.

**Popcorn:** Heat with a small amount of butter-flavored oil; add salt if needed; roll in or sprinkle with grated cheese and serve piping hot.

**Potato chips:** Freshen in oven or under broiler. Sprinkle with grated Parmesan or American cheese. Serve hot garnished with paprika. Vary by using sweet potato chips (p. 399).

**Peppers:** Dice uncooked red or green bell peppers and use as a garnish.

**Soup dumplings:** Prepare dumplings (p. 108), using half the recipe; drop from a teaspoon into boiling soup, bouillon, or consommé; cover utensil; boil slowly 10 minutes without removing lid and serve.

**Sour cream:** Add to spinach soup and to borsch.

**Toast cubes, or croutons:** Make of whole-wheat, wheat-germ, or rye bread and serve as both a garnish and an accompaniment to any soup.

*"Buttered" toast cubes:* Sauté bread cubes in butter-flavored fat; sprinkle lightly with parsley or minced chives or fresh herbs.

*Cheese croutons:* Melt slowly ½ cup shredded or cubed American cheese in ⅛ cup butter-flavored oil; quickly dip bread cubes into it, arrange on baking sheet, and reheat in oven just before serving. May be made in advance. Bread cubes may also be sautéed quickly and sprinkled generously with grated cheese while hot.

*Garlic croutons:* Sauté gently 1 clove garlic in butter-flavored fat; discard garlic and sauté bread cubes.

## SOUP STOCK

Using hatchet and hardwood board, chop the following into small pieces:

**2 pounds or more of accumulated, assorted bones, pieces of cartilage, gristle, meat scraps**

Or use uncooked bones sawed or chopped into small pieces, or both accumulated bones and fresh ones.

Select a large soup kettle with flat base and tight-fitting lid; put over high heat and add:

**chopped accumulated bones, cartilage, meat trimmings, and/or fresh bones**

If fresh bones are used and dark stock is desired, keep heat high and sear 10 to 15 minutes; turn frequently, and brown as many surfaces as possible; do not allow fat to smoke.

Pour off any fat rendered from meat scraps; add:

| | |
|---|---|
| **2 quarts water** | **2 teaspoons salt** |
| **4 tablespoons vinegar** | |

Cover kettle and boil very slowly for 3 to 4 hours. If odor of vinegar can be detected at the end of this period, uncover kettle and boil vigorously for a few minutes until vinegar has evaporated; add water if needed to make approximately 2 quarts stock.

Meanwhile chop quickly in wooden chopping bowl:

| | |
|---|---|
| **accumulated vegetable parings** | **leftover vegetable scraps from** |
| **leftover salads and salad scraps** | **plates** |
| **from plates** | **leftover vegetables impossible to** |
| | **use in other ways** |

Bring stock to a rolling boil and add:

| | |
|---|---|
| **chopped parings and leftovers** | **1 whole cayenne or chili tepine,** |
| **¼ to ½ teaspoon crushed black or** | **minced or pierced with a tooth-** |
| **white peppercorns** | **pick** |

Force the chopped vegetables down into stock and cover utensil; reduce heat and boil slowly 15 minutes. Wipe out chopping bowl with paper.

Remove stock from heat; if it is convenient, let soak ½ hour or longer; strain stock through cloth to remove all bone splinters; wring dry of juices and discard bones and parings.

If stock is not to be used immediately, pour it into a jar and chill; remove fat before using stock.

Use stock for brown sauces (p. 162), jellied meats (p. 224), soups, bouillons, consommés.

*Variations:*

In case hard-cooked eggs are desired, wash eggs, reduce heat to simmering, and cook 20 minutes in stock.

Cook in stock heart or tongue to be served cold, reheated, or added to soup.

If the odor of vinegar does not disappear quickly, add 2 or more crushed eggshells.

When stock is prepared in pressure cooker, sear bones first to develop flavor; add water, 2 tablespoons vinegar, salt; steam under pressure 30 minutes; cool under cold water, remove lid, boil until vinegar evaporates. Add vegetables and steam 3 to 5 minutes under pressure; remove from heat.

**Beef stock for jellied bouillons, consommés, aspics:** Purchase 2 pounds or more of ribs, backbones, or any bones from young but matured beef. Brown thoroughly and prepare as in basic recipe. If stock is not a firm jelly when chilled, reheat and add 2 to 4 teaspoons gelatin soaked in ½ cup water.

**Chicken stock:** Purchase 2 pounds or more chicken feet. Cover with boiling water and boil 5 minutes; drain and discard water, remove skin and claws, and chop bones into ½-inch pieces. Omit searing; otherwise proceed as in basic recipe. Delicious stock which costs almost nothing can be made from chicken feet. Vary by using bones from fried, stewed, or roasted chicken as well as the feet.

**Clear soup stock:** To clear stock for making jellied meats, reheat strained stock and add several shells from raw eggs or the uncooked white of 1 egg; stir well, simmer 5 minutes, and strain. Small particles stick to raw egg white and are held fast as soon as it cooks.

**Dark soup stock:** Include beef scraps from plates or trimmings; brown the meat well; or sear with the bones 2 tablespoons finely chopped raw liver.

**Light soup stock:** Use fresh veal or lamb bones; chicken legs, or leftover chicken, turkey, rabbit, veal, and pork bones; do not sear. Omit any vegetable scraps which may give a dark color.

**Stock for bisques:** Stock for bisques, or thick soups containing vegetables and meat, is prepared from the bones of wild game. Prepare as in basic recipe and make into bouillon, consommé, or soup by using recipes for chicken or beef.

**Stock for fish bisques:** Prepare as directed on page 323.

**Stock of uncooked meat and fresh bones:** Purchase beef shank or an oxtail; ask butcher to cut oxtail or to saw shank into 1-inch pieces; sear. When meat is almost tender, put chopped vegetable parings into cloth bag and boil in stock. Squeeze juices from parings and discard bones, returning meat to soup.

Bouillons and consommés are merely variations of seasoned soup stock. A bouillon is usually made of brown stock and delicately seasoned. A consommé is made from one or more kinds of bones and highly seasoned. Both are customarily served clear. Their delightful odors and meat extracts stimulate the flow of the digestive juices. When they are properly made, their virtue lies in the fact that they supply vitamins and minerals without calories. Bouillons and consommés should be served far more frequently than they usually are.

## BEEF CONSOMMÉ

Remove fat from **1 quart stock** made from assorted beef bones; heat and add:

| | |
|---|---|
| pinch each of marjoram, thyme, and basil | 1 to 2 tablespoons minced chives or tops of green onions |
| 1 small clove garlic | 1 to 3 drops Tabasco |

Stir well and simmer 10 minutes. Taste for seasoning and discard garlic; garnish with extremely thin slices of lemon topped with a dash of paprika. Serve with wheat-germ crackers.

*Variations:*

If stock is not clear, add with seasonings 1 to 3 crushed shells of uncooked eggs; pour directly into soup plates by passing through fine strainer; add chives or onion tops after straining.

If more calories are desired, cook soup dumplings (p. 108) in consommé. Add any diced leftover meat.

**Beef bouillon:** Omit garlic, Tabasco, and two herbs.

**Chicken bouillon:** Season chicken stock with a pinch of thyme or sage; add yellow coloring. Serve with cheese puffs filled with melted cheese and garnish with nutmeg or tiny wedges of red apple. Vary by serving with dumplings (p. 108) or by seasoning each serving with ½ teaspoon lemon rind or by sprinkling with Parmesan cheese.

**Consommé with egg:** Omit chives and garlic; remove from heat and add 2 well-beaten eggs; stir, cover utensil, and let stand 5 minutes; garnish with minced canned pimento or thin rings of fresh pimento.

**Jellied bouillon with chicken:** Omit herbs and garlic; clear chicken stock with eggshells and season with a pinch of sage, chervil, basil, or thyme; add yellow coloring, and strain into molds or flat pan to chill; when it starts to set, add a small amount of leftover chicken. Serve with lemon sections and soy crackers.

**Jellied consommé:** Prepare stock as directed on page 310; season as in basic consommé recipe. Clear with eggshells, strain into shallow pan, chill, cut into small cubes before serving. Vary by pouring into molds over slices of lemon or hard-cooked egg. Garnish lightly with ground parsley and Parmesan cheese; serve with rye crackers.

**Onion soup:** Sauté until transparent in 2 tablespoons fat from soup stock 4 to 6 thinly sliced onions; do not brown; add ½ teaspoon salt and 1 quart stock; make 1 slice toast for each person, cover with grated Parmesan, melt under broiler; put toast into soup plate and pour soup over it. Garnish with paprika.

**Tomato jellied bouillon:** Prepare stock for jellied bouillon (p. 310), using 1 quart tomato juice instead of water; season with basil, Tabasco, white peppercorns; add red coloring. Pour into molds or a shallow pan, chill, and unmold or cut into cubes. Garnish with chives or Chinese garlic and serve with toasted almonds or peanuts.

Soups of meat and vegetables may be served as the first course, especially when the entree is low in protein. What more could one want for dinner, however, than a delicious, piping-hot soup with enough for second and third helpings, a green salad tossed while the soup is heating, fresh bread, butter, and milk? Such a dinner is a favorite of mine even for winter entertaining. Perhaps the most nutritious and to many the most delicious of these soups is that made of ground meat, cooked only by the heat of the soup itself. This soup is also excellent to make when no stock is available and time is limited. Compared to the old overcooked varieties of soups, one taste of ground meat soup is convincing evidence of the soundness of quick-cooking vegetables, meats, and herbs. Long cooking should be used only for soup stocks.

Since the following soups are planned to be served as one-dish meals, each recipe is on the basis of 2½ quarts.

## GROUND MEAT AND VEGETABLE SOUP

Combine and heat in soup kettle:

| | |
|---|---|
| 1 to 2 tablespoons fat from top of soup stock | 2 chopped stalks celery |
| | 2 chilled, unpeeled, diced carrots |
| 1 minced clove garlic | 1 chilled, unpeeled, diced potato |
| 1 or 2 chopped onions | |

Cover utensil; keep heat high until vegetables are heated through; then sauté gently without browning until they are almost tender, or about 10 minutes; add and heat quickly:

| | |
|---|---|
| 2 quarts soup stock made of assorted bones | ½ teaspoon crushed black peppercorns |
| 2 teaspoons salt | pinch each of marjoram, thyme, and savory |
| ¼ crushed bay leaf | |

Simmer stock 10 minutes without boiling; add and stir rapidly:

| | |
|---|---|
| 1 pound finely ground beef heart | 2 tablespoons ground parsley |

Taste for seasoning. Serve immediately without further heating. Accompany with hot soy crackers sprinkled with grated American cheese.

*Variations:*

Omit 2 cups of the soup stock and use 2 cups tomato juice or canned or diced fresh tomatoes.

If no stock is available, sear 3 tablespoons ground meat in fat until well browned; proceed as in basic recipe, using vegetable-cooking water instead of stock.

Add 1 diced pimento; season with basil or orégano, no other herbs.

Mix with small amount of stock and add ¼ cup soy or peanut flour, or ½ cup soy grits.

Instead of the beef heart use any of the following: ground veal, pork, or lamb hearts; ground round steak or hamburger; ground beef liver frozen or quickly sautéed before grinding in order to prevent loss of juices; ½ pound each ground soup meat and chopped or ground veal or lamb kidneys; 1 lamb kidney, 1 slice liver, small piece of beef heart; if kidneys are especially enjoyed, add thinly sliced kidneys without other meat. Follow herb guide (p. 28) and vary seasonings with kind of meat used.

Substitute the following vegetables for any vegetable in basic recipe: turnips, kohlrabi, celery root, green pepper, tomatoes, corn, rutabagas, string beans, broccoli, cabbage, beets, green peas, a few shredded leaves of any greens; cook all vegetables the shortest time possible to make them tender.

**Browned-beef soup:** Buy 1 pound thinly sliced round steak; dredge with whole-wheat flour, pound thoroughly, and brown in fat taken from stock; remove, sauté vegetables, and proceed as in basic recipe; cut steak into narrow strips 1½ inches long and add 2 minutes before serving. Garnish with Chinese garlic and serve with rye crackers.

**Browned-liver soup:** Proceed as in browned-beef soup, using sautéed baby beef, veal, or lamb liver; substitute 2 cups canned or fresh diced tomatoes for part of stock and add a pinch of basil and/or orégano. Garnish generously with chives and serve with garlic croutons.

**Chicken gumbo:** Select a stewing chicken, disjoint, dredge with whole-wheat flour, and brown well in bacon drippings; add 3 cups each water and fresh or canned tomatoes, 1 tablespoon salt, 3 tablespoons vinegar; simmer 2 hours; add ½ cup brown rice, ½ teaspoon crushed white peppercorns; simmer ½ hour; add 3 cups sliced okra, 1 thinly sliced onion; simmer 10 to 12 minutes and stir in 3 tablespoons ground parsley. Serve with hot wheat-germ rolls and tossed green salad.

**Chicken or turkey soup:** Use stock prepared from chicken feet, bony parts of stewing chicken, or turkey carcass; cook in stock ½ cup brown or all-vitamin rice; proceed as in basic recipe, adding celery, carrots, onion, yellow coloring, ground parsley, pinch of sage; omit other herbs and vegetables. Add 1 or 2 cups diced chicken or turkey and leftover dressing when available.

**Clam chowder made with tomatoes:** Dice 2 slices bacon with scissors, pan-broil in soup kettle, drain off part of the fat; add and sauté carrots, celery, onion and potato, omitting garlic and herbs; add crushed white peppercorns, salt, 2 cups tomato purée, 5 cups soup stock or vegetable-cooking water; immediately before serving add 2 cups or more minced fresh or canned clams and 2 tablespoons ground parsley. Vary by adding 1 cup fresh or frozen corn with clams.

**Heart or tongue soup:** Cook beef, veal, lamb, or pork heart or tongue in soup stock while stock is being prepared; remove, skin the tongue, and dice; prepare soup as in basic recipe or any variation; add diced heart or tongue before serving.

**Italian meat soup:** Prepare stock of shank or oxtail; when meat is almost tender, add crushed black peppercorns, herbs, garlic, and onions; instead of vegetables of basic recipe add 1 cup fresh peas, 1 or 2 diced zucchini, 1 chopped leek, 4 shredded leaves curly or green cabbage; cook about 10 minutes. Serve as soon as vegetables are tender; sprinkle generously with Parmesan cheese.

**Oxtail soup:** Prepare stock as directed on page 311 for stock of bones and meat; reheat stock with meat from an oxtail; add vegetables and seasonings as in basic recipe or any variation.

**Pepper-pot soup:** Cook 1 or 2 pounds tripe while preparing stock, remove when tender, and cut with scissors into narrow strips; brown thoroughly 2 or 3 slices diced salt pork; drain; add vegetables, stock, tripe, seasonings of basic recipe, and 2 diced green peppers.

**Soup with meat balls:** Use 2 cups ground heart, lean beef, or veal; add 1 egg, ½ cup wheat germ, ⅓ cup each powdered milk and ground parsley; add salt, pepper, grated onion; mix well, mold into balls 1½ inches in diameter; prepare soup as in basic recipe and drop in meat balls 8 minutes before serving.

Vegetable purées are soups thickened by the bulk of the vegetables themselves. The conventional method of preparing them is to overcook the vegetables until they are mushy and colorless, and to pass them through a colander, a technique so tedious and so destructive of flavor, to say nothing of nutritive value, that they are rarely served except as a form of barbaric punishment for sick persons and innocent babes. If the fresh chilled vegetables are quickly shredded or passed through a meat grinder, then short-cooked, and combined with piping-hot and well-seasoned stock, the resulting soup is worth adding to the weekly menu. Since these soups are designed for light lunches or the first course of a dinner, the recipes are on the basis of approximately 5 cups.

Vegetables for purées may be quickly sautéed before the stock is added or may be cooked directly in the stock. Since an advantage of purées is to supply an abundance of vitamins and minerals with few calories, I have chosen the latter method for the basic recipe.

## MIXED-VEGETABLE PURÉE

Quickly pass through the food grinder the following chilled vegetables being careful to save all juices:

| | |
|---|---|
| 1 each carrot, onion, turnip, green pepper, pimento | several sprigs of parsley |
| | few leaves of cabbage, spinach, |
| 2 stalks celery with leaves | mustard |

Add ground vegetables to:

1 quart rapidly boiling soup stock

Boil 1 minute, reduce heat, add:

| | |
|---|---|
| pinch each of basil, savory, mar-<br>joram | 1 teaspoon Worcestershire<br>1 teaspoon salt |

Taste for seasoning; simmer no longer than 8 minutes. Serve with wheat-germ crackers.

*Variations:*

When vegetables are ready to be ground, heat in large frying pan 2 or 3 tablespoons fat from the top of soup stock and add 2 drops butter-flavoring; grind vegetables directly into hot fat, heat quickly, sauté 5 minutes, add stock and seasonings. Serve as soon as hot. Chop or pass through food grinder any leftover vegetables or meat and add in time to heat.

If no soup stock is available, use 1 quart vegetable-cooking water and before salting add 2 or more beef or chicken bouillon cubes or 2 teaspoons meat extract.

Add ¼ to ½ cup soy grits to any purée.

If the purée is prepared for persons needing high-calorie diets, sauté vegetables in 4 tablespoons margarine, butter, or fat taken from soup stock; mix with 1 cup soup stock ½ cup soy, peanut, or wheat-germ flour; add 5 minutes before serving. Accompany with cheese puffs (p. 435).

Make purées of any of the following vegetables alone or combined: onions, spinach, carrots, peas, green peppers, celery, celery root, tomatoes, leeks, zucchini, pimentos. Add ground parsley to all purées just before serving.

**Buckwheat-tomato purée:** Add to 3 cups boiling stock ½ cup whole unwashed buckwheat; simmer 5 minutes; add 2 cups tomato juice or purée, 1 each chopped or ground onion, green pepper, and carrot; pinch of basil; simmer 10 more minutes. Whole unpolished barley or all-vitamin rice may be substituted for buckwheat.

**Spinach-parsley purée:** Boil 1 bunch each shredded spinach and parsley and 1 shredded onion 3 minutes in 1 quart beef stock; add 1 teaspoon salt and 1 cup tomato purée or Spanish-style tomato sauce; serve as soon as heated through. Cut hard-cooked eggs lengthwise and put two halves into each soup plate before serving. Garnish with 2 tablespoons sour cream or yogurt topped with dash of paprika. This is a delicious soup.

## VEGETABLE SOUPS WITHOUT MEAT

Dice, shred, or cut into fingers the following chilled vegetables and sauté in butter-flavored fat or fat from stock:

2 unpeeled carrots                      2 or 3 stalks celery
1 or 2 onions or leeks                  1 unpeeled potato

Add:

¼ teaspoon crushed black pepper-        pinch each of basil, marjoram, and
   corns                                   savory
¼ crushed bay leaf

Cover utensil, keep heat moderate, and do not brown; when vegetables are tender, add and heat quickly:

1 quart soup stock or vegetable-        1 teaspoon salt
   cooking water                        2 tablespoons parsley
¼ cup soy or peanut flour shaken
   with a small amount of stock

As soon as soup is hot, serve with cheese popcorn or hot roasted peanuts.

*Variations:*

If no stock is available, use vegetable-cooking water and before salting add 2 beef bouillon cubes or 2 teaspoons beef extract. Add diced leftover vegetables.

Instead of any of the vegetables in basic recipe add one or more of the following diced or shredded vegetables: string beans, turnips, rutabagas, kohlrabi, cauliflower, zucchini, broccoli; fresh or frozen peas or corn; fresh or canned tomatoes. Add vegetables only in time to cook tender.

Add ½ cup soy grits to basic recipe or any variation.

**Borsch, or Russian beet soup:** Sauté in fat from soup stock **1 cup each unpeeled beets and carrots cut into thin fingers, ½ cup diced onions;** cook 10 minutes; add and stir in well **4 tablespoons whole-wheat pastry flour;** then add **2 cups shredded green cabbage;** cook 8 minutes longer; add **1½ teaspoons salt, 1 quart soup stock or vegetable-cooking water;** just before serving add **1 cup tomato purée** and serve quickly before cabbage loses color. Put **2 tablespoons sour cream or yogurt** into each soup bowl.

Corn soup: Pan-broil 2 slices bacon and remove when crisp; add and sauté vegetables of basic recipe, omitting herbs; add 1 cup tomatoes, 2 cups stock or vegetable-cooking water, 2 cups fresh or canned corn, 1 diced pimento, diced crisp bacon, parsley, soy or peanut flour. Serve as soon as heated.

Okra soup: Sauté in bacon drippings with other vegetables of basic recipe 2 cups diced okra, 1 chopped green pepper; add 1 cup fresh or canned tomatoes or purée and stock, salt, soy flour, parsley.

Rice-tomato soup: Cook ½ cup brown or all-vitamin rice in 4 cups boiling vegetable-cooking water or soup stock; add salt, crushed peppercorns, soy flour, 1 cup tomatoes, pinch each of basil and savory, and vegetables of basic recipe except potatoes. Vary by substituting for rice whole buckwheat, unground wheat, or unpolished whole barley.

Cream soups are excellent served at lunch, as a first course for dinner, or as a one-dish meal provided additional protein is supplied by other foods. These soups are easy to make and require only about 10 minutes of working time. Powdered milk should be added to all cream soups in order to improve flavor and richness as well as nutritive value. It is important that cream soup not be boiled, particularly after powdered milk is added.

## CREAM OF CHICKEN SOUP

Combine and heat to boiling:

| | |
|---|---|
| 1 quart chicken stock | ¼ teaspoon crushed white pepper- |
| pinch each of sage and thyme | corns |
| 1 teaspoon salt | |

Add and cook 8 minutes:

| | |
|---|---|
| ½ cup chopped celery | 1 or 2 diced carrots |
| 1 cup fresh or frozen peas | 2 diced pimentos (optional) |

Shake or beat until smooth and add:

| | |
|---|---|
| 1 cup chicken stock or fresh milk | 3 tablespoons whole-wheat pastry |
| ½ cup powdered milk | flour |
| | 1 drop yellow coloring |

*Cover and* simmer 10 minutes; *do not boil;* taste for seasoning, garnish with nutmeg or paprika. Serve with hot sweet potato or yam chips.

*Variations:*

When available, add 1 or more cups diced chicken.

Omit flour; add ½ to 1 cup toasted whole-wheat-bread crumbs, left-over mashed potatoes, or beat 1 or 2 whole eggs with powdered milk; add to basic recipe or any variation.

Substitute 1 can chicken soup for chicken stock and prepare half the recipe; or omit stock and before salting add with other ingredients 2 or 3 chicken bouillon cubes to 1 quart fresh milk.

Add to vegetables in basic recipe, or substitute for one or more, any of the following: shredded string beans, chopped onion or leek, diced cucumber, diced celery root, diced zucchini or summer squash, chopped green or red bell pepper, fresh paprika.

**Chicken-cucumber soup:** Omit vegetables of basic recipe; cook 5 minutes in **chicken stock 2 sliced or diced cucumbers;** proceed and season as in basic recipe; add **1 drop green coloring.** Garnish with **thin slices of orange.** Serve with toasted almonds.

**Chicken-mushroom soup:** Before adding other ingredients sauté **fresh mushrooms** in fat taken from stock or add **1 can sliced mushrooms** to soup or substitute **1 can condensed mushroom soup** for flour and fresh milk. Omit or include vegetables of basic recipe.

**Clam chowder made with milk:** Blend **3 tablespoons** each whole-wheat pastry flour and margarine or butter; add slowly and heat **1 quart whole milk;** simmer 10 minutes and add the powdered milk, salt, paprika, and peppercorns of basic recipe, **2 cups or more minced fresh or canned clams;** omit the other ingredients of basic recipe. Serve as soon as heated to simmering; garnish with **ground parsley.** Serve with whole-wheat-bread sticks sprinkled with cheese.

**Turkey soup:** Prepare like the basic recipe, using stock from turkey carcass.

Cream vegetable soups should be thickened with powdered milk and the bulk of the vegetables themselves. Instead of overcooking the vegetables until mushy and then puréeing them, shred, chop, or grind the chilled vegetables and sauté them or cook them in milk. Cream soups prepared in this manner have a delightful freshness and need only to be heated before being ready to serve. If the soup is to be served as the principal dish of the meal, double the following recipes.

## CREAM OF VEGETABLE SOUP

Use metal utensil for making soup and sauté in **butter-flavored cooking fat:**

1 chopped onion or leek

When onion is transparent, add, *cover utensil,* and heat to simmering:

| | |
|---|---|
| 3 cups fresh milk | 1 teaspoon Worcestershire (optional) |
| 1½ teaspoons salt | |
| ¼ teaspoon freshly ground black peppercorns | 1 to 4 drops Tabasco |

When milk is hot, add the following and simmer 3 to 6 minutes:

| | |
|---|---|
| 1 to 2 cups shredded, ground, or grated vegetable | 1 or 2 diced pimentos if color is needed |

*Keep utensil covered as much as possible.* Beat until smooth and add 5 minutes before serving:

| | |
|---|---|
| 1 cup fresh milk | 1 cup powdered milk |

Serve as soon as heated through; above all, *do not boil;* taste for seasoning, stir in **2 to 4 tablespoons ground parsley,** and garnish with **paprika, chives,** or **thin strips of fresh or canned pimento.**

*Variations:*

Add ½ cup soy grits to any cream soup.

Beat ¼ to ½ cup soy or peanut flour or 1 or 2 whole eggs with fresh and powdered milk.

Add 1 or 2 cups of any of the following chilled and shredded, mashed, ground, or grated vegetables: carrots, celery, celery root, corn, fresh or leftover lima beans, onions, spinach or equal parts of parsley and spinach, mustard greens, kale, chard, mustard-spinach, or other greens or mixed greens. Vary by adding bits of crisp bacon to spinach soup or soups of other greens.

Season any cream soup with one or more of the following: a generous dash of nutmeg or mace; 1 minced clove garlic sautéed with onion; mustard, celery, or dill seeds; a few leaves of fresh or a pinch of dried basil, tarragon, or thyme.

If soup is to be the principal dish of the meal, double recipe; slice 1 hard-cooked egg into each soup bowl.

Avocado soup: Prepare as in basic recipe, using white peppercorns; add
½ cup diced ham or chicken if available. Just before serving add 2 mashed
ripe avocados. Garnish with thin orange slices. Serve with whole-wheat
cheese wafers.

Clam chowder made with vegetables: Pan-broil 3 slices salt pork cut
into bits with scissors; drain; add and sauté with onion of the basic recipe
2 cups diced unpeeled potatoes; when vegetables are almost tender, add
milk, salt, peppercorns, and powdered milk as in basic recipe; add 1 pint
canned or minced fresh clams and serve as soon as heated through. Garnish with parsley.

Corn chowder: Pan-broil 4 slices diced bacon; drain off most of the
fat; proceed and season as in basic recipe, sautéing with onion 1 or 2 diced
unpeeled potatoes; add 2 cups canned, frozen, or fresh corn; heat only
to simmering; just before serving add 2 cups thick tomato purée. Do not
boil. Serve as a one-dish meal with cheese croutons, tossed salad.

Cream of leek and potato soup: Sauté lightly 2 chopped leeks or sweet
onions and 4 diced potatoes; proceed as in basic recipe; add 1 to 2 teaspoons caraway or dill seeds; beat ¼ teaspoon paprika and 2 egg yolks
with fresh and powdered milk. Serve with hot rye-bread cubes rolled in
grated cheese. This is one of my favorite soups.

Cream of mock-oyster soup: Pass through meat grinder enough salsify,
or oyster plant, to make 2 cups; prepare and season as in basic recipe,
adding ¼ teaspoon crushed dill or celery seeds or paprika. Serve with
toasted peanuts.

Cream of mushroom soup: Omit onion of basic recipe; sauté 1 or 2
cups sliced fresh mushrooms; proceed as in basic recipe. Garnish with
dash of mace or nutmeg. Serve with whole-wheat-bread sticks.

Cream of oyster soup: Drain liquid from 1 pint oysters into 3 cups whole
milk; heat; add salt, white peppercorns, 2 tablespoons each grated onion
and margarine or butter; chop the oysters and add with powdered milk.
Serve with whole-wheat crackers.

Oyster chowder: Sauté in butter-flavored fat 2 diced potatoes, 1 stalk
celery, 1 leek or sweet onion; add milk and proceed as in cream of oyster
soup.

Cream of potato soup: Proceed and season as in basic recipe, cooking
4 or 5 finely diced potatoes in hot milk; add 1 teaspoon chopped dill or
dill sauce or 1 or 2 teaspoons dill or caraway seeds. Vary by seasoning
with celery salt.

Cream soup of mixed vegetables: Grind and sauté for 5 minutes 1 each
carrot, stalk celery, small onion, green pepper, turnip, potato; proceed
and season as in basic recipe; garnish with dash of nutmeg.

**Cream of pea soup:** Run **2 cups fresh chilled peas** through the meat grinder; proceed and season as in basic recipe; cook peas only 3 minutes. Garnish with **slice of orange.** Serve with toasted almonds. This is truly a delicious soup.

**Cream of pea-leaf soup:** Gather **young leaves from pea vines;** grind enough to make **1 cup,** and prepare as in basic recipe; add **Worcestershire, 2 tablespoons each diced pimentos and lemon juice.** In center of each serving place **1 tablespoon chili sauce.** Serve with hot potato chips.

**Cream of pea soup made of split peas:** Simmer **1 cup dried split peas** in **3 cups vegetable-cooking water** until almost tender, or about 1 hour; add **crushed white peppercorns, 2 teaspoons salt, 1 or 2 chopped onions;** when onions are tender, add fresh and powdered milk, **3 tablespoons margarine or butter, 2 drops green coloring,** Worcestershire. Garnish with grated lemon or orange rind.

**Cream of tomato soup:** Add to sautéed onion **1 pint tomato purée or diced fresh or canned tomatoes, 2 whole cloves, peppercorns and salt, 1 or 2 teaspoons sugar, pinch of basil;** in separate utensil heat to simmering the fresh milk and stir in fresh and powdered milk; just before serving add tomatoes to hot milk so slowly that protein can neutralize acid and prevent curdling. If no powdered milk is available, mix **1 cup fresh milk** with ½ **cup soy or peanut flour** before adding tomatoes. *Do not add* soda. Garnish with **ground parsley.** Serve with garlic croutons.

**Cream of watercress soup:** Put enough chilled **watercress** through meat grinder to make **1 cup;** prepare and season as in the basic recipe; add ¼ **teaspoon nutmeg.**

Delicious bisques, or rich soups thick with vegetables, can be made of almost every variety of fish and are often enjoyed even more than the popular chowders. They take only a few moments to prepare. When one tastes soup of fish which is blended with onions, celery, garlic, tomatoes, and herbs without being overcooked, one realizes that fish bisques are a treat already missed overlong. By all means add them to your menus. The collars of large fish, and the portion directly behind the gills which is left from cutting steaks, may be purchased at almost no cost and are excellent for making bisques. Since fish scales are largely a form of connective tissue, they can be used in making stock. If ⅓ pound sea food or fish is allowed per person, these soups become excellent for one-dish meals.

## FISH BISQUE

Purchase **1½ or 2 pounds of collars** from red snapper, salmon, halibut, or other fish.
Steam on a rack above:

**1 quart boiling vegetable-cooking water**

Time carefully and steam 2 to 3 minutes for each inch of thickness; remove and flake the meat; drop bones and skin, including scales, into water used for steaming; add:

| | |
|---|---|
| **¼ to ½ teaspoon crushed white peppercorns** | **2 teaspoons salt** |
| **½ crushed bay leaf** | **1 tablespoon vinegar** |

Boil slowly about 15 to 20 minutes.
Meanwhile pan-broil in utensil to be used for making soup:

**2 slices bacon, cut into bits**

Dice fine or shred the following chilled vegetables and cook with bacon:

| | |
|---|---|
| **2 each carrots and onions** | **1 each green pepper and pimento** |
| **2 stalks celery and shredded celery leaves** | **1 minced clove garlic** |

When vegetables are almost tender, strain boiling fish stock directly over them; add:

**2 cups additional vegetable-cooking water**

Immediately before serving add:

| | |
|---|---|
| **flaked fish** | **3 tablespoons ground parsley** |
| **1 teaspoon dill sauce** | |

Taste for salt; garnish with **thin slices of lemon** sprinkled with **paprika.** Serve with rye or soy crackers.

*Variations:*
Prepare the recipe with flounder, barracuda, fresh cod, tuna, or any favorite fish.
If no skin or bones are available for making stock, add seasonings, 1 tablespoon lemon juice, and vegetable-cooking water to bacon and vegetables; add diced raw or flaked canned fish just before serving. If canned tuna is used, drain the oil before adding to bisque.

Add ¼ to ½ cup soy grits to basic recipe or any variation.

Shake with ½ cup vegetable-cooking water, and add just before serving, ½ cup powdered milk or ¼ cup soy or peanut flour.

Make bisques with the following combinations of vegetables, using any amounts desired: celery, carrots, potatoes with fresh dill; onions, peas, carrots; carrots, cabbage, celery, potatoes; tomatoes, celery, corn; string beans, carrots, pimentos; leeks, carrots, potatoes.

**Bisque of canned salmon:** Sauté vegetables; add seasonings, **1 quart vegetable-cooking water or any stock, 2 cups fresh or canned tomatoes;** immediately before serving add **2 cups flaked canned salmon.** Garnish with **diced pimento.** Serve with cheese popcorn.

**Bisque with mushrooms:** Omit garlic, onions, and green pepper; sauté **1 cup fresh or canned mushrooms** with other vegetables; proceed as in basic recipe. Garnish with **thin lemon slices or ground parsley.** Serve with whole-wheat crackers.

**Bisque of shellfish:** Use **2 cups fresh or canned shrimp, crabs, lobster, or fresh oysters;** instead of fish stock use **vegetable-cooking water.** Proceed and season as in basic recipe or any variation. Serve with toasted cheese sticks.

**Bisque of smoked fish:** Use any smoked fish; omit salt and bacon; sauté vegetables in **bacon drippings;** use **vegetable-cooking water** instead of fish stock. Serve with assorted finger salads.

**Tomato bisque:** Instead of 2 cups vegetable-cooking water use **2 cups tomato purée or canned tomatoes;** season with **orégano or basil.**

Since legumes are rich in protein, split-pea, bean, and lentil soups should be served frequently, especially if the budget is limited. The proteins they contain lack some of the essential amino acids; therefore when these soups are served as the principal dish of the meal, meat or other adequate protein should be added to them.

Although bean, lentil, and split-pea soups are customarily prepared with ham bone, delicious soups can be prepared with pigs' feet, pork bones, or accumulated bones, or without bones. If the skin from cured ham or bacon is cooked with the soup, or if smoke-flavoring is used, the popular ham flavor is added. Since the bones are cooked with the legumes, and since splinters left from chopping are difficult to remove, the bones should be sawed or left whole. Vinegar causes legumes to become tough; hence calcium cannot be extracted from the bones unless previously prepared stock is used.

## NAVY-BEAN SOUP MADE WITH HAM BONE

Use bone left from baked or steamed ham or cured shoulder.
Trim off all edible meat scraps and save; saw bone into 1-inch pieces.
Sear by pan-broiling cartilage, gristle, and bones until well browned, or
10 to 15 minutes; add skin removed from ham.
Drain off fat; add and bring to boiling:

**2 quarts water**

Wash quickly, drain, and add without soaking:

**2 or 3 cups white navy beans**

Cover utensil, lower heat, and simmer about 2 to 3 hours; add:

¼ to ½ teaspoon crushed black peppercorns  
½ cup soy or peanut flour shaken with 1 cup water  
⅓ crushed bay leaf

⅛ teaspoon marjoram, savory, and/or basil  
1 or 2 chopped onions  
1 small whole cayenne pepper or chili tepine, minced or pierced with a toothpick

Simmer 20 minutes longer, or until beans are tender; mash about half
the beans; taste for salt and add more if needed.

Discard bones, cartilage, skin, cayenne or chili pepper; add **ham scraps,**
if any, and garnish lightly with **chives.** Serve with garlic croutons.

*Variations:*

Add ½ cup soy grits to any bean, lentil, or split-pea soup.

Vary by adding any one of the following seasonings when beans are
almost tender: 2 teaspoons Worcestershire; ½ teaspoon paprika, curry
powder, dry mustard, or celery or caraway seeds; 1 chopped green pepper,
pimento, fresh paprika, or chili pepper; 3 drops Tabasco; 1 minced clove
garlic or garlic pierced with a toothpick and discarded before serving; 1 or
2 thinly sliced carrots or kohlrabi; 1 chopped stalk celery or 1 tablespoon
Chinese garlic.

**Bean soup made with cooked pork bones or assorted bones:** Do not
sear or chop bones; cook with beans; discard the bones; add **3 teaspoons
salt** and seasonings as in basic recipe; just before serving season to taste
with **smoke-flavoring.**

**Bean soup without bones:** Cook beans in **vegetable-cooking water** with
skin from cured pork; or when beans are almost tender, add **diced bacon
or ham or bacon drippings and smoke-flavoring;** season as in basic recipe.

**Bean soup made with pigs' feet:** Have butcher cut pigs' feet in half lengthwise; sear thoroughly and proceed as in basic recipe; season with **smoke-flavoring;** add **1 tablespoon salt.**

**Black-bean soup:** Substitute **2 cups black beans** for the navy beans; proceed as in basic recipe; season with ¼ **teaspoon savory.**

**Chili soup:** Prepare as for chili with meat (p. 200), adding soup stock to give the consistency desired. Serve with toasted bread sticks or tortillas.

**Kidney-bean soup:** Prepare as in basic recipe; season with **pinch each of basil, thyme, and savory, 1 teaspoon each Worcestershire and dry mustard, 1 chopped onion, 1 minced clove garlic.** Add ½ **pound sliced wieners.** Garnish with **green-onion tops** cut with scissors.

**Leftover baked or boiled bean soup:** Pan-broil ½ **pound bulk pork sausage or 2 slices bacon or ham;** remove ham or bacon if used, but let sausage remain in utensil; drain, leaving 2 or 3 tablespoons fat; sauté lightly **1 chopped onion, 1 stalk celery, 1 diced carrot;** mash beans and add to vegetables; add **1 cup tomato purée and** enough **stock or vegetable-cooking water** to give the consistency desired; add **smoke-flavoring to** taste, **4 or 5 drops Tabasco, diced bacon or ham** if used. Taste for salt; serve with **1 tablespoon chili sauce** in center of each serving.

**Lentil soup:** Cook as in basic recipe **2 cups lentils** with assorted bones; remove bones by passing soup through a colander; rinse utensil used for making soup, and pan-broil ½ **pound pork sausage;** drain off part of the fat and sauté lightly with sausage **1 minced clove garlic, 1 finely diced carrot, 2 chopped onions;** add **salt, peppercorns, bay leaf, 1 teaspoon each Worcestershire and caraway seeds;** add puréed lentils and simmer 10 minutes; add **3 tablespoons ground parsley.** Serve with whole-wheat crackers. Vary lentil soup by preparing and seasoning like any bean soup; by adding sliced wieners or other sausage, or 1 to 2 cups tomato purée; or by seasoning with ½ teaspoon curry powder.

**Lima-bean soup:** Prepare as in basic recipe or any variation; use **2 cups dried lima beans.** If assorted bones are used, pan-broil **1 or 2 slices ham or bacon;** remove; sauté onions, **2 each finely chopped stalks celery and carrots;** dice ham or bacon and add to soup with vegetables and **1 cup tomatoes.** Season as in the basic recipe, garnish with **nutmeg and/or chives.**

**Minestrone, or Italian soup:** Cook **2 cups black-eyed beans** as in basic recipe, using fresh beef shank; when beans are almost tender, add **1 cup tomatoes, 2 teaspoons salt, 2 teaspoons fresh or** ½ **teaspoon dried basil, 1 cup broken whole-wheat spaghetti;** simmer 15 to 20 minutes; meanwhile sauté lightly in **bacon drippings 1 chopped onion or 4 to 6 green**

onions with tops, 2 cloves garlic, 2 sliced summer squash or zucchini, 12 to 15 thinly sliced string beans, ½ to 1 cup green peas. Immediately before serving combine vegetables with beans, add ¼ cup ground parsley, and sprinkle generously with grated Parmesan cheese.

Pinto-bean soup: Cook beans until tender in stock made from assorted bones; when beans are almost tender, dice and brown 2 slices salt pork; add seasonings of basic recipe, 2 cups tomato purée, smoke-flavoring to taste, pinch of orégano, and/or 1 teaspoon cumin seeds. Garnish with orange slices. Serve with rye crackers.

Split-pea soup I: Follow basic recipe or any variation, using split peas instead of beans. Cook 40 minutes before seasoning. Add 1 teaspoon Worcestershire. Garnish with thin slices of orange or lemon sprinkled with paprika. Serve with wheat-germ crackers. Vary recipe by adding 2 chopped stalks celery and/or pimentos; or omit other herbs and season with 2 or 3 teaspoons dill or caraway seeds. For me, caraway seeds added to bean, lentil, or split-pea soup make the difference between mediocrity and sheer delight.

Split-pea soup II: Cook 2 cups peas in vegetable-cooking water for 40 minutes; add 2 or 3 diced carrots, 1 chopped onion or leek, 2 or 3 stalks celery, 3 tablespoons bacon drippings, 2 teaspoons salt, generous amount of cayenne, ¼ teaspoon thyme. Simmer 10 minutes longer; mash the peas thoroughly. Vary by adding 6 to 8 sliced wieners 5 minutes before serving.

In a large family, preparing vegetable-cooking water, or extracting vitamins and minerals from vegetable parings, should be almost a daily procedure. If your family is small, extract from the parings every 3 or 4 days. If a cloth sugar sack is used to hold the parings, they can be squeezed free of juices and no extra dishes need be washed. The bag can be rinsed and used repeatedly. The wooden chopping bowl should be wiped out with paper. The entire procedure should take no more than 5 minutes of actual working time.

Your first reaction will probably be that such water will not be used. When the habit of using vegetable-cooking water is once formed, one usually finds that the supply is not sufficient. Furthermore, when a mother must prepare a baby's formula calling for water and canned milk, what could be more healthful to use than vegetable-cooking water?

## VEGETABLE-COOKING WATER

Put into a wooden chopping bowl and chop quickly:

accumulated vegetable parings          leftovers impossible to use in other
leftover salad and salad scraps from       ways
    plates

Put chopped vegetables into a cloth bag, such as a 10-pound sugar sack. Tie securely. Meanwhile heat to boiling:

### 1 cup water for each cup vegetables to be used

Force chopped vegetables down into water; cover utensil and boil 10 minutes; if convenient, allow parings to soak ½ hour or longer.

Wring bag dry of all juices; discard parings and rinse bag; wipe out chopping bowl with paper.

Pour vegetable-cooking water into a wide-mouthed jar and keep in refrigerator; use for stews, gravies, aspics, soups, vegetable-gelatin salads; add to tomato-juice cocktails.

# CHAPTER 18

## KEEP THE FLAVOR AND NUTRITIVE VALUE IN YOUR VEGETABLES

The principal weakness in American cooking lies in the preparation of vegetables. As they are customarily cooked, much of their flavor and 50 to 90 per cent of many nutrients are lost before they reach the table. These losses are largely avoidable. Surely the stoical eating of waterlogged, tasteless boiled vegetables is proof that Americans have character.

Vegetables to be cooked should be handled in the same manner as salad vegetables. Ideally they should be gathered immediately before being cooked. If you must purchase them, try to reach the market in the morning and choose vegetables which are trimmed the least. With a few exceptions, such as potatoes, dry onions, and corn on the cob, wash and dry them immediately. Chill and put them into a dark place as quickly as possible to stop enzyme action. If they are left at room temperature and in the light, much folic acid, vitamin $B_2$, and 50 per cent or more of the vitamin C in most fresh vegetables can be lost in a few hours.

The greatest culinary crime is soaking. Boiling, or soaking as vegetables are softened, is a form of soaking at its worst. Vitamins C, P, and the many B vitamins pass out of the vegetables and dissolve in water as quickly as sugar dissolves in coffee. Studies have shown that when whole vegetables are boiled (soaked) only 4 minutes, 20 to 45 per cent of the total mineral content and 75 per cent of the sugars they contain pass into the water. Since vegetables are frequently soaked both before and during cooking for much longer periods, as much as 75 to 100 per cent of the sugars, minerals, and water-soluble vitamins are often lost. The color of the water left after beets are washed slowly or boiled indicates how easily and quickly substances can pass out of vegetables, even though unpeeled. The losses are accelerated when vegetables are soaked after being peeled, chopped, sliced, or shredded, and particularly after the cell walls are softened by cooking.

During World War II, scurvy, resulting from a total lack of vitamin C, appeared in English communities where cabbage, a rich source of this vitamin, was a principal food. Part of the vitamin had been destroyed needlessly; the remainder had been discarded in the cooking water. The cumulative loss of vitamins and minerals brought about by soaking and boiling is unquestionably a causative factor in numerous illnesses and diseases. From the point of view of nutrition, the chief purpose in recommending vegetables is to supply vitamins and minerals; any form of soaking largely defeats that purpose. It is nothing less than disgraceful in a country where animals have been fed scientifically for more than a quarter of a century that people are served vegetables which have been carelessly soaked before and during cooking.

When nutritive value is lost, flavor is also lost. All vegetables contain aromatic oils which give them their characteristic odor and flavor; since they are not true oils, they readily dissolve in water. Minerals add a certain saltiness to the taste of vegetables. Vegetables also contain sugars which cause them to be sweet if they are properly prepared and cooked. If you want your vegetables to be delicious, do not let them soak during slow washing or by letting water cling to them after they are washed; cook them by any other method than boiling.

Next to soaking, the greatest nutritive loss is caused by peeling vegetables. In root vegetables, the minerals, which are concentrated under the skin, are discarded when the vegetable is peeled. In sautéed parsnips, steamed eggplant, and French-fried potatoes, for example, the peeling adds flavor. If a vegetable is chopped, shredded, or diced, the only person who knows whether or not it is peeled is the one who has done the work. In case you spend 20 minutes daily peeling vegetables, in the course of a year you will have spent 121 hours, or 15 entire working days—an astounding waste of time. The waste of food value is even more startling. The average family throws away annually potato parings alone equivalent in iron to 500 eggs, in protein to 60 steaks, and in vitamin C to 95 glasses of orange juice. *Make it a rule to peel vegetables only when the skin is tough, bitter, or too uneven to be thoroughly cleaned.*

Provided vegetables are not soaked, the saving of vitamins C and $B_2$ during preparation and cooking depends largely on preventing enzyme action and excluding oxygen and light. Enzymes are inactive when cold and are destroyed by heat. Vitamin C is destroyed only in the presence of oxygen, and vitamin $B_2$ only in light. Prepare chilled vegetables so quickly that they will not reach room temperature. If you must prepare vegetables before time to cook them, put them back into the refrigerator. Unless they are chilled, cut them as little as possible. The peel, if left on, can prevent contact with oxygen and hence preserve vitamin C. In order to destroy the enzymes rapidly, heat all vegetables as quickly as possible. Preheat the oven or the utensil to be used, have the utensil filled with steam, which displaces oxygen, and try not to lift the lid during cooking.

After the enzymes are made inactive by heat, destruction of vitamin C continues slowly unless there is contact with alkali. Minerals in hard water harm vitamin C during cooking; the addition of soda destroys it rapidly; and contact with iron and copper-containing utensils causes instant and complete destruction. Although vitamin A in yellow and green vegetables and fruits is usually not harmed in cooking, the vitamin A in butter and margarine is quickly destroyed by heat; if these fats are used for seasoning, they should be added after the vegetables are cooked. The destruction of vitamin $B_1$ is slow unless the vegetables are cooked at a temperature above boiling, like those which are fried or cooked under pressure; the shorter the cooking time, the less the loss of vitamins $B_1$ and C. Vitamin $B_2$ is harmed during cooking only when glass utensils are used or the vegetable is cooked without being covered. Folic acid, the anti-pernicious anemia vitamin, is quickly destroyed by heat; yet the other B vitamins, unless at a temperature above boiling, and vitamins E, K, and P appear not to be harmed.

Many of the aromatic oils which give vegetables their delightful taste volatilize and are lost in proportion to the cooking time. If the best flavor and the most nutrients are to be retained, cook vegetables for the shortest time necessary to make them tender. Since chopping, shredding, and dicing shorten the cooking time, these procedures are recommended provided the vegetable is chilled, is not soaked, or is not ruined in appearance.

Frozen vegetables retain their nutritive value during freezing and storage, although 50 per cent of the vitamin C may be lost before they are frozen. After they are thawed, losses occur more quickly than in fresh vegetables. With the exception of corn on the cob, these vegetables should be put on to cook while still frozen. They cook in approximately half the time required for fresh vegetables.

Since salt attracts moisture, when a vegetable is salted at the beginning of cooking, its juices, which carry vitamins, minerals, sugars, and flavors, are drawn out. For example, studies have shown that spinach salted during cooking loses 47 per cent of its iron content and only 19 per cent when unsalted. Except when vegetables are cooked in a sauce, they should be salted just before being served.

If vegetables are properly prepared and cooked, their natural colors are preserved. Discoloration before cooking can be prevented by keeping them thoroughly chilled and by avoiding all contact with copper-containing equipment. Green vegetables contain plant acids which react chemically during cooking with the coloring matter, changing it to olive-gray. If the vegetable is cooked quickly and overcooking is avoided, little acid is freed, and the bright color is preserved. The white and red vegetables, such as turnips, cauliflower, celery root, purple cabbage, and red onions, discolor or turn dark upon contact with alkali. The minerals in hard water quickly destroy the attractiveness of such vegetables. Even when knives and cooking utensils are carefully rinsed, enough alkaline minerals from soap are left on them to discolor these vegetables, especially purple cabbage. If you must use hard water in cooking, add a drop or two of vinegar to it and rinse the cooking utensils with water containing a little vinegar. Proteins have the capacity of combining with both acids and alkalies; hence discoloration can be prevented and the green colors be intensified by cooking vegetables in milk or with any protein.

All liquids in which vegetables have been cooked should be used, regardless of the amount. The less liquid left from cooking them, the more concentrated are the nutrients in it. When cooked vegetables are soft in texture and only a little water has been used in cooking them, this water, carrying nutrients and flavor, is usually absorbed back into them. If vegetables are not absorbent and all the water is evaporated the nutrients are dried to the pan and are lost; in this case, a tablespoon of liquid should be added before serving.

If a meal is delayed after the vegetables are ready to serve, they should be quickly chilled and reheated later, thus preventing continued loss of vitamin C. Women have been warned repeatedly that serious nutritive losses occur when foods are reheated; not infrequently leftover vegetables are thrown away because "all the vitamins are destroyed by reheating." The losses referred to, however, are largely those caused by soaking, or boiling, already soft vegetables. Although reheating should be avoided whenever possible, little loss need occur if the vegetable is quickly reheated in fat or only a small amount of liquid, if the temperature is kept low, if oxygen is replaced by steam, and if light is excluded. Canned vegetables should be reheated in the liquid in which they are canned and all the liquid should be used.

The recipes advising that vegetables be purposely and unnecessarily cooked twice should certainly be discarded. Most cookbooks seem to abound in such recipes: parsnips, green peppers, or carrots to be boiled, drained, and then baked or fried; vegetables to be boiled, drained, and then creamed or made into casserole dishes or soufflés. When two processes are used in cooking a vegetable, the second is permissible only if no cooking liquid from the first process is discarded and if longer cooking is necessary to make a vegetable sufficiently tender to be palatable.

*Make it a rule to cook vegetables in the shortest time possible, guarding carefully against overcooking.* The shorter the cooking time, the more delicious the flavor of the vegetables. In order to prevent overcooking and to have the family ready to eat dinner the minute the vegetables are done, serve a first course of salad, soup, or appetizers. With a few exceptions, the vegetables can then be put on to cook when the family comes in to wash up for the meal or immediately before the first course is eaten.

Your ability as a cook is shown not by the desserts you make, but by the quantity and variety of vegetables your family demands.

## METHODS OF COOKING VEGETABLES

It has often been pointed out that there is no objection to boiling vegetables, or cooking them covered with water, if the water is rapidly boiling before the vegetable is dropped into it; if it is quickly reheated to boiling; if the vegetable is not overcooked; and if all the cooking liquid is used. Such a statement is true, but the catch is that all the liquid is not used. For twenty-five years housewives have been urged to save the water left from boiling vegetables, and many have tried; yet probably not one housewife out of the millions in the entire country has actually done it. Since the nutritive losses are so great and it is impractical to use all cooking water unless the amount is small, vegetables should be cooked by any other method than boiling.

If health is to be produced and nutritive losses are to be kept to a minimum, a good cooking method should meet the following requirements: to destroy enzymes quickly, the initial heating must be rapid; to prevent loss of vitamin C, contact with oxygen should be avoided by leaving the vegetable unpeeled, by covering cut surfaces with oil, or by displacing the oxygen in the utensil with steam; the vegetable should be cooked the shortest time necessary to develop tenderness; every drop of liquid which touches the vegetable should be used. If these rules are observed and any vegetable to be cut is first thoroughly chilled, probably 95 per cent of all nutrients can be retained.

Perhaps the best method of cooking vegetables is the so-called waterless method. All fresh vegetables contain 70 to 95 per cent water, which is sufficient for cooking them if the heat is controlled so that no steam escapes. The utensil used must have a tight-fitting lid and must distribute heat evenly to the sides and the lid; thus the vegetable cooks by heat coming from all directions. Although vegetables may be cooked without any added water, a tablespoon or two should usually be put into the preheated utensil in order to replace oxygen by steam and thus protect vitamin C. The success of the method depends upon keeping the heat low after the first few minutes, so that no steam escapes. Since the vegetables can be cooked largely over a simmer burner, waterless-cooking equipment pays for itself in saving fuel; it pays for itself many times over in promoting health.

Steaming in the new type of pressure cooker is excellent provided the cooking time is checked with stop-watch precision. Since directions are included with the equipment, I have not given them in the recipes. Only a few tablespoons of water need be used, and it should be brought to boiling before the vegetable is put into the utensil. As soon as the cooking time has expired, the utensil should be cooled immediately. All liquid used should be served with the vegetable or added to soup stock. During steaming, moisture continually condenses on the surface of the vegetable; since sugars, minerals, vitamin C, and the B vitamins can dissolve into the moisture, considerable nutritive loss occurs unless the liquid is used, especially if the vegetable is diced or otherwise cut. The disadvantage of the method is that vegetables overcook quickly. In this case a large proportion of vitamins C, $B_1$, $B_2$, and niacin can be destroyed; the sulfur compounds in the strong-flavored vegetables break down; if the vegetables contain protein, its health-building value is harmed; aromatic oils are driven off quickly and flavor is lost. Since the old type of pressure cooker is difficult to cool, vegetables prepared in it are almost invariably overcooked.

If steaming is done without pressure, the vegetables should be left uncut and unpeeled whenever possible so that a minimum of surface is exposed to moisture. If the vegetable is cut, only the amount of water necessary to prevent burning should be used; this water should be served with the vegetable. Since steam held above boiling water is exactly the same temperature as the water, the vegetables cook in the same time required for boiling. When no cooking liquid is discarded, the vegetables need not be placed on a rack above the water.

If no equipment is available for waterless cooking or pressure steaming, vegetables can be cooked with little nutritive loss in the top of a double boiler. A few tablespoons of water are put into the utensil and brought to a rolling boil; the vegetables are added and steamed over high direct heat until the enzymes are destroyed, the oxygen is replaced by steam, and most or all of the water has evaporated. The vegetables are then placed over boiling water to finish cooking. Since they cannot burn, they need no watching. The temperature in the top of the double boiler ranges from 206° to 210° F., at which vegetables cook as quickly as at boiling temperature after they are once heated through.

Since every housewife owns a frying pan, sautéing is a practical method of cooking vegetables largely in their own juices. No more than 2 tablespoons of fat need be used. The vegetable should be stirred thoroughly with the hot fat so that all cut surfaces can be sealed from oxygen, juices can be sealed in, and direct contact with moisture can be prevented. It is important that no drops of water cling to the vegetable; otherwise the fat will not adhere to it. When contact with moisture and air is prevented, the natural colors are preserved or even intensified. If a bulky leafy vegetable, such as spinach or shredded cabbage, is being cooked, the best method is to use the salad bowl and toss it with oil just as you would a salad. When the cooking time is longer than 5 minutes, 1 or 2 tablespoons water may be added to produce steam. The frying pan should be covered with a tight-fitting lid and the heat reduced as soon as the vegetable is heated through. If the heat is controlled, the vegetable will cook without shriveling or browning. This method is a variation of waterless cooking rather than of frying.

Another excellent method of cooking vegetables is to simmer them in milk. The nutrients in vegetables dissolve less readily into milk than into water. If the vegetable is thoroughly stirred with the milk, protein coats the surfaces and neutralizes the acids or alkalies which cause discoloration; thus the color is preserved and often intensified. Vegetables cooked in milk are milder and sweeter than those cooked in water. The milk itself is so delicious that there is little danger of its being discarded. Cooking should be done at a simmering temperature, or about 200° F., which destroys the enzymes quickly and cooks the vegetable in approximately the time required for boiling. If a simmering temperature is maintained, the milk will not boil over, scorch, or curdle. If the temperature cannot be controlled, the top of the double boiler can be used; the vegetable should be heated quickly over direct heat and then cooked over boiling water. Only ½ cup milk is needed if the utensil holds in steam, but if a tight-fitting lid is not available, the vegetable may be covered with milk. The milk should be saved and used again or made into cream soup. As a means of including more milk in the diet, keep cream sauce on hand and add it frequently to vegetables cooked in milk.

Broiling is an excellent method of cooking vegetables but is used far too little. The initial heating is rapid, the vegetables cook quickly, and no moisture need touch them. Unless the cooking time is extremely short, the vegetable should be brushed or tossed with oil to prevent contact with oxygen and unnecessary loss of vitamin C. The success of the method lies in keeping the heat moderate or low after the vegetable is once heated through; otherwise it shrivels and becomes unattractive.

Although fried vegetables are often frowned upon as being "bad for you," frying meets the requirements of an excellent method provided the vegetables are first thoroughly chilled. The initial heating is rapid, and the cooking time is short. The vegetable cooks in its own juices. Contact with oxygen is prevented by fat and steam. If the frying is done in vegetable oil, vitamins $B_6$, E, K, and essential fatty acids are supplied. If large amounts of these substances are needed, one of the easiest ways to obtain them is by eating fried vegetables. If the heat is kept moderate so that shriveling is prevented, carrots, beets, parsnips, turnips, and many other vegetables can be delicious when fried. The only disadvantages of the method are the extra calories and the possibility of destroying some of the B vitamins if the temperature becomes too high.

Although baking is far superior to boiling as a method of cooking vegetables, vitamin C is largely destroyed because of slow initial heating, long cooking, and exposure to oxygen if the vegetables are peeled. The loss can be minimized but not prevented if peeled vegetables are oiled and put into a preheated oven. Whenever possible, whole vegetables to be baked should first be quickly steamed or put under the broiler until they are heated through and the enzymes are destroyed; then they should be transferred to the preheated oven. In this way the cooking time can be shortened about a third. If vegetables are to be sliced and baked in a casserole, the liquid used should be hot, the casserole and the oven preheated, and, to prevent contact with oxygen, the casserole tightly covered to hold in steam; otherwise sufficient liquid should be used to cover the vegetables.

When utensils with tight-fitting lids are not available, cooking in parchment paper is an excellent method. Since the vegetables cook in their own juices, almost no nutritive loss occurs except partial destruction of vitamin C caused by slow heating. The vegetables should be diced to shorten the cooking time, the paper tied tightly around them to prevent dead-air space from retarding the penetration of heat, the water brought to rapid boiling before they are put into it, and the timetables relied on to indicate doneness.

The example of vegetable cookery at its worst is probably the tasteless, overcooked, puréed vegetables fed to babies and invalids. The purpose of puréeing vegetables is to break them into small pieces so that the nutrients can be absorbed into the blood readily and completely. Although the purpose in serving them is supposedly to build health, this purpose is defeated, since many nutrients are destroyed by cooking at high temperature, overcooking, and exposure to oxygen while the vegetable is being puréed. If you must prepare food for a baby, a person who must stay on a smooth diet, or one who cannot chew well, chop the carefully prepared vegetable after it is cooked, or grate, shred, or grind the chilled unpeeled vegetables and steam or sauté them quickly. Vegetables prepared in this manner are unusually sweet; since they cook in a few minutes, almost no flavor or nutritive value is lost. Persons who dislike beets, for example, almost invariably enjoy them when they are shredded and cooked quickly.

When so many excellent methods of cooking vegetables are available, the only housewife who would cook them by boiling is one who is indifferent to producing health in herself and her family.

Since vegetable cooking is so simple, I have deviated from using basic recipes and have summarized the cooking methods recommended under each vegetable. Every method, however, is given in detail several times.

## GLOBE ARTICHOKES

Cut off inedible tips of:

**4 large chilled artichokes**

Tuck into each:

¼ crushed bay leaf                    bits of minced garlic
pinch of basil

Put petal end down into:

**½ cup boiling vegetable-cooking water**

Cover utensil and steam 20 to 30 minutes, or until tender; drain and
save liquid; sprinkle artichokes with salt. Serve hot with melted butter,
or chilled with mayonnaise or any uncooked sauce (p. 168).

*Variations:*

It utensil does not distribute heat, steam on a rack above water.

Before cooking, tuck into the artichoke leaves ground parsley, chopped
onion or green-onion tops, celery leaves, chives, or crushed black peppercorns.

Cook artichokes in soup stock or juices around a pot roast or Swiss
steak.

Steam without seasoning; serve with Hollandaise sauce or remove
leaves from center of whole steamed artichoke and serve hot filled with
cheese sauce (p. 163) or creamed chicken (p. 216), garnish with paprika
or ground parsley; or chill, fill with shrimp or fish cocktail, and serve as
an appetizer; or fill with chicken or fish salad.

Cut into halves, cook in ½ cup hot milk or enough milk to cover;
drain off milk and use for cooking other vegetables.

**French-fried artichokes:** Use cooked or canned artichoke hearts; dip
in batter (p. 183) and French-fry at 350° F. until brown.

**Stuffed artichokes:** Prepare dressing of **1 minced clove garlic, 2 tablespoons each chopped celery and onion, ½ teaspoon salt, 2 tablespoons
bacon drippings, crushed peppercorns, pinch of basil, ¾ cup whole-wheat-
bread crumbs;** stuff between artichoke leaves; steam on a rack above
water; sprinkle with **paprika** and brown slightly under broiler.

Jerusalem artichokes, tubers of the sunflower family, are so similar in appearance and taste to new potatoes that most persons
quickly learn to enjoy them. These artichokes are rich in sugar

and must be washed rapidly if their delightful taste is to be retained. Get acquainted with them and serve them often. They become tough if cooked at high temperature or overcooked. Raw Jerusalem artichokes, which have the texture of cabbage stalks, are particularly delicious in salads.

## JERUSALEM ARTICHOKES SIMMERED IN SHALLOW MILK

Slice, dice, or cut into halves:

1 pound chilled unpeeled artichokes

Drop into:

¼ cup hot milk

Stir to cover all surfaces with milk protein; cover utensil and simmer 6 to 10 minutes; add:

1 teaspoon salt                    2 tablespoons ground parsley

Garnish with **paprika**.

*Variations:*

Steam whole in waterless-cooking utensil or pressure cooker; or simmer in enough milk to cover.

Add 1 small chopped onion and/or 1 clove garlic before steaming; discard garlic before serving; or add chives or green-onion tops cut with scissors.

Remove from heat and add ½ cup diced American cheese; cover utensil until cheese is melted; stir; garnish with parsley.

Steam with any vegetable which cooks in the same time, such as fresh or frozen peas or diced carrots or turnips.

Thicken milk by adding cream sauce; add 1 diced pimento, or after removing from heat add ½ cup diced American cheese.

**Broiled Jerusalem artichokes:** Cut unpeeled artichokes into fingers, mix with 1 tablespoon oil, and put on oiled baking sheet; keep heat high until browning starts, or about 2 minutes; turn with pancake turner, brown the other side, lower heat, and cook 6 or 8 minutes.

**Fried Jerusalem artichokes:** Slice unpeeled artichokes and fry 8 to 10 minutes in preheated bacon drippings or oil; turn 2 or 3 times during cooking; or sauté without browning in 1 tablespoon each fat and water.

## ASPARAGUS COOKED IN MILK

Allow ⅓ pound asparagus per serving.
Break off ends where stalks snap easily; tie stalks into bunches for individual servings or keep parallel in utensil.
Drop chilled asparagus into:

**2 cups hot milk, or enough to cover**

Use a cooking thermometer and heat milk quickly to 200° F.; adjust heat, cover utensil, and simmer 8 to 10 minutes, or until tender; pour off milk and use for cream soup made of tough ends of stalks.
Add:

**½ teaspoon salt**

*Variations:*

Dice asparagus and cook in ½ cup milk.
Put asparagus on hot serving platter or plates, sprinkle with shredded American or Parmesan cheese, and garnish with paprika.
Steam asparagus in or above ¼ cup boiling water; or stand stalks in small amount of water in top of double boiler and steam.
**Asparagus patties:** Follow recipe for zucchini patties (p. 370); cut asparagus into ¼-inch pieces.
**Asparagus sautéed in batter:** Cut asparagus of irregular sizes or lengths into ½-inch pieces, drop into batter made by mixing **1 egg, 3 tablespoons milk, 1 teaspoon salt, ¼ cup wheat germ;** let stand for 10 minutes; drop from tablespoon onto a hot pan brushed with bacon drippings or oil; brown quickly on both sides; cook 6 to 8 minutes.
**Asparagus soufflé:** Add **2 cups ground raw asparagus** to plain or cheese soufflé (p. 209).
**Creamed asparagus:** Cook in **1 cup milk;** thicken by adding **cream sauce;** do not cut asparagus unless lengths and sizes are irregular.
*With cheese:* Cook asparagus in heat-resistant baking dish; wipe edges of dish after adding cream sauce; cover top with **toasted whole-wheat-bread crumbs and ½ cup shredded American cheese;** cover utensil until cheese is melted.
**Sautéed asparagus:** Heat 1 tablespoon bacon drippings or oil in frying pan; add asparagus stalks, a few tablespoons of water; cover utensil and steam 12 to 15 minutes; keep heat low to prevent shriveling.

The bean sprouts most often sold, or the sprouts of the mung bean, should be little more than heated through. If they are overcooked even a few minutes, the water they contain dries out and they become shriveled and tasteless. If soybean sprouts are used, they should be cooked about 5 minutes longer than the mung sprouts.

## STEAMED BEAN SPROUTS

Wash, drain, and whirl dry:

**2 cups bean sprouts**

Add to:

**2 tablespoons boiling water**

Steam only long enough to heat through, or about 4 minutes. Season with ½ teaspoon salt and dash of paprika.

*Variations:*

Steam in ¼ cup milk instead of boiling water, thicken with cream sauce, add ground parsley, diced pimento, or dash of nutmeg.

**Bean sprouts with tomatoes:** Pan-broil 1 slice bacon and drain on paper; add 1 diced fresh or ½ cup canned tomatoes, 2 tablespoons chopped onion, ½ diced green pepper, crushed peppercorns, ½ teaspoon salt; simmer 5 to 8 minutes; add and heat bean sprouts; break bacon into small pieces and add with 1 teaspoon soy sauce just before serving.

## CRISP SHREDDED BEETS

Shred:

**4 to 6 chilled unpeeled beets**

Put into preheated frying pan with:

**1 tablespoon water or lemon juice      2 teaspoons bacon drippings or oil**

Stir, cover utensil, and cook over moderate heat for 5 minutes. Add and stir:

**½ teaspoon salt**

Serve piping hot but crisp.

*Variations:*

Put beets into casserole brushed with oil; cook for 7 minutes in hot oven at 400° F.

Omit fat and cook beets in 2 tablespoons milk or 1 tablespoon each water and vinegar or lemon juice.

**Baked beets:** Brush medium-size unpeeled beets with oil, put under broiler or over boiling water, and heat rapidly for 10 minutes; transfer to moderate oven, at 350° F., and cook until tender, or about 30 minutes; cut petal-fashion and sprinkle with salt, paprika, and butter or margarine.

**Beets cooked with tops:** See page 379.

**Beets simmered in milk:** Dice 4 to 6 medium unpeeled beets in ¼-inch cubes or cut into fingers; put into utensil with ¼ cup hot milk and ¼ teaspoon crushed black peppercorns; stir beets to moisten all surfaces with milk protein; cover utensil, lower heat, and simmer 8 to 12 minutes; sprinkle with ½ teaspoon salt.

*With herbs:* Just before serving add 1 tablespoon chopped mint, dill, chives, fresh basil, chervil, or 2 tablespoons ground parsley.

*With sour cream:* Just before removing from heat add ½ cup sour cream or yogurt.

**Broiled beets:** Cut 4 or 5 raw unpeeled beets into shoestring strips; toss with 1 tablespoon French dressing, put on oiled baking sheet and set 2 inches from broiler; keep heat high for about 2 minutes and turn with pancake turner; after 2 more minutes lower heat and cook 8 to 12 minutes. If beets are no more than 1 inch in diameter, oil and broil whole.

**Sautéed beets:** Slice 6 to 8 unpeeled beets; sprinkle lightly with lemon juice or vinegar; put into heated frying pan with 2 tablespoons bacon drippings or oil; except for initial heating, keep heat low; turn with pancake turner occasionally; cover utensil and cook 10 to 15 minutes, or until tender; sprinkle with salt and pepper; or cook in 2 teaspoons fat and 2 tablespoons water; cover and steam.

**Spiced beets:** Cut 6 unpeeled beets into fourths, fingers, or cubes; put into hot utensil with 4 tablespoons boiling water, 1 tablespoon vinegar, 3 each cloves and cassia buds; cover and steam 12 to 18 minutes; add 1 teaspoon blackstrap molasses, 1 teaspoon salt; or cook all seasonings with water and add diced beets steamed without being peeled.

*With herbs:* Omit spices and steam beets with vinegar, water, 1 tablespoon oil, ¼ crushed bay leaf, 1 minced clove garlic; or just before serving add molasses and salt, 1 teaspoon chopped fresh mint, tarragon, or savory leaves.

Bell peppers should be eaten as frequently as possible because of their content of vitamins A and C. Since the vitamin C content doubles as the pepper becomes red, use ripe ones when available. Ripe bell peppers may be cooked in any way suggested for fresh pimentos (p. 365).

## SAUTÉED BELL PEPPERS

Dice into bite size:

**4 to 6 bell peppers, preferably red**

Put into:

**2 tablespoons bacon drippings**

Stir well, cover utensil, keep heat moderate, and cook 8 to 10 minutes; sprinkle with **salt and pepper.** Serve while still slightly crisp.

*Variations:*

Simmer peppers in ¼ cup milk or ½ cup medium cream sauce; add ½ cup cubed cheese before serving.

Sauté peppers with an equal amount of sliced onions and 1 clove garlic; discard garlic before serving.

## SAUTÉED CARROTS

Cut into fingers or slice crosswise:

**6 to 8 chilled unpeeled carrots**

Put into:

**1 or 2 tablespoons hot butter-flavored oil or bacon drippings**

Stir well and add:

**1 tablespoon water**

Cover utensil, heat quickly, and reduce to moderate heat; turn occasionally and brown only slightly; cook for 10 to 15 minutes.

Season with:

**½ teaspoon salt**                              **freshly ground black peppercorns**

*Variations:*

Dice carrots; sauté without browning; add ½ teaspoon black molasses or brown sugar.

Sauté with carrots 2 diced unpeeled apples or 1 or 2 sliced onions or raw potatoes.

To prepare carrots to be served with a roast, slice in half lengthwise and sauté in fat dipped from dripping pan; sauté small whole onions and potatoes cut in half lengthwise with carrots; allow about 20 minutes for cooking.

**French-fried carrots:** Cut unpeeled carrots into fingers; fry in bacon drippings at 285° F. for 8 minutes, or until tender; drain and salt.

**Sautéed mixed vegetables:** Slice 1 onion, 1 green or red bell pepper or pimento, 1 or 2 each unpeeled carrots, turnips, potatoes; sauté together, turning frequently; sprinkle with salt and pepper. At college, a group of us used to live on this dish when we were broke; we called it "fried stew."

## BAKED CARROTS AND APPLES

Slice in alternate layers into a heat-resistant casserole:

| | |
|---|---|
| 4 or 5 chilled unpeeled carrots, cut into quarters lengthwise | 1 to 3 unpeeled apples, quartered and then sliced |

Top with dots of margarine or butter; sprinkle with:

| | |
|---|---|
| 1 teaspoon salt | 3 tablespoons hot water |
| 1 teaspoon grated lemon rind | |

Cover casserole, steam 5 or 10 minutes, then bake in hot oven at 400° F. for 15 to 20 minutes, or until tender; or cook until tender over direct heat.

*Variations:*

Omit lemon rind; top with whole-wheat-bread crumbs, bake until tender, and sprinkle with ½ cup grated or cubed American cheese; garnish with paprika; leave uncovered in oven until cheese melts.

## STEAMED CARROTS

Use waterless-cooking utensil or top of double boiler.
Cut into fourths lengthwise:

6 chilled unpeeled carrots

Drop into:

1 tablespoon boiling water

Add:

¼ teaspoon crushed black peppercorns

Cover utensil, heat quickly, then simmer over direct heat or boiling water for 12 to 15 minutes. Add:

½ teaspoon salt

Serve at once.

*Variations:*

Add ¼ teaspoon minced mint leaves after cooking 10 minutes.

Dice carrots and cook with diced celery, chopped or grated onion, or fresh or frozen peas.

Cook in ½ cup soup stock or milk or milk thickened with cream sauce; at beginning of cooking add crushed white peppercorns and pinch of thyme.

Steam whole unpeeled carrots on rack above boiling water; season with butter or margarine and 2 tablespoons parsley; or transfer to flat baking dish, sprinkle with ¾ cup shredded cheese; melt under broiler; or chill, cut into fingers, mix with French dressing or mayonnaise, serve cold.

**Broiled carrots:** Cut carrots into fingers ⅛ inch thick and toss with 1 tablespoon butter-flavored oil; place on baking sheet and broil at moderate heat until browning starts, or about 4 minutes; turn with pancake turner; lower heat, cook until tender, or about 10 minutes; season with salt and pepper.

**Carrots simmered in milk:** Cut carrots in half and drop into enough hot milk to cover, or about 2 cups; simmer 10 to 15 minutes; drain off milk and save; season carrots with salt, pepper, paprika.

**Shredded carrots:** Shred unpeeled carrots; cook 5 minutes in small amount of milk, water, or **1 tablespoon French dressing** or bacon drippings; or bake in preheated oiled casserole; **¼ cup or more shredded cheese** may be added.


## GREEN CELERY WITH LEAVES

Use outer green celery stalks and leaves; dice stalks into ¾-inch pieces and shred leaves.

Add approximately:

**2 cups diced stalks to ½ cup simmering milk**

Stir well to cover all surfaces with milk protein.

Cover utensil, heat quickly, and simmer 8 to 10 minutes; add:

**shredded celery leaves**

Stir well and cook 2 minutes. Season with:

**½ teaspoon salt**                              **dash of cayenne**

Garnish with **strips of canned pimento.**

*Variations:*

When celery is tender, remove from heat and add ½ cup cubed American cheese or ⅛ cup Parmesan cheese; serve as soon as cheese melts.

**Broiled celery:** Dice celery into ½-inch pieces and toss with 1 tablespoon oil; broil on baking sheet at high temperature 2 minutes, turn, and cook 2 minutes longer before lowering heat; broil until tender, or about 12 minutes; add salt and paprika.

**Celery cooked in soup stock:** Cut in half lengthwise the base of 2 small bunches of celery, leaving the stalks about 5 inches long; drop into ¾ cup boiling soup stock; cover utensil and cook 12 to 15 minutes, or until tender; remove to serving platter, add cream sauce to thicken stock, boil 1 minute, and pour over celery.

**Celery with cheese:** Steam celery cut as specified above in vegetable-cooking water; put into flat baking dish, add salt, and cover with 1 cup grated cheese; sprinkle with paprika; melt cheese under broiler without browning it.

**Celery with tomatoes:** Sauté lightly 1 each chopped onion and green pepper; add 1 cup canned tomatoes, pinch of basil, ¾ teaspoon salt, crushed black peppercorns; heat to boiling; cut in half lengthwise the base of 2 small bunches of celery, leaving stalks 4 to 6 inches long; wash, drop into hot tomatoes, and cook until tender, or about 15 minutes.

**Creamed celery:** Cook diced celery in ½ cup milk; thicken with cream sauce; after removing from heat add ½ cup American cheese. Serve on toast and garnish with paprika.

**Marinated celery:** Cut stalks 3 inches long; steam, chill, and marinate in French dressing; serve chilled for hot-weather dinners.

**Sautéed celery:** Cut into 1-inch pieces; sauté slowly in bacon drippings, margarine, or butter; sprinkle with paprika.

Celery root, or celeriac, is a bulbous root 4 to 6 inches in diameter covered with rough skin. Since it cannot be cleaned thoroughly, it must be peeled. The texture of cooked celery root is similar to that of potatoes; its taste resembles that of celery, but it is milder and sweeter. The stalk and leaves, which are stronger in flavor than celery, are excellent for seasoning. Since celery root discolors easily, it should be chilled thoroughly and dropped into hot liquid immediately after being peeled and cut. When quickly prepared and simmered in milk, it is snowy white and so delicious that people usually enjoy its taste the first time they eat it.

## CELERY ROOT

Heat to simmering:

### ½ cup milk

Add and stir:

### ¼ teaspoon crushed white peppercorns

Meanwhile peel and quickly dice or cut into fingers ½ inch thick:

### 1 or 2 celery roots, or about 2 cups

Drop celery root into hot milk; stir thoroughly, cover utensil, heat rapidly, and simmer over direct heat or in double boiler 12 to 15 minutes; add:

### ½ teaspoon salt

Garnish with **paprika.**

*Variations:*

Add 2 tablespoons ground parsley or 1 tablespoon chopped chives.

Add ½ cup shredded celery-root leaves 5 minutes before serving. Use other leaves for soup stock or tossed salads, or dry in a slow oven and save for general seasoning.

Increase milk to ¾ cup; thicken with cream sauce; add a few diced pimentos, ground parsley, or a dash of nutmeg.

**Baked celery root:** When oven is being used, cut small celery roots in half without peeling them; brush the cut surface with oil; bake until tender, or 20 to 25 minutes, and remove skin; salt and garnish with paprika; or steam until hot, then bake.

**Chilled celery root:** Cut into halves and steam until tender; chill, peel, dice, and marinate with ¼ cup French dressing or mayonnaise.

**Mashed celery root:** Cook as in basic recipe until tender; pass through hot ricer or food mill; add salt, butter, and milk left from steaming.

**Sautéed celery root:** Peel and slice celery root crosswise; cut slices into quarters; moisten with 1 tablespoon lemon juice; sauté over low heat in bacon drippings; sprinkle with salt and paprika.

Chayote is a variety of squash with pale-green meat and a soft edible seed. Small tubers, which taste much like sweet potatoes, grow on the roots; they can be cooked like sweet potatoes or served in salads. The tender leaves and raw young fruit are also excellent in salads.

## SAUTÉED CHAYOTE

Pan-broil until crisp:

### 1 slice bacon

Meanwhile cut **1 or 2 chilled chayotes** lengthwise into quarters without removing seed; if peel is tender, leave unpeeled; hold quarters together and slice crosswise in ¼-inch pieces.

Remove bacon to paper; put chayote into:

### 1 tablespoon hot bacon drippings

Keep heat high until chayote is heated through; leave utensil uncovered to allow moisture to evaporate, turn frequently, and serve while still slightly crisp, or in about 8 minutes.

Season with:

**½ teaspoon salt**                             **freshly ground black peppercorns**

*Variations:*

Sauté with chayote chopped or sliced onion, green pepper, pimento, or celery.

Slice chayote crosswise ¼ inch thick; dip in egg stirred with 2 tablespoons milk and in whole-wheat-bread crumbs; fry in shallow or deep fat; season with salt and freshly ground peppercorns.

Cut into wedges lengthwise; steam with small amount of water or cook in waterless-cooking utensil or in top of double boiler; season with salt and paprika.

**Baked chayote:** Cut chayotes into halves lengthwise, brush all surfaces with oil, and bake in a moderate oven for 20 to 30 minutes, or until tender; season with salt and pepper; garnish with ground parsley; or steam until hot, then bake.

**Broiled chayote:** Cut chayotes into ½-inch slices crosswise, brush with oil, broil on baking sheet 10 to 12 minutes; season with salt and pepper.

**Chayote with cheese:** Add ½ cup cubed American cheese to chayote steamed in its own juices, in milk, or in cream sauce; garnish with ground parsley and paprika.

**Creamed chayote:** Heat ½ cup each milk and cream sauce, add sliced chayotes, cook until tender; salt.

Cucumbers selected for cooking are usually too large for salads. Although many people will frown at the suggestion of cooked cu-

cumbers, others find them delicious. If you have never eaten
cooked cucumbers, try them and see whether you have been
missing something.

## SAUTÉED CUCUMBERS

Cut large chilled cucumber into halves lengthwise; discard seeds; remove peel only if it is hard. Hold halves together and slice quickly into
¼-inch slices.

Meanwhile heat in frying pan:

**1 tablespoon oil, butter-flavored fat, or bacon drippings**

Add and stir:

| | |
|---|---|
| sliced cucumber | generous dash of paprika and nutmeg |
| ½ teaspoon salt | 1 tablespoon chopped chives |

Keep heat high to evaporate juices from cucumber.
Serve as soon as transparent, or in about 5 minutes.

*Variations:*

Pan-broil 1 slice bacon until crisp; remove; brown 1 clove garlic and
discard; sauté cucumbers in bacon drippings; cut bacon into bits and
add just before serving.

Sauté cucumbers with any one of the following vegetables: bell peppers,
fresh pimentos, celery, turnips, carrots, onions, or potatoes; if vegetable
requires longer to cook, add cucumbers 5 minutes before serving.

Cook cucumber with scrambled eggs; sauté as in basic recipe; add eggs,
stir, season, and cook over low heat until eggs are firm.

Cut cucumbers into rings; steam in preheated waterless-cooking utensil
or top of double boiler; heat quickly, turn heat low and cook 5 minutes;
season with salt, pepper, and butter or 1 teaspoon lemon juice or dill
sauce.

**Creamed cucumbers:** Dice cucumbers and cook in ½ cup milk; thicken
with cream sauce; season with ½ teaspoon salt and ⅛ teaspoon paprika.
Vary by adding any one of the following: ½ cup diced cheese; chopped
fresh herbs or chives; capers; sliced stuffed olives or diced ripe olives;
ground parsley; minced raw onion or canned pimento.

**Mashed cucumbers:** Steam sliced cucumbers in hot top milk until quite
tender, or about 10 minutes; mash; season with salt, freshly ground black
peppercorns, margarine or butter, paprika.

## STUFFED CUCUMBERS

Slice **2 chilled unpeeled cucumbers** in half lengthwise and remove seeds; put cut side down in frying pan with:

**1½ tablespoons hot oil or bacon drippings**

Heat through quickly, lower heat, cover utensil, and let cook 5 to 8 minutes; meanwhile chop fine or dice:

| | |
|---|---|
| **1 onion** | **2 stalks celery** |
| **1 chilled green or red bell pepper or fresh pimento** | **2 wieners** |

Put mixed vegetables and wieners in frying pan, place cucumbers on top of vegetables, cover utensil, and sauté for 5 to 10 minutes.

Remove cucumbers to serving platter, season with **salt and pepper,** put mixed vegetables on top. Garnish with **ground parsley and paprika.**

*Variations:*

Add leftover vegetables or other fresh vegetables.

Omit wieners and pan-broil 2 strips bacon until crisp; remove bacon, cut into pieces with scissors, and mix with vegetables just before serving.

Prepare cucumber halves as in basic recipe; sauté until tender, or 10 to 15 minutes; serve filled with creamed fish (p. 188), creamed chicken (p. 216), or any creamed vegetable.

Edible-pod peas should be grown in every garden in America. If properly cooked, they are brilliantly green and almost as crisp as raw cabbage stalk. Immature pods of most varieties of peas may be cooked and eaten.

## EDIBLE-POD PEAS SIMMERED IN MILK

Remove ends and strings from:

**1 pound chilled edible-pod peas**

Put into:

**½ cup hot milk**

Stir well, heat quickly to simmering, cook 8 to 10 minutes; add:

**½ teaspoon salt**

Serve at once.

*Variations:*

For babies, invalids, or persons who have difficulty in chewing, put chilled peas through the food grinder immediately before cooking; if peas are ground before cooking time, chill quickly in ice tray.

Cut carrots into thin sticks and cook with edible-pod peas; season with salt and paprika.

About 8 minutes before serving add and cook peas with vegetable stew or in gravy around Swiss steak.

**Creamed edible-pod peas:** Heat ½ cup top milk and add ½ cup or more cream sauce, ½ teaspoon salt, crushed white peppercorns; stir in chilled peas and simmer 12 minutes.

**Steamed edible-pod peas:** Steam the peas above ¼ cup water; or cook by waterless method or in top of double boiler with 1 tablespoon boiling water. Serve hot; or chill, mix with French dressing, and serve on a bed of lettuce.

## EGGPLANT WITH ONION

Cut quickly into ½-inch slices:

### 1 chilled unpeeled eggplant

Use utensil for waterless cooking or cook in top of double boiler; put eggplant into:

**2 tablespoons boiling water          1 teaspoon vinegar**

Cover utensil, heat quickly, and simmer 15 minutes.

Meanwhile chop fine in chopping bowl:

### 1 raw onion

Add steamed eggplant to raw onion and chop to any desired texture; season to taste with salt, freshly ground peppercorns, cayenne.

Garnish with ground parsley. Serve hot, or chilled as a relish.

*Variations:*

Chop with onion 1 stalk raw celery or 1 tomato, fresh pimento, or ripe bell pepper; or add ¼ cup French dressing.

Add onion and cook with eggplant cut into 1-inch cubes.

## EGGPLANT CREOLE

Pan-broil until crisp:

### 2 slices bacon

Remove bacon, drain off part of the fat, and sauté lightly:

**1 chopped onion**                    **1 diced green or red bell pepper**

Add and heat to boiling:

### 2 peeled diced or 1 cup canned tomatoes

Meanwhile cut into ½-inch cubes:

### 1 large or 2 small chilled unpeeled eggplants

Add eggplant to other vegetables, stir well, heat quickly, and simmer 12 to 15 minutes; add:

**bacon cut in small pieces**          **1 teaspoon salt**

Serve at once.

*Variations:*

Omit bacon and green pepper; just before serving add ½ cup diced American cheese.

**Eggplant in casserole:** Prepare as in basic recipe, using heat-resistant casserole; when tender, sprinkle with ½ cup **toasted whole-wheat-bread crumbs, ¾ cup cubed American cheese, paprika;** cover utensil until cheese is melted.

**Eggplant with rice:** Omit bacon; brown ½ cup **all-vitamin or brown rice in bacon drippings,** add 1 cup tomato juice or soup stock, and simmer until almost tender before adding eggplant and other ingredients; or add **1 cup leftover steamed rice** to basic recipe.

## FRIED EGGPLANT STICKS

Cut **1 chilled unpeeled eggplant** lengthwise into 1-inch sticks; dip in:

**1 egg stirred with**                 **2 tablespoons milk**

Roll in:

### salted wheat germ or whole-wheat-bread crumbs

Let dry for 10 minutes or more; fry in:

### 3 tablespoons preheated bacon drippings or butter-flavored fat

Cover utensil, turn frequently, cook until golden brown on all sides.

*Variations:*

Cut eggplant crosswise into ½-inch slices; fry as in basic recipe until well browned, sprinkle generously with nippy cheese and paprika; or serve with cheese, sautéed onions, fried tomato slices, or diced leftover meat between matching slices of eggplant.

Cook 1 clove garlic with eggplant and discard before serving.

**Broiled eggplant:** Cut eggplant crosswise into slices ½ inch thick; dip in egg and crumbs or brush with butter-flavored oil; put on oiled baking sheet and broil at moderate heat until browned, or about 6 to 8 minutes; turn and brown the other side; if slices are not tender, lower heat to finish cooking; sprinkle with salt and paprika or grated cheese.

*Eggplant grill:* Brown both surfaces of eggplant slices quickly at high heat; place **1 slice tomato and ½ strip bacon** on top of each slice; lower heat and broil slowly until bacon is crisp; sprinkle with **salt and ground parsley.**

**French-fried eggplant:** Prepare 1-inch sticks as in basic recipe or dip in batter (p. 183); fry in deep bacon drippings at 325° F. until brown.

## EGGPLANT WITH CHIVES

Dice into ½-inch cubes:

**1 chilled unpeeled eggplant**

Use utensil for waterless cooking or top of double boiler; put eggplant into:

**1 or 2 tablespoons boiling water**      **¼ teaspoon crushed black pepper-**
    **seasoned with**                            **corns**

Cover the utensil, heat quickly, and simmer 10 minutes.
Add and stir:

**2 tablespoons chopped chives or**      **dash of paprika**
  **Chinese garlic**                              **2 tablespoons ground parsley**
**¾ teaspoon salt**

*Variations:*

Omit chives and season eggplant with 2 tablespoons tomato catsup or ¼ teaspoon onion or celery salt, smoke-flavoring, or a dash of nutmeg.

Mash after steaming and serve with margarine or butter.

After removing from heat add ¾ cup cubed American cheese; stir, cover utensil, and serve as soon as cheese is melted.

**Baked eggplant:** If oven is being used, put diced eggplant into preheated casserole with ½ cup boiling soup stock, ¼ teaspoon crushed black peppercorns, pinch of savory, ½ teaspoon salt; stir, cover, and bake 20 minutes at 350° F.

**Chilled eggplant:** Cut into cubes or leave in slices; steam and chill; add seasonings of basic recipe and ¼ cup French dressing; serve for hot-weather dinners.

**Eggplant with bacon:** Pan-broil 1 strip bacon and cook with it 1 clove garlic; remove bacon, discard garlic, and sauté cubed eggplant; cover utensil, heat rapidly, and cook until tender, or about 10 minutes; add bacon broken into bits, 2 tablespoons each chopped pimentos and ground parsley. Vary by cooking with 2 or 3 link sausages cut into ½-inch pieces.

**Leftover eggplant:** Put in flat baking dish, cover with cheese, and heat in oven; if vegetable was steamed in own juices, marinate with French dressing and serve chilled; or add 1 tablespoon whole-wheat flour and 1 egg to 1 cup eggplant, stir well, and fry as patties.

**Steamed eggplant:** Steam small whole unpeeled eggplants above ½ cup water until tender, or about 20 minutes; split lengthwise, fluff pulp with a fork, and season with butter or margarine, salt, paprika, and chives or parsley. If oven is being used, bake whole unpeeled eggplant until tender.

## STUFFED EGGPLANT

Cut 1 large unpeeled eggplant in half or leave whole; steam in or above ½ cup water until almost tender, or about 15 to 20 minutes.

Remove center of eggplant, leaving shell ⅛ inch thick; chop pulp fine, adding water left from steaming; in utensil used for steaming sauté in bacon drippings:

| | |
|---|---|
| 1 finely chopped onion | ½ chopped green pepper or 1 stalk celery |

Add, stir, and heat through:

| | |
|---|---|
| ½ cup diced leftover beef | leftover diced carrots or other vegetables |
| 1 teaspoon minced fresh or pinch of dry sage | ½ to 1 cup dry whole-wheat-bread crumbs |
| 1 teaspoon salt | |
| chopped eggplant | |

Put stuffing in eggplant shells, sprinkle top with **paprika**, and place in shallow baking dish; bake in preheated oven at 350° F. for 10 minutes.

*Variations:*

Use lamb, ham, chicken, turkey, or diced wieners instead of beef.

Omit meat and dry crumbs; add 2 or 3 slices stale whole-wheat bread softened with ½ cup milk and pinched into bits.

A few minutes before serving cover top of eggplant with grated cheese.

## GREEN STRING BEANS

String and shred lengthwise:

### 1 to 1½ pounds chilled green beans

Drop into a preheated utensil with:

### 2 tablespoons bacon drippings

Stir well; cook over direct heat or in top of a double boiler for 10 to 15 minutes, or until just tender; stir in:

### ½ teaspoon salt                    2 tablespoons parsley

Serve immediately.

*Variations:*

Cook beans with 1 finely chopped onion, ¼ teaspoon mustard or celery seeds, or a pinch of basil.

Cook beans in 2 tablespoons each water and bacon drippings or oil; season with celery salt or smoke-flavoring; or brown 1 clove garlic in fat and discard before serving.

Just before serving add any one of the following: 3 tablespoons chives or Chinese garlic; 1 small grated raw onion, chopped leek, or diced pimento; 2 tablespoons mayonnaise or Thousand Island dressing; ½ cup cubed American or pimento cheese.

**Creamed string beans:** Cook beans in ½ cup milk; when tender, thicken with **cream sauce; salt** and season with **paprika, dash of celery salt, nutmeg,** or chopped pimentos; or add ½ cup cubed or shredded **American cheese** and 1 tablespoon ground parsley just before serving; or instead of cream sauce add ½ cup condensed tomato soup; season with a pinch of basil.

**Chilled string beans:** Cook as in basic recipe; chill and marinate in ¼ cup French dressing, mayonnaise, Thousand Island dressing, or any sauce of yogurt or sour cream (p. 168). Serve on bed of lettuce.

String beans simmered in milk: Shred beans, add to ½ cup hot milk, and heat to simmering; stir frequently to cover surfaces with milk protein; simmer 12 to 15 minutes; add ½ teaspoon salt; or simmer in enough milk to cover; drain milk and save.

String beans with sour cream: Cook as in basic recipe until tender; add 3 tablespoons canned mushrooms and ½ cup sour cream or yogurt. Serve immediately.

String beans with tomatoes and cheese: Prepare beans as in basic recipe; sauté with beans 1 chopped onion and add ½ cup canned or fresh, peeled, and diced tomatoes; after removing from heat add ½ cup diced or shredded cheese.

Succotash: Prepare 1 pound beans as in basic recipe; when almost tender, add 1 to 2 cups fresh, canned, or frozen corn; serve as soon as corn is heated through.

## QUICK-COOKED STRING BEANS

Use this recipe when beans are too well developed to be tender without long cooking.

Pan-broil until crisp:

**1 slice bacon**

Meanwhile run through the meat grinder, using large knife:

**1 to 1½ pounds chilled green string     1 small onion
beans**

Remove bacon when crisp, drain off some of the drippings, and add ground beans with 1 clove garlic; stir, cover utensil, heat rapidly, then simmer slowly without added moisture until beans are tender, or 6 to 8 minutes.

Discard garlic, add bacon broken to bits, and season with:

**¾ teaspoon salt**

*Variations:*

Stir ground string beans in preheated casserole with ¼ cup hot milk. salt, cover utensil, and cook over direct heat or in hot oven for 10 minutes;

Just before serving add 2 tablespoons ground parsley or ½ cup cubed American cheese.

Add 2 cups ground raw beans and ¾ teaspoon salt to cheese soufflé (p. 209).

**Creamed string beans:** Thicken ½ cup hot milk with cream sauce; stir well, add ground string beans, crushed white peppercorns, and ½ teaspoon salt; simmer 6 to 8 minutes; serve without other seasonings or add dash of nutmeg, cheese, or chopped pimentos.

Have you ever tasted string beans prepared in the old-fashioned way by boiling them with salt pork for 5 or 6 hours before they are served? On a blindfold test, it is doubtful whether a person unfamiliar with this recipe could possibly identify them as string beans. If you have eaten such beans until the taste is enjoyed, yet wish to serve beans with a semblance of their original vitamin content, try using the following recipe.

## GREEN STRING BEANS AND SALT PORK

Fry fat from:

### 2 slices diced salt pork

Meanwhile slice lengthwise:

### 1 to 1½ pounds chilled string beans

Add beans, stir well, and add:

### 2 tablespoons water

Cover utensil and heat beans quickly; simmer for 10 to 12 minutes. Before serving, taste for salt.

*Variations:*

Use bacon or 2 or 3 tablespoons bacon drippings instead of salt pork; or use 2 tablespoons butter-flavored oil; brown a clove of garlic in oil and discard before adding water and beans. Cook beans with a pinch of basil or ½ teaspoon caraway, celery, or mustard seeds; or just before serving stir into beans 1 chopped raw onion or leek or 3 tablespoons chives or Chinese garlic.

Kohlrabi, a rich source of vitamin C, is a cross between turnip and cabbage. It is somewhat similar to turnip in appearance except that the bulb grows above the ground. Its meat is sweet and has the delightful crispness of raw cabbage stalk, making it a "must" for salads; the crispness may be retained by short-cooking. Young kohlrabi leaves are excellent for tossed salads; they may be cooked alone or with other greens. The taste is so similar to cabbage and turnip that it is readily enjoyed. Kohlrabi should be grown in every garden.

Since kohlrabi discolors quickly, it is most attractive when steamed with milk.

## KOHLRABI STEAMED WITH TOPS

Cut tops from 5 to 7 chilled young kohlrabi bulbs; peel and dice bulbs; put immediately into:

½ cup simmering milk

Stir to cover all surfaces with milk protein; cover utensil and simmer 8 to 10 minutes.

Meanwhile shred tops into ¼-inch strips; add tops to diced kohlrabi, stir thoroughly, and simmer about 5 minutes.

Just before serving add:

½ teaspoon salt

*Variations:*

Steam either tops or diced bulbs separately or with other greens or diced vegetables.

Steam or bake whole unpeeled kohlrabis; peel before serving; cut petal-fashion; serve with salt, paprika, and margarine or butter.

**Broiled kohlrabi:** Peel kohlrabi bulbs and cut into ¼-inch fingers, using a knife dipped in vinegar; toss with 1 tablespoon oil and put on baking sheet; broil at moderate heat until browning starts, or about 5 minutes; turn with pancake turner, lower heat to finish cooking.

**Chilled kohlrabi:** Cut peeled kohlrabi bulbs into fingers, steam in small amount of water; chill quickly; marinate in Thousand Island or French dressing for 2 or 3 hours before serving.

**French-fried kohlrabi:** Fry kohlrabi fingers in oil or bacon drippings heated to 275° F. After fat is once hot, keep heat low to prevent shriveling; cook 8 to 10 minutes.

**Kohlrabi with cheese sauce:** Cut peeled kohlrabis into halves or wedges; simmer until tender in top milk and thicken with cream sauce; remove from heat, add ½ cup cubed American cheese, ¼ teaspoon salt; stir; garnish with ground parsley, paprika.

**Kohlrabi with tomatoes:** Sauté lightly in bacon drippings 1 minced clove garlic, 1 chopped onion, 2 cups sliced kohlrabi; add 1 cup canned or diced fresh tomatoes, ¼ teaspoon crushed black peppercorns, ¼ teaspoon salt; cook until kohlrabi is tender, or 10 to 12 minutes. Vary by adding 1 chopped ripe bell pepper or pimento, a pinch of basil.

**Sautéed kohlrabi:** Slice kohlrabi bulbs and sauté in 1 or 2 tablespoons bacon drippings; turn occasionally; keep heat moderate to prevent shriveling.

**Steamed kohlrabi:** Cut kohlrabi bulbs into fingers and steam in small amount of water and ¼ teaspoon vinegar; stir well to prevent discoloring; season with salt and paprika. Vary by adding ½ cup cubed cheese or 1 tablespoon mayonnaise or French dressing.

## STUFFED MUSHROOMS

Unless mushrooms are sandy, try to keep water from touching them. Brush them first with a soft dry brush, then go over them carefully with a damp cloth.

Remove stems from **12 medium-size mushrooms** and chop stems with:

| | |
|---|---|
| 1 slice onion | 1 stalk celery |
| 2 or 3 sprigs parsley | 3 tablespoons leftover chicken |

Add and mix:

1 tablespoon oil

Stuff mushroom caps, sprinkle top with **crumbs,** put into heated oiled casserole; cover and bake in hot oven at 425° F. for 10 to 12 minutes; remove casserole lid and bake 4 minutes longer.

*Variations:*

Use any leftover meat, such as diced turkey, ham, or beef instead of chicken; or use cooked pork sausage or diced wieners.

Omit stuffing, toss with oil, bake uncovered in flat baking dish; or cook in covered casserole with 1 tablespoon hot water; sprinkle with salt and freshly ground white peppercorns.

**Broiled mushrooms:** Toss chilled mushrooms in oil; place on oiled baking sheet with stems down; set 2 inches from broiler at moderate heat for about 5 minutes; turn stem ends up and lower heat after 3 minutes to finish cooking; sprinkle with salt and pepper; serve stems up to prevent loss of juices.

French-fried mushrooms: Drop mushrooms into 1 egg mixed with 2 tablespoons milk; roll in whole-wheat-bread crumbs or wheat germ; let stand 10 minutes or longer and fry in hot fat at 300° F. until golden; or stuff as in basic recipe and fasten pairs together with toothpicks before frying.

Sautéed mushrooms: Sauté whole or diced mushrooms in preheated pan with 1 tablespoon oil; cover utensil and simmer 6 to 8 minutes, or until tender.

## SAUTÉED OKRA

Cut crosswise into ⅛-inch slices:

2 cups chilled okra

Add to:

1 tablespoon bacon drippings

Stir well and add:

1 tablespoon hot water

Cover utensil, heat rapidly, and simmer until tender, or about 10 minutes; add and stir:

½ teaspoon salt                    1 tablespoon ground parsley
generous dash of paprika

*Variations:*

Cut okra crosswise into ½-inch pieces; toss on wax paper with ½ cup yellow corn meal; fry until golden in ¼ cup bacon drippings.

Sauté with okra ½ cup finely diced celery, 1 chopped onion, green or red bell pepper, or fresh or canned pimento; or just before serving add 2 tablespoons chopped chives, Chinese garlic, or green-onion tops, 1 teaspoon mixed fresh herbs, or 1 tablespoon mayonnaise.

Cook with 1 tablespoon water in waterless-cooking utensil or top of double boiler; season with salt, pepper, and margarine or butter.

Cook okra with eggplant as in any of the recipes on pages 352-355.

Okra with tomatoes: Sauté lightly 1 chopped onion, 2 diced stalks celery; add 1 cup canned or diced fresh tomatoes or purée, 2 cups sliced okra, 1 teaspoon salt, ¼ teaspoon crushed black peppercorns, pinch of basil; simmer 10 minutes. Before serving, ½ cup cubed cheese may be added.

Oyster plant, or salsify, is a slender root somewhat like parsnip. The tender leafy tops may be chopped and added to tossed salads, used in making soup stocks, or quickly cooked with other greens. The root should be cooked with carrots, parsnips, turnips, and other vegetables until its bland taste is enjoyed.

## OYSTER PLANT WITH TOMATOES

Cut **6 to 8 chilled scraped oyster plants** into fourths, then into fingers 2½ inches long. Put immediately into:

**1 cup boiling tomatoes**                    **¼ teaspoon crushed black pepper-corns**

Stir well to cover all surfaces with acid from tomatoes; cover utensil and steam until tender, or about 10 to 15 minutes.
Add:

**½ teaspoon salt**                           **dash of cayenne**

Taste for seasonings and serve.

*Variations:*

Add chopped onion, celery, and/or ripe pepper or pimento to the tomatoes.

Omit tomatoes and cook in ¼ cup vegetable-cooking water to which are added 1 teaspoon vinegar, 1 clove, 1 cassia bud; evaporate off most of the water before serving.

Just before serving stir in 2 tablespoons ground parsley or ½ cup cubed or grated nippy cheese; cover utensil until cheese melts.

Dice or cut into ¼-inch slices and cook with 1 tablespoon hot water in waterless-cooking utensil or top of double boiler; season with ½ teaspoon salt and 1 tablespoon ground parsley or chives.

**Chilled oyster plant:** Steam with small amount of water, chill quickly, and marinate with Thousand Island or French dressing or any sauce of sour-cream or yogurt base. Serve on bed of lettuce.

**Creamed oyster plant:** Cut oyster plants into fingers and cook in ½ cup top milk until tender; thicken with **cream sauce**; add salt, pepper, pinch of basil, 1 teaspoon Worcestershire, or ¼ cup cubed American cheese; or omit cream sauce, cook in milk, and season with salt and cayenne.

**Mock oysters:** Steam unpeeled oyster plant until almost tender; peel and cut into ¾-inch pieces; dip in batter (p. 183) and fry in shallow fat or in deep fat at 350° F. until golden.

**Sautéed oyster plant:** Slice chilled scraped oyster plant crosswise or cut into fingers; sauté in 1 tablespoon each hot fat and water; cover utensil, heat quickly, then cook slowly until tender, or about 10 minutes. Salt.

Parsnips are often disliked because of the abominable method of cooking them in water. They are most delicious if not touched with water after they are thoroughly washed. Even when they are steamed, a large amount of sugar quickly dissolves out; if overcooked only a few minutes, the pulp becomes waterlogged and mushy. Parsnips cook quickly; hence recipes which advise cooking them twice should be avoided. Since the sugar in parsnips burns easily, the heat should be kept low after they have been heated through.

## SAUTÉED PARSNIPS

Cut **4 to 6 chilled unpeeled parsnips** into fingers ¼-inch thick and about 2 inches long; drop into:

**2 tablespoons hot butter-flavored oil or bacon drippings**

Stir well, cover, and heat rapidly; lower heat and cook very slowly 10 to 12 minutes; stir 2 or 3 times and let brown only slightly. Season with:

**½ teaspoon salt**

*Variations:*

A few minutes before serving add 1 to 3 teaspoons dark molasses; stir well.

Cut small parsnips in half lengthwise; sauté with 2 tablespoons each bacon drippings and water, keeping heat extremely low.

**Baked parsnips:** Cut unpeeled parsnips into fingers and put into preheated oiled casserole; add **1 teaspoon salt** and **1 tablespoon hot water;** cover and bake in preheated oven at 350° F. for 10 to 15 minutes, or until tender. If sweet parsnips are enjoyed, add **1 tablespoon dark molasses** before baking. Or select thick short parsnips; leave whole and unpeeled; brush with oil and bake slowly in moderate oven until tender, or about 30 minutes.

*With cheese:* Cut parsnips lengthwise into halves or fourths; bake in covered casserole until almost tender; remove cover to finish cooking; salt, and sprinkle generously with cheese and paprika.

**Broiled parsnips:** Dice or cut into fingers, toss with butter-flavored oil, place on oiled baking sheet; broil under moderate heat until browning starts, turn with pancake turner, brown other side slightly; lower heat to finish cooking; after initial heating keep heat low to prevent shriveling.

**Chilled parsnips:** Cut unpeeled parsnips into fingers; cook in waterless-cooking utensil or top of double boiler; or steam whole parsnips on rack above water. Chill quickly, dice if whole, and marinate in mayonnaise or French dressing; garnish with paprika.

**French-fried parsnips:** Cut chilled unpeeled parsnips into fingers and fry in deep fat at 280° F. Watch temperature carefully; cook about 8 minutes, or until tender.

**Fried parsnips:** Slice parsnips across and fry like raw fried potatoes in 2 tablespoons fat; keep heat low, turning frequently to prevent burning; cover and cook only until tender, or about 10 minutes; season with salt and serve.

Peas should be washed unhulled and not be touched with water unless absolutely necessary. Any peas which require washing should be kept separate from the others and washed in a sieve under running water. When peas are kept at room temperature, enzymes quickly change sugar into starch, thereby causing loss of flavor; if they cannot be cooked immediately, they should be chilled quickly in an ice tray or frozen. Be particularly careful not to overcook them.

## PEAS SIMMERED IN MILK

Add **2 cups chilled or frozen peas** to:

**¼ cup hot milk**

Stir well to cover surfaces with milk protein; cover utensil, and simmer until tender, or about 2 minutes for frozen peas, 7 minutes for fresh peas. Season with:

**½ teaspoon salt**

*Variations:*

Just before serving add 2 teaspoons ground parsley, ¼ teaspoon chopped mint leaves, or 1 diced canned pimento.

Cook in 1 tablespoon hot water in waterless cooker or top of double boiler.

**Creamed peas:** Cook as directed in top milk; thicken milk with cream sauce; salt.

**Peas with other vegetables:** Simmer peas in milk or cream sauce with one of the following vegetables: chopped celery, leeks, or pimentos; diced celery root, turnips, kohlrabi, summer squash, or carrots. If the other vegetable takes longer to cook, add peas 7 to 10 minutes before serving.

**Soufflé of fresh peas:** Unless using leftover peas, grind 1 or more cups uncooked fresh or frozen peas and add to soufflé (p. 209).

Pimentos and all varieties of sweet peppers should be used in quantity as a food as well as a seasoning or garnish. Enough sweet peppers should be grown to be used daily while fresh and to be canned for winter use. Two small pimentos equal a glass of orange juice in vitamin C. When cooked, they should be served piping hot, but still slightly crisp.

## TART PIMENTOS

Remove seeds and stems from:

### 5 or 6 chilled pimentos

Slice into rings ¼ inch thick; drop into:

**2 tablespoons boiling water**          **3 each whole cloves and cassia buds**
**1 tablespoon vinegar**

Stir or shake utensil until all surfaces are covered with vinegar, to prevent change of color; cover utensil, heat quickly, and simmer 5 minutes; season with:

### ½ teaspoon salt

*Variations:*

Cook pimento in ¼ cup sour cream or hot milk, stirring to cover all surfaces with milk protein.

**Broiled pimentos:** Toss chilled pimento rings in oil and place on oiled baking sheet; put under moderate heat 2 inches from broiler; broil 3 minutes on each side. Broil alone or with slices of tomato, eggplant, leeks or sweet onions.

**Creamed pimentos:** Dice 1½ cups chilled pimentos or use equal amounts pimentos and peas, finely diced carrots, diced potatoes, or green peppers; cook in ½ cup hot top milk and thicken with cream sauce. Vary by adding ½ cup cheese after removing from heat; or omit cream sauce and simmer in milk.

**Stuffed pimentos:** Stuff raw pimentos with **fresh, frozen, or canned corn**; cover each pimento with **2 tablespoons grated cheese** and cook in hot oven 10 minutes. Or stuff with leftover reheated **macaroni, fried rice,** or **eggplant**; cover with grated cheese and garnish with **paprika.** Serve as soon as hot.

## SUMMER SQUASH WITH CHEESE

Slice or cut into 1-inch pieces:

**6 to 8 chilled unpeeled summer squash**

Sauté squash in **2 tablespoons bacon drippings or oil** with:

| | |
|---|---|
| 1 chopped onion | 1 clove garlic pierced with toothpick |
| 1 chopped chilled green pepper or pimento | pinch of savory or basil |
| 1 small stalk celery diced | ¼ teaspoon crushed black peppercorns |

Stir well, cover utensil, heat quickly, then simmer 10 minutes.
Discard garlic, remove from heat, and add:

| | |
|---|---|
| 1 teaspoon salt | ½ cup diced **American cheese** |

Stir well and put into serving dish.
In the utensil used for squash, heat quickly:

| | |
|---|---|
| ¾ cup canned or diced fresh tomatoes | ¼ teaspoon salt |

Pour tomatoes over squash.

*Variations:*

Instead of summer squash use small crookneck squash or zucchini in preceding or following recipes.

Instead of savory or basil season with a dash of powdered coriander or with chopped fresh dill, sage, chives, marjoram, or mixed herbs.

Omit other ingredients and steam squash with 1 tablespoon water, using waterless-cooking utensil or top of double boiler; or steam with diced onion, celery, or pimento; season with salt and paprika.

Omit tomatoes and add with cheese ½ cup sour cream or thick commercial yogurt.

**Baked summer squash:** Split unpeeled summer squash petal-fashion into 6 parts, cutting toward the stem end; put into a low baking dish and brush surfaces with **oil or soft bacon drippings;** set in preheated oven at 400° F. and bake 10 to 15 minutes; sprinkle with **salt;** garnish with **chopped chives or ground parsley and paprika.**

*With sauce:* Bake squash and serve covered with cheese sauce (p. 163) or tomato sauce (p. 166).

**Broiled summer squash:** Choose large summer squash and cut crosswise ¼ inch thick, saving smaller parts for tossed salad; toss slices in oil, dip in **whole-wheat-bread crumbs,** and put on oiled baking sheet; broil 'nder moderate heat until brown on both sides; sprinkle each slice with **grated cheese** and put a **slice of small tomato** on top; broil tomato 3 to 6 minutes without turning.

**Creamed summer squash:** Cut 1½ pounds squash into 1-inch wedges; stir into ¾ **cup hot top milk;** simmer 10 to 12 minutes; when squash is tender, thicken with **cream sauce;** add **1 teaspoon salt.** Vary by adding ½ cup cubed American cheese and 2 tablespoons diced canned pimentos; cover until cheese melts; or omit cream sauce and simmer in ½ cup milk seasoned with margarine or butter.

**Sautéed summer squash:** Quarter squash and slice; add **2 cups squash** to **1 tablespoon butter-flavored** oil or bacon drippings; add **pinch of thyme or dash of celery salt, crushed white peppercorns;** stir well, cover the utensil, lower heat when squash is heated through, and simmer 8 to 10 minutes; **salt.**

*With other vegetables:* Sauté 1 cup each squash and one of the following vegetables: chopped onions, green pepper, sliced carrots, kohlrabi, turnips, or potatoes.

*Sautéed with bacon:* Pan-broil 1 strip bacon with 1 clove garlic; remove bacon when crisp and discard garlic; sauté sliced squash until tender; add bacon cut into small pieces, ½ teaspoon salt.

**Steamed summer squash:** Steam whole unpeeled squash; cut petal-fashion, serve with salt, paprika, margarine or butter; or cut into wedges, steam in a small amount of water until nearly tender; set lid of utensil to one side and evaporate off moisture before serving. Cook until barely tender.

**Summer squash fried in batter:** Cut squash into small wedges; stir 1 to 2 cups wedges into a batter of 1 egg, 2 tablespoons milk, ½ teaspoon salt, ¼ teaspoon celery or 1 teaspoon dill seeds, ¼ cup each soy grits and wheat germ or whole-wheat-bread crumbs; allow to stand in refrigerator at least 10 minutes; pour from tablespoon into hot butter-flavored fat or bacon drippings; fry at moderate temperature until well browned.

*Fried in crumbs:* Cut squash into ¼-inch rounds; dip into 3 tablespoons evaporated milk mixed with ½ teaspoon salt, then into wheat germ or whole-wheat-bread crumbs; fry in 2 tablespoons hot butter-flavored fat; turn when golden brown; serve garnished with thin slice of leek or sweet onion.

*Fried with tomatoes:* Dip large slices of squash into milk and crumbs; fry, salt, and put on serving platter; use same utensil to fry tomatoes rolled in crumbs or wheat germ; put thin slices of leeks or sweet onions on slices of squash and cover with tomatoes.

## TOMATOES WITH GREEN ONIONS

Loosen skin on **4 or 5 fresh tomatoes** by piercing with large fork and holding over high heat; peel, dice, and put into heat-resistant casserole.

Cook over direct heat 5 minutes and add:

**8 to 10 green onions cut into ½-inch pieces**

**½ teaspoon salt**

**¼ teaspoon crushed black peppercorns**

pinch of basil or orégano

**1 to 3 teaspoons blackstrap molasses**

Simmer 5 to 8 minutes; move lid to one side to let juice evaporate; remove from heat and sprinkle surface with:

**¼ cup toasted whole-wheat-bread crumbs**

**½ cup cubed American cheese**

Serve as soon as cheese melts.

*Variations:*

Instead of fresh tomatoes use 2 cups canned tomatoes and 1 or 2 chopped leeks or dry onions; or omit onions.

Add with onions chopped ripe bell pepper or pimento, celery, okra, eggplant, corn, kohlrabi, or mixed vegetables.

Omit onions and herbs; cook in saucepan; just before serving crumble 2 slices whole-wheat bread into tomatoes.

Leave tomatoes whole; put into hot oiled casserole, sprinkle with seasonings and crumbs; cook in hot oven 12 to 15 minutes; add cheese and paprika; serve when cheese has melted.

**Broiled tomatoes:** Peel 2 or 3 firm tomatoes and cut into ¾-inch slices; sprinkle slices with bits of raw diced bacon; broil on oiled baking sheet under moderate heat until tender, or about 8 to 10 minutes; or omit bacon and sprinkle with grated Parmesan cheese; garnish with ground parsley. Vary by rolling in 4 tablespoons whole-wheat-bread crumbs mixed with ½ teaspoon salt, freshly ground black peppercorns, and a pinch of basil; dot top with bacon drippings.

**Creamed tomatoes:** Peel and dice 3 or 4 tomatoes or use 1½ cups canned tomatoes; add ½ teaspoon salt, 2 whole cloves, crushed black peppercorns, 2 teaspoons dark molasses, pinch of basil; cook about 10 minutes with high heat to evaporate off part of the juice; beat together 1 cup cream sauce and ¼ cup powdered milk; heat in separate utensil and add tomatoes slowly to sauce just before serving.

**Sautéed tomatoes:** Cut 3 or 4 firm unpeeled ripe or green tomatoes into ½-inch slices; dip in evaporated or fresh milk and whole-wheat-bread crumbs, wheat germ, or any cereal-flake crumbs mixed with ½ teaspoon each salt and cumin or caraway seeds; sauté in 2 tablespoons hot butter-flavored oil or bacon drippings 8 to 10 minutes, or until golden brown on both surfaces. Vary by marinating sliced tomatoes with 2 tablespoons French dressing for ½ hour; dip in seasoned crumbs and sauté slowly; put tomatoes on platter, heat juices drawn out by marinating, and serve over tomatoes as sauce.

**Stuffed tomatoes:** Hollow out centers of 4 large unpeeled tomatoes; chop tomato pulp with 1 chilled green pepper, 1 small onion; add ¼ teaspoon each chopped basil and tarragon or pinch of each dry herb, ½ teaspoon salt, ground black peppercorns; heat stuffing quickly in flat baking dish over direct heat; put stuffing into tomatoes, sprinkle with cheese or buttered crumbs, and bake in moderate oven at 350° F. for 10 to 15 minutes. Vary stuffing by adding fresh or canned corn, leftover chopped vegetables, whole-wheat macaroni, steamed rice, or baked beans; leftover diced meat or flaked fish; diced wieners; or stuff with spinach and parsley cooked with bacon (p. 376).

Vegetable marrow is a member of the squash family which resembles summer squash. Prepare both vegetable marrow and zucchini by recipes given for summer squash (p. 366). Since these squashes contain a large amount of moisture, the flavor is more delightful if part of the juices is allowed to evaporate.

## ZUCCHINI PATTIES

Chop in chopping bowl:

4 chilled unpeeled zucchini    4 green onions or 1 dry onion or
              leek

Add and stir:

2 eggs         ¼ cup wheat germ or whole-wheat-
1 teaspoon salt       bread crumbs
freshly ground black peppercorns

Drop from tablespoon onto grill or frying pan brushed with butter-
flavored oil or bacon drippings.
Brown on both sides; cover and sauté 5 to 8 minutes.

*Variations:*

Use summer or crookneck squash instead of zucchini.
Add to patties any one of the following: 1 tablespoon catsup; 1 teaspoon
Worcestershire; 1 diced pimento, green pepper, or celery stalk; 2 tablespoons ground parsley or powdered milk.
Slice 2 or 3 leftover pork sausages or wieners and add to chopped zucchini and eggs. Sauté as in basic recipe.
Add to zucchini diced leftover vegetables or a small amount of any unfamiliar vegetable, such as kohlrabi, Jerusalem artichoke, vegetable marrow, okra, oyster plant.

## STUFFED BAKED ZUCCHINI

Cut lengthwise:

2 large zucchini

Scoop out pulp, leaving shells no thicker than ¼ inch; make dressing
by chopping together:

squash pulp        2 stalks celery
1 onion

Sauté the chopped vegetables in **bacon drippings** until onion is transparent; add and mix well:

2 tablespoons ground parsley  ¼ cup wheat germ, soy grits, or
pinch of savory or basil     whole-wheat-bread crumbs
             ½ teaspoon salt

Stuff dressing into zucchini shells; put into baking dish with 2 table-spoons water; place strips of bacon on top and put into moderate oven at 350° F. for 15 minutes, or until bacon is browned.

*Variations:*

Add to stuffing any diced leftover meat or vegetables. Leave zucchini whole, remove centers with an apple corer, stuff, and bake.

In preparing zucchini, follow recipes for cooking summer squash (pp. 366–368).

### SERVE AN INTENSELY GREEN VEGETABLE DAILY

Since intensely green leaves offer the greatest concentration and the widest variety of vitamins and minerals of all the vegetables, they should be eaten daily. A half cup of cooked beet or turnip tops or tampala, for example, supplies approximately 19,000 units of vitamin A, or carotene, while beet and turnip roots contain none. If handled properly before cooking, heated rapidly to destroy enzymes, and quick-cooked in their own juices, green leaves lose little nutritive value in cooking. Although the daily quota of greens may be eaten in tossed salads, cooking condenses them so that a small serving equals an amount impossible to eat raw; hence the quantity of nutrients obtained from cooked leaves may be many times greater than from raw ones.

Leafy vegetables are often disliked because of the texture rather than the taste. A long string from a chard or beet leaf sometimes wraps itself around a tooth while the leaf to which it is attached is already tugging away from the stomach in a sort of fishing tackle arrangement. Except for extremely tender or small leaves, such as New Zealand spinach and watercress, or those containing almost no stringy parts, such as mustard-spinach, it is wise to shred all leaves and especially all stalks before cooking them. Mature greens, such as large beet and turnip tops, can be cooked palatably provided they are shredded carefully before cooking or chopped after cooking.

The flavor of greens can be controlled largely by the method of cooking. Plant acids cause many of the more mature greens to have a pungent and sometimes bitter flavor. The flavor becomes mild when these acids are neutralized by proteins. If you wish to change a pungent flavor into a mild one, cook the greens in milk, cream sauce, batter, or a soufflé. The milder the taste desired or the stronger the flavor to start with, the greater is the amount of protein which should be used in cooking. If this procedure is used, very mature and bitter greens can become delicious. If the greens are to be cooked in water, as in preparing liquid for a baby's formula, boil a washed egg with the greens so that the calcium in the eggshell will neutralize the oxalic and phytic acids in the greens.

As much as ½ cup or more of water may cling to greens after they are washed. If carelessly allowed to remain on the leaves, this water quickly dissolves out sugars, iron, vitamin C, and many other nutrients; the water also dissolves out acids which cause the green to change to an unappetizing olive-gray and which leave the teeth-on-edge feeling experienced after eating improperly cooked spinach. Immediately after being washed, greens should be whirled in a thin cloth bag until dry. When carefully dried greens are allowed to cook in their own juices without added moisture, the heat should be kept low or they should be stirred constantly until the plant juices have changed to steam.

Certain recipe books advise cooking spinach in three or more quarts of water in order to extract the oxalic acid. Unfortunately such treatment dissolves most of the vitamins and minerals. During cooking, the oxalic acid in spinach combines with calcium in the vegetable cells, forming calcium oxalate. This salt does not dissolve in the digestive juices and therefore cannot enter the blood. Although no thought need be given to extracting it, spinach must not be relied upon as a source of calcium. Whenever possible, cook spinach in a little milk or season it with calcium-rich lemon juice to supply added calcium.

The recipes for cooking green leafy vegetables can be used interchangeably; any greens may be substituted for those in the basic recipes. In these recipes I have suggested greens most often available rather than those I consider most delicious. I urge you to prepare your favorite greens by each of these recipes, then gradually combine the less familiar leafy vegetables with old favorites. When available, each of the green leafy vegetables listed on the next page should be served frequently.

beet tops *
broccoli leaves *
Brussels sprout leaves
cabbage, outer green leaves
carrot tops, when immature *
cauliflower leaves, young outer or tender inside leaves
celery leaves
celtuce
chayote leaves
chicory, or witloof
Chinese cabbage *
Chinese celery *
Chinese mustard
dandelion, thick-leafed cultivated variety *
endive, or escarole *
kale *
kohlrabi leaves

lettuce, Bibb or dark-leafed *
lettuce, mature or going to seed
mustard greens *
mustard-spinach *
New Zealand spinach *
parsley *
pea leaves *
radish tops *
rhubarb chard, green leaves *
rhubarb chard, red leaves †
rutabaga tops
savoy cabbage, loose outer leaves *
sorrel *
spinach
Swiss chard *
tampala *‡
turnip tops *
watercress *
wild greens *

* Greens of outstanding nutritive value.
† May be prepared by any recipe given for purple cabbage (p. 385).
‡ Similar to spinach in texture, but more tender and sweet; the flavor of the celery-like stalks resembles that of artichoke.

## CREAMED RHUBARB CHARD

Prepare:

**1 to 1½ cups thick cream sauce (p. 161)**

Meanwhile cut into ¼-inch shreds:

**1 or 2 bunches of well-whirled rhubarb chard and stalks**

When available, use part green and part red leaves.

Add chard to cream sauce, stirring until all leaves are covered with sauce; simmer 6 to 8 minutes, stirring occasionally.

If juices from chard have not thinned cream sauce to desired consistency, add a small amount of milk; before serving add:

**½ teaspoon salt**

Garnish with **paprika**.

*Variations:*

Add a dash of nutmeg or mace and/or 1 small grated onion or leek.

Instead of plain cream sauce prepare caraway, celery, cheese, dill, egg, mock Hollandaise, olive, pimento, or piquant sauce (p. 163), using thick cream sauce as base instead of medium cream sauce; cook chard in sauce or with any vegetable or combination of vegetables listed on page 373.

Combine any of the following vegetables with chard: 1 cup or more shredded greens of any kind; or shredded green, purple, Chinese, or savoy cabbage.

Instead of chard use any greens listed on page 373 or any combination of greens.

Remove from heat, stir in ½ cup cubed or grated cheese; cover utensil until cheese melts; or garnish with sliced or sieved hard-cooked eggs.

Prepare in baking dish over direct heat; when vegetable is heated through, sprinkle top with whole-wheat-bread crumbs and grated cheese; finish cooking in oven.


## MUSTARD GREENS WITH SALT PORK

Dice with scissors:

### 1 or 2 slices salt pork

Pan-broil until crisp. Cut into ¼-inch shreds:

### 1 to 2 bunches chilled mustard greens

Put into hot fat; stir well; keep heat moderate and turn constantly until mustard has wilted; lower heat and steam 4 to 6 minutes. Taste for salt. Sprinkle with freshly ground peppercorns and serve.


*Variations:*

Instead of mustard greens use any greens listed on page 373 or any combination of greens.

Cook greens in 2 tablespoons bacon drippings instead of salt pork; or pan-broil 1 or 2 slices bacon; remove when crisp and cook greens; add ½ teaspoon salt; cut bacon to bits and add before serving.

Omit salt pork and cook with greens ½ to 1 cup diced leftover ham or 2 or 3 sliced wieners.

**Mixed garden greens:** Gather assorted leaves from garden, such as broccoli, outside leaves of cabbage, and young tops of carrot, radish, and kohlrabi; add a small amount of fresh herbs or horseradish leaves for seasoning. Shred and cook with salt pork or bacon.

**Wild greens:** Gather such wild greens as lamb's-quarters, curly and sour dock, tender poke sprouts, dandelions, deer's-tongue, peppergrass, and wild turnip, lettuce, and mustard greens; cook with salt pork as in basic recipe.

## NEW ZEALAND SPINACH SAUTÉED IN BATTER

Beat to a smooth batter:

| | |
|---|---|
| 1 egg | ¾ teaspoon salt |
| ½ cup fresh milk | ¼ teaspoon crushed peppercorns |
| ½ cup powdered milk | 1 grated onion |
| ¼ to ½ cup wheat germ | 1 teaspoon Worcestershire |

Cut into ¼-inch shreds enough chilled New Zealand spinach leaves and stems to make **1½ tightly packed cups;** stir shredded spinach into batter and set in refrigerator for 10 minutes.

Drop batter with spinach from tablespoon onto a hot grill brushed with:

**bacon drippings or butter-flavored oil**

Sauté slowly until brown on both sides; garnish with paprika.

*Variations:*

Shred spinach with other greens, using ¾ cup each.

Add finely chopped celery, fresh pimento or red bell pepper, or a few leaves of fresh tarragon, basil, or marjoram, or a pinch of dried herbs.

Instead of spinach use any greens listed on page 373.

**French-fried New Zealand spinach:** Drop the batter with spinach from a teaspoon into hot bacon drippings or other deep fat at 300° F.; drain on absorbent paper; serve garnished with paprika.

When shredded or ground parsley is cooked, so many of its aromatic oils escape that it has a mild pleasant taste; it can therefore be used in large quantities with other greens without its flavor predominating. The following recipe is one of my favorites. I have never known anyone to dislike it. It is particularly delicious with raw grated onion added just before serving. Even my husband, who hates cooked greens, will eat generous amounts when prepared in this manner. Frankly, I never discard the garlic, a habit which seems to horrify many people. To be a solitary garlic-eater, however. is as bad as being a solitary drinker.

## PARSLEY AND SPINACH WITH BACON AND GARLIC

Pan-broil in a large utensil:

**1 or 2 slices bacon**

Remove bacon when crisp; keep heat moderate; cook in **2 tablespoons bacon drippings:**

| | |
|---|---|
| **1 clove garlic** | **2 bunches shredded spinach** |
| | **1 bunch shredded parsley** |

Stir until wilted; cover utensil, reduce heat to simmering, and cook 4 to 6 minutes; discard garlic and add:

| | |
|---|---|
| **½ teaspoon salt** | **bacon broken to bits** |
| **freshly ground black peppercorns** | |

Stir well and serve.

*Variations:*

Sauté with bacon or add raw to cooked greens 1 chopped onion and/or ½ chilled green pepper or 1 pimento or 1 stalk celery; or heat ⅓ cup canned or fresh tomatoes or tomato purée or chili sauce in a separate utensil; combine with greens immediately before serving.

Instead of parsley and spinach use any greens listed on page 373 or any combination of greens.

When radish tops are cooked, the prickles on the leaves soften quickly and cannot be noticed. The taste is mildly peppery and somewhat similar to that of the roots. The greens are usually enjoyed the first time they are eaten.

## RADISH TOPS AND KALE WITH SOUR CREAM

Cut into ¼-inch shreds:

| | |
|---|---|
| **1 bunch chilled kale** | **tops from 1 or 2 bunches radishes** |
| | **or about 20 to 30 roots** |

Put shredded greens into hot flat-bottomed utensil over moderate heat; stir or turn leaves with a pancake turner continually until almost wilted; reduce heat to simmering, cover utensil, and cook 4 to 6 minutes.

Add:

### ½ teaspoon salt

Put greens into hot serving dish; heat slightly in the same utensil:

**½ to 1 cup sour cream or yogurt     ⅛ teaspoon salt**

Pour heated cream or yogurt over greens and serve.

*Variations:*

Add 3 tablespoons capers or sliced stuffed olives.

Cook with greens a few leaves of fresh horseradish, parsley, or other herbs, or ½ teaspoon caraway, dill, celery, or mustard seeds.

Instead of radish tops and kale use any greens listed on page 373 or any combination of greens.

**Chilled greens:** For hot-weather dinner or buffet, chill cooked greens quickly and toss with sour cream or marinate in French dressing.

**Greens with cheese:** Omit sour cream; add ½ cup diced American cheese after greens have been taken from the heat; cover utensil until cheese is melted.

Both mustard-spinach and tampala should be grown in every garden. Mustard-spinach has the delightful flavor of mustard greens, yet the tenderness of immature spinach. Tampala leaves are as tender as spinach and taste much the same except that they are sweeter and usually better liked. Both vegetables have a lower content of oxalic acid than spinach has. Since tampala grows some two feet high, it is much easier to wash than is spinach; fewer nutrients are lost because of the faster washing.

The recipe which follows is my favorite for cooking all green leafy vegetables as well as shredded cabbage.

## SAUTÉED MUSTARD-SPINACH AND TAMPALA

Gather equal amounts of mustard-spinach and tampala or purchase 1 bunch of each. Wash thoroughly but quickly; whirl until free from all moisture. Shred, or if only small leaves are used, leave whole. Put into salad bowl and add:

### 1 to 3 tablespoons peanut or corn oil, or other salad oil

Toss 30 times if 1 tablespoon of oil is used, 20 for 2 tablespoons, 10 for 3 tablespoons, or toss until all surfaces glisten with oil.

Put tossed leaves into hot utensil over moderate heat; turn frequently until heated through; cover utensil, lower heat, and steam 3 minutes without added moisture.

Do not salt until immediately before serving.

*Variations:*

Rub salad bowl well with crushed garlic or cook minced garlic or chopped green onions with greens.

Instead of mustard-spinach and tampala use shredded cabbage or any greens listed on page 373 or any combination of greens.

One of the best ways of including greens in the smooth diet is to use them in a soufflé. Unless leaves are of a soft texture, they should be shredded or ground before being added to the soufflé. Leaves from pea vines, although quite sweet, are very delicious.

## SOUFFLÉ OF GROUND LEAVES FROM PEA VINES

Gather green leaves from garden peas during or after bearing.
Beat until smooth:

**1 cup thick cream sauce** (p. 161)       **1 teaspoon salt**
**½ cup powdered milk**

Add:

**¼ teaspoon crushed white pepper-**       **1 grated onion**
**corns**                                  **3 tablespoons chopped pimento**
**1 teaspoon Worcestershire**              **4 egg yolks**

Meanwhile run through the meat grinder enough chilled leaves from pea vines to make **1 cup**; stir into cream sauce. Beat stiff:

### 4 egg whites

Fold egg whites into other ingredients. Pour into oiled loaf pan and bake in preheated slow oven at 300° F. for 45 to 50 minutes.

*Variations:*

Make soufflé of ½ cup ground pea leaves with ½ cup ground parsley, chard, kale, broccoli, or shredded tender greens.

Instead of leaves from pea vines use 1 cup of any ground greens or 2 cups of any shredded greens. When shredded leaves are used, stir into hot cream sauce before adding other ingredients.

## STEAMED BEET TOPS WITH BEET ROOTS

Dice into ¼-inch cubes:

**4 to 6 chilled unpeeled beet roots**

Drop into:

**½ cup hot milk**

Add:

**¼ teaspoon crushed black peppercorns**

Stir to cover all surfaces with milk protein; cover utensil, reduce heat, and simmer 8 to 10 minutes, or until beets start to be tender.

Meanwhile cut into ¼-inch shreds:

**chilled beet tops**

Add leaves to beet roots; stir well, cover utensil, and steam 6 to 8 minutes.

Season with ½ teaspoon salt.

*Variations:*

If leaves are extremely large, cut into ⅛-inch shreds and increase milk to ¾ cup; or if roots are no more than ½ inch in diameter, cook roots and tops together without shredding leaves. Cook 1 chopped onion with beet roots.

Omit peppercorns and sprinkle lightly with nutmeg or mace.

**Combined roots and leaves:** Follow the same procedure using roots and green tops of kohlrabi, turnip, celery root, or young rutabagas.

**Grated beet roots with tops:** Combine grated unpeeled beet roots and shredded tops or grated carrots or turnips with shredded greens; cook in 1 tablespoon butter-flavored fat or ½ cup milk; cover utensil and steam.

Watercress should be served cooked not only because of its outstanding nutritive value and small bulk after being heated, but because it grows wild in such abundance in many parts of the country. Care must be taken that the stems are cut into small pieces; otherwise they become tough and stringy. When watercress is cooked only a few minutes, its peppery flavor is well retained. If the watercress has just been washed and is still wet, omit the milk in the following recipe.

## WATERCRESS WITH MUSHROOM SAUCE

Stir and heat to simmering:

¼ cup milk                              1 can condensed mushroom soup

Meanwhile shred into ¼-inch pieces:

2 bunches chilled watercress

Drop into hot sauce and mix thoroughly; simmer 5 minutes, or until tender. Taste for salt. Garnish with **paprika.**

*Variations:*

Cook diced fresh or canned pimento or ripe bell pepper with watercress.

Instead of mushroom soup use 1½ cups leftover cream gravy; add a dash of nutmeg or mace.

Instead of watercress use any greens listed on page 373.

## TURNIP TOPS

Shred across the veins:

chilled tops of about 10 to 12 turnip roots

Put into hot utensil without added moisture.

Cover utensil, keep heat moderate, and stir frequently as leaves wilt; reduce heat to simmering and cook 5 to 10 minutes; add just before serving:

½ teaspoon salt                        1 tablespoon chopped chives, leeks,
freshly ground black peppercorns           or raw, sweet onion
2 tablespoons French dressing or
  mayonnaise

Stir well and serve.

*Variations:*

Omit French dressing and serve with margarine or butter.

Instead of turnip tops use any greens listed on page 373.

**With vinegar sauce:** Turn greens into hot serving dish; put into utensil **1 tablespoon water, 1 teaspoon sugar, 3 tablespoons vinegar, 2 or 3 sliced green onions and tops;** pour boiling sauce over greens and serve immediately.

## THOSE "STRONG-FLAVORED" VEGETABLES

Although vegetables such as onions, cabbage, cauliflower, ruta-bagas, turnips, and Brussels sprouts are spoken of as being strong-flavored, the flavors referred to do not exist in the raw fresh vegetables, nor do they develop when the vegetables are properly cooked. Such flavors are produced only when sulfur compounds found in these vegetables are broken down. The breakdown may be brought about by enzymes during long storage or slow initial heating; by plant acids allowed to soak out of the vegetable during cooking; or by heat when the vegetable is overcooked, especially at a high temperature. Since some of the sulfur compounds are volatile, odors escaping during cooking indicate that the vegetables are being overcooked or cooked at too high a temperature. When the sulfur compounds are broken down, gases are formed from them during digestion; the person who eats improperly cooked vegetables may suffer from discomfort and digestive disturbances.

Housewives are often advised to cook these vegetables in large amounts of water and to leave the utensil uncovered so that the volatile compounds can escape. After the cooking liquid is discarded, the vegetables—odorless, tasteless, vitaminless, and mineralless—are ready to be served. When these vegetables are put into water, the plant acids soak out and bring about the rapid breakdown of the sulfur compounds. More than any other type of vegetables, the sulfur-containing vegetables should be washed with the utmost speed and dried thoroughly and quickly. They should not be touched unnecessarily with water. Since enzymes can bring about the breakdown of the sulfur compounds, thorough chilling and quick initial heating are particularly important.

Experiments have shown that almost no sulfur compounds break down when these vegetables are cooked 8 to 10 minutes at a temperature not above boiling. If the chilled vegetable is shredded or diced, it can be thoroughly cooked in this time. When longer cooking is desired, as when cauliflower is to be cooked whole, the vegetable should be cooked in milk, which can neutralize the plant acids and thus prevent the breakdown of the sulfur compounds. Cooking in milk is the ideal method of preparing these vegetables for babies, invalids, and persons with digestive disturbances; it has the added advantages of preserving color and of ensuring that the temperature will be kept low.

If vegetables which contain sulfur are cooked in a pressure cooker, the cooking time should be checked with a stop watch; if they are sautéed or fried, the heat should be kept low and the vegetable cooked only a short time. When acids are neutralized or are not soaked out, when the cooking temperature is kept low and the cooking time held to the minimum, these vegetables are surprisingly sweet and mild-flavored. No fresh vegetable which is properly prepared and cooked can be called strong-flavored.

## BROCCOLI WITH CREAM SAUCE

Use **1 pound chilled broccoli;** cut bud ends into ¾-inch pieces; shred leaves and chop smaller stalks; peel any large stalks and cut into fingers ¼-inch thick or keep for salad.

Meanwhile heat to 200° F., using cooking thermometer:

### 1 or 2 cups cream sauce

Stir in broccoli, being careful to cover all surfaces with sauce; keep heat high until 200° F. is reached; reduce heat, cover utensil, and simmer, stirring occasionally until broccoli is barely tender, or about 10 minutes.

Add and stir:

½ teaspoon salt                              ¼ teaspoon celery salt (optional)

Pour into serving dish and garnish with **paprika.**

*Variations:*

Omit cream sauce and heat 1 cup fresh milk shaken with ¼ cup powdered milk; stir well to cover all surfaces with protein; control temperature carefully.

Prepare recipe in casserole; cook over direct heat; when tender, sprinkle with whole-wheat-bread crumbs, 1 cup cubed cheese, paprika; or bake in a preheated oven at 350° F. for 15 minutes.

Omit celery salt and just before serving add any of the following: 3 tablespoons diced canned pimento; ½ cup cubed nippy or pimento cheese; a dash of nutmeg or mace; 2 tablespoons lemon juice, ½ teaspoon grated lemon rind; 1 teaspoon Worcestershire. Or before cooking add to milk 1 grated onion, 1 teaspoon fresh or ⅛ teaspoon dried basil, marjoram, or savory; ½ teaspoon caraway, dill, mustard, or celery seeds.

**Broccoli simmered in deep milk:** Cook uncut broccoli in enough milk to cover, or 2 to 3 cups; simmer until tender; drain milk and save; season.

**Broccoli soufflé:** Add to plain or cheese soufflé (p. 209) **2 cups ground broccoli;** season with **cayenne pepper,** 1/4 **teaspoon celery salt, 1 grated onion, 1 minced clove garlic.**

Quick-cooked broccoli: Cut **1 clove garlic** in half and sauté lightly in **butter-flavored oil or bacon drippings;** discard garlic; cut broccoli into small pieces, add to fat, stir well, and add **2 tablespoons water;** heat quickly, cover utensil, and cook 4 to 5 minutes.

**Steamed broccoli:** Leave broccoli stalks uncut; stand upright in utensil containing 1/2 cup boiling vegetable-cooking water; steam until tender, or about 15 minutes. Serve with Hollandaise or cheese sauce (p. 163).

Brussels sprouts may be prepared by the recipes given for broccoli, cabbage, or cauliflower.

## BRUSSELS SPROUTS WITH MUSHROOM SAUCE

Heat to 200° F., using a cooking thermometer:

**1 can condensed mushroom soup**          1/2 **cup milk**

Add:

**1 pound chilled whole Brussels sprouts**

Stir well to cover all surfaces with sauce; heat to 200° F., cover utensil, and simmer until just tender, or 10 to 12 minutes.

Taste for salt and garnish with **paprika or ground parsley.**

*Variations:*

If especially soft texture is desired, cut each sprout into halves or fourths.

Cook in parchment paper, steam with a small amount of water, simmer in deep or shallow milk, or cook in waterless-cooking utensil or top of double boiler with 1 tablespoon hot water.

**Creamed Brussels sprouts with celery:** Cream like broccoli (p. 382); add with raw sprouts 1/2 cup chopped stalk and shredded celery leaves.

**Sautéed Brussels sprouts:** Brush frying pan with butter-flavored fat; add Brussels sprouts cut in half; stir well and add 1 tablespoon hot water; cover utensil and cook 5 to 6 minutes over low heat. Season with 1/2 teaspoon salt and garnish with paprika. Or toss whole sprouts with oil before steaming.

Savoy and Chinese cabbage and collards may be prepared by any recipe used in cooking ordinary cabbage. Since they are nutritionally superior to the lighter-colored variety, they should be served more frequently when available.

## STEAMED CABBAGE

Dry well after washing and shred fine on kraut cutter:

> ½ head chilled cabbage

Add to:

> 2 tablespoons boiling water

Cover utensil, heat rapidly, and reduce heat; simmer 8 minutes.
Season with ½ teaspoon salt.

*Variations:*

Add 1 or 2 teaspoons caraway seeds.

Cook shredded cabbage in ½ cup milk; or cut head into sixths without removing stalk and cook in deep milk.

**Creamed cabbage:** Heat 1 cup medium cream sauce, ½ teaspoon salt, dash each of cayenne and celery salt; add chilled shredded cabbage; stir thoroughly and simmer 8 minutes. **Cubed American cheese and/or 2 tablespoons diced canned pimento** may be added before serving; or **diced fresh pimento** may be cooked with cabbage.

*Scalloped cabbage:* Prepare creamed cabbage in heat-resistant casserole, cooking over direct heat; when cabbage is tender, stir in ¼ cup toasted whole-wheat-bread crumbs and ¾ cup cubed American cheese; sprinkle surface with toasted crumbs, cheese, and paprika; cover utensil until cheese melts; or combine all ingredients and bake 15 minutes in moderate oven.

**Cabbage chop suey:** Chop together ½ head chilled cabbage, 4 stalks celery, 1 chilled green pepper, 1 large onion; sauté with low heat in bacon drippings for 10 minutes; add and stir in ½ teaspoon each soy sauce and salt, dash of paprika. Serve with steamed or fried brown rice.

**Sautéed cabbage:** Cook shredded cabbage with 1 tablespoon each hot water and oil or bacon drippings; cover utensil and cook over low heat 8 minutes; or sauté like mustard-spinach (p. 377).

*With bacon:* Pan-broil 2 slices bacon, remove when crisp, and sauté shredded cabbage until tender; salt, and sprinkle chopped bacon over each serving.

**With purple cabbage:** Cook equal parts shredded green and purple cabbage as in the basic recipe or any variation. Purple cabbage should be shredded finer than green cabbage so that both will be tender at the same time; if carefully prepared, this combination is both beautiful and delicious.

**With sauerkraut:** Combine and cook together 8 minutes without added moisture approximately **2 cups each sauerkraut and chilled shredded cabbage;** if sour taste is not enjoyed, add ½ teaspoon sugar. Vary by seasoning with 1 or 2 teaspoons caraway seeds.

Unless carefully prepared, purple cabbage changes color more quickly than does any other vegetable. Knives and equipment to be used in shredding and the utensil in which it is to be cooked should be rinsed with a cup of water containing 1 teaspoon vinegar. Cook purple cabbage preferably in glass or enamel rather than in aluminum. Purple cabbage should be served slightly crisp; if a soft texture is desired, shred it paper-thin for quick cooking.

## PURPLE CABBAGE WITH APPLE

Shred paper-thin, cutting shreds into lengths of 3 to 4 inches:

**½ head chilled purple cabbage**

Heat to boiling:

**¼ cup water**

Add:

| | |
|---|---|
| **shredded cabbage** | **dash of nutmeg** |
| **2 diced tart apples** | |

Cover utensil, heat quickly, and steam 12 to 15 minutes.
Season with ½ teaspoon salt.

*Variations:*

Omit apples and nutmeg; sauté until transparent 1 chopped onion in 1 tablespoon bacon drippings; add cabbage, stir well, and add 1 teaspoon vinegar or 1 tablespoon French dressing or lemon juice.

**Purple cabbage with sour cream:** Cook shredded purple cabbage in ½ cup heated sour cream; season with ½ teaspoon salt and ½ teaspoon caraway or cardamom seeds; simmer 12 to 15 minutes without allowing temperature to go above 200° F. Mix in **1 tablespoon ground parsley** and serve.

Sautéed purple cabbage: Pan-broil 1 slice bacon, remove when crisp; add 2 tablespoons each vinegar and water and ¼ teaspoon crushed black peppercorns; add shredded cabbage and stir to cover surfaces with acid; season with ½ teaspoon salt; before serving add bacon cut into small pieces.

Spiced purple cabbage: Boil 2 to 3 minutes ¼ cup water, 1 tablespoon vinegar, 4 each cassia buds and whole cloves, 1 tablespoon brown sugar; add shredded cabbage, stir well, and steam 12 to 15 minutes.

## CAULIFLOWER PATTIES

Put quickly through meat grinder, making sure vegetables are chilled:

| | |
|---|---|
| 2 peeled tomatoes | 1 clove garlic |
| 1 dry onion or 2 or 3 green onions and tops | 1 small green pepper or pimento |
| | 1 small raw cauliflower broken into pieces |

Add to the vegetables and stir in:

| | |
|---|---|
| ½ cup powdered milk | 1 teaspoon salt |
| 2 eggs | freshly ground black peppercorns |
| 1 cup grated or shredded American cheese | |

Drop from tablespoon onto hot grill brushed with butter-flavored oil or bacon drippings; keep heat low; cover utensil and brown slowly; turn when browned; cook 5 to 6 minutes on each side.

*Variations:*

Omit eggs and sauté ground vegetables for 6 minutes; after removing from heat, add cheese, salt, and pepper; or bake in preheated casserole in hot oven at 400° F.

Add ground carrot, kohlrabi, parsley, spinach, turnip, or any vegetable desired; or add any diced leftover vegetables to patties just before frying.

Omit eggs, powdered milk, and ground green peppers; sauté ground vegetables in 1 tablespoon bacon drippings for 5 minutes; pack into chilled green peppers or pimentos, sprinkle with cheese, and heat in moderate oven at 325° F. for 10 to 15 minutes.

**Cauliflower simmered in milk:** Cook entire cauliflower head in enough fresh or reconstructed milk (p. 451) to cover; simmer at 200° F. for 20 minutes, or until just tender; place cauliflower on serving platter; prepare 1½ cups medium cream sauce (p. 161), using milk left from cooking cauliflower; add to sauce ½ cup shredded cheese or 2 egg yolks and dash of nutmeg. Vary by cooking broken cauliflower in ½ cup hot milk; stir to cover all surfaces with milk protein; simmer 10 minutes, or until tender, and season with salt, paprika, and margarine or butter.

**Cauliflower with tomatoes:** Sauté 1 clove garlic and 1 chopped onion in 1 tablespoon bacon drippings; discard garlic and add ¼ teaspoon crushed black peppercorns, 1 teaspoon salt, ¾ cup canned or raw diced tomatoes or tomato purée; bring to boiling and add raw cauliflower broken into pieces; stir well and add 1 teaspoon fresh or pinch of dry basil, orégano, or thyme; cover utensil and cook 10 minutes; serve sprinkled with Parmesan cheese. Bell pepper, pimento, or celery may be sautéed with garlic, or ground parsley may be added before serving.

**Creamed cauliflower:** Break raw cauliflower into 2-inch pieces and add to ¾ cup hot milk; stir thoroughly, cover utensil, heat quickly, and simmer at 200° F. for 12 minutes; thicken milk with cream sauce; season with ½ teaspoon salt and freshly ground black peppercorns. Before serving add any one or more of the following: 2 tablespoons chopped canned pimento or sliced stuffed olives; ½ cup sliced canned mushrooms; ¾ cup cubed cheese; 4 tablespoons ground parsley; or garnish with 2 sliced or sieved hard-cooked eggs.

**Fried cauliflower:** Use leftover cauliflower which has been steamed or simmered in milk; dip in batter (p. 183) mixed with an equal amount of shredded cheese; fry in deep fat at 350° F. until light brown, or 2 to 3 minutes.

**Leftover cauliflower:** Remove centers from 4 peeled tomatoes; place in baking dish, sprinkle with salt and pepper, put a piece of cauliflower in each tomato; cover with 1½ cups thick cream sauce and sprinkle generously with cheese and paprika; bake in hot oven at 400° F. for 10 to 15 minutes.

**Steamed cauliflower:** Break cauliflower into 2-inch pieces and rinse with 1 cup water containing 1 tablespoon vinegar; steam about 10 minutes, or until just tender, using the least water necessary to prevent burning; serve with salt, paprika, and margarine or butter, or with Hollandaise (p. 164) or cheese sauce (p. 163).

Leeks might be described as overgrown green onions. Their flavor is similar to that of green onions or sweet dry onions, except that they are more mild, sweet, juicy, and, to most people, more delicious. Any person who enjoys the flavor of onions in small amounts will probably be enthusiastic about leeks.

Leeks may be prepared by recipes given for onions. As much as 2 to 3 inches of the green leaves should be used. Leeks are especially delightful when cooked in milk and served with Hollandaise or cheese sauce.

Onions are almost invariably overcooked, and as a result their delightful fresh flavor is sacrificed. They should be served while still slightly crisp, or cooked only until translucent. Dry onions contain about 15 per cent sugar. If they are peeled only after they are cooked, no sugar is lost and they are far sweeter and more delicious than when prepared by the usual methods.

## BROILED ONIONS

Select flat white or purple onions no more than 1 inch thick but as large as available; do not skin or cut.

Set on the broiler rack 2 inches from heat; keep heat as high as possible without burning skin; broil 8 to 10 minutes; turn, lower heat, and continue broiling until tender, or about 10 minutes longer; remove from heat; peel off skin and outside layer.

Cut petal-fashion toward root; sprinkle with salt and paprika.

*Variations:*

When oven is being used, bake whole unpeeled onions 20 to 30 minutes, or until tender; remove skin just before serving.

**Broiled onion slices:** Cut large onions into ½-inch slices; set on oiled baking sheet, brush top surface with oil, and place 2 inches from broiler under moderate heat; when they start to brown, or in about 6 minutes, turn with pancake turner; brown the other side slightly and lower heat to finish cooking; sprinkle with salt and paprika.

**Creamed onions:** Select small white onions, peel, and simmer at 200° F. in ½ cup hot milk until almost tender; add ¾ teaspoon salt, 1 cup cream sauce, ¼ teaspoon paprika; or add ¼ cup diced green pepper or pimentos before cooking, or 2 tablespoons parsley or ½ cup cubed cheese before serving. If it is more convenient, steam unpeeled onions on rack above water until tender; peel and drop into hot cream sauce.

*Creamed green onions:* Cut off tops of 2 bunches green onions, retaining 2 inches or more of green; keep parallel and drop into 1 cup simmering milk; add ¼ teaspoon crushed white peppercorns; simmer at 200° F. until barely tender, or 10 to 12 minutes; put onions on serving plate, thicken milk with cream sauce; season with 1 tablespoon mayonnaise, ¾ teaspoon salt, ¼ teaspoon paprika; pour sauce on onions without covering green tops and white base; garnish with parsley sprigs or pimento strips.

*Scalloped onions:* Prepare creamed whole or sliced onions in heat-resistant casserole over direct heat; when onions are tender, sprinkle with ½ cup each toasted whole-wheat-bread crumbs and cubed American cheese; garnish generously with paprika. Cover utensil until cheese melts.

**French-fried onion rings:** Cut onions into ½-inch slices, separate into rings, and dip in batter (p. 183); fry a few rings at a time in hot fat at 300° F. for 2 to 4 minutes; drain on brown paper. Vary by mixing shredded cheese with batter. With onions fry rings of chilled green pepper, fresh chili pepper, or pimento.

**Onion casserole:** Slice **4 large onions** and put into hot casserole containing **2 tablespoons each water and bacon drippings or oil;** cover casserole and bake in preheated moderate oven until transparent, or about 15 minutes; sprinkle with **½ teaspoon salt, ¼ cup ground parsley, and ½ cup cubed or grated cheese;** turn off heat and leave in oven until cheese melts. If mild flavor is desired, omit water and add ½ cup top milk.

**Onions cooked in sour cream:** Add small white onions or ⅓-inch rings of red and white onions to 1 cup heated sour cream; simmer at 200° F. until tender, or about 10 to 12 minutes; add ½ teaspoon salt and dash of cayenne.

**Spiced red onions:** Slice large red onions ⅓ inch thick and separate into rings, or alternate slices of white and red onions; add to **1 tablespoon each vinegar, water, bacon drippings;** season with **3 whole cloves and 3 cassia buds or small piece of cinnamon bark;** heat quickly, then simmer 8 to 10 minutes. Serve while rings are slightly crisp.

**Steamed onions:** Set dry unpeeled onions on rack above boiling water; steam until tender, or 15 to 20 minutes; peel, sprinkle with salt and paprika. Vary by putting cooked peeled onions in flat baking dish; sprinkle with toasted crumbs, grated cheese, paprika; heat slowly under broiler until cheese melts.

**Stuffed onions:** When chopped onions are to be used in other cooking, cut out centers from large onions, leaving the skin and 4 to 6 outside, meaty layers; when 4 shells or more accumulate, fill with heated stuffing of leftover diced carrots or other vegetables, diced leftover meat, chopped pepper or pimento, and celery; add salt and pepper; or prepare half the meat-loaf recipe (p. 134) and use for stuffing; cover with tomato sauce or cream sauce (p. 162); bake in hot oven 15 to 18 minutes.

## RUTABAGAS

Peel **1 to 3 chilled rutabagas** and cut into wedges or fingers ½-inch thick; dice old and fibrous rutabagas into small cubes; drop into:

### ½ cup hot milk

Stir to cover all surfaces with milk protein; cover utensil, heat rapidly, and simmer for 15 minutes, or until tender, stirring occasionally; season with:

**½ teaspoon salt**                              **margarine or butter**
**dash of cayenne**

*Variations:*

Cook rutabagas by any recipe suggested for turnips (p. 391).

Mash rutabagas by pressing through a hot colander or ricer; season as in basic recipe or add a dash of nutmeg.

Before serving add to rutabagas 1 tablespoon chopped chives, green-onion tops, or Chinese garlic, or 3 to 4 tablespoons ground parsley.

A few minutes before serving add ½ cup thick cream sauce; season with ground parsley or diced pimento and paprika.

Cut rutabagas into quarters and steam until tender; season as in basic recipe.

**Baked rutabagas:** Leave young and tender rutabagas whole; otherwise cut into halves or quarters; do not peel; brush all surfaces with oil and bake in preheated oven at 350° F. for 40 to 50 minutes, or until tender; or steam until they start to be tender; finish cooking in oven. Serve like baked potatoes.

**French-fried rutabagas:** Cut peeled rutabagas into fingers; cook in fat at 240° F. for 10 minutes, or until almost tender; increase heat to 300° F. until golden brown, or about 1 minute.

**Leftover rutabagas:** Beat **1 egg** slightly and add **½ teaspoon salt, 1 or 2 cups mashed rutabagas;** shape into patties, roll in whole-wheat flour, and sauté at low temperature.

## SAUERKRAUT WITH CARAWAY SEEDS

Put into utensil for waterless cooking or top of double boiler:

**1 tablespoon water**                          **1 pound sauerkraut**
**1 to 2 teaspoons caraway seeds**

Stir well, cover utensil, and simmer 8 minutes.
Taste for salt.

*Variations:*

Pan-broil ham; heat sauerkraut quickly in same utensil without added moisture.

Cook sauerkraut with an equal amount of shredded green or purple cabbage.

**Sauerkraut with apples:** Omit caraway seeds and add **2 diced unpeeled red apples, 1 tablespoon ham or bacon drippings or dash of smoke-flavoring, ½ teaspoon black molasses, dash of nutmeg.** Serve while apples are still slightly crisp.

**Sauerkraut with tomatoes:** Sauté in **1 tablespoon bacon drippings 1 each chopped onion and celery stalk;** add **½ cup canned or diced fresh tomato;** heat to boiling, and stir in sauerkraut. Cut **2 or 3 wieners** into ½-inch pieces and add 2 minutes before serving; or stir in **1 cup cubed mild cheese.**

**Sauerkraut with wieners:** Prepare sauerkraut as in basic recipe; lay wieners on top of sauerkraut, serve as soon as heated through.

Use yellow, or golden ball, turnips in preference to white turnips. After they are washed and wiped dry, try not to touch them with water.

## CRISP SHREDDED TURNIPS

Shred **4 to 6 chilled unpeeled turnips** and put immediately into:

**2 tablespoons hot top milk**

Stir well, cover utensil, and cook 5 minutes; season with:

**½ teaspoon salt**          **freshly ground black peppercorns**

Serve while slightly crisp.

*Variations:*

Salt grated turnips and cook in oiled hot casserole in preheated oven 6 to 8 minutes; or sauté in 2 teaspoons bacon drippings with ½ clove garlic; discard garlic; salt.

**Baked turnips:** If oven is being used, select whole baby turnips or flat ones no more than 1½ inches thick; toss or brush with oil and heat rapidly by steaming 5 minutes or by putting under broiler for 10 minutes; bake until tender, or about 10 to 15 minutes. Serve like baked potatoes.

**Creamed turnips:** Cut unpeeled turnips into quarters; simmer at 200° F. in ¾ cup top milk seasoned with crushed white peppercorns until almost tender, or about 15 minutes, add cream sauce, dash of nutmeg.

**French-fried turnips:** Cut unpeeled turnips into fingers and fry in deep bacon drippings at 240° F. for about 6 minutes; when starting to be tender, heat fat to 300° F. for browning; drain on paper; sprinkle with salt and paprika.

**Mashed turnips:** Cut unpeeled turnips into 4 to 6 wedges each and steam in ½ cup top milk until tender; pass through hot colander or food mill; season with margarine or butter, salt, pepper, and milk left from cooking them.

**Sautéed turnips:** Slice 4 to 6 chilled unpeeled turnips; sauté in butter-flavored oil or bacon drippings over low heat; cover utensil, turn frequently, and cook 8 to 10 minutes; season with ½ teaspoon salt and dash of paprika; or sauté sliced turnips with carrots, kohlrabi, onions, green peppers, pimentos, rutabagas, or potatoes. In combining vegetables, those which require a longer cooking time should be cut into thinner slices than others.

**Scalloped turnips:** Using slicer, cut chilled unpeeled turnips into paper-thin slices; cook in casserole in ½ cup hot milk seasoned with ½ teaspoon salt and ¼ teaspoon crushed black peppercorns; sprinkle with crumbs, shredded cheese, paprika; cover casserole and bake in preheated oven at 400° F. for 10 to 15 minutes, or until just tender.

**Steamed turnips:** Steam whole unpeeled turnips 10 to 18 minutes, or until tender; cut petal-fashion and season with salt, paprika, ⅓ cup grated cheese.

**Turnip pancakes:** Mix 2 cups shredded turnips or 1 cup each shredded turnips and carrots with 2 tablespoons each minced onion and ground parsley; stir in 4 tablespoons powdered milk, 1 egg, 4 drops Tabasco, ½ teaspoon salt; drop from spoon and sauté slowly in bacon drippings until brown on both sides.


## RESPECT THE POTATO

Since millions of people eat potatoes daily, it is especially important to form habits of cooking them so that their nutrients are retained. Aside from calories, the contribution white potatoes can make to health, if allowed to do so, is the cumulative amount of vitamin C and iron they offer, although they contain other vitamins and minerals as well. A medium-size potato supplies an average of 33 milligrams of vitamin C, or approximately the amount in a glass of tomato juice, and 1.5 milligrams of iron, the amount in an egg. During the winter months, potatoes may be the chief source of these nutrients for many families. Yet both iron and vitamin C are often extracted or thrown away before the potatoes reach the table.

View critically, for example, the atrocious but common method of preparing mashed potatoes for Sunday dinner. The potatoes are often peeled in the early morning and left swimming in water at room temperature while the family goes to church. This water is usually poured off and more water is added before the potatoes are put on to boil; this water is also thrown away. Yet even un-peeled potatoes have been found to lose 83 per cent of their iron and 100 per cent of their vitamin C if boiled 20 minutes.

If you wish to retain the nutritive value, prepare potatoes like any other fresh vegetable which contains iron and vitamin C. Scrub them thoroughly with a brush and dry them immediately. If they are to be peeled, sliced, diced, or grated, chill them in ad-vance to inhibit enzyme action when the cut surface is exposed to the air; thus discoloration and loss of vitamin C are prevented. If old potatoes need to be freshened, put them into the refrigera-tor pan for 24 hours; keep enough crisped potatoes ahead for one or two meals. When potatoes must be cut in advance of cooking, put them in a utility bag in the refrigerator without added mois-ture. Avoid peeling them for most uses. Heat them as quickly as possible, and use all the liquid in which they have been cooked.

Mashed potatoes prepared by steaming them unpeeled and then passing them through a hot colander have far more flavor than those which have been peeled and boiled. When equipment for waterless cooking is available, potatoes can be baked on top of the range more easily and more economically than in an oven. This is explained by Method I, which follows.

To avoid needless destruction of nutritive value, do not cook potatoes twice except to use leftovers. Potatoes to be French-fried or pan-fried, for example, should be uncooked.

Although sweet potatoes and yams are not rich in vitamin C or iron, they supply from 3500 to 5000 units of vitamin A per serv-ing. When they are available, use them interchangeably with white potatoes.

## BAKED POTATOES

There are three methods of baking potatoes, of which the slow but customary oven method is the least desirable.

Select 4 to 6 medium-size potatoes, preferably long slender ones; scrub and dry them; brush surface with oil or soft fat.

Method I: Put potatoes into a preheated utensil designed for waterless cooking; cover utensil, keep heat moderate for 6 minutes, then set over simmer burner until potatoes are tender, or 20 to 30 minutes; set lid of utensil to one side during the last 5 minutes of baking.

Method II: Set oiled potatoes under the broiler near moderate heat for 10 to 15 minutes, turning to heat all sides; finish baking in moderate oven at 350° F. for 15 to 20 minutes.

Method III: Place in hot oven at 425° F. and bake until tender, or 40 to 45 minutes.

Remove from utensil or oven and make two crosswise gashes on top of each potato; pinch to open gashes, insert a piece of margarine or butter in each potato, sprinkle with salt, freshly ground peppercorns, and paprika. Serve at once.

*Variations:*

Bake large potatoes until nearly tender; split lengthwise and spread each half with 1 teaspoon prepared mustard; sprinkle with salt, Worcestershire, 1 teaspoon grated onion, whole-wheat-bread crumbs, chopped leftover bacon or grated cheese; finish baking until tender.

**Baked new potatoes:** Place small new unpeeled potatoes in waterless-cooking utensil or flat baking dish with 2 tablespoons butter-flavored fat; bake over direct heat or in oven until tender, or from 15 to 25 minutes; shake utensil twice during baking to rotate potatoes in fat.

**Baked sweet potatoes or yams:** Prepare and bake by any method suggested in basic recipe; yams cook in about half the time required for white or sweet potatoes.

*Glazed sweet potatoes or yams:* Bake or steam unpeeled sweet potatoes or yams until nearly tender; cut in half lengthwise, place in flat baking dish; brush with dark molasses, dot with margarine or butter; bake until tender in moderate oven.

**Stuffed sweet potatoes or yams:** Cut 4 hot baked sweet potatoes or yams in half lengthwise; fluff pulp with a fork, add ½ teaspoon salt and top milk or crushed pineapple; garnish with paprika, dot with margarine or butter, reheat under broiler.

When white potatoes are stuffed immediately after being baked, oxygen is whipped into them; the baking time is needlessly prolonged, and vitamin C has little chance of escaping destruction. Use stuffed potatoes largely as a means of making leftover baked potatoes interesting. If the pulp is chilled before being mashed, little loss of vitamin C occurs except that destroyed during reheating. However, by all means do not bake more potatoes than are needed at one meal just to have some to stuff at a later time. No vegetable should be heated twice if it is possible to avoid doing so.

## STUFFED WHITE POTATOES

Cut in half lengthwise:

### 2 or more baked potatoes

Scoop out pulp, mash, and mix with:

| | |
|---|---|
| ½ cup shredded yellow cheese | ½ teaspoon salt |
| 4 tablespoons top milk | freshly ground peppercorns |
| 2 tablespoons ground parsley | |

Pack mixture into skins; sprinkle with **paprika** and put in hot oven at 400° F. for 10 minutes.

*Variations:*

Mix with potato pulp any one or more of the following: 1 minced clove garlic; 1 or 2 teaspoons caraway seeds; 1 teaspoon Worcestershire; 1 grated onion or finely chopped green-onion tops; chopped and lightly sautéed celery, mushrooms, or green peppers; sliced stuffed olives; anchovies; diced canned pimento; 2 teaspoons minced fresh dill, dill seeds, or dill sauce; diced leftover vegetables or meat.

Omit milk and add 2 tablespoons mayonnaise or ¼ cup cream sauce; combine with cream sauce 2 tablespoons chives or Chinese garlic or ¼ cup chopped almonds.

Omit cheese and milk; combine with potato pulp any leftover creamed ham, chicken, dried beef, fish, or vegetables.

**Hash-browned potatoes:** Dice leftover white or sweet potatoes or yams, preferably unpeeled; season with **salt and pepper**; sauté quickly in **bacon drippings**; add **chives, minced green-onion tops, or diced leftover meat or other vegetables.** See also page 403.

**Leftover baked sweet potatoes or yams:** Cut leftover sweet potatoes or yams lengthwise into slices and brush with **dark molasses;** place in alternate layers in shallow oiled baking dish with **pineapple slices or thick applesauce;** sprinkle applesauce lightly with **grated lemon rind, nutmeg, or cinnamon;** bake in moderate oven until heated through.


## BROILED POTATOES

Cut into ⅛-inch sticks:

### 3 or 4 chilled unpeeled potatoes

Toss in salad bowl with:

### 1 tablespoon oil

Place on oiled baking sheet and broil at moderate temperature until top is browned, or about 6 minutes; turn with pancake turner and brown the other sides; lower heat and cook until potatoes are tender; sprinkle with:

### ½ teaspoon salt

*Variations:*

Instead of white potatoes use yams or sweet potatoes.

Cut potatoes lengthwise into ⅛-inch slices; brush surfaces with oil; broil as in basic recipe; garnish with chives and paprika or chopped fresh dill.

**Broiled sweet potatoes or yams:** Cut chilled unpeeled sweet potatoes or yams lengthwise into ⅛-inch slices; brush top surface with **oil or soft bacon drippings** and broil as in basic recipe; season with **salt and smoke-flavoring or grated orange rind;** or after cooking a few minutes, brush surfaces with **dark molasses** and add **dash of nutmeg.**

*With bananas:* When slices of sweet potatoes or yams are almost tender, cut bananas in two lengthwise, then in half, and put one section of banana on each slice of potato; brush with molasses and broil until well browned.

**Broiled sweet potatoes or yams on skewers:** Cut chilled unpeeled sweet potatoes or yams into ¾-inch cubes; arrange on skewers with cubes of raw apple; brush with oil and broil on oiled baking sheet until almost tender; on ends of skewers put cubes of baked ham, fresh or leftover lamb, or pineapple; continue broiling with low heat until potatoes are tender.

## CREAMED WHITE POTATOES

Leave small new potatoes whole; cut chilled large ones into 1-inch sections or cubes.

Heat to simmering:

¾ cup milk

Add and stir:

**8 or 10 new potatoes or 3 or 4 large ones, preferably unpeeled**

Cover utensil and simmer until potatoes are tender, or 12 to 15 minutes; add:

½ teaspoon salt                1 tablespoon chives cut with scis-
1 cup cream sauce              sors

Serve sprinkled with **paprika.**

*Variations:*

Omit chives and add to milk any one or more of the following: ½ to 2 teaspoons caraway, dill, or celery seeds; grated onion; a pinch of thyme or basil; crushed peppercorns; or season with ½ teaspoon paprika, 1 teaspoon Worcestershire, 5 drops Tabasco, or 1 teaspoon minced fresh dill or dill sauce.

Omit cream sauce and simmer potatoes in ½ cup milk; garnish with ground parsley and paprika; or cook potatoes in chicken stock instead of milk; add cream sauce and a pinch of sage.

Instead of plain cream sauce use dill, caraway, pimento, egg, cheese, piquant, mock Hollandaise, or other cream sauce (p. 162).

## AMERICAN FRIED POTATOES

Slice thin:

4 to 6 chilled unpeeled white potatoes

Heat:

3 or 4 tablespoons bacon drippings or butter-flavored fat

Drop potatoes into fat; fry over moderate heat, turning frequently until almost tender; add:

½ to ¾ teaspoon salt           freshly ground black peppercorns

Cook until tender and well browned, or about 15 minutes.

*Variations:*

Brown 1 clove garlic in fat and discard before adding potatoes; fry with potatoes 1 or 2 sliced dry onions or green onions with tops; or season with ¼ teaspoon celery salt or 1 or 2 teaspoons caraway seeds.

Instead of white potatoes slice chilled unpeeled sweet potatoes or yams and fry as in basic recipe; keep heat moderate to prevent shrinking. Fry in fat left from ham or pork chops when available. Vary by frying diced apples with sweet potatoes; or cut sweet potatoes lengthwise into ½-inch slices and fry with pineapple slices or rings of cored unpeeled apple.

**Fried leftover potatoes:** Slice potatoes; keep heat high and cook the shortest time necessary for browning; sprinkle with ground parsley.

**Fried whole potatoes:** Use small new white potatoes; leave unpeeled; shake utensil during frying to keep potatoes well greased; cook 8 to 15 minutes; when tender, salt and add 1 tablespoon each chopped chives, ground parsley, or mixed fresh herbs, such as tarragon, basil, marjoram, sage.

**Potato patty shells:** Fry shredded white or sweet potatoes or yams without browning until nearly tender; arrange against sides and on bottom of deep muffin pans, pressing firmly to pan; bake in hot oven at 450° F. for 10 minutes; serve filled with creamed peas, spinach, or other vegetables or with creamed shrimps or ham.

**Potatoes to be served with a roast:** When a roast is cooked at low temperature, potatoes, carrots, and onions baked around it require almost 2 hours to become tender; as a substitute, cut peeled or unpeeled potatoes and carrots in half lengthwise and fry with whole peeled onions in ¼ cup or more of fat dipped from the dripping pan; keep heat moderate and turn as surface browns; cook with utensil covered 20 to 25 minutes; sprinkle with salt, pepper, paprika; serve around roast.

**Spanish-fried potatoes:** Fry with white potatoes 1 minced clove garlic, 1 each chopped green pepper, onion, fresh or canned pimento; ½ cup cooked diced ham may be added.

## FRENCH-FRIED POTATOES

Chill **3 or 4 large potatoes** thoroughly; do not peel.
Heat to 360° F., using cooking thermometer:

### 2 to 3 cups bacon drippings or butter-flavored oil

Put wire basket in oil to heat; when thermometer reading is about 340° F., cut unpeeled potatoes into sticks ⅓ inch thick; lay on heated basket and put in hot fat; watch thermometer carefully and do not allow temperature to exceed 325° F. after the potatoes are added; if fat becomes too hot, potatoes shrivel.

Fry until golden brown, or 8 to 10 minutes; drain on absorbent paper, sprinkle with salt, and serve immediately.

*Variations:*

Cut potatoes into shoestrings, slices, or lattice slices; fry at 360° F. until brown.

Use whole unpeeled new potatoes the size of large marbles; fry until tender, or about 7 minutes; drain, salt, and sprinkle with ground parsley.

**French-fried leftover potatoes:** Use leftover steamed or baked white or sweet potatoes or yams; cut lengthwise into fingers; fry at 375° F. for 3 to 5 minutes.

**French-fried sweet potatoes or yams:** Cut raw chilled unpeeled sweet potatoes or yams into fingers; fry at 300° F. until brown, or about 6 minutes for yams, 15 for sweet potatoes; watch temperature carefully to prevent shriveling; drain and salt.

**Potato chips:** Using slicer, cut 1 chilled unpeeled white or sweet potato or yam into extremely thin slices; fry at 360° F. until brown, or 3 to 5 minutes; drain on paper, salt, and proceed with next potato. Chips of sweet potatoes or yams are delicious, especially if served hot.

## MASHED POTATOES

Scrub, chill, and cut into pieces 1 inch thick:

### 3 to 5 unpeeled potatoes

Drop into:

½ cup steaming top milk seasoned with     ¼ teaspoon crushed black peppercorns

Cover utensil and simmer 10 to 15 minutes, or until tender.

Meanwhile heat colander or food mill by setting it on utensil holding potatoes; press potatoes through colander or food mill as soon as they are tender.

Add:

½ to ¾ teaspoon salt     top milk left from steaming
2 tablespoons margarine or butter

Beat vigorously with a heated eggbeater; taste for seasonings and serve at once.

*Variations:*

Whip into mashed potatoes 2 or 3 tablespoons ground parsley.

Instead of white potatoes use sweet potatoes or yams.

Cook and mash together equal quantities of potatoes and rutabagas or winter squash; cut squash or rutabagas into smaller pieces than potatoes; season as in basic recipe.

Steam whole unpeeled potatoes on rack above boiling water or cook without added moisture in waterless-cooking utensil; proceed as in basic recipe.

If equipment with a tight-fitting lid is not available, simmer potatoes until tender in enough hot milk to cover; drain milk into a wide-mouthed jar and save.

## LEFTOVER MASHED POTATOES

Stir into **1 or 2 cups leftover mashed potatoes:**

**2 tablespoons parsley**

Make into patties and roll in:

**whole-wheat-bread crumbs or whole-wheat flour**

Heat grill and brush with bacon drippings. Brown patties quickly on both sides, cooking only 6 to 8 minutes.

*Variations:*

Add leftover flaked fish with 1 teaspoon chopped dill or dill sauce, or diced leftover ham, chicken, or other meat with a pinch each of savory and basil.

Add ½ cup shredded cheese; while patties are browning, sauté 1 chopped onion; put browned patties on serving platter, heat with onion 1 cup tomato purée; salt and serve over patties.

**Potato puffs:** Beat **1½ cups mashed potatoes with 2 egg yolks, ¼ cup each fresh milk and powdered milk, ½ teaspoon salt, 3 diced pimentos;** fold in **2 stiffly beaten egg whites;** put into flat oiled baking dish, sprinkle with **cheese and paprika,** and bake at 350° F. for 15 minutes. Vary by adding flaked salmon or other fish or diced meat, 1 to 3 teaspoons each chopped onion and fresh dill or dill sauce.

*Fried potato puffs:* Combine ingredients, press lightly into balls, roll in crumbs, and brown quickly in deep or shallow fat.

In most potato casserole dishes, the sliced or diced potatoes are placed in a cold casserole, cold liquid is added, and the potatoes are baked uncovered for an hour or more; so much surface is ex-

posed to oxygen and the dry heat penetrates so slowly that vitamin C is largely destroyed. If you do not have a heat-resistant
casserole which can be used on top of the range, have the liquid
hot before adding the potatoes and keep the casserole covered
throughout most of the baking time.

## SCALLOPED POTATOES

Combine in casserole and heat to simmering over direct heat or in
moderate oven:

| | |
|---|---|
| 1 cup top milk or evaporated milk | ¼ teaspoon crushed white pepper- |
| ¾ teaspoon salt | corns |

Slice thin and dust with 2 tablespoons whole-wheat flour:

### 3 cups chilled unpeeled potatoes

Add potatoes to hot milk; cover casserole and simmer over direct heat
10 to 15 minutes; or bake in moderate oven at 350° F. for 20 to 25 minutes; remove cover, sprinkle with whole-wheat-bread crumbs and paprika; brown under broiler.

*Variations:*

Omit flour and stir cream sauce with milk at the beginning of cooking
if oven is to be used, or when potatoes are tender if casserole is used on
top of range.

Just before putting casserole under broiler, sprinkle top with ½ cup
shredded cheese; add or omit crumbs; broil at an extremely low heat.

Instead of in milk cook potatoes in ¾ cup chicken stock seasoned with
a pinch of sage, or ¾ cup ham stock seasoned with 1 teaspoon chopped
dill or dill sauce or dill or caraway seeds; thicken with cream sauce.

Omit 1 cup of potatoes and use 1 cup thinly sliced carrots, turnips,
kohlrabi, onions, celery root, or salsify.

Add 2 tablespoons ground parsley, chopped pimento, or green pepper.

Cook potatoes in 1 cup tomatoes instead of milk; add 1 chopped onion,
green pepper, or celery stalk, 1 minced clove garlic, 2 tablespoons bacon
drippings, a pinch of basil. Before putting casserole under broiler vary
by adding diced leftover meat, flaked fish, or crisp bacon cut to bits.

Omit flour and salt; cook white or sweet potatoes in 1 can condensed
mushroom soup diluted with ¼ cup milk; add peppercorns, ¼ teaspoon
paprika.

**Sweet potato or yam casserole:** Heat in casserole ¾ cup pineapple juice, 2 tablespoons dark molasses; add unpeeled sweet potatoes or yams cut lengthwise into ¼-inch slices; cover casserole; simmer over direct heat or bake in moderate over 15 to 20 minutes until almost tender; cover with pineapple slices, dot with bacon drippings, and brown under broiler. Vary by broiling thin slices of ham lightly over sliced pineapple.

**Sweet potatoes or yams with apples:** Alternate sliced sweet potatoes and thinly sliced apples in an oiled heat-resistant casserole; sprinkle layers with salt, cinnamon, grated lemon rind; add 2 tablespoons each hot water and bacon drippings, margarine, or butter; simmer over direct heat until tender, or about 15 minutes. Brown top under broiler.

Potato salad should be served, not as a substitute for a salad, but as a cooked vegetable. The nutrients it supplies are entirely different from those furnished by green leaves and uncooked fruits and vegetables. The same is true of other so-called salads made of cooked vegetables.


## POTATO SALAD

Steam until tender in or above a small amount of water:

### 4 to 6 unpeeled potatoes

Chill quickly, peel, and slice; combine and heat to boiling:

| | |
|---|---|
| ⅓ cup vinegar | 1 chopped onion |
| ⅓ cup water left from steaming | ½ teaspoon freshly ground black |
| ¾ teaspoon salt | peppercorns |

Pour over sliced potatoes and let stand until absorbed, stirring 2 or 3 times; chill; add:

| | |
|---|---|
| ½ cup chopped celery | ¼ cup or more of mayonnaise or |
| 2 to 4 tablespoons ground parsley | cooked dressing |

Mix well, let stand in refrigerator until ready to serve, and turn onto nest of lettuce or watercress.

*Variations:*

Add any one or more of the following: 1 diced red unpeeled apple; 1 or 2 chopped green peppers or fresh or canned pimentos; 2 or 3 sliced hard-cooked eggs; 2 or 3 tablespoons sliced stuffed olives; 1 diced cucumber; 1 minced clove garlic; 1 tablespoon chives or minced fresh dill or dill sauce; or 1 or 2 teaspoons dill or caraway seeds heated with vinegar.

**Hot potato salad:** Steam potatoes; mash (p. 399) or peel and slice; dice **2 slices bacon,** fry until crisp; add and heat to boiling **¼ cup vinegar, ¼ cup each chopped onions and celery, ¾ teaspoon salt, dash of cayenne, 2 tablespoons water;** combine sauce with hot potatoes; garnish with ground parsley and sliced hard-cooked egg.

One of the most delightful ways of preparing potatoes is to shred and quick-cook them. The cooking time is so short that almost no flavor or nutritive value is lost, and so much surface is exposed that if high heat is used, a large proportion of the sugar caramelizes, making the taste delicious. Potatoes prepared in this way should take the place of the customarily overcooked hash-browned potatoes.

## HASH-BROWNED POTATOES

Heat until extremely hot:

### 4 to 6 tablespoons bacon drippings or oil

Quickly shred directly into fat:

### 4 unpeeled thoroughly chilled potatoes

Keep heat high and turn frequently; cook until golden brown, or about 5 to 8 minutes.
Add:

**½ teaspoon salt**                    **¼ teaspoon celery salt**
**dash of paprika**

*Variations:*

Cook 1 or 2 shredded onions with potatoes.

Stir in any one of the following a few minutes before serving: chives, parsley, chopped fresh dill, green-onion tops cut with scissors, a few minced leaves of fresh marjoram, orégano, or sage.

Fry shredded sweet potatoes or yams as in basic recipe; omit celery salt.

**Baked shredded potatoes:** When oven is being used, put shredded potatoes into an oiled preheated casserole; add ½ teaspoon salt and freshly ground black peppercorns; cover and bake 7 to 10 minutes. Vary by combining potatoes with an equal amount of shredded turnips, carrots, parsnips, or rutabagas, or add 1 grated onion or finely chopped green pepper, pimento, and dill, or celery stalk; potatoes may be sprinkled with ½ cup shredded cheese.

**Creamed shredded potatoes:** Heat to simmering 1 cup cream sauce, ¾ teaspoon salt; 6 minutes before time to serve, stir in 2 cups shredded raw potatoes; cover utensil and simmer; garnish with ground parsley or chives and paprika. Vary by using any of the following sauces: caraway, celery, mustard, cheese, curry, dill, mushroom, olive, onion, or pimento (p. 162).

**Potato pancakes:** Grate 4 unpeeled chilled potatoes and 1 onion; add 1 tablespoon whole-wheat flour, 1 teaspoon salt; drop from spoon into 1 tablespoon hot oil or fat; brown quickly on both sides. Serve with applesauce.

*With vegetables:* Make pancakes of equal amounts of potatoes and turnips, carrots, parsnips, or rutabagas. Serve with chopped parsley.


## STEAMED POTATOES

Leave small unpeeled potatoes whole and cut large ones into halves lengthwise; drop into:

¼ cup boiling water

Cover utensil and cook 12 to 18 minutes, or until tender.

Serve with skins on or remove skins quickly and reheat potatoes for 1 minute in fat.

Sprinkle with ½ teaspoon salt, ground parsley, and freshly ground black peppercorns.

*Variations:*

If utensil does not distribute heat, steam potatoes on a rack above water.

Combine and heat 2 tablespoons each oil, chopped chives, and ground parsley, 3 tablespoons lemon juice, ½ teaspoon salt, freshly ground black peppercorns; pour sauce over steamed potatoes.

Sprinkle over hot potatoes 1 teaspoon chopped fresh orégano, thyme, and/or basil or dill.

Heat 1 cup or more of any cream sauce (p. 162); pour over potatoes; garnish with parsley.

Peel steamed potatoes and sprinkle with ½ cup grated cheese; add seasonings as in basic recipe.

**Leftover steamed potatoes:** Peel and slice cold steamed potatoes; sauté quickly in **bacon drippings** with **1 grated onion**; add **salt, freshly ground peppercorns, 1 tablespoon each chopped green pepper and ground parsley.** Vary by heating in ½ cup top milk or well-seasoned leftover gravy.

## POTATO SUBSTITUTES LEND VARIETY

There are a number of foods which may be substituted for potatoes in that they supply approximately the same number of calories per serving: dry beans, dry peas, lentils, rice, corn, whole buckwheat, unground wheat, bananas, and the more solid varieties of squash. None of these foods should be served with potatoes, not because the combination is harmful but because they are similar to potatoes in composition. They do not supply the same vitamins and minerals which could be obtained from the less starchy vegetables. The higher protein supplied by beans, lentils, peas, and grains than that supplied by potatoes is healthful.

Grains contain more phosphorus and sulfur than do potatoes, beans, and other vegetables. The presence of these minerals has caused rice, wheat, and corn to be spoken of as "acid-forming" foods in contrast to the "alkali-forming" vegetables which are rich in minerals such as potassium. These terms are misunderstood and overemphasized; no food should be foregone because it is "acid-forming." One should realize that phosphorus and sulfur are as essential to health as are alkaline minerals. When the diet is adequate in other respects, both types of minerals are amply supplied.

Several vegetables not listed with the following recipes, such as parsnips, rutabagas, and almost any fried vegetable, have approximately the same calorie content as potatoes and may be substituted for them. Foods prepared as meat extenders, such as dry beans, buckwheat, macaroni, spaghetti, rice, and unground wheat, can serve as a substitute for both meat and potatoes. When these foods are to be served in addition to meat, or purely as a substitute for potatoes, prepare them by the recipes given on pages 197 to 206, omitting the meats suggested.

## SAUTÉED BANANAS

Whenever possible, sauté bananas on a grill which has been used for pan-broiling ham, pork chops, or pork sausage; otherwise use 1 table-spoon bacon drippings seasoned with a small amount of smoke-flavoring.

Remove skins from:

**4 large firm bananas**

Put on hot grill; keep heat high and turn as each side is browned; when golden on all sides, or in about 6 minutes, sprinkle with salt. Serve with meat.

*Variations:*

Choose red bananas or plantains when available; cut plantains in half lengthwise and crosswise; after browning, cook 10 to 12 minutes with the utensil covered.

**Baked bananas:** Wrap each banana in a strip of bacon or a thin slice of boiled ham; put in shallow baking dish and bake in hot oven at 425° F. about 8 minutes, or until bacon or ham is light brown. If bacon is used, pan-broil it first with extremely low heat without browning.

**Bananas fried in batter:** Cut bananas in ¾-inch pieces and drop into batter (p. 183); fry in 4 tablespoons hot fat or French-fry at 350° F. until golden brown. Serve with lemon slices.

**Bananas with cheese:** Bake, sauté, or broil bananas and sprinkle with grated American or pimento cheese; vary by rolling in crumbs and grated cheese before broiling or baking.

**Broiled bananas:** Put bananas on oiled baking sheet; set 2 inches from broiler under high heat until lightly browned, or for about 2 minutes; turn and brown on all sides; sprinkle with **salt and paprika or nutmeg.**

**Glazed bananas:** Brush bananas lightly with **black molasses;** broil or bake; sprinkle lightly with **salt and cinnamon or nutmeg** and serve with **lemon slices.**

## RED BEANS MEXICAN STYLE

Wash quickly without soaking:

**1½ cups dry red beans**

Heat to boiling:

**2½ to 3 cups vegetable-cooking water or soup stock**

Add beans slowly to rapidly boiling liquid; reduce heat and simmer until beans are tender, or about 2 to 2½ hours, when they should be almost dry.

Add 15 minutes before serving:

| | |
|---|---|
| 1 finely chopped dry onion or 2 green onions and tops | 2 or 3 tablespoons oil or bacon drippings |
| 1 or 2 minced cloves garlic | 1 teaspoon salt |
| ½ teaspoon cumin seeds | |

Immediately before serving add:

¼ cup ground parsley

*Variations:*

Add chopped raw onion, and 1 chopped green pepper or fresh pimento just before serving.

If fresh red beans are used, follow same procedure but shorten cooking time to 30 or 40 minutes.

Omit cumin seeds and add ¼ teaspoon dry or 1 teaspoon fresh orégano or marjoram.

Omit oil and add 1 or 2 slices of diced bacon or salt pork when beans are almost tender.

Buckwheat has a delightful flavor and is well liked by almost everyone who tastes it. It is a good source of the B vitamins and should be served frequently. The more highly seasoned recipes are perhaps best for introducing it, but the simple ones soon become favorites. If any is left over, it may be served as a cereal.

## STEAMED BUCKWHEAT

Heat to boiling:

2 cups soup stock, vegetable-cooking water, or water

Add so slowly that boiling does not stop:

1 cup unwashed whole buckwheat       1 teaspoon salt

Boil rapidly 1 minute; cover utensil, lower heat, and simmer 12 to 15 minutes; remove lid of utensil and let steam escape, so that each grain is fluffy and separate.

Serve with a small amount of **margarine or butter.**

*Variations:*

Add buckwheat to 2 tablespoons hot fat; stir well and add liquid so slowly that it boils immediately; add 1 each chopped onion and green pepper, ¼ teaspoon crushed black peppercorns; proceed as in basic recipe.

Just before serving add 2 diced canned pimentos and 1 can mushrooms, or cook with buckwheat fresh or frozen peas or diced carrots; add diced leftover vegetables in time to heat through.

Corn on the cob is a delightful but long mistreated vegetable. Ideally it should be brought from the garden immediately before time to cook it. If bought at the market, it should be kept in the coldest part of the refrigerator and not husked until immediately before cooking. When the husks are removed, enzymes quickly change much sugar to starch, causing loss of flavor. Corn should be washed quickly in running water and dried immediately to prevent the sugars from being dissolved. Corn is almost invariably overcooked. It becomes tough if heated to boiling temperature longer than 2 or 3 minutes. Allow it only to heat through; the less it is cooked after it is hot, the more delightful its flavor.

## CORN ON THE COB

Take off outer husks, leaving 1 or 2 layers to prevent corn from drying out during cooking. Fold these husks back, remove silks, bad spots, and wash quickly·

### 4 to 6 ears of corn

Replace husks and put ears into hot oven at 400° F.; roast 10 to 12 minutes, or until just heated through.

Remove husks before serving if corn is to be eaten immediately; leave husks on second servings.

*Variations:*

If frozen corn on the cob is used, thaw completely at room temperature before putting it on to cook; steam on rack above water.

Put bed of husks in bottom of waterless-cooking utensil; husk corn, put into preheated utensil, and cook without added moisture 6 to 8 minutes.

**Broiled corn:** Prepare corn as in basic recipe, leaving 1 or 2 layers of husks on cob; set on broiling rack or baking sheet under moderate heat; broil 4 to 5 minutes on each side if corn is chilled, or less if warm.

**Leftover corn:** Hold cob upright and cut downward, being careful not to cut too near cob; scrape cob with blunt edge of knife; use corn in salad, reheat to simmering in a little top milk, or add to string beans, carrots, peas, or other vegetables just before serving.

**Steamed corn:** Leave on 1 or 2 layers of husks so that condensed steam cannot touch corn during cooking; set on a rack above rapidly boiling water; cover utensil and steam 4 to 6 minutes; if corn is husked, steam only 3 to 5 minutes; serve immediately. Steam 2 or 3 minutes longer if corn is thoroughly chilled.

If corn must be cut from the cob before time to cook it, put it into an ice tray and keep near freezing temperature to prevent the sugar from changing to starch. Canned or dried corn may be prepared by any of the following recipes. Dried corn should be soaked overnight in milk, 1 cup milk being used for each cup corn; it should be heated in the same milk.

## CORN COOKED IN MILK

Quickly cut from cob, scraping cob with knife to get fluid from base of kernels:

**2 cups corn**

Keep chilled until 3 minutes before serving; then add to:

**⅓ cup simmering top milk**

Stir, heat rapidly to simmering; cover utensil, lower heat, simmer 2 minutes; add:

**½ teaspoon salt**                                     **freshly ground white peppercorns**

*Variations:*

If frozen corn is used, put into hot milk while still frozen; simmer 3 to 4 minutes.

**Corn baked in milk:** When oven is being used, preheat casserole with **2 tablespoons top milk**; add **2 cups corn and ½ teaspoon salt**; cover casserole and heat in moderate oven 5 to 8 minutes.

*With cheese:* Put corn, top milk, and seasonings into flat preheated baking dish and cover with grated cheese; heat in oven until cheese is melted, or about 8 to 10 minutes.

Corn fritters: Stir 1 cup canned corn and liquid or fresh corn with 2 egg yolks; combine in sifter ½ cup whole-wheat flour, ¼ cup powdered milk, 1 teaspoon salt, ⅛ teaspoon paprika; sift into eggs and corn; fold in 2 stiffly beaten egg whites; drop from teaspoon into deep fat at 350° F. and fry until delicately brown, or about 5 minutes; drain on paper towels.

*Corn and pepper fritters:* Add to fritter batter 1 finely diced stalk celery, 1 chopped chilled green pepper or 3 tablespoons canned or fresh pimento; add any leftover vegetables, such as peas or carrots. Vary by frying in shallow fat.

Corn patties: Beat well 1 egg, ½ cup each powdered milk and fresh milk, ⅛ teaspoon each paprika and dry mustard; add ½ cup wheat germ, 1 cup corn, ½ teaspoon salt; drop from teaspoon onto hot grill and sauté until brown on both sides.

Corn pudding: Heat to simmering in heat-resistant casserole 1½ cups fresh milk; meanwhile beat together 3 eggs, ½ cup each fresh milk and powdered milk, 1¼ teaspoons salt, ¼ teaspoon crushed black peppercorns; stir into milk and add 2 cups fresh, frozen, or canned corn; bake uncovered in slow oven at 325° F. for 35 minutes, or until firm. If pudding is to be given to infants, invalids, or persons suffering from digestive disturbances, purée the canned corn or remove chilled corn from cob by grating.

Corn soufflé: Add 2 cups fresh, canned, or frozen corn to plain soufflé (p. 209).

Creamed corn: Heat to simmering 1 cup cream sauce, ½ teaspoon salt, ¼ teaspoon crushed white peppercorns; add 2 cups corn; stir, cover utensil, and simmer 3 minutes, or until heated through.

Scalloped corn: Chop together 1 medium onion, 1 chilled green pepper and/or 1 fresh pimento or 3 tablespoons canned pimento; sauté for 3 minutes in heat-resistant casserole brushed with butter-flavored fat; add 1 teaspoon salt, ¼ teaspoon each paprika and dry mustard, and 1 cup cream sauce; simmer and add 2 cups corn; heat 5 minutes; cover with toasted whole-wheat-bread crumbs; garnish with paprika, dot lightly with margarine or butter.

Smothered corn: In utensil which retains heat melt 1 tablespoon butter-flavored oil or other fat; remove from heat, add corn, stir; cover utensil and let stand until corn is heated through, or 5 to 7 minutes.

## RICE COOKED IN MILK

Put in a wire strainer and wash quickly under running water, shaking to dry immediately:

### 1 cup brown or all-vitamin rice

Heat until almost boiling:

**1½ cups whole milk**                    **1 teaspoon margarine or butter**

Add rice to hot milk so slowly that the temperature of the milk does not drop; keep heat high for 2 or 3 minutes, then reduce to simmering.

Simmer 30 to 40 minutes if brown rice is used, 15 to 20 if all-vitamin rice is used, adding more milk if needed; add:

**1 teaspoon salt**                    **pinch of saffron or dash of nutmeg**

Garnish with **sprigs of parsley.**

*Variations:*

When rice is almost tender, add ½ to 1 cup strained crushed pineapple; pack into oiled ring mold and finish cooking in oven; turn out on platter and serve curried lamb (p. 102) or chicken (p. 96) in center of mold.

Add and cook with rice 1 cup fresh peas or ½ cup each diced raw carrots and celery or other fresh vegetables; or 5 minutes before serving stir in diced leftover meats and/or vegetables, or a can of mushrooms.

Instead of milk cook rice in soup stock, using chicken or ham stock when available; season with ¼ teaspoon crushed white peppercorns and ½ cup finely minced onion, and/or sliced mushrooms. Use this recipe for cooking wild rice.

Cook rice in top of double-boiler over direct heat 5 to 8 minutes; place over boiling water and cook until tender.

Omit saffron or nutmeg; just before serving stir in finely chopped chives or green onions or 3 tablespoons minced raw celery or finely chopped parsley.

**Baked rice:** Prepare rice as in basic recipe, using heat-resistant baking dish over direct heat; simmer 10 to 20 minutes; add ¼ **bay leaf, salt, and 1 each chopped green pepper, green onion, pimento;** put in moderate oven to finish cooking.

**Rice cooked with tomatoes:** Add rice to 1½ **cups rapidly boiling tomato juice or 2 cups tomato purée;** season with ¼ **teaspoon crushed black peppercorns, 2 tablespoons oil or bacon drippings, 1 minced clove garlic, 1 finely chopped onion, ¼ crumbled bay leaf.**

## LEFTOVER RICE PATTIES

Mix **1 cup leftover rice** with:

¼ cup each fresh milk and powdered milk

1 egg

1 tablespoon each minced chives
and ground parsley

pinch of savory and thyme

¼ teaspoon salt

freshly ground black peppercorns

Make into small cakes or drop from spoon into:

**1 tablespoon hot butter-flavored oil or bacon drippings**

Sauté until golden brown on both sides.

*Variations:*

Make rice into balls, roll in whole-wheat-bread crumbs, fry in deep fat.

Add any one of the following: ¼ to ½ cup wheat germ or precooked
soy grits (p. 196); 2 tablespoons soy flour; ¼ cup American or pimento
cheese; diced pimento or grated onion.

Instead of fresh milk use catsup or chili sauce; omit thyme and add a
pinch of basil; 1 to 3 teaspoons debittered brewers' yeast may be added.

Whole unground wheat is an excellent food which should be
served far more often than it is, especially to growing children or
to any person whose calorie requirements are high. Families who
are accustomed to eating it are often enthusiastic to the extreme.
Its chewiness, which may seem objectionable at first, becomes its
charm.

## STEAMED UNGROUND WHEAT

Put **1 cup unground wheat** in a wire strainer and wash quickly under
running water; add to:

**2 to 3 cups boiling water, soup stock, or tomato juice**

Cover utensil, reduce heat to simmering, and cook until tender, or 2
to 3 hours; uncover utensil during last of cooking and evaporate any remaining moisture; add:

**1 teaspoon salt**                              **1 tablespoon margarine or butter**

Serve with chicken or other meat and country gravy.

*Variations:*

Cook in pressure cooker 25 to 30 minutes, using 2 cups liquid to 1 cup wheat.

When wheat is almost tender, add 1 or 2 tablespoons bacon drippings, 1 minced clove garlic, 1 chopped onion or ½ cup sliced mushrooms.

A few minutes before serving add ½ cup or more cream sauce, salt, ground white peppercorns, diced canned pimento; or add leftover gravy, 2 tablespoons minced onion, a pinch of sage. Vary by using seasoned cream sauces (p. 162). Cook in chicken stock with crushed white pepper corns until wheat is almost tender; add salt, ½ cup diced celery, 1 cup raw or frozen peas, 1 chopped pimento, a pinch each of thyme and basil.

Cook in tomato juice; when wheat is almost tender, add ¼ teaspoon cumin seeds, a pinch of orégano, 1 each chopped green pepper and onion, 1 minced clove garlic.

Although fresh soybeans contain no starch, they are rich in sugar. Many varieties are so sweet that they taste like new peas. They should be washed before being hulled. To prevent the protein from becoming tough, do not submit them to temperatures higher than simmering. Fresh lima beans may be cooked by the same recipe.

## FRESH SOYBEANS OR LIMA BEANS

Add **2 to 3 cups fresh chilled soybeans** or **lima beans** to:

½ **cup hot milk**

Stir to cover beans with milk protein; cover utensil, heat quickly, then simmer 15 to 20 minutes.

Add:

½ **teaspoon salt**

Garnish with **paprika.**

*Variations:*

Steam soybeans or lima beans in vegetable-cooking water or soup stock, or cook without added moisture.

Until a taste for soybeans is acquired, steam a few of them with fresh lima beans.

After removing soybeans from heat, add chopped canned pimento and ½ cup melted cheese.

Season steamed soybeans with one or more of the following: chopped chives, onions, celery, pimento, green-onion tops, crisp bacon or bacon drippings, smoke-flavoring, minced garlic, ground parsley, or sliced stuffed olives.

**Chilled soybeans:** Quickly chill cooked soybeans and marinate in French dressing. Serve cold or add to salads.

**Creamed soybeans or lima beans:** Prepare beans as in basic recipe, using top milk; a few minutes before serving add cream sauce.

Winter squashes include all the solid squashes: banana, Danish, acorn, Hubbard squashes, crookneck and straightneck squashes, green warted squashes, and Boston marrow, or basket pumpkin. All these squashes and pumpkin can be prepared by the following recipes. Since squashes are difficult to peel, it is usually easier to cook them unpeeled and cut off the peel before they are served or to serve them unpeeled. The cooking time varies somewhat with the type of squash.

## BROILED WINTER SQUASH

Wash the peel, remove seeds and stringy parts, and cut into serving sizes:

1½ to 2 pounds squash

Set peel side down on rack above a small amount of boiling water; cover utensil and steam 10 to 15 minutes, or until squash is slightly tender; set on baking sheet and sprinkle with:

salt                                         celery salt or nutmeg
freshly ground black peppercorns

Dot with **bacon drippings.**
Broil a few minutes and brush with **dark or blackstrap molasses.**
Continue broiling under moderate heat until squash is brown and tender, or about 10 to 15 minutes.

*Variations:*

Instead of browning under broiler, bake in moderate oven at 350° F. until tender, or about 20 minutes; if squash was not steamed, brush with oil and molasses; salt; bake for 50 minutes.

**Acorn squash:** Cut in half and prepare as in basic recipe; before placing under broiler or in oven, put into each half **1 tablespoon molasses, 2 tablespoons top milk or evaporated milk, 1 teaspoon butter or margarine.**

*Stuffed acorn squash:* Steam until squash is almost tender; salt and stuff with crumb dressing (p. 155) or with 2 tablespoons each shredded cheese and chili sauce; sprinkle top with crumbs if cheese is used; bake until tender. Vary by serving baked squash filled with creamed chicken, ham, peas, or other leftover creamed meat or vegetables.

**Mashed squash:** Steam squash until tender; scrape out pulp with a spoon, mash, season with **margarine or butter, salt, paprika.** Vary by adding any one of the following: 1 teaspoon minced fresh basil or mint leaves; 2 tablespoons ground parsley; ½ cup crushed pineapple with 1 tablespoon molasses; ½ cup uncooked or steamed raisins, dash each of nutmeg and cinnamon.

*Leftover mashed squash:* Put into flat oiled baking dish, cover with thick applesauce or with 2 strips bacon; bake in moderate oven until heated through and bacon is crisp. Vary by folding into squash 1 or 2 beaten eggs, ½ cup each fresh and powdered milk.

**Sautéed squash:** Cut into strips, peel, and slice or dice; sauté in oil or bacon drippings, using moderate heat and turning frequently until almost tender; set lid of utensil to one side to allow moisture to evaporate; cook about 15 minutes; add ½ teaspoon salt and any one of the following: ¼ teaspoon celery salt; 1 tablespoon chives, Chinese garlic, or 2 tablespoons ground parsley; 2 tablespoons dark molasses, dash of nutmeg and/or cinnamon. Vary by sautéing with squash 1 chopped onion, stalk celery, green pepper or pimento, or minced clove garlic.

**Steamed squash:** Cut squash into strips, peel, and dice into 1-inch cubes; put into preheated utensil with 1 or 2 tablespoons boiling water; cook over simmer burner or in top of double boiler until tender, or about 15 to 20 minutes; season with **salt, margarine or butter, and cayenne or black molasses.** Set lid of utensil to one side to let moisture escape during last 5 minutes of cooking.

# CHAPTER 19

## MAKE YOUR OWN BREADS

Whenever anyone asks me how to build up the health of a growing child, a convalescent, or an invalid, how to add more protein, calcium, iron, or B vitamins to the diet, how to work more wheat germ, brewers' yeast, or blackstrap molasses into foods, or simply how to have fun at cooking, my answer is, "Make your own breads." There are many excellent whole-wheat breads on the market, but none can compare in nutritive value or, to my way of thinking, in flavor with those which you can make at home.

Any bread which is customarily sweetened can be made with blackstrap molasses, a by-product of the sugar industry. Cane juice, like any other vegetable juice, contains many vitamins and minerals. When it is boiled down into dark molasses, the nutrients not harmed by heat are concentrated to about thirty times that of the original juice. Pure sugar is then crystallized out and removed, leaving in the remaining molasses, known as blackstrap, minerals and heat-stable vitamins some ten times more concentrated than in ordinary dark molasses. A tablespoon of blackstrap supplies as much calcium as does a glass of milk and as much iron as do 9 eggs. This molasses also supplies generous amounts of all the B vitamins except vitamin $B_1$ and folic acid, which are harmed by boiling. Ordinary dark molasses has great nutritive value compared with refined sugar, which contains no vitamins or minerals, or with raw sugar, which contains only an insignificant amount of a few minerals; blackstrap molasses, in comparison with sugar, can be considered a miracle food.

People usually enjoy the taste of yeast in bread; hence debittered brewers' yeast can be added to bread together with bakers' yeast, thus supplying generous amounts of some ten or more B vitamins. Brewers' yeast is pasteurized as it is dried, and cannot make bread rise; it must not be confused with fresh bakers' yeast.

Aside from being one of the richest known sources of the B vitamins, brewers' yeast supplies as much protein in a heaping tablespoon as does an egg.

Experiments have been carried out at Cornell University in which from a few tablespoons to as much as a half cup of brewers' yeast was added to breads, biscuits, cookies, spice cakes, meat loaves, tomato sauces, and other foods. These foods were served at a cafeteria to unsuspecting persons who gave no indication that the taste was different in any way. When food of unknown ingredients is prepared and served to you, however, the situation is different indeed from that in which you prepare food yourself. If your taste is keen and your imagination vivid, and if you add yeast with misgivings, the food may easily be ruined for you; for this reason I have suggested adding only small amounts of yeast to only a few recipes. The desire to attain perfect health must come from within yourself; it cannot be forced upon you. I do urge you, however, to start by adding a teaspoon of brewers' yeast to all products you bake and to well-flavored foods and sauces, then to increase the amount gradually. It will pay dividends in terms of vigor and more attractive appearance.

The protein content of breadstuffs can be increased not only by yeast but also by adding powdered milk, wheat germ, and soy, peanut, and cottonseed flour; these products contain five to ten times as much protein as does wheat flour. Wheat germ, like brewers' yeast, is a concentrated source of the B vitamins; it also supplies iron and vitamin E, needed before vitamin A can be utilized. Although bread usually contains little calcium, it becomes an appreciable source of this mineral when made with blackstrap molasses and powdered milk. Thus bread can be made a rich source of the nutrients most often lacking in the American diet: calcium, iron, B vitamins, and protein.

Contrary to popular opinion, whole-grain flour is far superior nutritionally to fortified flour. At least twelve substances essential to health have been largely removed during the refining of fortified flour and have not been put back: many B vitamins, vitamin E, several minerals, and much of the protein. Only three substances are added to the "enriched" wheat flour: two-thirds as much vitamin $B_1$ and one-third as much iron and niacin as are found in whole-wheat flour. "Enriched" flour is one of the most misleading terms ever used. It would be as logical to consider yourself enriched by a burglar who ransacked your home but left you a few possessions. The detrimental effect on health of using "enriched" breadstuffs rather than the whole-grain products can accumulate in the course of months and years to be tremendous indeed. The following table shows clearly the superiority of whole-grain and high-protein flours over the refined products, and the value of certain highly nutritious foods which may be added to bread.

Until a few generations ago the only flour available was unrefined, and all bakery products were made of whole-grain flours. Similarly, you can make any breadstuffs with unrefined flour. After you become accustomed to the texture and the full nutty flavor of whole-grain breadstuffs, those made of white flour seem by contrast as tasteless as cotton or corrugated paper. The whole-wheat pastry flour which I use is so finely ground that the starch coats the bits of bran, causing the products made from it to be almost as white as those prepared from refined flour. Whole-wheat pastry flour should be used for biscuits, cakes, pie dough, and quick breads. Yeast breads, however, must be made of hard-

FOOD VALUES

| Food | Measurement | Weight in Grams | Protein in Grams |
|------|-------------|-----------------|------------------|
| Whole-wheat flour | 1 cup | 113 | 12 |
| Fortified flour | 1 cup | 113 | 10 |
| White flour | 1 cup | 113 | 10 |
| Soy flour | 1 cup | 113 | 37 |
| Peanut flour | 1 cup | 113 | 59 |
| Cottonseed flour | 1 cup | 113 | 57 |
| Wheat-germ flour or wheat germ | ½ cup | 100 | 24 |
| Milk, dried, skim | ½ cup | 100 | 53 |
| Milk, evaporated | ½ cup | 100 | 8 |
| Milk, fresh, whole | ½ cup | 100 | 4 |
| Blackstrap molasses | 1 tablespoon | 20 | 1 |
| Dark molasses | 1 tablespoon | 20 | 0 |
| Cane syrup | 1 tablespoon | 20 | 0 |
| Brewers' yeast | 1 tablespoon | 15 | 4 |

* The pellagra-preventing B vitamin.

wheat, or high-protein, flour rich in gluten; such flour may also be finely ground.

The merits of soy flour are becoming well known. A flour which I have enjoyed using even more is that made from peanuts; I have never tested a recipe using peanut flour which I considered a failure. The flour is light in color, and if all fat has been removed from it, it has no distinctive flavor. Cottonseed flour, or cottonseed meal ground into a flour, has high nutritive value and no disagreeable flavor, but its color resembles that of burned mustard. Although it can be used interchangeably with soy or peanut flour, I have suggested using it principally in recipes where its color would be covered by molasses. However, out of some fifteen samples of pie dough which my assistants and I prepared and many friends tasted, that made of cottonseed flour was considered the most delicious and its color was not thought to be unappetizing. Wheat germ ground into flour can be obtained, and produces a finer texture in biscuits, cakes, and pastries than does wheat germ itself. For convenience I have listed wheat germ or wheat-germ flour with ingredients to be sifted, although obviously wheat germ cannot be sifted; if you use it, add it after sifting in the other ingredients.

OF BREAD INGREDIENTS

(Minerals and Vitamins in Milligrams)

| Calcium | Iron | Thiamin (Vitamin B$_1$) | Riboflavin (Vitamin B$_2$) | Niacin * |
|---|---|---|---|---|
| 45 | 5.0 | 0.48 | 0.16 | 5.5 |
| 20 | 3.3 | 0.32 | 0.15 | 1.5 |
| 20 | 1.0 | 0.08 | 0.03 | 0.8 |
| 200 | 7.4 | 0.65 | 0.37 | 8.2 |
| 65 | 10.0 | 0.6 | 0.3 | 18.9 |
| .... | .... | 1.18 | 1.15 | 9.6 |
| 750 | 7.5 | 2.60 | 0.75 | 24.2 |
| 1930 | 1.9 | 0.55 | 2.61 | 19.2 |
| 250 | 0.5 | 0.06 | 0.39 | 3.6 |
| 150 | 0.2 | 0.03 | 0.27 | 1.8 |
| 259 | 9.6 | 0.05 | 0.06 | 6.1 |
| 40 | 1.4 | 0 | 0 | 0.5 |
| 2 | 0 | 0 | 0 | 0 |
| 11 | 0.3 | 2.25 | 1.00 | 6.4 |

Since whole-wheat, soy, peanut, and cottonseed flours, wheat germ, and rice polish contain a small amount of fat which can become rancid, purchase no more than you will probably use in a month's time unless you can keep them in a cool place. Be sure to purchase these products directly from the mill, where they are freshly made, or from a store where the turnover is rapid; rancid flour is as unpleasant as the fresh product is delicious. During the summer months it is better to put the flour into a shallow pan and heat it in a slow oven to 185° F. The heating prevents weevils from hatching, helps to prevent rancidity by destroying enzymes, yet does not harm the vitamins. Wheat germ or wheat-germ flour to be added to yeast bread should first be cooked or slightly toasted; if the enzymes it contains are not destroyed, they digest starch and protein in the dough while it is rising and cause it to become runny.

The success of making yeast breads depends on the gluten content of the wheat flour used and the amount of stirring. When the dough is stirred, the bits of gluten, or protein, in each particle of flour stick together and become elastic and rubberlike. The process is similar to chewing gum, which is crumbly when first put into the mouth but becomes elastic as it is chewed. When bread rises, it is the stretching of the elastic gluten which holds in the bubbles of carbon dioxide liberated by the yeast, thereby allowing the loaf to be light. The more the dough is stirred and the more gluten the flour contains, the larger the loaf and the lighter the bread. When substances lacking gluten, such as sugar, powdered milk, soy, peanut, or cottonseed flour, or brewers' yeast, are added to bread, they prevent the bits of gluten from sticking together; it is as if you tried to chew gum with your mouth full of peanuts. If you wish yeast bread to be light, substances lacking gluten should be added after the dough has been thoroughly stirred. In making all bakery products, your choice of flour and the amount of stirring depend upon whether or not you wish the gluten to be elastic. When you wish tenderness without lightness, as in pie dough or cookies, use pastry flour low in gluten and stir it little.

Bakers' yeast, or compressed yeast, is a plant. Treat it as you would a potted geranium. Yeast, like a geranium, grows best at

80 to 85° F., or the temperature of a warm summer day. Just as a geranium would not grow in cold weather or would be killed if put into a hot oven, so does yeast stop growing when chilled and is killed if overheated. If yeast dough is allowed to rise too much or if it is not kept sufficiently warm while the yeast is growing, the dough becomes sour. Unless you desire sour bread, stir or knead down the dough each time it has doubled in bulk; keep it near 85° F. or else chill it so completely that the yeast cannot grow. Since eggs and fat inhibit the growth of yeast, they are added to refrigerator rolls to prevent them from souring.

How quickly bread rises depends on the amount of bakers' yeast used in making it. If three cakes of yeast are added to waffles, for example, they will be ready to bake as soon as they are prepared. If only one cake is used, time must be allowed for it to grow into the equivalent of several cakes. The longer yeast is allowed to grow, the more the yeast plants multiply, the more tiny bubbles of carbon dioxide are liberated, and the finer is the texture of the bread. When convenient, therefore, allow the dough to rise three or four times. Since speed is often considered an advantage, however, I have stressed it in the recipes.

Keep on hand a carton of quick-rising dry yeast (which works like fresh compressed yeast yet needs no refrigeration) and add as many packages to a recipe as time demands. The more yeast used, the greater the nutritive value of the bread. Keep your bread-making flexible, however, and vary the recipes to suit your convenience. If you are in a hurry, combine your ingredients and bake the bread two hours later. If it suits your schedule better, stir down the dough each time it doubles in bulk, set it in the refrigerator when you are busy or away, and make it into loaves and bake it when you get around to it; or use only half of the flour and make a sponge, let the yeast grow, stir it down or chill it, then add the other ingredients and do your beating at a later time.

Yeast bread will keep moist for many days if a cooked cereal, such as wheat germ cooked in milk, is added to the dough. The cooked starch holds moisture in the bread, somewhat as apple-sauce does when added to a cake. Make a point of adding any leftover cereals to bread. If you use only a little bread, keep the baked loaves fresh by wrapping in wax paper and storing in the refrigerator.

During baking, a loss of vitamin $B_1$ occurs in the crust. If you make several loaves of bread at one time, put them side by side in a large pan so that the minimum amount of crust will be formed. Toasting causes a loss of from 5 to 25 per cent of the remaining vitamin $B_1$, the loss being in proportion to the degree of brownness. Contrary to popular opinion, therefore, untoasted bread is nutritionally superior to toast. As a matter of improving flavor and freshening stale bread, however, light toasting is justified. As to the belief that hot breads are "bad for you," I can find neither a basis for it nor a person who ever became ill from eating them.

When soda is used in making breadstuffs, it causes the destruction of 25 per cent or more of vitamin $B_1$ and harms several other B vitamins. Avoid using soda in baking. Even baking powder, which contains soda, causes some destruction of these vitamins; therefore use yeast instead of baking powder whenever possible. Yeast greatly improves the flavor of such foods as cornbread, hotcakes, waffles, and muffins. Since protein neutralizes the alkali which harms the vitamins, add powdered milk, wheat germ, and flour rich in protein to all products made with baking powder. When ingredients high in protein are included, buttermilk and sour milk may be used with baking powder or yeast without soda; the protein neutralizes the excess acid. Do not expect such recipes to be successful, however, if you omit powdered milk or other ingredients rich in protein.

If you have a home freezing unit, fresh bread and other bakery products not to be used immediately may be frozen as soon as they have cooled to room temperature. You can keep such products frozen for months and when thawed they will taste as if they had just been taken from the oven.

In all baking, the flours should be sifted before they are measured. An extra flour sifter permanently attached to a closet door is a convenience. Keep two or more paper plates with your baking equipment and sift the flour into them; they can be formed into a funnel when transferring flour to a measuring cup. If you are an experienced cook who does not bother with sifting, at least stir the flour thoroughly with a spoon before measuring it, and use approximately ⅞ cup flour for each cup called for. Unless the flour is thoroughly stirred, 1 cup unsifted flour will often measure 1½ cups after being sifted.

Since it is much easier to draw hot water from the tap than to take time to scald fresh milk, I have suggested using water in the following yeast-bread recipes; the powdered milk included is equivalent to many times the fresh milk which could be used.

There is the same satisfaction, the same pleasant sense of accomplishment, in making yeast breads as in canning fruit. In fact, breadmaking can easily become a hobby which your family will not let you give up.

## TWO-HOUR BREAD

Before gathering other ingredients, stir:

| | |
|---|---|
| 2 packages or cakes crumbled bakers' yeast into | 2 cups warm water |

Add at leisure:

| | |
|---|---|
| ⅓ cup blackstrap molasses | 3½ cups sifted hard, or high-protein, whole-wheat flour |
| 2 tablespoons butter-flavored shortening (optional) | |

Stir until ingredients are combined, then beat 300 strokes. Do not be frightened by the beating; it takes only a few minutes. If an electric mixer is used, mix at low speed for exactly 10 minutes; gluten can be broken down by overbeating. Combine and sift in:

| | |
|---|---|
| 1½ cups sifted hard, or high-protein, whole-wheat flour | ½ cup powdered milk |
| | 1 tablespoon salt |

Stir well but do not knead; cover bowl, set in a warm place at 85° F. or in warm water at 110° F. Check the temperature with cooking thermometer. Let rise until double in bulk, or about 45 minutes.

Stir dough until of original size and transfer to an oiled 5- by 8-inch bread pan; brush surface with oil, shaping loaf with pastry brush; or turn onto floured wax paper, knead lightly, and shape into a loaf; place in pan and brush with oil.

Let rise until double in bulk, or about 30 minutes. Put into moderately hot oven at 385° F. and bake 45 to 50 minutes, or until golden brown.

If soft crust is desired, brush loaves lightly with top milk or soft butter-flavored fat after taking from pan; set on wire rack to cool.

*Variations:*

Instead of 1 cup whole-wheat flour use 1 cup of any of the following or ½ cup of any 2 of the following: soy, peanut, cottonseed, buckwheat, rye, or lima-bean flour; rice polish; toasted wheat germ or wheat-germ flour; yellow corn meal; add to dough after it has been beaten. Use in basic recipe or any variation.

Add to basic recipe or any variation 2 to 4 tablespoons debittered brewers' yeast or ½ cup soy grits.

After beating and before sifting in remaining dry ingredients add 1 cup wheat germ which has been simmered 5 minutes in 1 cup milk; or add 1 cup of any leftover cooked whole-grain cereal.

Use 1 cake of yeast; let dough rise 3 or more times, being particularly careful to keep it warm and to stir it down each time it doubles in bulk; make into loaves when convenient, let rise, and bake. Or make dough in the evening, keep in refrigerator overnight, remove and let rise, and bake the following morning. Or add 2 cups whole-wheat flour to water, yeast, and molasses; keep warm, stir down whenever it is double in bulk or set in refrigerator overnight; when convenient, add other ingredients and beat.

**Apricot-nut bread:** Just before making into loaves, stir in ½ cup each ground dried apricots and broken walnuts or pecans; sift in ⅛ cup sugar with powdered milk.

**Bran bread:** After beating dough stir in 1 cup each bran and seedless raisins.

**Buckwheat bread:** After beating dough add 1½ cups buckwheat flour instead of wheat flour; or add 1 cup cooked buckwheat (p. 407) to basic recipe. This is my favorite bread.

**Date-nut bread:** Add ¼ cup sugar with molasses; after beating dough add 1 cup each chopped dates and broken walnuts.

**Potato bread:** After beating dough stir in 1 cup cooked or leftover mashed or riced potatoes.

**"Reducing" bread:** Omit fat; add **4 tablespoons vinegar;** after dough has been beaten, instead of wheat flour sift in 1¼ cups low-fat soy, peanut, or cottonseed flour, ¼ cup debittered brewers' yeast, ¾ cup powdered milk; add 1 cup wheat germ cooked 5 minutes in ½ cup water. This bread is heavy, and so rich in protein that 1 slice is extremely filling; hence it is excellent to use for reducing diets.

**Rye bread:** Instead of 2 cups of wheat flour use **2 cups rye flour;** stir in 1½ **cups rye flour** after beating dough; add **2 or 3 tablespoons caraway seeds or grated rind of 2 oranges** to water and molasses if desired. Shape like commercial rye bread and bake on baking sheet.

Sour rye bread: Omit molasses and fat; use 2½ cups each whole-wheat flour and rye flour; add 1½ cups rye flour after beating dough. Let dough rise in a cool place overnight to sour. Shape like rye bread, bake on baking sheet. This is a heavy bread but extremely delicious.

Wheat-germ bread: Instead of wheat flour stir in after beating dough 1½ cups toasted wheat germ, wheat-germ flour, or wheat germ and middlings; or simmer 1½ cups wheat germ in 1 cup milk for 5 minutes and add to basic recipe after beating dough.

## WHEAT-GERM ROLLS

Before gathering other ingredients, stir:

| | |
|---|---|
| 1 package or cake crumbled bakers' yeast into | 1 cup warm sweet or sour milk, buttermilk, yogurt, or water |

Add:

| | |
|---|---|
| ¼ cup butter-flavored shortening | 1 egg |
| 1½ teaspoons salt | ¾ cup toasted wheat germ |
| 3 tablespoons blackstrap molasses | |

Sift in:

| | |
|---|---|
| 2½ cups hard, or high-protein, whole-wheat flour | ⅓ cup powdered milk |

Stir until ingredients are combined, then beat 200 or more strokes; or beat exactly 10 minutes in electric mixer.

Cover bowl, set in a warm place at 85° F. or in warm water at 110° F. until double in bulk, or about 1 hour; make into rolls at once or stir and chill in refrigerator 1 to 8 hours before using; if time permits, let rolls rise slowly in refrigerator until double in bulk, or about 2 hours.

Bake in moderate oven at 350° F. for 20 to 25 minutes, or until golden brown. This recipe makes twenty 2-inch rolls.

*Variations:*

To make Parker House rolls, cut with biscuit cutter, brush top with oil, crease center with knife, and fold in half. For dinner rolls, cut with small biscuit cutter, make circle of thumb and forefinger of left hand, push dough through circle, squeezing cut edges together; set close together on oiled baking pan. For 3-leaf-clover rolls, place 3 small balls of dough in oiled muffin tin. Make scones by rolling dough into two 9-inch circles; cut each into 10 pie-shaped wedges and roll each wedge from outside toward center.

Make rolls of part of the dough, put the remainder into a utility bag, keep in refrigerator overnight; when dough is doubled in bulk, knead without removing from bag.

Instead of ½ cup whole-wheat flour stir in after beating dough ½ cup rye, buckwheat, soy, peanut, or cottonseed flour, or rice polish; or add 2 tablespoons brewers' yeast.

**Cinnamon buns:** Add 2 tablespoons sugar to rolls; make in shape of buns; mix 1 tablespoon cinnamon with uncooked icing (p. 522); brush on rolls while hot.

**Cinnamon rolls:** Use half the dough; roll ¼ inch thick, brush with soft butter-flavored shortening and black molasses; sprinkle with cinnamon and 2 tablespoons sugar; roll like jelly roll, cut in 1-inch pieces, and set close together in baking pan. Vary by sprinkling with broken walnuts, pecans, raisins, or chopped pitted prunes before rolling; use or omit cinnamon.

**Coffee cake:** Add ¼ cup sugar and ½ cup raisins to dough; after dough rises, roll it ⅛ inch thick and place on flat baking pan; brush surface with black molasses and sprinkle lightly with cinnamon, nutmeg, 2 tablespoons sugar, ½ cup nuts; press nuts into dough; bake when double in thickness or let rise in refrigerator overnight; bake 18 to 20 minutes.

**Modified English muffins:** Roll dough ½ inch thick, cut with large biscuit cutter; let rise 15 or more minutes; lift with pancake turner to hot grill and sauté slowly in butter-flavored fat until brown on both sides, or about 12 minutes.

**Orange roll:** Stir or knead into half the dough 3 tablespoons sugar and grated rind of 2 oranges; form dough into 3 long pieces and braid; bake as soon as double in bulk or let rise in refrigerator overnight and bake for breakfast.

**Raised doughnuts:** Add ½ cup sugar, 1 teaspoon each nutmeg and cinnamon; after dough rises, roll ½ inch thick and cut with doughnut cutter; let rise to double in bulk and fry in deep fat at 360° F. for about 5 to 7 minutes. Makes 25 doughnuts.

**Refrigerator rolls:** Use ½ cup shortening, 3 eggs, 2 teaspoons salt, 3¼ cups flour; add with other ingredients 3 to 6 tablespoons sugar; transfer dough to oiled utility bag; leave in refrigerator 12 hours or longer before using; when double in bulk, knead without removing from bag.

*Butterhorns:* Prepare like refrigerator rolls; roll in form of large scones, then shape into semicircles; arrange far apart on baking sheet, sprinkle with sugar and shaved almonds; press nuts into dough before letting it rise.

*Rusks:* Make like refrigerator rolls; roll in form of scones.

**Spiced almond rolls:** Add ¼ cup sugar, 1 cup chopped almonds, ½ teaspoon almond extract, ¼ cup finely diced citron, ¼ teaspoon ground cardamom, 1 teaspoon cinnamon. Form dough into long loaf, place on baking sheet, then make into a circle like a huge doughnut; cut outside margin at 2-inch intervals with scissors.

Pancakes, waffles, muffins, and cornbread are not only more delicious when made with yeast instead of baking powder but can be made just as quickly and easily. The delightful aroma which fills the house when these foods are baking is justification enough for using yeast.

If pineapple, banana, nuts, crisp bacon, or diced ham is added to pancakes or waffles, there is less temptation to eat them with syrup, honey, and other concentrated sweets. Whenever possible, serve waffles with creamed chicken or tuna, thick applesauce, or crushed fresh strawberries, apricots, or peaches. The crushed and sweetened fresh fruit is also delicious on pancakes. The next time you have wheat-germ pancakes, try fresh or frozen raspberries on them; I believe you will come back for a second serving.

## PANCAKES

Before gathering other ingredients, stir:

| | |
|---|---|
| 1 to 3 packages or cakes crumbled bakers' yeast into | 1½ cups warm water, warm sweet or sour milk, sour cream, buttermilk, or yogurt |

Add:

| | |
|---|---|
| 1 tablespoon blackstrap molasses or sugar<br>2 whole eggs | 2 tablespoons bacon drippings, butter-flavored oil, or soft shortening |

Sift into liquid:

| | |
|---|---|
| 1 cup whole-wheat pastry flour<br>½ cup wheat germ or wheat-germ flour | ⅓ cup powdered milk<br>1 teaspoon salt |

Stir with 50 strokes; bake immediately, or let rise in a warm place 30 minutes or longer, or set in refrigerator overnight.

Drop from tablespoon onto moderately hot griddle; bake slowly; turn when upper surface is full of bubbles and brown the other side. Serve with applesauce, apricot purée, or crushed and sweetened fresh fruit.

*Variations:*

Instead of flour and wheat germ use 1½ cups wheat germ and middlings; or use ½ cup whole-wheat flour and ½ cup rice polish, yellow corn meal, or rye, buckwheat, soy, or peanut flour. Add 1 teaspoon caraway seeds with rye flour if desired.

Add any of the following: ½ cup well-drained crushed pineapple, fresh or canned blueberries, or mashed banana; ¼ cup peanut butter; diced leftover ham, or crushed walnuts or pecans; bits of crisp bacon; or 1 cup pan-broiled bulk sausage.

**Baking-powder hotcakes:** Omit yeast; sift 2 teaspoons double-acting baking powder with dry ingredients; add moist ingredients; use in basic recipe or any variation.

**Buckwheat pancakes:** Instead of wheat flour use 1 cup buckwheat flour; add 3 tablespoons each blackstrap molasses and brewers' yeast.

Since waffles are so frequently served for late breakfasts or Sunday guest suppers, I have purposely kept the recipe a large one making 8 waffles.

## WAFFLES

Before gathering other ingredients, stir:

| | |
|---|---|
| 1 package or cake crumbled bakers' yeast into | 2 cups warm water, warm sweet or sour milk, buttermilk, or yogurt |

Add:

| | |
|---|---|
| 2 tablespoons dark molasses or sugar | 1 teaspoon salt |
| 3 egg yolks | ⅓ cup butter-flavored shortening |
| | 1 cup wheat germ |

Sift in:

| | |
|---|---|
| 1¼ cups whole-wheat pastry flour | ⅓ cup powdered milk |

Stir well, let rise in a warm place for 2 hours or longer, stirring down each time batter has doubled in bulk; just before baking, beat stiff and fold in:

**3 egg whites**

Bake on hot waffle iron. Serve with applesauce or crushed sweetened berries.

*Variations:*

Use 3 or more packages or cakes yeast; bake immediately or let rise 30 minutes; or use 2 packages or cakes yeast and let rise 1½ hours.

If more convenient, prepare waffle batter, let rise once or twice, stir down, and set in refrigerator overnight; remove from refrigerator 30 minutes before baking; stir egg yolks into batter just before folding in whites.

If any batter is left over, keep in refrigerator; thin slightly with milk and bake as pancakes.

Omit flour and wheat germ and use 2¼ cups wheat germ and middlings; or instead of ½ cup flour use ½ cup yellow corn meal, rice polish, or soy, peanut, or cottonseed flour; or add 1 or 2 tablespoons brewers' yeast.

Use 2 tablespoons fat and add 6 tablespoons peanut butter.

Add ½ to 1 cup of any of the following: ground or crushed walnuts or pecans; finely diced ham; leftover mashed potatoes or cooked rice; drained crushed pineapple or chopped and well-drained cooked apricots or prunes; diced banana; fresh or drained canned blueberries; or combine pineapple or banana with nuts, ham, or bits of crisp bacon.

**Baking-powder waffles:** Omit yeast; sift with dry ingredients 3 teaspoons double-acting baking powder; instead of water use sour milk, buttermilk, or yogurt. Do not add soda. Use baking powder with basic recipe or any variation. Compared with yeast waffles, these are scarcely worth the effort of making.

**Buckwheat waffles or pancakes:** Omit whole-wheat flour and use 1¼ cups buckwheat flour; bake as waffles or add ½ cup fresh milk and bake as hotcakes.

**Corn meal waffles:** Use 3 tablespoons fat; instead of water add yeast to lukewarm sour milk, buttermilk, or yogurt; omit flour and add 1¼ cups coarsely ground yellow corn meal.

**Gingerbread waffles:** Use 1½ cups sour milk, yogurt, or buttermilk and increase molasses to ⅔ cup; add with dry ingredients 2 tablespoons sugar, 1 teaspoon each ginger and cinnamon. Serve with whipped cream or ice cream.

**Raised pancakes:** Add ½ cup more liquid to basic recipe or any variation; bake on grill heated only to moderate temperature until brown on both sides.

**Rye waffles:** Use buttermilk; instead of whole-wheat pastry flour use 1¼ cups unrefined rye flour; add grated rind of 2 oranges or 1 teaspoon caraway seeds as desired.

**Wheat-germ waffles:** Instead of whole-wheat flour and wheat germ, use only wheat-germ flour—2¼ cups. This is my favorite.

## RAISED CORNBREAD

Before gathering other ingredients, stir:

1 to 3 packages or cakes crumbled          1 cup warm water, warm sweet or
  bakers' yeast into                         sour milk, buttermilk, or yogurt

Add:

1 egg                                      3 tablespoons bacon drippings
1 to 3 tablespoons sugar or honey

Sift in and stir well:

1 cup yellow corn meal                     ¼ cup powdered milk
½ cup whole-wheat pastry flour             ½ cup wheat germ or wheat-germ
1 teaspoon salt                              flour

Pour into oiled 8- by 8-inch pan or into muffin tins until half full; put
immediately into oven or let rise in a warm place 30 minutes or longer.
Bake in moderate preheated oven at 350° F. for 30 minutes.

*Variations:*

Add ¼ to ½ cup soy grits.
Instead of wheat germ add ½ cup soy or peanut flour.
Add ¼ to ½ cup ground parsley, grated carrots, or finely chopped
celery. Grated carrots give cornbread a beautiful color.
If fluffy cornbread is desired, let batter rise 2 or 3 hours or set in refrigerator overnight; add egg white stiffly beaten just before putting in oven.
**Baking-powder cornbread:** Omit yeast; sift with dry ingredients 3 teaspoons double-acting baking powder; bake in hot oven at 425° F. for 20
to 25 minutes.

## RAISED MUFFINS

Before gathering other ingredients, stir:

1 to 3 packages or cakes crumbled          1 cup warm water, warm sweet or
  bakers' yeast into                         sour milk, buttermilk, or yogurt

Add and stir slightly:

3 tablespoons black molasses or            3 tablespoons bacon drippings or
  sugar                                      soft butter-flavored shortening
1 egg

Sift in:

| | |
|---|---|
| 1 cup whole-wheat pastry flour | ⅓ cup powdered milk |
| ½ cup wheat germ or wheat-germ flour | 1 teaspoon salt |

Stir with no more than 30 strokes. Drop from tablespoon into oiled muffin tins until half full; bake immediately or let rise until double in bulk.

Bake at 350° F. for 20 minutes. This recipe makes 12 large muffins.

*Variations:*

Omit ½ cup of wheat flour and add ½ cup rice polish or soy, peanut, cottonseed, buckwheat, or rye flour; or add 1 or 2 tablespoons brewers' yeast, or ¼ cup soy grits.

Add ½ cup of any of the following: walnuts, pecans, raisins, chopped dates, ground dried apricots, shredded carrots, finely diced raw apple, chopped drained cooked prunes, or thick applesauce; or add ¼ cup ground parsley, 1 tablespoon grated onion, or a pinch of marjoram, basil, or thyme.

**Baking-powder muffins:** Omit yeast; sift with dry ingredients 3 teaspoons double-acting baking powder; bake at 425° F. for 15 minutes. Use with basic recipe or any variation.

**Blueberry muffins:** Use ⅓ cup sugar, omitting molasses; before stirring add 1 cup fresh or well-drained canned blueberries.

**Bran muffins:** Increase salt to 1¼ teaspoons; add 1 cup bran or bran flakes, ½ cup raisins and/or nuts.

**Cheese muffins:** Omit molasses or sugar and fat; blend 1 cup grated cheese with dry ingredients. Vary by adding ground parsley and/or 1 teaspoon dill or caraway seeds. Cheese muffins with dill are delicious.

**Corn meal muffins:** Use ¾ cup each whole-wheat pastry flour and coarse yellow corn meal, omitting wheat germ, or use ¾ cup each yellow corn meal and wheat-germ flour; use sugar rather than molasses if flavor of corn meal is particularly enjoyed. These are delicious muffins.

**Oatmeal muffins:** Add 1 cup quick-cooking raw rolled oats or ½ to 1 cup leftover cooked oatmeal.

**Orange muffins:** Use sugar; add grated rind of 2 oranges.

**Pineapple muffins:** Omit molasses, sugar, and liquid; add 1½ cups crushed pineapple and juice.

**Rice muffins:** Add ½ to 1 cup cooked brown or all-vitamin rice and ½ cup raisins or chopped dates.

**Rye muffins:** Omit wheat germ; use ¾ cup each wheat and rye flour; add 1 or 2 tablespoons caraway seeds or grated orange rind.

## BAKING-POWDER BISCUITS

Sift into a mixing bowl:

1½ cups whole-wheat pastry flour     4 teaspoons double-acting baking
½ cup wheat germ or wheat-germ       powder
   flour                             ¼ cup powdered milk
1¼ teaspoons salt

Add and cut in with pastry cutter:

     4 tablespoons chilled butter-flavored lard or shortening

Add and stir with 25 strokes:

     ¾ cup fresh or sour milk, buttermilk, or yogurt

Turn onto floured canvas or wax paper; knead 10 times; pat 1 inch thick
and cut with biscuit cutter.

Place close together on oiled baking sheet; bake in hot oven at 450° F.
for 12 to 15 minutes.

*Variations:*

Instead of ½ cup whole-wheat flour use ½ cup rice polish or soy, peanut, rye, or buckwheat flour; knead 20 times.

Cut dough with doughnut cutter; serve covered with creamed ham,
tuna, or chicken.

Add any of the following: 1 or 2 tablespoons brewers' yeast; ¼ to ½
cup finely shredded parsley; ¼ teaspoon thyme, basil, or marjoram; 3
tablespoons finely diced pimentos, celery, or grated onion; 2 teaspoons or
more poppy, sesame, or caraway seeds. Don't miss parsley or herb biscuits; they are delicious.

**Cheese biscuits:** Use 2 tablespoons shortening; blend with dry ingredients ¾ cup grated nippy cheese, preferably Cheddar.

**Cobblers:** Sift 4 tablespoons sugar with dry ingredients; mix 3 cups
sweetened sliced fresh or canned fruit or berries with 2 or 3 tablespoons
whole-wheat pastry flour; put in bottom of shallow baking dish, cover
with dough rolled ¼ inch thick, and bake as in basic recipe; if fruit, such
as apples, will not cook in 15 minutes, steam first until almost tender.

**Drop biscuits:** Use 1¼ cups milk; drop from spoon onto oiled baking
sheet or into muffin tins.

**Fruit or nut biscuits:** Before adding fat mix with dry ingredients ½
cup chopped dates, seeded raisins, ground dried apricots or peaches, or
broken walnuts, pecans, or other nuts; if desired, sift with flour 2 tablespoons sugar and ¼ teaspoon each cinnamon and nutmeg.

**Peanut-butter biscuits:** Use 2 tablespoons shortening; cut in with shortening ¼ cup peanut butter; add 1 tablespoon blackstrap molasses with milk.

**Sour-cream biscuits:** Use 2 tablespoons shortening; add 1 cup sour cream instead of milk.

Many women tell me that they do not make steamed bread because they have nothing to steam it in. All you need is any covered utensil large enough to hold two pint cans. The cans may be those in which fruits or fruit juices have been purchased. If you haven't a rack, jar lids may be used to keep the bread away from the direct heat.

### STEAMED BROWN BREAD

Before gathering other ingredients, stir:

| | |
|---|---|
| 1 to 3 packages or cakes crumbled bakers' yeast into | 2 cups warm sweet or sour milk, buttermilk, or yogurt |
| | ¾ cup blackstrap molasses |

Sift in:

| | |
|---|---|
| 1 cup whole-wheat pastry flour | ¼ cup powdered milk |
| 1 cup yellow corn meal | ¼ cup brewers' yeast |
| ⅔ cup wheat germ or wheat-germ flour | 1 teaspoon salt |

Drop in before stirring:

| | |
|---|---|
| 1 cup raisins or chopped dates or | ½ cup each raisins and broken walnuts or pecans |

Stir 40 strokes; pour into 2 oiled pint cans; cover tightly with lid or wax paper held on with string or rubber band; start cooking immediately or let rise ½ hour or longer.

Set on rack in cooking utensil; add water to the depth of 2 inches; cover utensil and steam slowly for 2 hours.

*Variations:*

Instead of corn meal add 1 cup rice polish or rye, buckwheat, soy, peanut, or cottonseed flour.

Add ½ to 1 cup soy grits or bran flakes to basic recipe or any variation.

**Baking-powder brown bread:** Omit yeast; sift 3 teaspoons double-acting baking powder with dry ingredients; add molasses and cold fresh or sour milk.

## NUT BREAD

Before gathering other ingredients, stir:

| | |
|---|---|
| 1 to 3 packages or cakes crumbled bakers' yeast into | 1¼ cups warm water, warm sweet or sour milk, buttermilk, or yogurt |

Add:

| | |
|---|---|
| 3 tablespoons butter-flavored oil or soft shortening | ⅓ cup dark or blackstrap molasses or sugar |

Sift in:

| | |
|---|---|
| 1¼ cups sifted whole-wheat pastry flour | ½ cup wheat germ or wheat-germ flour |
| ½ cup soy or peanut flour | 1½ teaspoons salt |
| | ⅓ cup powdered milk |

Before stirring, add:

½ to 1 cup broken walnuts, pecans, or other nuts

Stir 40 strokes. Line bottom of loaf pan with wax paper and brush with oil; pour batter into pan and start baking immediately, or let rise 30 minutes or longer before and after pouring into pan.

Bake in moderate oven at 350° F. for 15 minutes; lower heat to 300° F. and continue baking 45 minutes.

*Variations:*

Instead of nuts add ½ cup soy grits soaked in ¼ cup milk and 1 teaspoon black-walnut flavoring.

Add 2 tablespoons brewers' yeast to basic recipe or any variation calling for molasses; omit 2 tablespoons of flour.

Instead of soy or peanut flour use ½ cup rice polish, yellow corn meal, or rye, buckwheat, or cottonseed flour; or omit wheat germ and soy or peanut flour and use 1 cup wheat germ and middlings. If color of cottonseed flour is objectionable, use only with dark molasses.

**Apricot-nut bread:** Use sugar instead of molasses; mix with dry ingredients ½ to 1 cup ground dried apricots; use 1½ cups liquid; or omit water or milk and add 1 cup and 2 tablespoons cooked dried apricots beaten with rotary beater to a purée.

**Baking-powder nut bread:** Sift with dry ingredients 3 teaspoons double-acting baking powder; omit yeast; add other ingredients and bake as directed for yeast bread; use in basic recipe or any variation.

**Banana-nut bread:** Use sugar; instead of liquid add 1¼ cups mashed bananas; add grated rind of ½ lemon; use or omit nuts.

**Bran-nut bread:** Add 1 to 2 cups bran or bran flakes and ½ cup raisins.

**Date-nut bread:** Add 1 cup finely chopped dates; or add dates to banana-nut bread or other variations.

**Orange-nut bread:** Add ½ teaspoon orange flavoring (optional), grated rind of 2 oranges, and 2 drops orange coloring. This bread is delicious with either molasses or sugar.

**Peanut-butter bread:** Omit fat and nuts; blend ¾ cup peanut butter with dry ingredients, using pastry cutter; add other ingredients; use molasses.

**Pineapple-nut bread:** Instead of other liquid use 1¼ cups crushed pineapple and juice; add grated rind of ¼ lemon.

**Spiced honey-nut bread:** Instead of molasses or sugar use ⅓ cup honey; sift 1 teaspoon each nutmeg and cinnamon with dry ingredients.

**Prune-nut bread:** Instead of water or fresh or sour milk use 1½ cups pitted cooked prunes and juice; chop prunes or leave whole.

Cheese puffs are surprisingly easy to make. They are a delightful accompaniment to any soup or salad. They may be prepared in advance and stored for days. Keep them on hand to use when meals must be prepared in a hurry or to add a festive touch when guests drop in unexpectedly.

### CHEESE PUFFS

Heat to simmering:

½ cup milk                          ¼ cup butter-flavored shortening

Meanwhile sift flour before measuring, then sift into milk:

½ cup whole-wheat pastry flour      ⅛ teaspoon salt

Cook the batter, stirring constantly, until it leaves the sides of the pan and forms a large ball, or about 2 minutes. Remove from heat and beat in one at a time with rotary beater:

2 eggs

If convenient, chill 30 minutes or longer; otherwise bake immediately; chilling causes the puffs to be larger. Heap teaspoons of the batter on an oiled baking sheet 1½ inches apart, making high 1- or 2-inch mounds.

Put into a hot oven at 425° F. and bake until puffs have expanded and the peaks show a delicate brown, or about 6 minutes; lower temperature to 325° F., open oven door 1 minute, then bake slowly for 15 to 20 minutes.

Cut a gash in side of each puff and fill with cream cheese or grated American, pimento, or Jack cheese; season cheese with dill, dill sauce, or dill seeds, caraway seeds, or chopped ripe or stuffed olives as desired. Return to oven for 5 minutes, or until cheese has heated. Serve at once.

This recipe makes twenty 1-inch puffs or eight to ten 2-inch puffs.

*Variations:*

Store puffs in a paper bag in a cool place; fill with cheese or other filling; reheat in a moderate oven, and serve.

Instead of cheese, fill puffs with creamed or curried shrimps, chicken, lamb, ham, or other meats.

**Cream puffs:** Chill puffs; fill with sweetened whipped cream, chilled cake filling (p. 524), chiffon-pie filling (p. 534), or ten-minute-pie filling (p. 537); cover with icing (p. 522) as desired. Serve for dessert.

## CHAPTER 20

## COOK CEREALS QUICKLY

If the achievement of health is to be the goal, the labels of cereals should be carefully read and only those made of whole grain should be purchased. Any cereal to be used in feeding an infant or an invalid should be unrefined but finely ground. Refined but "enriched" cereals, like "enriched" flour, cannot compare nutritionally with the whole-grain products.

Formerly it was sometimes recommended that cereals be cooked 2 or 3 hours in order to change the starch into dextrin, a process which normally takes place when starch is digested. Later studies showed that starch is quite completely digested even when heated only to 180° F., far below boiling. Furthermore, cooking cereals a long time or at high temperatures decreases the health-building quality of the protein and causes partial destruction of several of the B vitamins. Even cereals to be given to a baby as its first solid food should be cooked in the shortest possible time. With the exception of unground wheat, they should not be cooked under pressure. Cooking them over direct heat is preferable to the slower process of cooking in a double boiler. Although the shorter cooking time is better, little loss of vitamin $B_1$ occurs when cereals such as steel-cut oats are cooked without pressure 10 or 15 minutes.

Reheating cereals causes an additional loss of B vitamins. Try to prepare only the amount of cereal which will be eaten at one meal. The practice of cooking cereal in the evening and reheating it for breakfast is not wise. If there is little time to prepare breakfast, use short-cooking cereals which cook as quickly as any cereal can be reheated.

Whenever possible, cereals should be cooked in milk rather than in water. Bring the milk to scalding temperature over direct heat before adding the cereal. If water is used, it should be brought to a rolling boil, salted, and the cereal added so slowly that boiling does not stop. Cereals containing much starch, such as rice, whole buckwheat, and oatmeal, do not become gummy when added slowly to boiling liquid, because the starch on and near the surface is cooked before it can dissolve out into the cooking water and thicken it into a paste.

Of all cereals, wheat germ contributes most to health. Wheat germ and middlings, which are often milled together, may be cooked alone as a cereal; the taste is so similar to that of familiar cereals that it is often enjoyed the first time it is eaten. A taste for pure wheat germ usually has to be developed. If it is new to your family, start by adding only ½ teaspoon to a serving of any cereal and increase the amount gradually as the taste becomes more familiar. When once the taste is enjoyed, pure wheat germ can be used alone as an uncooked cereal, toasted and eaten with uncooked cereal, or cooked 5 minutes, preferably in milk.

A number of cereals not generally used are excellent and usually enjoyed. For example, steel-cut oats have not been submitted to the high temperature necessary before oats can be rolled; they are therefore nutritionally superior to rolled oats and deserve wider use. In order to increase the protein intake, soy grits, or cracked soybeans, can be mixed with any cereal to be cooked. They are enjoyed alone as a cooked cereal after a taste for them has been developed. Whole buckwheat is especially appreciated by anyone who enjoys buckwheat pancakes. Triple-cleaned, unground wheat, purchased at stock-feed stores, makes an excellent cereal. Any whole-wheat cereal, however, has a considerably lower vitamin and protein content than wheat germ has, because of its large percentage of starch; it should not be thought of as being more valuable than wheat germ.

The old idea that a warm food is superior to a cold one is unfounded. From the point of view of nutrition, it makes no difference whether a food is hot or cold. If prepared cereal is made of the entire grain or contains a high proportion of the germ, it can be used interchangeably with cooked cereal. Cooked and chilled soy grits and toasted or untoasted wheat germ may be added to any prepared cereal. Cold cereals have the advantage of soaking up more milk than a hot cereal cooked in water.

Although cereals are excellent foods, they need not be eaten if iron, protein, vitamin E, and the B vitamins are amply supplied in the diet. Persons who have difficulty in maintaining their weight or those who wish to reduce can scarcely afford to include the calories supplied by eating cereals daily.

The iron, calcium, and B vitamins in cereal can be increased, and refined sugar, if eaten with cereal, can often be decreased if a small amount of dark or blackstrap molasses is added to the milk or water in which the cereal is cooked. The amount may be increased gradually as the taste becomes familiar.

## COOKING CEREALS

Heat to simmering:

### 2 cups fresh milk

Stir in so slowly that milk is not cooled:

**1 cup whole-grain cereal**         **1 teaspoon salt**

Add if sweet cereal is desired:

### ½ to 2 teaspoons dark or blackstrap molasses

Cover utensil and simmer until cereal is tender, or 5 minutes for wheat germ and middlings, pure wheat germ, ground wheat, soy grits, quick-cooking rolled oats; cook 10 minutes for untreated rolled oats or coarsely ground cereals; 15 minutes for whole buckwheat, all-vitamin rice, or steel-cut oats.

*Variations:*

If water is used instead of milk, bring to a rolling boil before adding cereal; use water for cooking unground wheat or brown rice; if utensil does not hold in steam, increase water to 3 cups for 1 cup wheat or brown rice.

Omit molasses or increase amount as flavor becomes appreciated.

# CHAPTER 21

## MILK DRINKS

Milk is such a valuable food that a quart daily should be drunk by each person, regardless of age. Almost every individual who does not drink milk shows signs of deficiencies of protein, calcium, and riboflavin, or vitamin $B_2$. People who do not use milk as a beverage have been found to have an average intake of only 0.3 gram of calcium daily; yet they wonder why they suffer from insomnia and are often highstrung and nervous. One should learn to enjoy the taste of milk and drink it with meals and between meals, as a substitute for water. People often remark, "I don't drink milk but I take calcium tablets," implying that calcium is a substitute for milk. Such a remark is like saying, "I do not have a car but I have a beautiful fender."

All fresh milk should be pasteurized or heated to 165° F., even that produced at home. Nothing is destroyed by pasteurization except an insignificant amount of vitamin C. "Pure, fresh milk" which is not pasteurized is responsible for thousands of deaths annually from undulant fever, septic sore throat, tuberculosis, and other milk-borne diseases.

When cold milk is exposed to light, riboflavin is gradually destroyed. *For example, if milk is left on the doorstep on a sunny day, 33 per cent of the vitamin is lost in 1 hour, 69 per cent in 2 hours.* When milk is heated, this vitamin is destroyed rapidly unless protected from light. *As much as 48 per cent of the vitamin is destroyed in 10 minutes when milk is heated in a glass utensil compared to 22 per cent when heated in an uncovered metal utensil; if heated in a covered metal utensil, no loss occurs.* If you cannot be at home when milk is delivered, arrange for the milkman to cover it with a box or a dark cloth. Cartons which do not admit light are preferable to bottles for delivering milk which cannot be taken in immediately. *Be particularly careful to use* opaque utensils rather than glass ones for preparing milk soups, custards, puddings, and milk drinks unless the pudding or custard is to be baked in a dark oven. *Keep these foods covered as much as possible not only during cooking but also while they are cooling.*

Although persons who rely entirely on milk drinks for their supply of milk rarely obtain sufficient amounts to produce a high degree of health, milk drinks are particularly valuable during illnesses and infections, and in the summer when parents must compete with the soft-drink industry if health is to be maintained. Ingredients should be kept on hand so that malted milks and milkshakes may be prepared at home. Since egg white should not be served uncooked, especially to children or ill persons, eggnogs should be cooked.

Contrary to popular opinion, skim milk contributes far more to health than does cream. The cream offers only calories and a small amount of vitamin A. Skim milk contains the nutrients in which people are so often deficient: protein, calcium, and riboflavin; it also supplies a variety of other minerals and small amounts of many B vitamins. Frequently mothers make the mistake of buying the richest milk possible for their children. The cream satisfies the appetite readily; instead of gaining, these children usually lose weight because they can eat so little other food. Often undigested fat from the rich milk combines with calcium, preventing this valuable mineral from reaching the blood; thus calcium deficiences occur. The combined fat and calcium form a hard soap in the intestines, causing constipation. Regardless of how thin a person may be, the emphasis should be on supplying him with milk protein, calcium, and the other nutrients in whole or skim milk rather than in cream. Since skim milk is filling, no food is so helpful to use in liberal quantities on a reducing diet as is skim milk.

In addition to milk served as a beverage, the more milk you can work into your cooking, the better health your family will probably enjoy. Whenever you can, use evaporated milk without diluting it. Add it to custards and ice creams; use it in gelatin desserts instead of whipped cream. Since half the water has been evaporated, it supplies (if not diluted) twice the amount of nutrients found in fresh milk. Its taste, if disliked, can be disguised with lemon juice and flavorings.

Few foods can offer so much to your family's health as can powdered skim milk, officially known as skim-milk solids. The popular use of this one food alone could easily prevent the widespread deficiencies of protein, calcium, and riboflavin. It is nothing less than ironical that in America, where these deficiencies cause untold loss of energy and efficiency, millions upon millions of pounds of powdered milk of the highest quality are produced annually; are sold at a nominal cost; are all but unknown except commercially; are used for making plastics while teeth are extracted and nerves are jagged. It is ridiculous that powdered milk is not on every kitchen shelf and used daily by every family. The people in foreign countries who have long enjoyed using American powdered milk are amazed when they hear that we scarcely know of its existence.

There are two types of powdered milk. Roller-processed milk, which is dried between hot rollers and ground to a powder, has a slightly brown cast, settles out when made into beverages, and is unsatisfactory to use except for baking. Spray-processed milk, which is dried by being sprayed into compressed air, has the texture of face powder. It is beautifully white with a faint suggestion of green caused by its concentration of riboflavin. Its odor, which is almost nonexistent, somewhat resembles sweet dried coconut. Its flavor is mild and delicate.

The one thing to remember about powdered milk is that it *must be kept in a tightly closed container*. Powdered milk is a hydrophyl, or water-lover. The fresh powder contains less than 2 per cent water, whereas flour, which you consider dry, is usually 13 per cent water. If left uncovered or in a paper bag, dried milk can absorb almost 10 per cent water in a single foggy or rainy day. Moist powdered milk becomes lumpy and is difficult to mix. The moisture causes decomposition of protein to set in; exposure to air allows the small amount of fat which the milk contains to become rancid; eventually a disagreeable odor and flavor develop. I recently used powdered milk which I had purchased 3 years ago and left in a mountain cabin; it was delicious and in excellent condition. Yet I have seen and certainly smelled powdered milk which could not possibly be used because it had been left open for a few days.

Powdered whole milk is much more expensive than is skim milk. Since it contains about 30 per cent butterfat, it becomes rancid quickly. If extra calories are desired, it is much cheaper to add margarine, butter, or cream to products prepared with powdered skim milk than to purchase dried whole milk. All recipes in this book have been tested with spray-processed powdered skim milk. I heartily recommend the same product to you.

If powdered milk is new to you, purchase only a few pounds at a time. Get it directly from a dairy in vacuum-packed or tightly sealed tin cans. I hope that eventually all milkmen will deliver it. Keep it in an airtight container protected from light. I keep my supply for immediate use in a canister. If it takes on a peculiar odor or taste, feed it to the dog; it's still too valuable to throw away.

Less than ½ cup of powdered skim milk contains all the nutrients of a quart of fresh skim milk. The addition of only a tablespoon to a serving of food makes a worth-while contribution. Do not use it as a substitute for fresh milk. *Use it in addition to fresh milk as a means of producing a higher degree of health.* In case a person refuses to drink fresh milk, then certainly he should obtain his milk requirement from foods containing powdered milk. Although powdered milk adds to the deliciousness of cream soups, milk drinks, custards, and cream sauces, reconstructed milk, or ½ cup of powdered milk stirred into a quart of water, is usually not considered palatable when drunk alone. The taste is flat, like that of boiled water. The value of powdered milk lies in its concentration, not its dilution.

There is something about nutrition which causes people, once sold on its value, to go overboard. A few weeks ago a friend whose child was refusing to drink milk and was showing definite protein and calcium deficiencies borrowed powdered-milk recipes from me. Reasoning that if a little was good more would be better, she doubled the quantities specified and found herself in difficulty. Since powdered milk is almost 8 per cent minerals—most foods contain less than 1 per cent—adding excessive amounts to food produces a salty or chalky taste. Since it is 37 per cent protein, if added in concentrated amounts to hot foods which are allowed to boil, the protein toughens and separates, giving a curdly appear-

ance, to say nothing of sticking to the pan. Use the amount specified in the recipes. Surely it is apparent that I have recommended
as much as is compatible with taste and texture.

A form of milk about which you will hear much in the future is
the Bulgarian-culture milk, yogurt. People who eat yogurt enough
to develop a taste for it almost invariably become enthusiastic
about it, often notice a marked pick-up in health following its use,
and therefore try to force it on their friends. This milk has long
been the principal food of the Bulgarians and is considered responsible for their unusual health. These people are noted for retaining the characteristics of youth to a late age, for their outstanding vigor and virility even into advanced age, and for unusually long lives. The 1930 census showed that there were more
than 1600 Bulgarians over 100 years old to every million of population compared with only 9 persons in America. It's a safe guess
that 90 per cent of the American centenarians are anything but
spry, whereas the Bulgarian oldsters are said to be romping around
like mere 60-year-olds. Moreover, it is said that baldness and white
hair are almost unknown in Bulgaria.

Yogurt culture was brought to America by the famous Rosell
Institute of the La Trappe Monastery in Canada. The yogurt itself is now sold by many markets and dairies. Inexpensive yogurt
culture, which is a vigorous strain of bacteria, is shipped to all
parts of the country by mail. Yogurt can be prepared at home by
adding to warm milk either yogurt culture or already prepared
yogurt, which contains the bacteria. As long as the milk is kept
warm, the bacteria grow, thriving on milk sugar and breaking it
down into lactic acid. As the acid is formed, it causes the milk to
thicken and become like junket or a soft custard. At this stage the
yogurt should be chilled immediately to stop bacterial growth;
otherwise so much acid will be liberated that the milk curds will
become hard and separate from the whey, and the product will
be too sour to be palatable.

Chilled yogurt is usually enjoyed when served with sweetened
fruit or with black molasses and cinnamon; it may be eaten as a
dessert, a midmeal, or an evening snack. Commercial yogurt is
often used as a salad dressing and is especially valuable as a substitute for oil dressings when a low-calorie diet is desired. Yogurt

sherbet is particularly delicious, and the valuable bacteria are not harmed by freezing. When homemade yogurt is beaten and served as a beverage, most people cannot distinguish it from buttermilk. If it is properly made, its flavor is similar to that of pineapple juice mixed with fresh milk. The taste of yogurt should be described as "clean"; it leaves your mouth feeling refreshed after it is eaten.

Yogurt is nutritionally superior to sweet milk in many ways. The milk protein in yogurt is partially broken down by the bacteria; some of the calcium dissolves in lactic acid. If digestion is below par, the protein and calcium from yogurt are more available to the body than are these substances in sweet milk. The bacteria in yogurt thrive in the intestines, whereas bacteria found in ordinary sour milk and buttermilk are killed at 90° F., or below body temperature. The yogurt bacteria living in the intestines break down milk sugar into lactic acid; since the bacteria which form gas and cause putrefaction cannot live in lactic acid, they are largely destroyed. It is for this reason that persons suffering from digestive disturbances and allergies usually find yogurt especially beneficial. The yogurt bacteria appear to synthesize, or make, the entire group of B vitamins in amounts sufficient for both themselves and their host; thus the person who uses yogurt liberally has a "B-vitamin factory" in his intestines. Evidence is accumulating which indicates that this source of B vitamins, thought to be largely responsible for the vigor, long lives, and lack of baldness and gray hair among the Bulgarians, may be of tremendous importance to health.

If yogurt is new to you, do not expect to enjoy it immediately. Cultivate a taste for it gradually, then serve it frequently. When health is below par, it is often advisable to drink as much as a quart of yogurt daily, substituting it entirely for fresh milk. Since the bacteria are killed by heat, there is no nutritional advantage in using yogurt in cooking. I do use it, however, as a substitute for buttermilk or sour milk in baking, because I enjoy its flavor more.

Surveys have shown that about 90 per cent of the milk purchased in many school cafeterias is chocolate milk. Since chocolate contains theobromine, a stimulant similar to caffeine, experiments have been undertaken to study the effect of chocolate milk on growth. Compared with animals given the identical diet except for plain milk, animals fed chocolate milk absorbed less calcium and phosphorus; their growth was retarded, and their bones were much smaller and more fragile. The fact that chocolate seriously interferes with the absorption of calcium is more harmful than the stimulating effect of the drug it contains. Since calcium deficiencies are already widespread and tooth decay is rampant, mothers are indeed unwise to entice their children to drink milk by making it into cocoa. Neither small children nor adolescent youngsters, whose calcium requirement has skyrocketed because of rapid growth, should be served chocolate. If chocolate and cocoa are used in spite of their detrimental effect, extra powdered milk should be added to all products containing them in order to supply additional calcium. For this reason I have included a recipe for making cocoa. I assure you that I am just as sorry as you are that chocolate and cocoa are not valuable foods.

In cooking for your family, use a combination of all types of milk: fresh milk, evaporated milk, powdered milk, buttermilk, and yogurt; use them all liberally.

Of all the milk drinks, none can compare in nutritive value to caramel milk. Few persons find it objectionable, and many declare that it is delicious.

### CARAMEL MILK

Shake or beat until smooth:

| | |
|---|---|
| 1 cup fresh milk | 3 drops vanilla and/or maple flavoring |
| 4 tablespoons powdered milk | oring |
| 2 teaspoons blackstrap molasses | pinch of salt |

Serve for midmeals or to anyone needing extra iron, calcium, or protein.

*Variations:*

Add 1 or 2 tablespoons vanilla ice cream.

Shake or beat 1 egg with other ingredients; heat to simmering; serve hot.

Add ½ to 1 teaspoon debittered brewers' yeast; increase the amount gradually to 1 tablespoon as flavor becomes familiar.

## VANILLA MILKSHAKE

Shake or beat until smooth:

| | |
|---|---|
| 1 cup chilled fresh milk | ⅛ teaspoon vanilla flavoring |
| 4 tablespoons powdered milk | ½ to 1 cup vanilla ice cream |
| 2 or 3 teaspoons sugar | |

Pour into chilled glass and serve.

*Variations:*

Add any one of the following: crushed fresh strawberries; mashed banana; crushed pineapple; apricot purée; date pulp; orange juice and grated rind or orange extract; crushed and sweetened loganberries or raspberries.

Instead of vanilla flavoring use almond or a drop each of almond and lemon; lemon and banana; black walnut, maple, peach, or pineapple flavorings.

Use any fruit ice cream or sherbet.

Omit ice cream and add 3 tablespoons sweetened whipped evaporated milk.

## PINEAPPLE FLOAT

Beat or shake together until smooth:

| | |
|---|---|
| 1 cup pineapple juice | 4 tablespoons powdered milk |

Pour into a glass and add:

4 tablespoons vanilla ice cream or whipped cream

*Variations:*

Omit pineapple juice and use any of the following juices: apricot, pear, loganberry, strawberry, raspberry, boysenberry, black cherry, grape, peach, or orange; use juices from canned fruits when available.

Omit ice cream and add evaporated milk whipped with lemon juice and sweetened to taste.

## MALTED MILK

Shake together or beat until smooth:

| | |
|---|---|
| 1 cup fresh milk | 1 or 2 teaspoons sugar |
| 1¼ tablespoons malted milk | 6 tablespoons powdered milk |
| ½ to 1 teaspoon debittered brewers' yeast | ½ to 1 cup ice cream |
| | ¼ teaspoon vanilla |

Pour into chilled glass and serve.

*Variations:*

Add ¼ cup crushed pineapple, strawberries, or other fruit purée or juice.

Omit sugar and add 1 teaspoon or more blackstrap or dark molasses; add vanilla, maple, or rum flavoring.

Omit ice cream, heat to simmering, and sprinkle generously with nutmeg.

Instead of vanilla use almond, maple, banana, peach, or pineapple flavoring. Use flavorings with fruit to accentuate natural flavors.

## ORANGE SHAKE

Combine in a quart jar in the order given

| | |
|---|---|
| 2 cups chilled orange juice | 2 teaspoons sugar |
| ½ cup powdered milk | 1 drop vanilla |

Stir slightly, then shake until smooth; chill thoroughly or add 3 tablespoons crushed ice.

*Variations:*

Instead of orange juice use the following juices: apricot, pear, strawberry, raspberry, boysenberry, loganberry, black cherry, peach, grape, pineapple; omit vanilla except for apricot and peach shake; add 1 tablespoon lemon juice to berry and pineapple shake; omit sugar when juices from canned fruits are used. Don't miss Concord grape shake; it is delicious.

So many friends helped me test milk drinks that the kitchen was practically converted into a soda fountain, and every recipe including each variation was tested in one day. We had even the milkman, the postman, and an expressman in as tasters. Although yogurt was new to most of the group, each of the following yogurt drinks was pronounced delicious. The one which we expected to enjoy the least, yogurt with Concord grape juice, we voted the best of them all.

## RASPBERRY YOGURT

Shake or beat until smooth:

| | |
|---|---|
| 1 cup chilled juice from canned raspberries | ⅓ cup powdered milk |

Add and beat slightly:

1 cup yogurt

Pour into chilled glasses and serve.

*Variations:*

Instead of raspberry juice use 1 cup of any of the following juices: apricot, orange, Concord grape, pineapple, prune, pear, peach, strawberry, or other berry juice; sweeten to taste.

Use fresh milk instead of yogurt in basic recipe or any variation.

## EGGNOG

Shake or beat until smooth:

| | |
|---|---|
| 1 cup fresh milk | 4 tablespoons powdered milk |
| 1 egg | pinch of salt |
| 3 teaspoons sugar | |

Simmer *in a metal utensil* 5 minutes, or heat to 160° F.; *keep covered as much as possible;* do not boil; remove from heat and add:

⅛ teaspoon vanilla

Serve hot sprinkled with nutmeg.

*Variations:*

Use 2 teaspoons sugar and add 1 teaspoon or more dark or blackstrap molasses; increase vanilla to ¼ teaspoon or add maple, rum, or brandy flavoring.

Omit vanilla and add 1 tablespoon brandy or rum.

## COCOA

Mix together:

2 tablespoons sugar                    ½ cup powdered milk
2 tablespoons cocoa                    pinch of salt

Add and beat until smooth while heating *in a metal utensil:*

### 1 cup fresh milk

When smooth, add and stir well:

### 3 cups fresh milk

Cover and heat to simmering, or to 185° F.; do not boil. Remove from heat and add:

### 1 teaspoon vanilla

Serve at once.

*Variations:*

If fresh milk is not available, heat cocoa, sugar, and salt with 3 cups water; beat until creamy ¾ cup powdered milk with 1 cup water; add 5 minutes before serving.

For rich cocoa, use 3 cups fresh milk; 5 minutes before serving add 1 cup evaporated milk. For foamy cocoa, use 3½ cups fresh milk; whip ½ cup chilled evaporated milk and stir in just before serving. The evaporated milk adds to both texture and flavor.

Omit cocoa; drop into warm milk and stir until melted 1 square bitter chocolate; or omit sugar and use sweet chocolate.

Chill cocoa; pour into glasses and add ½ cup vanilla ice cream to each serving.

## POSTUM

Beat or shake until smooth:

¾ cup fresh milk                      3 tablespoons powdered milk

*Pour into a metal utensil, cover,* and heat to simmering; pour over:

### 1 teaspoon postum

Stir well and sweeten to taste.

*Variations:*

Omit fresh milk; shake 4 tablespoons powdered milk with ¾ cup water and heat to simmering.

Instead of postum use any other powdered coffee substitute.

The one drawback in using powdered milk in cooking is that it is difficult to mix with water. Time, energy, and space in the refrigerator can be saved by mixing concentrated proportions of powdered milk with water, then diluting it to the equivalent of fresh milk as it is needed. The concentrated milk may be added directly to cream soups, custards, milk drinks, and almost any food containing milk. If you have an electric beater, you will find this method of using powdered milk particularly satisfactory. I mix the powder by the cupful and keep it on hand at all times.

## RECONSTRUCTED MILK

To give the equivalent of 2 quarts of fresh milk, beat with rotary beater or electric mixer until smooth:

**1 cup cold water**                    **1 cup powdered whole or skim milk**

Dilute with:

**2 cups cold water**

Store in quart jar or milk bottle; before using, dilute again with 1 cup water for each cup of milk mixture; use this diluted milk instead of fresh milk for general cooking; if budget is too limited to allow sufficient fresh milk for drinking, mix equal parts of water, milk mixture, and fresh whole milk; serve as a beverage.

*Variations:*

To reconstruct only 1 quart milk, put 2 cups cold water into a quart jar; add ½ cup powdered milk, cover tightly, and shake until smooth; finish filling jar with water; or use 1 cup of mixture beaten as directed above and dilute with 3 cups cold water.

To save storage space, beat 2 cups each water and powdered milk until smooth; store in refrigerator without diluting; when making cream soups, soft custards, milk drinks, cream sauces, puddings, and other foods containing fresh milk, for each cup of fresh milk called for in the recipe, use ¾ cup fresh milk and ¼ cup undiluted powdered-milk mixture. Stir in the powdered-milk mixture 2 or 3 minutes before removing food from heat.

Although yogurt has been made for hundreds of years by persons who never heard of thermometers, it is much easier to make with a thermometer. Yogurt bacteria grow rapidly between the temperatures of 90 and 120° F. They are killed by high temperatures; below 90° F. they grow slowly if at all. The bacteria which produce ordinary sour milk multiply rapidly at warm room temperatures, or between 65 and 85° F., but are killed at 90° F. If you attempt to make yogurt and fail to keep the milk warm enough, you will have ordinary sour milk, not yogurt. The trick of making yogurt is in keeping the milk quite warm until it thickens.

## YOGURT

Pour into pottery bowl and mix well:

**1 quart pasteurized whole or skim       ¼ cup commercial yogurt
milk**

Fasten cooking thermometer to side of bowl or float dairy thermometer on surface; set in oven and heat slowly to 120° F.; turn off oven heat, cover milk to hold in heat, and let cool gradually to 90° F. Maintain temperature between 90 to 105° F. by reheating oven if needed until milk becomes the consistency of junket, or about 2 to 3 hours. Check consistency frequently during the last 30 minutes; chill immediately after milk thickens. Yogurt may be kept in the refrigerator 3 to 5 days.

Serve with black molasses and cinnamon, or beat slightly with rotary beater and serve as buttermilk, or mix with fruit juices or purées before serving.

Keep ¼ cup of this yogurt as a starter for preparing it again; beat yogurt until smooth before stirring it into milk; purchase fresh culture or commercial yogurt once each month.

*Variations:*

Double or triple recipe, making several quarts at one time.

If raw milk is used, heat to simmering and cool to 120° F. before stirring in yogurt starter or culture.

Instead of yogurt starter use pure yogurt culture; incubate 4 to 6 hours. Occasionally in hot weather it will require 8 or 9 hours for yogurt prepared with culture to thicken. Obtain fresh culture once each month; at other times use ¼ cup of the last yogurt prepared as a culture; incubate for 2 to 3 hours, preparing as in basic recipe.

Instead of preparing yogurt in the oven, heat milk in the top of a double boiler; set over hot water; reheat water when necessary to maintain temperature of milk at 105° F.; or pour cultured warm milk into jars or custard cups and set in warm water; or pour into a thermos bottle.

To prepare thick yogurt resembling that made commercially, combine yogurt starter or culture with 3 cups pasteurized milk and 1 large can (1½ cups) evaporated milk or 1 quart pasteurized milk shaken with ½ cup powdered skim milk. Serve as pudding with cinnamon or nutmeg and black molasses, make into sherbet (p. 509), or serve with raspberries, pineapple, or other fruit.

For salad dressings or as a base for sauces (p. 168) make yogurt with 1½ cups each fresh milk and evaporated milk.

For reducing diets prepare yogurt with pasteurized skim milk or ⅔ cup powdered skim milk shaken with 1 quart water; add 2 drops yellow coloring; prepare several quarts at one time; drink 1 quart daily as a substitute for buttermilk.

Prepare yogurt as in basic recipe, using any of the following milks or combinations of milks: homogenized milk; goats' milk; undiluted evaporated milk; ½ cup powdered milk and/or sweetened condensed milk with 1 quart fresh milk; ⅔ cup powdered whole or skim milk shaken with 3½ cups water and 1 large can evaporated milk; ½ cup each powdered milk and sweetened evaporated milk, 3 cups water. Obtain consistency and flavor desired by combining different amounts and types of milk.

If whey separates from milk curds, the incubation time has been too long, the temperature during incubation too high, or the yogurt not chilled quickly enough. Beat, sweeten to taste with black molasses, honey, or sweetened condensed milk, and serve as a beverage.

If yogurt does not thicken, temperature during incubation has been so high that the bacteria were killed or so low that the bacteria could not grow; incubation time may have been too short; you may have forgotten to add the starter or culture; or the starter or culture may have been old. Add more culture or starter, check temperature carefully, and incubate longer.

If yogurt has an unpleasant taste, molds and foreign bacteria are probably responsible. Sterilize all equipment in boiling water; be extremely careful to pasteurize milk; keep starter carefully covered and refrigerated

# CHAPTER 22

## EAT MORE FRUITS

Fruits should have an important place on your menus. Serve them daily for breakfast and midmeals, and frequently in salads and appetizers. The dessert superior to all others is fresh or canned fruit, served perhaps with nuts or cheese and whole-grain crackers.

If the nutritive value of fruits is to be retained during preparation and cooking, the same general rules must be followed as were given for preparing salads and cooking vegetables. Enzyme action should be kept to the minimum by refrigeration, by the exclusion of oxygen and light, by avoiding all contact with copper and iron, and by rapid heating in case the fruit is to be cooked. Fruit should be cooked in the shortest time possible.

The vitamin content of fruits increases until they are ripe. If fruits are gathered or purchased when underripe, leave them at room temperature, preferably in a dark place, until well ripened. With the exception of fruits having a heavy peel which protects the vitamins from oxygen, such as citrus fruits, bananas, and apples, put fruits into the refrigerator as soon as they have ripened. Purchase only the amount of ripe fruits which can be refrigerated, canned, or frozen immediately. If ripe fruits are left at room temperature, their vitamins A, $B_2$, and C are gradually destroyed. The destruction of these vitamins takes place rapidly when fruits are allowed to become overripe, especially if they are bruised. For example, guavas, one of the richest sources of vitamin C, contain 1600 to 2000 milligrams of this vitamin per pound when ripe but firm. If they are allowed to stand until overripe and soft, though only for a day, four-fifths of the vitamin is lost. On the other hand, if citrus fruits, protected by a thick peeling, are stored in a cool place, almost no loss of vitamin C occurs even after several months, provided the fruit stays in good condition.

Soft fruits, such as berries, should be put into the refrigerator unwashed and unstemmed. Any handling causes bruises which result in increased enzyme action and vitamin loss. Just before being used, the chilled berries should be washed so quickly that they will not reach the temperature of the water. If they cannot be served immediately, they should again be put into the refrigerator. Fruits which are sufficiently firm not to bruise may be washed before being chilled. No fruit should be peeled or cut until shortly before it is to be used; any exposure to oxygen increases loss of vitamin C.

Wash all fruits rapidly. If they are allowed to stand in water, considerable amounts of sugars, vitamin C, and the B vitamins dissolve out and are lost. Avoid soaking any fresh fruit. Instead of loosening the skin of tomatoes or peaches by soaking them in hot water, steam them a few minutes until the peel can easily be slipped off. Before cutting apples chill them to prevent discoloration. Do not put them into water afterward. Avoid using any knife which contains copper; such a knife will cause almost instant discoloration and complete loss of vitamin C in the discolored portions. Since acid retards enzyme activity, discoloration can be prevented by mixing cut fruit with a little lemon juice.

Trim fruits as little as possible. When fruits are not chilled, leave them in large pieces; the less surface exposed, the less nutritive value lost. Since fruits are usually served in the liquid in which they are cooked, little or no loss of minerals or heat-stable vitamins occurs during cooking.

Keep oranges from which juice is to be extracted in the refrigerator until chilled; then extract the juice quickly to prevent unnecessary contact with air. If the juice is not to be drunk immediately, squeeze the oranges lightly, being careful to get no oil from the skin into the juice. It is this oil which gives orange juice the off-taste after standing. Extract any juice left in the lightly reamed oranges and drink it. Store the juice in a closed container so full that no oxygen is closed in above the juice. As some juice is used, transfer the rest to a smaller container. No significant loss of vitamin C or of flavor occurs when fresh juice, treated in this way, is kept in the refrigerator for a few days. On the other hand, if the oranges are not chilled before squeezing, if air is sealed with the juice, or if the juice is left at room temperature, as much as 50 per cent of the vitamin C may be lost within an hour.

Since cooking destroys enzymes which bring about the vitamin loss, juices which have been cooked, such as canned tomato or grapefruit juice, retain their vitamin content much better than do fresh juices. Vitamin C in natural foods is the most easily destroyed of all vitamins, whereas synthetic vitamin C, containing no enzymes, is extremely stable. In extracting juices to be canned, such as tomato or grape juice, far less loss of vitamin C occurs if the raw fruits are first quickly cooked and the enzymes destroyed before the juice is extracted. Cider, even though made from apples rich in vitamin C, quickly loses its vitamin C content unless it is heated to destroy the enzymes immediately after it is made.

There is little loss of vitamin C during the cooking of sour fruits such as rhubarb, green apples, and plums, because the acids they contain inhibit enzyme action. Since steam heat penetrates food more quickly than does dry heat, steam or stew fruits in preference to baking them. When fruits are to be baked, put them into a hot utensil containing a small amount of boiling water, and heat them by putting into a preheated oven at a high temperature. Cook any fruit only until tender. After the enzymes are destroyed, the shorter the cooking time, the less the nutritive loss.

All fruits contain three sugars: glucose, fructose, and sucrose, or table sugar. The less water used in cooking fruits, the less of these sugars is soaked out. Little sugar need be added for sweetening if the fruits are cooked with the minimum amount of water. Whenever it is practical, allow cooked fruits to cool before adding sugar to them. If fruits are sweetened during cooking, the acid in the hot fruit causes the added table sugar to break down into glucose and fructose. These two sugars are far less sweet than is table sugar; hence almost twice the amount must be added to give the same degree of sweetness. If sugar is added at the last of the cooking, less sugar is required than at the beginning; yet this amount is considerably more than is needed when the fruit is chilled. Persons wishing to reduce or to maintain their weight can sweeten fruits with saccharin or eat fruits canned in water and sweetened with saccharin before being eaten. Sugar need not be added during canning to keep fruits from spoiling.

When you buy dried fruits, choose apricots and peaches which have been sulfur-dried, and figs and prunes which are sun-dried. There is no loss of vitamin A when fruits are dried with sulfur, and some vitamin C is retained. Since sulfur-dried apricots are an outstanding source of vitamin A, use them more frequently than other dried fruits. Sun-drying results in a complete loss of vitamin C and an appreciable loss of vitamin A, the amount lost being proportional to the loss of color. Sulfur-drying, however, destroys some of the vitamin $B_1$. Since figs and prunes contain vitamin $B_1$ but little vitamin A, sun-dried ones are nutritionally superior to those which have been sulfured.

Dried fruits should be washed quickly. They may be cooked without being soaked, and since they absorb moisture quickly from steam, they need not be covered with water. Dried fruits contain about 75 per cent sugar. If prepared with only the amount of water needed to soften them, they retain so much of the natural sugar that further sweetening is usually unnecessary. If they are to be soaked, under no circumstances should the water used for soaking be thrown away.

The peel and seeds of many fruits, if used, can contribute delicious flavors. For example, unpeeled pears which are steamed, baked, or canned, have a more appetizing color, a more delicious flavor, and a firmer texture than those which are peeled. Not only is the flavor of applesauce improved but far less nutritive loss occurs when it is prepared by first steaming the unpeeled apples and then pressing them through a colander than when they are peeled and boiled. Delicious fruit sauces can be prepared if such fruits as apricots, peaches, and pears which are too small to be of value whole are steamed and passed through a colander. Apricot, nectarine, and peach pits add flavor when cooked with the fruits.

There is little loss of nutrients when fruits are frozen or during the time they are stored after they are frozen. Losses may have occurred before the fruit was frozen unless scientific rules for food preparation were observed. When frozen foods are thawed, however, loss of vitamin C takes place rapidly. Serve frozen fruits as soon as they have thawed.

Since certain unavoidable losses occur when fruits are cooked, serve raw fruits in preference to cooked ones whenever possible.

## APPLES

Adopt the Italian and French custom of serving a bowl or basket of raw apples for dessert, supplying each person with a fruit knife and small plate. Serve with any one of the following:

Camembert, Roquefort, Swiss, American, Jack, or other cheeses.

Unhulled walnuts, peanuts, or paper-shell almonds or pecans; heat nuts 10 minutes in moderate oven and serve hot; supply a nutcracker for each person.

Toasted and salted almonds, pecans, peanuts, or other nuts.

Salted and buttered popcorn or cheese popcorn (p. 548); have popcorn hot, apples chilled.

Caraway or poppy seeds; heat seeds in oven 10 minutes and serve hot.

Remove cores and cut chilled red apples into slices ½ inch thick; spread with Camembert or cream cheese; sprinkle with caraway or poppy seeds.


## STEWED WHOLE APPLES AND OTHER FRUITS

Wash quickly, dry, and core:

#### 4 or more large chilled apples

Remove peel from upper fourth of apples; put peeled side down into:

#### ½ cup boiling water

Heat through quickly; reduce heat and simmer until tender when pierced with a toothpick, or about 10 minutes; turn apples peeled side up and sprinkle with:

¼ cup sugar                                    cinnamon, nutmeg, or grated lemon
                                                          rind

Brown under broiler and serve with top milk, sour cream, yogurt, whipped evaporated milk, or whipped cream. These apples appear to be baked, yet are cooked much more quickly and with less nutritive loss.

*Variations:*

Before putting apples on to cook, fill centers with raisins or nuts mixed with raisins; or just before putting apples under the broiler fill with broken walnuts, pecans, almonds, or other nuts, or mincemeat.

**Apricots, nectarines, peaches, and other fruit:** Do not remove pits; put whole, unpeeled fruit into preheated utensil containing 1 or 2 tablespoons boiling water, or just enough to prevent sticking; steam until tender, or 6 to 10 minutes. Skins may be removed from peaches and apricots after steaming; sprinkle with ¼ cup sugar; chill. The less water used in cooking the fruit, the more delightful the flavor will be when they are served.

**Cinnamon apples:** Add to water used for stewing apples 6 each cloves and cassia buds or a small piece of cinnamon; prepare apples and cook as in basic recipe; remove apples and add to remaining liquid ½ cup water, ¼ cup sugar, and 1 drop red coloring; simmer until sugar is dissolved; soak 2 teaspoons gelatin in ¼ cup water and dissolve in hot liquid; chill until it starts to congeal, brush over apples, pour remainder into centers. Serve with meat or as dessert. Instead of cloves and coloring, add 2 tablespoons cinnamon drops.

*Mint apples:* Omit cloves and cassia buds and add green coloring and 2 drops peppermint oil; proceed as for cinnamon apples.

**Fruit with custard sauce:** Steam whole unpeeled peaches or apricots, or unpeeled pears cut in half and cored; remove from heat, pit apricots or peaches, and sprinkle lightly with sugar; serve covered with soft custard (p. 493), pouring custard into centers of apricots or peaches.

**Glazed fruit:** Steam whole unpeeled pears or peaches; core pears from the blossom end, leaving stems on; pit and peel peaches after steaming; prepare and apply a glaze as directed for cinnamon apples, omitting spices.

**Stewed whole pears:** Stew whole unpeeled pears with cores removed from blossom end; stuff with broken nuts or raisins or nuts and raisins mixed, or with chopped candied or preserved ginger. Just before removing from heat sprinkle with ¼ cup sugar and 1 teaspoon grated lemon rind; chill and serve. Vary by stewing without added seasonings; serve with apricot or plum sauce.

*Pears with orange sauce:* Cut unpeeled pears in half and remove cores; stew in 1 cup boiling orange juice; remove pears and sweeten juice with ½ cup sugar; add 1 teaspoon grated orange rind; pour syrup over pears and chill.

**Stuffed peaches:** Stew whole unpeeled peaches; cool, remove pits and skins; stuff with broken walnuts or pecans; or remove pits before stewing and stuff with raisins or nuts and raisins mixed.

**Whole fruit with crumbs:** Stew whole unpeeled apples, peaches, apricots, or pears as in basic recipe; sweeten and chill; roll in graham-cracker crumbs to which 1 or 2 drops almond extract are added. Serve with whipped evaporated milk or cream.

## APPLESAUCE AND OTHER FRUIT SAUCES

Wash quickly and quarter:

### 2 pounds tart cooking apples

Do not peel or remove cores if fruit is in good condition; put apples into saucepan containing:

### ½ cup boiling water

Heat quickly, reduce heat, steam until soft, or about 15 minutes; press apples through colander or food mill.

Unless fruit is to be served immediately, chill thoroughly before sweetening to taste.

Season to taste with **dash of nutmeg, cinnamon, or small amount of lemon juice or grated lemon or orange rind.** If flavor of the apples is excellent, add no seasonings.

*Variations:*

While applesauce is still hot, add 3 or 4 tablespoons cinnamon candies; or 1 drop red coloring if sauce is seasoned with cinnamon, yellow coloring with lemon juice or grated lemon rind.

Add 3 or 4 tablespoons uncooked or lightly toasted wheat germ to applesauce just before serving; add wheat germ to any fruit sauce.

Follow the procedure of the basic recipe and make fruit sauces of small pears, peaches, apricots, plums, or other fruit; if apricots or peaches are extremely small, do not remove pits before steaming.

## BAKED APPLES AND OTHER FRUIT

Wash quickly, dry, and core:

### 4 large chilled apples, preferably red

Set in baking dish and put in center of each:

### 1 tablespoon sugar

Sprinkle lightly with:

### cinnamon, nutmeg, or grated lemon rind

Add:

### ¼ cup boiling water

Put into a preheated hot oven at 400° F. and bake until tender when tested with a toothpick, or 15 to 20 minutes.

Serve hot or chilled with top milk, sour cream, yogurt, or whipped cream.

*Variations:*

Fill centers of apples with mincemeat or with cinnamon drops, broken nuts, raisins, or nuts and raisins mixed.

Bake peaches, pears, apricots, or other fruits, following suggestions for seasoning listed under stewed whole fruits.

## FRIED APPLES

Use tart, slightly green apples; core and slice or dice the pulp from:

**6 to 8 chilled unpeeled apples**

Put into frying pan with:

**2 tablespoons bacon drippings or butter-flavored fat**

Keep heat high, turn apples frequently, and brown well; if they are not tender by the time they are browned, cover utensil and steam until tender. Add 5 minutes before taking up:

**¼ cup brown sugar (optional)**          **⅛ teaspoon salt**

Serve with meat.

*Variations:*

Core and cut apples into rings ⅛ inch thick; brown on both sides in fat, sprinkle lightly with sugar and nutmeg. Serve with ham or pork.

Fry cling peaches as in basic recipe. Serve with meat.

**Stewed apples:** Prepare as for frying, cutting each piece into bite sizes; do not peel; cook in waterless-cooking utensil with 2 tablespoons boiling water; cool and sweeten to taste. If waterless equipment is not available, heat apples through in top of double boiler over direct heat and finish cooking over boiling water.

*Spiced apples:* While apples are cooking, add 4 to 6 cloves, a small piece of cinnamon or 6 cassia buds or 1 tablespoon cinnamon drops. Add red coloring as desired.

Serve bananas when yellow skin is dotted with brown spots. Combine with other fruits in fruit cup and compotes, serve sliced, whole, or cut in half lengthwise and sprinkled lightly with pow-

dered sugar and lemon or orange juice. Since baking is a slow
process, broil bananas in preference to baking them.


## BROILED BANANAS

Peel:

### 4 ripe bananas

Set in low oiled baking dish, brush surface with **blackstrap molasses,**
and broil with moderate heat until well browned, or about 10 minutes;
turn and brown the other side, or about 6 to 8 minutes.

Sprinkle with **nutmeg, cinnamon, or lemon juice;** serve hot.

*Variations:*

Serve with orange juice, grated lemon or orange rind, or stewed raisins
seasoned with lemon rind.

Omit molasses, broil, and sprinkle with small amount of powdered
sugar and grated orange rind.

Remove skin from half of each banana; broil unpeeled side first, turn,
brush with molasses, and finish broiling.


Wash raspberries, youngberries, blackberries, strawberries, and
similar soft berries not earlier than ½ hour before they are to be
served. Sprinkle lightly with granulated or powdered sugar and
serve with top milk. Larger berries may be sliced or cut in half.
Serve firm, attractive strawberries without stemming them, especially if you desire to avoid the calories in cream and sugar.

When washing blueberries and huckleberries, discard those which
come to the top of the water; worms have usually eaten the center
of such berries, making them light. Chill berries thoroughly and
serve with top milk and sugar. Stew berries by adding 2 cups berries to ¼ cup boiling water; lower heat and steam until berries
are tender, or about 5 to 7 minutes. Chill before adding sugar to
taste.


Chill melons thoroughly before serving. Cut as desired. Serve
small melon halves in chopped ice but do not allow ice to touch
edible parts.

## CANTALOUPE CUP

Cut cantaloupe or other small melon in half, making sawtooth edge; remove seeds; cut thin slice from bottom of each half so that it will rest securely on plate. Fill center with one of the following:

| | |
|---|---|
| diced pineapple, sliced peaches, or other fruit | strawberries |
| | mixed diced fruits |
| unstemmed black cherries | ice cream |

Garnish with **mint leaf or maraschino cherry** if diced fruit is used.

*Variation:*

Make rings of small melons by cutting center portion into 1-inch slices; fill centers of rings with mixed diced fruits, strawberries, cherries, or ice cream.

## FESTIVE WATERMELON BOWL

Cut chilled watermelon in half lengthwise; remove pulp; dice into 1-inch cubes, discard seeds, and combine pulp with the following:

| | |
|---|---|
| sliced peaches or apricots | diced honeydew or casaba melon |
| halved and seeded purple grapes | diced pineapple slices |

Place mixed fruit in watermelon rind. Garnish with **fresh green leaves.**

Wash cherries quickly; chill and serve without stemming. If stewing is desirable, cook in 2 tablespoons water; chill before adding sugar to taste.

## BLACK CHERRIES WITH BRANDY

Put into heat-resistant casserole or metal serving dish:

**1 can black cherries**

Heat quickly to boiling; add:

**¼ cup brandy**

Ignite brandy; serve flaming cherries alone or over vanilla ice cream.

*Variation:*

Instead of cherries use canned apricots, peaches, or pears.

## DRIED FRUITS

Drop into **2 cups boiling water:**

**1 pound dried prunes, apricots, apples, raisins, peaches, pears, or figs**

Cover utensil, reduce heat to simmering, and cook until fruit is tender, or about 12 to 15 minutes. Chill.

Let fruit soak in cooking liquid overnight; sweeten to taste.

*Variations:*

Add bits of lemon or orange rind to prunes, apples, pears, or figs during cooking. Add to cooking water ½ teaspoon each cloves and cassia buds or stick of cinnamon; use for prunes, pears, peaches, or apples; add red coloring to spiced apples, green coloring to spiced pears.

Sweeten prunes and raisins with 2 or 3 tablespoons blackstrap molasses; add at the end of cooking.

Add to dried pears during cooking 2 tablespoons diced preserved or candied ginger.

### CANNED FRUITS

Canned fruits are excellent to serve alone as desserts. If you wish to make them more festive, serve them with one or more of the following:

Whipped and sweetened evaporated milk or whipped cream.

Sour cream or thick yogurt.

Sprinkle generously with broken walnuts, pecans, crushed peanuts, or other nuts.

Sprinkle with moist shredded coconut; or mix coconut with a small amount of water and food coloring; dry before sprinkling over fruit.

Quarter 2 or 3 marshmallows and add to each serving of fruit.

Since guavas are such a rich source of vitamin C, use as many of them as possible. Add them to appetizers, fruit cups, fruit salads, and gelatins containing mixed fruits. Can them when available, using either the cold-pack or open-kettle method. Slice chilled peeled guavas and serve with lemon sections or mix with lemon juice; sweeten to taste.

## STEWED GUAVAS

Peel and slice:

### 2 cups chilled guavas

Heat to boiling:

**2 tablespoons water**                    **1 tablespoon lemon juice**

Add the guavas, cover utensil, and steam 5 to 8 minutes. Chill and sweeten to taste.

*Variations:*

Omit water and lemon juice and stew guavas in ¼ cup orange juice; chill, sprinkle with grated orange rind and sugar to taste.

Boil for 5 minutes with ¼ cup water 6 each cloves and cassia buds; add guavas and 1 drop red coloring.

Stew guavas with an equal amount of sliced peaches, pears, or other fruit.

The large California persimmons are an excellent source of vitamin A. If you have facilities for quick freezing, obtain them in season and freeze enough to use throughout the year. Persimmons are delicious when served unthawed. Prepare persimmons and serve in any of the following ways:

Cut unpeeled persimmons petal-fashion, leaving base intact; separate the sections slightly, sprinkle with shredded coconut or lemon juice, or garnish center with mint leaves or grated lemon rind.

Cut either chilled or frozen unpeeled persimmons crosswise into ½-inch slices; serve alone garnished with mint or with sour cream or yogurt.

Cut chilled or frozen persimmons into thin slices; alternate persimmon slices with orange slices.

Freeze very ripe persimmons; immediately before serving shred and serve in sherbet glasses; garnish with green maraschino cherries.

Shred frozen persimmons and mix with shredded coconut and broken walnuts, almonds, or pecans.

Add 1 cup mashed or shredded persimmon pulp to ice cream (p. 505), custard (p. 493), or Bavarian cream (p. 503).

Dice and mix with other fruits in preparing fruit cup, or slice and use in fruit compote.

Fresh uncooked pineapple contains protein-digesting enzymes. Persons whose digestion is below par often benefit by eating it uncooked. Following are suggestions for serving pineapple:

Spread slices of fresh or canned pineapple with sour cream or yogurt if sour cream is prepared at home, sour with yogurt bacteria.

Alternate slices of orange or California persimmon with slices of pineapple.

Peel fresh pineapple, slice, and serve uncored with fruit knives and forks; sprinkle lightly with powdered sugar.

Split whole chilled pineapple in half lengthwise; remove pulp, core, and dice; sprinkle with sugar and serve from shell with leaves still intact; or mix diced pineapple with fresh strawberries, raspberries, melon cubes, sliced peaches, diced unpeeled apple, or other fruit; serve from the half shell.

Split whole chilled pineapple; mix diced pulp with slices of stoned dates and/or shredded coconut, or with walnuts, pecans, or almonds.

Remove pulp from whole pineapple by cutting off top 1 inch below leaves, inserting knife near bottom, revolving it without cutting edges, and cutting out entire center in one piece; slice, sprinkle with powdered sugar, return slices to shell; serve with leaves as if uncut; or dice pulp and mix with fresh fruit; sweeten to taste and serve from shell.

To make an elaborate fruit platter for a buffet, set in center of platter whole pineapple with pulp sliced as directed above; cut skin of oranges petal-fashion; pull back and separate the orange sections; sprinkle with powdered sugar; surround pineapple with oranges and lay chilled bananas around edge. Just before serving, remove skin from top of bananas, brush with lemon juice, and sprinkle with powdered sugar. Scatter unstemmed black cherries or strawberries over platter.

## STEAMED RHUBARB

Cut into 1-inch pieces without peeling.

### 1½ pounds rhubarb

Add to:

### 1 or 2 tablespoons boiling water

Cover utensil, keep heat low, and steam 16 to 18 minutes. Chill thoroughly and add:

### ½ cup sugar

Stir well and let sugar dissolve before serving.

*Variations:*

If utensil with tight-fitting lid is not available, heat rhubarb in top of double boiler over direct heat and finish cooking over boiling water.

If low-calorie diet is desired, sweeten rhubarb to taste with saccharin.

**Cooked cranberries:** Cook like rhubarb, using ¼ cup boiling water; chill thoroughly before sweetening.

## FRUIT ASPICS

Soak 5 minutes in saucepan:

**1 tablespoon gelatin in**                    **½ cup fruit juice**

Heat gelatin slowly until dissolved; add:

**1½ cups plum, apricot, loganberry, pineapple, peach, or other berry or fruit juice or purée**

If fruit is not tart, add:

**1 or 2 tablespoons lemon juice**

Pour into chilled mold; chill until firm, unmold. Serve with meat.

*Variations:*

If juice is extremely tart, add a small amount of sugar.

Make aspic of prune or apple purée or 1 cup each prune purée and applesauce to which are added a few chopped or broken walnuts, pecans, or almonds when gelatin starts to congeal.

Make purées and juices of small fruits or fruits which are too soft to be attractive when cooked whole; can in generous amounts to be used for aspics.

Chill fruit until it starts to congeal before putting into mold; whip 1 cup chilled evaporated milk, add 3 tablespoons lemon juice, ¼ cup each sugar and powdered milk; stir into aspic, pour into mold, chill, and serve for dessert.

Pour aspic into flat baking dish; chill, cut into cubes, and serve.

## FRUIT COMPOTES

A fruit compote is a combination of two or more fresh or canned fruits. The fruit is cut as little as possible and served from an attractive bowl at the table. Dark-colored juices should be drained before the fruits are combined. Use fresh fruits of contrasting colors or combine fresh with canned fruits. For additional vitamin C, add rose-hip extract or sliced guavas to compotes if they are available. Following are suggestions for compotes:

Canned apricots, fresh or frozen strawberries.
Apricot halves, preferably fresh, drained canned black cherries.
Large dices of casaba or honeydew melon, canned or stewed purple plums.
Pineapple cubes or slices, fresh or canned peach halves, fresh or frozen raspberries.
Canned unpeeled pear halves, orange slices; drain 1 cup canned black cherries and scatter over top of compote just before serving.
Cubes of chilled cantaloupe; layer in bowl with canned or fresh grapefruit sections, sliced pineapple, or fresh youngberries.
Canned figs, orange slices, seeded purple-grape halves.

Fruit cup makes an ideal dessert usually enjoyed by everyone. It is essentially the same as an appetizer of mixed fruits except that the fruit is diced in larger, or bite, sizes. When canned fruits are used, add them to oranges, grapefruit, diced unpeeled apples, or other fresh fruits. Combine the fruits, sweeten slightly, and allow to stand at least 15 minutes before serving so that the flavors blend. When rose-hip extract or fresh or canned guavas are available, add them for additional vitamin C. If calcium requirements are not fully met, add calcium-rich lemon juice (p. 239).

## FRUIT CUP

Wash and cut into fourths:

**6 or 8 fresh or canned apricots**

Add:

| | |
|---|---|
| 1 or 2 diced oranges | 2 or 3 tablespoons calcium-rich |
| 1 sliced banana or 2 sliced peaches | lemon juice |
| ½ cup strawberries or other fresh | sugar to taste |
| or canned berries | |

Mix well and set in refrigerator; serve in sherbet glasses.

*Variations:*
Use any combination of fresh and canned fruit, follow suggestions for fruit appetizers (p. 261).

Add ½ cup broken walnuts, pecans, chopped almonds, or other nuts.
Add ½ to 1 cup moist shredded coconut or 6 to 8 marshmallows cut
into quarters with scissors.

**Fruit cup with custard:** Prepare fruit cup using 3 cups fruit, such as
diced canned pineapple, fresh unpeeled pears or red apples, seedless grapes
or canned cherries; add ¼ pound quartered marshmallows; put into a
shallow dish, cover top with soft custard (p. 493), using half the recipe
and seasoning custard with 2 tablespoons lemon juice; let chill overnight
until marshmallows absorb fruit juices; cut into cubes and serve.

Commercial gelatin desserts supply no vitamins or minerals; yet
they readily satisfy the appetite. They contain coloring, flavoring,
a small amount of inadequate protein, about 90 per cent water as
they are usually prepared, and at least 100 calories of sugar per
serving. In order to make them nutritionally valuable, generous
amounts of fruits should be added. One package of flavored gelatin will hold 2 cups or more of diced fruits and nuts.

## FRUIT GELATIN

Heat to boiling:

### 1¾ cups water

Dissolve in water and stir well:

### 1 package raspberry gelatin

Chill until it starts to congeal; add:

| | |
|---|---|
| ½ cup canned cherries, cut in half | 1 cup sliced peaches |
| ½ cup seedless grapes | ¼ cup walnuts or pecans |

Stir well, pour into chilled ring mold, chill until firm; unmold and serve
with center filled with whipped evaporated milk flavored with vanilla or
whipped cream.

*Variations:*

Put gelatin in loaf bread pan, unmold, slice; or mold in flat baking dish,
chill, cut into cubes.

Use lime, lemon, orange, or other fruit gelatins; instead of water use
pineapple, apple, or clear grapefruit juice.

Add guavas or 2 or 3 tablespoons each rose-hip extract and calcium-rich lemon juice, using juice or extract instead of equal amount of water.

Use sliced or diced bananas, apricots, plums, fresh or frozen berries, pears, or other fruits instead of those suggested; the total amount of fruit should measure 2 to 2¼ cups.

## FROZEN FRUIT PURÉES OR JUICES

Use canned puréed fruit or applesauce; or beat soft fresh, stewed, or canned apricots, pitted plums, prunes, peaches, or other fruits until puréed; or use plum, loganberry, pineapple, grapefruit, or other fruit juices. If purées or juices are extremely tart, add a small amount of sugar; if they are sweet, add 2 or 3 tablespoons lemon juice.

Put into freezing compartment:

**2 or 3 cups fruit juice or purée**

Stir or beat 3 or 4 times as juice or purée freezes; serve in sherbet glass with meat course. Serve frozen applesauce or pineapple juice with ham or pork; plum, peach, or apricot with beef; apricot, grapefruit juice, or loganberry juice with lamb.

*Variations:*

If frozen purée or juice is desired for dessert, sweeten to taste, using more sugar than for a meat accompaniment.

Add calcium-rich lemon juice or rose-hip extract.

Season applesauce or prune purée with a dash of nutmeg or cinnamon; add 1 drop red coloring to applesauce.

Shake with juice or beat into purée ¼ cup powdered milk; sweeten to taste with sugar and serve for dessert.

## FRUIT SNOW

Heat to boiling:

**1 cup apple, apricot, plum, prune, peach, or other fruit purée**

Meanwhile beat until stiff:

**2 egg whites**

Fold egg whites into hot fruit; add **sugar and lemon juice** to taste. Cool slowly, then pour into serving dishes, chill, and serve.

*Variations:*

Add before folding in egg whites ½ cup broken or chopped walnuts, pecans, or other nuts.

**Fruit whip:** Chill ½ cup evaporated milk in ice tray until crystals form around edges; whip; add **4 tablespoons each lemon juice, powdered milk, and sugar, 1 teaspoon vanilla or ¼ teaspoon lemon extract;** fold into **2 cups thick sweetened and chilled fruit purée,** such as prune, plum, apple, apricot, or into mashed chilled bananas; prepare no earlier than ½ hour before time to serve. Add 1 or 2 drops red coloring to apple whip, green coloring and diced candied ginger to pear whip.

*Fruit sherbet:* Freeze any fruit purée slowly to a soft mush and then fold in whipped evaporated milk; finish freezing until firm.

## CHAPTER 23

## MAKE CANNING AND PICKLING YOUR HOBBY

Unless you have a freezing compartment sufficiently large to hold fruits for daily use throughout the winter, by all means can quantities of fruits. Whether you grow your own fruits or must purchase them, home-canned ones are far less expensive and usually much more delicious than commercially canned fruits. When gallons of fruits and fruit juices are stored away, larger quantities are eaten and a higher degree of health is assured. Put apricots first on your list of "musts"; the vitamins A and $B_2$, copper, and iron which they supply are needed during the winter months. Hardy apricot trees which can withstand Canadian winters have been developed. If you live in a rural district or if your back yard has space available, by all means set out a few of these trees and grow sufficient apricots for home canning. Do not assume, however, that plums, pears, apples, and fruits low in vitamin A are not worth canning; they offer other vitamins and many minerals. Fruits are so easy to can that dozens of quarts may be put up in a single day.

Do not overlook canning quantities of fruit juices and sauces. Use small fruits and those which are too ripe to be attractive when canned whole; the strawberries too small to bother to stem; small or unattractive cherries, apricots, peaches, and pears. Such fruits can be purchased at wholesale markets at little cost; when home-grown, they are frequently not used. I make it a point to go to the wholesale market late on Saturday mornings. The ripe fruit, which is just right for canning but which cannot be held over the week-end, can often be purchased at a fraction of the usual cost.

Make sauce not only of apples but of pears, peaches, nectarines, apricots, and plums. Do not miss making delicious loganberry juice or luscious golden apricot purée; or guava juice, which

472

supplies approximately ten times the amount of vitamin C in orange juice. Can enough juices so that each member of your family may have a glass or two daily; serve juices at any meal or midmeal. Use both juices and purées in making gelatin desserts, ice creams, appetizers, milkshakes and other milk drinks, and punches, as well as tart sherbets and aspics to accompany meats. Juices and sauces are excellent to have on hand at any time, especially during illness. Few foods surpass them if you must plan meals for a baby, an elderly person, or anyone who must stay on a smooth diet. When fruits are used for making jams and jellies, their nutritive value is counterbalanced by the excessive amounts of refined sugar added to them. It seems strange to me that applesauce, which is really a purée, should be so popular and other fruit purées rarely served. I use quantities of all fruit purées, particularly apricot and plum. One of my favorite ways of eating wheat germ is to stir it into a dish of apricot purée. All sauces I expect to use during the year I can at one time.

The same rules for preserving nutrients in cooking fruits and vegetables should be applied in canning. The foods should be washed without a moment's unnecessary soaking. Loosen the skins of peaches and tomatoes by steaming them a few minutes rather than by soaking them in hot water. Do not use lye to remove the skins of peaches. It not only destroys vitamin C but may cause the fruit to become so alkaline that botulinus, or fatal food poisoning, may develop. Above all, avoid adding soda to any fruit. The atrocious recipes recommending that figs be soaked in soda have been responsible for deaths from botulinus throughout the country. Whenever it is possible, chill the fruit before cutting it. Syrup which is to be poured over the fruit should be boiling, so that enzymes will be quickly destroyed. The initial heating should be as rapid as possible.

Space permits only a short discussion of canning and pickling here. More detailed instructions and the directions for canning vegetables and meats may be obtained from your State Department of Agriculture. Many directions for canning which have been published have proved unreliable and have resulted in serious accidents and deaths; it is safest to rely on those put out by the government.

## CANNING JUICES AND SAUCES

The purpose of cold-pack canning, or cooking the fruit in the jars, is to prevent the fruit from mashing by being handled after it is cooked. When mashing is not a problem, the easiest method of canning fruits is the open-kettle method in which the juice or cooked fruit is brought to a boil, poured into clean jars, and sealed. Since the pasteurization point is 140° F., the jar is sterilized by the hot fruit or juice.

Tart sauces and juices should be sweetened just before being used rather than before they are canned.

## TOMATO JUICE AND PURÉE

Purchase inexpensive tomatoes, such as small ones or irregular sizes; wash quickly, remove decayed spots, and put into a large utensil; do not peel, quarter, or remove stem ends.

Set over high heat; use a large knife and cut through many tomatoes at one time, bringing knife from one side of utensil to the other, as if cutting a pan of fudge; mash tomatoes slightly to squeeze out juice. Add:

### 1 teaspoon salt for each quart of tomatoes

If seasoned juice is desired, add celery leaves, green pepper stalks and seeds, onion tops, a few sliced carrots.

Cover utensil; keep heat high and cook until tomatoes are tender, stirring occasionally to ensure even heating.

Press tomatoes through a cone-shaped colander; collect thin juice in one utensil; change utensils and keep thick purée separate.

Bring juice to a rolling boil; set jar in pan of warm water to prevent breaking; pour boiling juice into jar to ⅛ inch of top; wipe edge of glass, adjust rubber and lid, and seal.

Invert jar to sterilize lid. Let stand in a place free from draft. Do not move the jars until cool. If screw top is used, remove ring after 24 hours.

Use purée for making sauces (p. 481); or bring to a rolling boil, stirring frequently; pour into clean jars and seal.

*Variations:*

If rose hips are available, add to tomatoes or other fruit at the beginning of cooking; add a few guavas to any fruit.

Use the same procedure in making sauces and/or juices from the following fruits: apricots, apples, plums, berries, grapes, cherries, peaches, pears, nectarines, or yellow tomatoes. Use small or especially ripe fruits not desirable for other canning. Do not remove stems from strawberries or stones from small apricots or cherries. If clear berry, plum, or grape juice is desired, strain through a cloth after passing through colander. Do not peel, core, or cut apples except to remove damaged spots. Add only enough water at the beginning of cooking to prevent sticking.

Obtain cider as soon as possible after it is made; heat quickly to destroy enzymes, bring to a rolling boil, pour into clean jars, and seal.

To can tomatoes by the open-kettle method, loosen skins by steaming over boiling water; peel, remove stem ends, quarter; cook until tender in a covered utensil, or about 10 to 15 minutes; pour into clean jars and seal.

## COLD-PACK CANNING

In cold-pack canning the uncooked fruit is packed into clean jars, hot syrup is poured over it, and the fruit is cooked in the jar. The method of cooking cold-packed fruit in the oven has proved unsafe. The dry heat penetrates so slowly that the fruit is often not sterilized. Molds frequently grow on it, which cause the fruit juices to become so alkaline that botulinus sometimes develops. The number of botulinus organisms which could cover the tip of a pin can kill a person within a few hours.

The method of cooking fruit by setting the filled jars in hot water is cumbersome and difficult. By far the easiest way to cold-pack fruit, and a substitute for the hot-water bath, is to cook it by steam. Set the jars on a rack above boiling water in any large utensil which can be tightly covered. If the steam is held in, it is the same temperature as that of boiling water. Since the jar and lid are sterilized as the fruit cooks, the jars do not need to be sterilized previously.

Do not fasten the lids tightly until after the fruit is cooked; the steam inside the jars must be allowed to escape. When the lid is tightly fastened, the steam pressure often causes the jars to break or even explode, resulting in serious accidents from flying glass and scalding liquid.

If the top of the fruit discolors, enzyme action has occurred before the fruit was cooked. When discoloration occurs after the food is canned, it indicates that the fruit was not sufficiently cooked to destroy the enzymes. If the fruit comes to the top of the jar, the syrup used is heavier than the fruit or much juice has been cooked out of the fruit, causing it to be light. These conditions do not mean that the fruit is spoiled. If the syrup becomes cloudy or mold develops, discard the fruit without tasting it. Botulinus gives no warning odor, color change, or taste.

Vary the cooking time and the syrup used according to the condition of the fruit. Use a somewhat longer cooking time when fruit is unusually solid or put into the jars so compactly that little or no hot syrup can be added. Use heavier syrup for very sour fruits or those tightly packed. Fruits may be canned without sugar and sweetened just before being used. Since sugar penetrates fruit slowly, it is more evenly distributed when added before the fruit is canned.

### COLD-PACK APRICOTS

Wash fruit quickly, cut into halves, and remove seeds, decay, and bruised parts; pack into clean jars to within 1 inch of the top. Put 3 or 4 pits in each jar for flavor.

Fill to within ½ inch of the top with boiling water or syrup; slip a silver knife down the inside edge of jar to allow liquid to be evenly distributed.

Wipe off glass edges and adjust rubber and lid; fasten lid with thumb and little finger; it must be loose enough to turn easily; if glass lid with wire clamp is used, do not spring the clamp.

Set jars on a rack above boiling water in a large utensil such as a turkey roaster, electric cooker, or washboiler; cover utensil. If lid does not fit tightly, put a towel or heavy cloth between utensil and lid, put weight on lid.

Bring water under rack to a rolling boil; start counting cooking time when water begins to boil; steam 16 minutes for pint jars, 20 minutes for quart jars, 30 minutes for half-gallon jars.

At the end of cooking period, fasten tops securely; leave jars upright; if ring tops are used, remove rings after 24 hours; store in a cool dark place.

*Variations:*

For sweet loosely packed fruits, make light syrup of 1 cup sugar to 3 cups water; make medium syrup of 1 cup sugar to 2 cups water, or heavy syrup of 1 cup each sugar and water; use heavy syrup for soft, tightly packed fruits or sour fruits.

Steam pint and quart jars of berries, precooked apples, precooked rhubarb, and small plums 15 minutes, half-gallon jars 24 minutes. Steam pints or quarts of cherries, freestone peaches, very ripe or small pears, or large plums 20 minutes, half gallons 30 minutes; steam quarts of fresh prunes, cling peaches, firm unpeeled pears, peeled grapefruit sections, and pints of tomatoes 30 minutes; half gallons of the fruits and quarts of tomatoes 40 to 45 minutes.

Follow basic recipe in canning berries, cherries, grapes, peaches, pears, and plums; loosen skins of tomatoes and peaches by steaming over boiling water. Leave high-quality pears unpeeled; put 2 or 3 pits in each jar of freestone nectarines or peaches.

**Canned apples:** Prepare 1 quart light syrup with 1 cup sugar to 1 quart water; bring to boiling; meanwhile wash, core, and remove bruised and wormy spots from apples; do not peel or touch with water after they are washed; dice, slice, or quarter and drop directly into boiling syrup; boil 4 minutes; pack into clean jars, fill with hot syrup, and steam 15 minutes; seal. Add red coloring and ½ teaspoon each cloves and cassia buds to each quart or a small piece of cinnamon as desired. Repeat the process as syrup is used, preparing only 2 or 3 pounds of apples at a time.

**Canned figs and guavas:** Figs and guavas are less acid than other fruits and should be canned with lemon juice; wash fruit, peel guavas, leave whole or slice directly into jars; pack figs without peeling them; add 4 tablespoons lemon juice for each quart jar, fill with hot syrup; steam guavas 20 minutes and figs 40 minutes for pint or quart jars. If no lemon juice is used, boil figs in syrup 4 minutes, steam 2 hours.

**Canned peppers:** Since peppers are such a rich source of vitamin C, can large amounts of them; use red bell peppers, fresh pimentos, and paprikas when available; wash, remove stem ends and seeds, cut into halves or quarters; pack into jars, add ½ teaspoon salt for each pint, fill with boiling water, and steam 55 minutes for pint or quart jars, or 40 minutes at 5 pounds pressure; or add 2 tablespoons vinegar and steam without pressure 40 minutes. If it is desirable to peel peppers, roast at 450° F. for about 6 minutes, or until peel loosens, or fry in deep fat at 400° F. for 2 minutes and chill immediately by dipping into ice water. Peel and can chili peppers without removing stem ends or seeds; use for chili relleno (p. 207).

**Canned rhubarb:** Wash, cut into 1-inch lengths, steam with 2 tablespoons water until soft, or about 15 minutes; pack boiling hot without adding water or sugar; steam 15 minutes, seal. After opening, sweeten to taste; let stand before serving.

**Canned tomatoes:** By far the easiest way to can tomatoes is to remove stem ends, pack solidly into jars, squeezing out enough juice to fill jar; add 1 teaspoon salt per quart and steam 45 minutes for quart jars, 60 minutes for half-gallon jars. After opening a jar of tomatoes, lift off and discard skins. If peeling before canning is desired, steam the washed tomatoes over boiling water, cool slightly, and remove skins; do not immerse in either boiling or cold water; pack solidly into jars; salt but do not add water.

## FREEZING FRUITS AND VEGETABLES

It is to be hoped that every family in America will soon have facilities available so that they can freeze and store home-grown or purchased fruits and vegetables. Since this process of preserving food is relatively new, it is particularly important that methods be used which allow the maximum nutritive value to be retained.

Fruits and vegetables to be frozen should be prepared and frozen with all possible speed to prevent loss of vitamin C. Fruits which discolor easily, such as apricots, and all vegetables retain greater nutritive value and better color and flavor if they are precooked, or blanched, to destroy enzymes before being frozen. Uncooked fruit should be cut sufficiently so that it can be solidly packed without air spaces between the pieces of fruit. Crushed or puréed raw fruit, for example, has been found to retain more vitamin C than whole or halved fruit because it packs more solidly.

If you must purchase your fruits and vegetables for freezing or if you must pack them and take them some distance to a plant for quick-freezing, purchase them in the early morning and prepare them immediately. If you have your own garden and freezing unit, you may spend a lazy day, taking a long nap in the afternoon; then gather the various foods at dusk after a sunny day, when the vitamin content has been found to be at its highest, and pack and freeze them in the cool of the evening.

## PREPARATION OF FRUITS FOR FREEZING

Wash fruit quickly without soaking; peel or stem; cut as for table use, preparing only 3 to 5 cups at one time; when facilities permit, chill before washing.

Loosen skins of peaches by steaming 5 minutes over boiling water.

Sweeten fruit to taste, using approximately ¼ cup sugar to each 3 cups sliced California persimmons, guavas, very ripe apricots; ½ cup sugar for 3 cups sliced peaches, nectarines, seeded black cherries, firm apricots, or sweet berries; ¾ cup sugar for sour cherries, gooseberries, or other sour berries. Mix fruit well with sugar, let stand in refrigerator until sugar is melted.

Pack fruit in square or rectangular containers; put on lid; label and date containers; if fruit cannot be frozen immediately, keep in very cold refrigerator. Molds and bacteria may cause fruits, particularly soft berries, to spoil before they are frozen.

Place in quick-freezing unit and freeze at −20° F. or at a lower temperature; store at 0° F. or below.

Before serving let fruit thaw slowly in refrigerator; serve immediately after thawing.

*Variations:*

Instead of mixing dry sugar with fruit, prepare a heavy syrup of 3 cups sugar to 1 quart water; heat until sugar is dissolved; store in refrigerator until thoroughly chilled. Place fruit in container and fill with cold syrup to 1 inch of the top; if any fruit floats, push down into syrup before sealing package.

**Frozen cooked fruits:** For any fruit which would be more palatable cooked than raw, such as cranberries, rhubarb, gooseberries, underripe peaches or apricots, steam in 2 or 3 tablespoons water until just soft, or 4 to 8 minutes; chill thoroughly, sweeten to taste, pack, freeze, and store.

**Frozen fruit purées:** Use overripe fruits or small unattractive berries, apricots, or other fruits. Chill thoroughly and mash or crush by passing through meat grinder; turn meat grinder slowly to avoid beating air into fruit. Sweeten to taste; pack, freeze, and store. Use for making ice cream, gelatin salads or desserts, sherbets, or serve as a sauce alone or over rice, ice cream, or baked custard. Prepare applesauce or apricot purée as for canning (p. 474); chill, pack, and freeze.

**Frozen fruit juices:** Prepare tomato, berry, grape, or any fruit juice as for canning (p. 474); chill thoroughly, pack into suitable containers, freeze, and store.

**Frozen vegetables:** Prepare vegetables as if for table use; wash quickly, cut, sort for sizes; break broccoli and cauliflower into sizes suitable for serving; slice string beans; wash fresh lima beans and peas before hulling. Prepare no more than 2 pounds of vegetables at one time. Place vegetables, in a cloth bag, such as a 10-pound sugar sack; set on a rack above rapidly boiling water in utensil with tight-fitting lid; shake bag so that vegetables are loose and steam can easily surround them. Steam asparagus, string beans, lima beans, broccoli, Brussels sprouts, cauliflower, and diced zucchini or summer squash 5 minutes; steam peas 2 minutes; steam spinach and other greens and corn to be cut from cob 3 minutes; steam artichokes and corn to be frozen on cob 8 minutes. Lift bag of vegetables and immerse immediately in ice water to which are added several teaspoons of salt; do not soak longer than 1 minute, or only long enough to chill. Drain. Pack in cellophane bags, seal with a hot iron, package, freeze, and store. Except for corn on the cob, put frozen vegetables on to cook while still frozen.

**Frozen vegetable purées:** Blanch vegetables as directed above; chill in ice water, drain, and pass through food chopper, using small knife; salt to taste, pack, freeze, and store. Use for soufflés and cream soups, mix with cottage cheese, or set in gelatin for salad. Prepare large amounts of these vegetables if you must cook for a person staying on a smooth diet, an elderly person, or a small baby. Put purées on to heat while still frozen.

## TOMATO CATSUP AND SAUCES

Few recipes need revising so much as do those customarily used for making catsup, chili sauce, and barbecue sauce. Instead of laboriously peeling the tomatoes and cooking them for 3 hours or more to evaporate off gallons of delicious juice, make these sauces of purée left from canning tomato juice (p. 474). By this procedure, no sauce need be cooked longer than a few minutes.

The nutritive value of any tomato sauce can be greatly increased by sweetening it with dark or blackstrap molasses. Catsup, chili sauce, and barbecue sauce are customarily sweetened with brown sugar, which contains black molasses; hence the flavor is a familiar one. Unfortunately the calcium in the blackstrap molasses slowly neutralizes the acid of the vinegar and tomatoes; therefore the molasses should be added only after the sauce is opened. Since botulinus cannot develop in food which is exposed to air, catsups and sauces combined with blackstrap molasses are safe to use as long as the molasses is not added before they are canned. Brewers' yeast may also be added to tomato sauces and its flavor disguised; it too should be added immediately before the sauce is used.

## CHILI SAUCE

Put through the meat grinder, using large knife:

| | |
|---|---|
| ½ cup celery | ½ cup green peppers, preferably |
| ½ cup onion | green chili peppers |
| 2 cloves garlic | |

Steam vegetables in a small amount of tomato juice until onion is transparent; add:

| | |
|---|---|
| 1 quart tomato purée | 1 tablespoon minced fresh or ½ |
| ½ cup vinegar | teaspoon dried basil and/or |
| 1 teaspoon crushed black pepper-corns | orégano |

Heat to a rolling boil; pour into a clean jar and seal; invert jar to sterilize lid.

Before using, mix well with a small amount of sauce and add:

| | |
|---|---|
| 4 tablespoons blackstrap molasses | 1 to 3 tablespoons debittered brewers' yeast (optional) |

Serve with meat or fish.

*Variations:*

If purée has not been salted, add 1 teaspoon salt.

For spiced chili sauce add ½ teaspoon each cinnamon, allspice, nutmeg, ¼ teaspoon ground cloves.

**Barbecue sauce:** Prepare as in basic recipe, adding the following ground and cooked vegetables to 1 quart purée: 1 cup each celery and onions; or ½ cup each celery, onions, green or red bell pepper, chili pepper, or pimentos; or omit onions and use 1 cup celery or ½ cup each celery and sweet peppers.

*Spiced barbecue sauce:* Add ½ teaspoon each cinnamon, allspice, nutmeg, ¼ teaspoon cloves.

**Italian sauce:** Add a pinch each rosemary, marjoram, savory, basil, orégano. Serve with ravioli, fish, and meat. Vary by adding 1 cup ground unpeeled carrots with other vegetables.

**Mexican sauce:** Add ½ cup each chopped bell and green chili peppers, ½ teaspoon cumin seeds; season with orégano; if only bell peppers are used, add 1 tablespoon chili powder.

**Tomato catsup:** Omit vegetables except garlic; add ¼ teaspoon ground cayenne, 1 teaspoon each ground mace, dry mustard, crushed celery seeds.

## PICKLING

Tomatoes, peppers, cabbage, and most of the fruits and vegetables used in making pickles and relishes are rich sources of vitamin C. The vinegar used in pickling retards the action of the enzymes which destroy this vitamin. Carefully prepared pickles, therefore, can be sufficiently rich in vitamin C to make an important contribution to health, especially in localities where few fresh fruits and salads are eaten during the winter.

When vegetables are soaked, whether in brine or in ice water, many vitamins and minerals are drawn out and discarded. The purpose of such soaking is to make the ingredients crisp and to prevent shriveling when sugar is added to them. The same purpose can be accomplished without loss of nutritive value if the vegetables are soaked in the pickling liquid to which is added a small amount of a calcium salt, calcium chloride. This salt is much more effective than is table salt and is used commercially to produce the delightful crispness of small cucumber pickles and gherkins. It may be purchased inexpensively at a drugstore, or any druggist can order it for you. Fifty cents' worth will probably last you five years or longer. Not only is this salt absolutely harmless but it adds to the nutritive value of the pickles.

The amounts of refined sugar customarily added to pickles are far too high to be compatible with ideal health. By decreasing the proportion of vinegar, as I have in the following recipes, less sugar is needed to overcome tartness. Try to develop a taste for tart rather than oversweet pickles.

Pickles and relishes are easy to make and are delightful accompaniments to almost any meat course. Do not fail to put up many jars of them.

Since peppers are one of the richest known sources of vitamin C, put up as many of them as you can. Use them in salads, aspics, appetizers, in seasoning meats and meat extenders, and in every way possible. Do not waste a drop of the liquid used in canning them; add it to aspics, juice appetizers, and sauces. Since the vitamin C content doubles as peppers ripen, can the red, or ripe, peppers in preference to green ones whenever they are available.

## PICKLED BELL PEPPERS, PIMENTOS, PAPRIKAS, AND OTHER SWEET PEPPERS

Bring to boiling the estimated amount of liquid needed, using the following proportion:

**1 cup vinegar**                  **1 cup water**

Remove stems and seeds from:

**red or green bell peppers, fresh pimentos, paprikas, or other peppers**

Cut peppers into halves or thirds and drop into boiling liquid; simmer 5 minutes and pack firmly into pint or quart jars; add to each quart:

**1 teaspoon salt**             **1 teaspoon sugar**

Finish filling jars with hot liquid; seal and store.

*Variations:*

Add to each jar ¼ bay leaf and 1 small clove garlic.

To remove skin from pimentos, paprikas, or fresh chili peppers, sear with high heat under broiler; wrap quickly in a towel, cool, and peel; or can as directed above and remove skin before using.

## BEET RELISH

Shred enough chilled unpeeled raw beets to make:

**4 cups when tightly packed**

Combine and heat to boiling:

**1 cup vinegar**             **1 to 3 tablespoons sugar**
**1 cup water**                **2 teaspoons salt**

Add beets to liquid, simmer 5 minutes; add and stir well:

**¼ to ½ cup ground horseradish**

Pack into clean jars and seal.

*Variations:*

Use 2 cups beets and 2 cups finely shredded carrots, cauliflower, cabbage, or ground broccoli.

Add 1 minced clove garlic and ¼ crushed bay leaf.


## RIPE TOMATO RELISH

Put through meat grinder, using largest knife:

| | |
|---|---|
| 6 ripe unpeeled tomatoes | 3 green or red bell peppers or pimentos, paprikas, or green chili peppers |
| 4 stalks celery | |
| 2 large onions or 4 leeks | |

Squeeze the juices from the ground vegetables and keep for immediate use.

Mix well and bring to boiling:

| | |
|---|---|
| 1 pint cider vinegar | 1 teaspoon freshly ground black peppercorns |
| ¼ cup mustard seeds | |
| 2 tablespoons salt | ½ teaspoon paprika |
| 2 tablespoons white or brown sugar | |

Add vegetables to boiling liquid, simmer 10 minutes without covering, pack into clean jars, and seal.

*Variations:*

Substitute green tomatoes for ripe; use ¼ cup sugar and add 1 tablespoon cinnamon stick or cassia buds, 1 teaspoon whole cloves; tie spices in a cheesecloth bag if you prefer.

Add 2 cups finely chopped green or purple cabbage to ripe or green tomato relish.

If sweeter relishes are desired, add blackstrap molasses to taste just before using; do not add molasses before canning.

Add to ripe or green tomato relish 1 cup raisins or currants; simmer 10 minutes and add 2 whole oranges ground with 1 lemon. Seal immediately.

Omit tomatoes and add 4 small ground cucumbers.

**Broccoli relish:** Use only 3 large tomatoes; add 4 ground stalks of broccoli.

**Cabbage relish:** Omit tomatoes and mustard seeds; add 1 finely shredded head cabbage, 1 teaspoon turmeric.

**Cauliflower relish:** Instead of the tomatoes grind and add 1 cauliflower and 2 to 4 carrots.

**Celery-horseradish relish:** Use white mustard seeds; increase celery to 2 cups when ground; add ½ cup horseradish, 2 teaspoons each whole cloves, cinnamon bark, allspice berries; stir in horseradish immediately before putting into jars.

**Cucumber relish:** Omit tomatoes and paprika; add 4 ground large cucumbers, ½ cup ground horseradish; increase sugar to ¼ cup.

**Corn relish:** Add 2 cups fresh corn to relish 2 minutes before putting into jars.

**Pepper relish:** Omit tomatoes and celery; use 6 green and 6 red peppers.

**Purple cabbage relish:** Omit tomatoes, celery, mustard seeds; instead of bell peppers use 4 fresh or canned pimentos; add 2 tablespoons celery seeds, 1 large or 2 small heads purple cabbage, ground or finely shredded.


## APPLE AND TOMATO CHUTNEY

Put through meat grinder, using large knife:

| | |
|---|---|
| 6 large ripe unpeeled tomatoes | 1 green or red bell pepper, pimento, |
| 6 red unpeeled apples | or paprika |
| 4 small onions | 1 cup seeded or seedless raisins |

Meanwhile boil together 5 minutes:

| | |
|---|---|
| 1½ cups white vinegar | 2 teaspoons salt |
| 2 tablespoons pickling spices tied in cloth | ¼ cup brown sugar |

Add fruits and vegetables to hot liquid, simmer 10 minutes, put into clean jars, and seal.

*Variations:*

Add ½ cup finely ground mint leaves; use white sugar; serve with lamb or mutton.

Add 1 cup ground or finely chopped celery.

**Apple chutney:** Omit tomatoes; use 8 to 10 apples, ripe bell pepper or pimento; add 2 tablespoons mustard seeds.

**Peach chutney:** Omit tomatoes and add pulp of 6 large cling peaches, or omit both tomatoes and apples and use 8 to 10 peaches; peel peaches by steaming over boiling water.

## CUCUMBER PICKLES

Wash cucumbers thoroughly with a cloth; combine in a pottery bowl or earthenware jar:

2 cups vinegar
1 cup water
1 tablespoon salt
¾ teaspoon calcium chloride

3 pounds small whole cucumbers, or as many as can be covered by liquid

Let soak overnight.
Drain liquid into saucepan and add:

4 tablespoons white or brown sugar
2 or 3 drops green coloring

seasonings suggested in variations, tied in cloth bag

Bring to boiling and add:

cucumbers

Simmer 10 minutes without boiling; pack into clean jars and seal.

*Variations:*

Add any of the following groups of seasonings: 1½ tablespoons mixed pickling spices; 1 tablespoon each white mustard seeds and crushed white peppercorns; 1 crushed bay leaf, 1 clove garlic, 2 whole cayenne peppers; 1 teaspoon each whole cloves and allspice berries, 1 stick cinnamon bark or 1 tablespoon cassia buds; 1 tablespoon each mustard seeds and cloves, 1 whole cayenne.

Cut cucumbers in half lengthwise if they are 3 or 4 inches long; cut larger cucumbers into fourths lengthwise or into chunks 1 inch long.

If liquid is left after canning pickles, add sliced cucumbers or chopped mixed vegetables, simmer 10 minutes, and seal.

*In the following variations, soak ingredients overnight in vinegar, water, calcium chloride, and salt in proportions given in basic recipe; add spices to vinegar; follow exact procedure of basic recipe except as noted.*

**Bread-and-butter pickles:** Use 2 quarts sliced cucumbers, 2 large sliced onions; add 3 tablespoons mustard seeds, 1 tablespoon celery seeds and ¼ teaspoon cayenne.

**Cauliflower pickles:** Break 1 small head cauliflower into pieces, dice stalk; add 2 tablespoons mustard seeds and 1 teaspoon ground turmeric. Vary by adding 2 sliced red or green bell peppers and/or 1 cup pickling onions or diced cucumbers.

**Dill pickles:** After soaking, put cucumbers directly into jars; omit sugar; heat with vinegar for each quart of pickles. 1 large sprig of dill or 1 tablespoon dill seeds, ½ teaspoon mustard seeds, ½ teaspoon crushed white peppercorns.

**Gherkins:** After soaking, pack into pint jars; add ¼ cup vegetable oil and 1 small clove garlic; heat liquid with ½ teaspoon each mustard seeds and crushed white peppercorns for each pint.

*Small onions:* Use same procedure as for gherkins.

**Mustard pickles:** Use large cucumbers; slice in strips lengthwise; add 2 sliced onions; mix together 2 tablespoons each whole-wheat flour and powdered mustard, 1 teaspoon each turmeric and celery seeds, and a little liquid used for soaking; stir into remaining liquid, cook 5 minutes before adding cucumbers.

*Mixed mustard pickles:* Use 1 cup each sliced cucumbers, thinly sliced carrots, whole pickling onions, chopped green tomatoes, chopped green and red bell peppers, cauliflower broken into small pieces; proceed as for mustard pickles.

**Pickled onions:** Omit cucumbers and use 1 quart pickling onions; add 1 tablespoon mixed pickling spices.

**Pickled watermelon rind:** Peel rind and dice into 1-inch cubes, using 4 to 6 cups, or as much as can be covered with liquid given in basic recipe; after soaking, add 1 to 2 teaspoons cloves and 1 stick cinnamon bark, and simmer until rind is transparent. If a tart pickle is desired, add ½ teaspoon mustard seeds; if a sweet pickle is preferred, increase sugar to ¾ cup and omit table salt.

## SPICED FRUIT

Use about **4 quarts fruit.** Wash quickly and drain.
Combine and simmer 10 minutes:

| | |
|---|---|
| 2 cups vinegar | 2 teaspoons whole cloves |
| 1 cup water | 3 or 4 sticks cinnamon, or ½ ounce |
| 1 cup white or brown sugar | |

Add the amount of fruit which can be covered by liquid; simmer until tender; pack firmly into clean jars, fill to the top with liquid, and seal.

Add fresh fruit to liquid and continue until liquid is used.

*Variations:*

**Pickled beets:** Steam whole beets until tender; slice, reheat in pickling syrup containing ¼ to ½ cup sugar and 2 teaspoons salt, and seal. Vary by omitting sugar and spices; add to each quart jar of pickles 1 teaspoon salt, 1 clove garlic, ½ bay leaf, 1 cayenne pepper, 2 tablespoons vegetable oil.

**Spiced apricots, crabapples, figs, and plums:** Leave fruit whole and unpeeled; pierce skins with fork to allow steam to escape; wash figs thoroughly but do not touch with soda.

**Spiced peaches:** Use cling peaches; loosen skins by steaming over water 5 to 8 minutes; use brown sugar instead of white. If crisp pickles are desired, add ¾ teaspoon calcium chloride to vinegar and water, and soak peeled peaches overnight. When peaches are out of season, use commercially canned peaches, adding peach juice instead of water.

**Spiced pears:** If pears are large, cut in half and core; leave small pears whole without coring; do not peel.

**Spiced prunes:** If fruit is for immediate use, simmer uncooked prunes 15 minutes in 1½ cups water, ½ cup vinegar, and ½ cup blackstrap molasses; add spices. If fruit is to be sealed and held, prepare as in basic recipe.


## UNLIMITED VITAMIN C FREE FOR THE EXTRACTING


A source of vitamin C, or ascorbic acid, which is fantastic in its concentration is that of rose hips, or rose apples. Rose hips are the seed pods left after ordinary garden roses bloom. The amount of vitamin C they contain varies with the species. They have been found to average 1200 to 1800 milligrams per half cup, or about 24 to 36 times the vitamin-C potency of fresh orange juice. Some species have been found to contain 96 times the vitamin-C content of citrus juices. The amount of vitamin C which goes to waste annually from rose hips is estimated to be thousands of tons.

Just as people used to go berrying, the nutrition-conscious person goes "rose-hipping." If you do not have a rose garden or if wild roses do not grow in your neighborhood, ask a less wise neighbor if you may trim her rose bushes. The vitamin-C content is at its highest when the rose hips are red, or in the late fall, but gather them at any time when you have a chance. The vitamin can be extracted by boiling them until they are tender and letting them stand while the vitamin passes into the cooking water. Since the extract is very mild in flavor, lemon juice or vinegar must be added both to prevent enzymes from destroying the vitamin and to keep botulinus from developing.

Try to can enough rose-hip extract so that each member of your family can have at least one tablespoon daily. Add it as a routine procedure to the breakfast juice. Put a small amount into gelatin salads and desserts, appetizers, meat sauces, soups, fruit cups, and sherbets. Since vitamin C plays such an important role in maintaining the health of the teeth and gums, and in promoting resistance to infections, allergies, and diseases, the use of even a small amount of rose-hip extract throughout the winter months can contribute a great deal indeed. During a time of illness, such extract is invaluable. Put up as much of it as you possibly can.

## ROSE-HIP EXTRACT

Gather rose hips; chill; remove blossom ends, stems, and leaves; wash quickly.

Meanwhile for each cup of rose hips bring to a rolling boil:

### 1½ cups water

Add:

### 1 cup rose hips

Cover utensil and simmer 15 minutes; if fresh, mash with a fork or potato masher; if dried, run hips through the meat grinder. Let stand in a pottery utensil 24 hours.

Strain off extract, bring to a rolling boil, add 2 tablespoons lemon juice for each pint, pour into jars, and seal.

*Variations:*

If extract is not to be prepared immediately, chill rose hips quickly to inhibit enzyme action; when they are thoroughly chilled, wash quickly, pare, and pass through the meat grinder before adding to water; simmer 5 to 10 minutes. Proceed as in basic recipe.

## CHAPTER 24

## MAKE YOUR DESSERTS CONTRIBUTE
## TO HEALTH

One of the most encouraging nutritional trends of today is that many mothers serve only fruits as desserts. The less frequently oversweet desserts are made, the sooner the family comes to care little for them; an improvement in health invariably follows.

The most objectionable feature of desserts is the amount of sugar they contain. The tremendous consumption of refined sugar in America has caused untold ill health. The more refined sugar eaten, the greater the need for several of the B vitamins; yet sugar satisfies the appetite so rapidly that the more sugar eaten, the less vitamins obtained. Without adequate B vitamins, sugar cannot be completely converted into energy, the blood sugar drops below normal, and a craving for sweets results. Naturally this craving is satisfied by eating still more sugar. Thus a vicious circle occurs which becomes ever worse.

Despite this vicious circle, commercial interests on every hand urge the use of more sugar, saying that it is necessary for quick energy. They fail to point out that sugar can be obtained from almost every food one eats; that a person who eats rather heartily can obtain as much as 2 cups of sugar in the course of a single day even though he does not taste refined sugar in any form; and that the quickest energy does not come from table sugar, which must be digested before it can enter the blood, but from fruits rich in glucose and fructose, both of which pass directly into the blood.

Many desserts serve no nutritional need. Such desserts are often made merely because the career of being a housewife and mother has not been considered of as much importance as that of the professional woman; hence mothers have not received the recognition they deserve and need. By preparing a "superior" dessert they achieve a feeling of importance. For example, many women get ego gratification by making a fluffier, whiter cake than any of their friends can make. The exclamations of praise and delight which greet the serving of the fluffy white cake give these women the recognition which every normal individual craves and needs. The woman who prepares such desserts rationalizes and believes in all sincerity that she makes them merely to give pleasure to others.

When cake, usually covered with rich icing, is served at dinner, the family is tempted to overeat; possibly they omit some wholesome food in order to have room for the cake. The concentrated fat-sugar-and-starch satisfies their appetites not only temporarily but for many hours afterward. Chances are that no one has much appetite for breakfast. The children probably go to school and the older members of the family to work with little or nothing to eat. By midmorning, however, their supply of stored sugar has been used up, and they become mentally and physically sluggish, think slowly, are inefficient, and make frequent mistakes. By this time, however, they are hungry and in the absence of better food may eat a candy bar or take a soft drink; the appetite for lunch is thus partially ruined. If oversweet desserts are served at each dinner, much the same sequence may take place day after day, and the cumulative effect on health is detrimental indeed. The family's total intake of vitamins and minerals is greatly decreased; pimply skins, sallow complexions, fatigue, irritability, low resistance to colds and other infections, and possibly abnormal weight follow.

The so-called breakfast problem which causes thousands of children to go to school and adults to go to work without an adequate breakfast is not so much a breakfast problem as a problem of eating oversweet desserts at dinner. Other factors enter, of course, such as too little time to eat in the morning, but the person who is hungry enough to enjoy breakfast usually makes sure there is time to eat it.

If a mother who has prepared oversweet desserts so long that her family demands them is sincere in wishing to produce ideal health, she silently sets out to break the dessert habit. She may serve a juice or fruit appetizer, a rather filling soup or a delicious salad before the dinner course so that there will be little room left for dessert. While she is thus increasing the bulk and health value of the meal, she may plan a simple dessert such as fruit cup or apricot sauce which will not tempt one to overeat.

When you serve desserts other than fruits, make them particularly nutritious to compensate for the disadvantages they offer. Plan your desserts to meet the individual needs of your family. If you have adolescent youngsters whose need for calcium has skyrocketed because of rapid growth, serve desserts crowded with evaporated and powdered milk. If your husband does hard physical work, make your desserts supply the B vitamins needed to give him energy and endurance. If grandmother cannot chew green salads with her false teeth, let her get iron and vitamin A from a dessert containing apricots. If you, like thousands of other women, are deficient in protein, make your desserts contribute to your protein intake. Even when you prepare desserts for special occasions such as holidays, birthdays, and guest dinners, take pride in making them contribute to health.

If you are one of the hundreds of thousands of people who are overweight and who avoid nutritious foods in an attempt not to gain more, and yet reward your "sacrifice" by eating desserts, set out to break the dessert habit. When you eat appetizers, soups, salads, meats, and vegetables deliciously prepared and attractively served, little room is left for desserts. Now and probably always desserts mean calories which your body does not need and must only store as fat. When desserts tempt you, remember that the fleeting delight of taste lasts perhaps 3 minutes, whereas fat often remains on the hips or abdomen for 30 years.


### SOFT CUSTARDS

One evening when I had served soft custard for dessert, a guest remarked, "I love custards but I never have them. They are so difficult and tedious to make." A friend and I who had been testing recipes burst out laughing. That day the friend had held the stop watch, checking the cooking time, while I made one custard after another: 3 minutes 45 seconds; 4 minutes 15 seconds, and so on. No custard had required 5 minutes to cook. If you make custards, by all means use a thermometer and make them quickly and safely. For a hurry-up dessert which can be chilled while dinner is being eaten, few desserts can compare with soft custards.

The most nutritious soft or baked custards—and junkets, ice creams, and other desserts—are those sweetened partly or wholly with dark molasses. Try them, particularly if you have children in the family.

## FIVE-MINUTE CUSTARD

Combine in a *metal* saucepan and stir well:

| | |
|---|---|
| ¼ cup sugar | ⅛ teaspoon salt |
| ½ cup powdered milk | |

Add and beat until smooth:

| | |
|---|---|
| ½ cup fresh milk | 2 whole eggs or 4 egg yolks |

Stir in after beating:

| | |
|---|---|
| 1½ cups fresh milk | few drops egg coloring |

Fasten cooking thermometer to side of saucepan; cook over moderate heat, stirring constantly until temperature reaches 175° F., or about 4 minutes; remove from heat and chill.

Before serving stir in **1 teaspoon vanilla.**

*Variations:*

Use 2½ cups fresh milk and add ¼ to ½ cup soy grits; add uncooked grits before cooking the custard, or toasted or quick-cooking grits just before serving.

Add 2 to 8 tablespoons wheat germ before serving.

If rich custard is desired, use 1 large can (1½ cups) evaporated milk and ½ cup fresh milk.

Before serving stir into custard ½ to 1 cup sliced canned or sweetened fresh apricots or peaches; well-drained crushed pineapple; sliced bananas; or fresh, frozen, or canned berries; omit vanilla or decrease to ½ teaspoon; add ½ teaspoon lemon extract with bananas and pineapple.

**Almond custard:** Omit vanilla; add ¼ teaspoon almond extract and ¼ cup chopped toasted almonds or soy grits.

**Caramel custard:** Use 3 tablespoons sugar and add 1 tablespoon dark or blackstrap molasses, or use 2 tablespoons each sugar and molasses, or omit sugar and add ¼ cup molasses; flavor with ½ teaspoon maple, brandy, or rum flavoring.

**Coconut custard:** Add ½ cup shredded coconut or coconut meal to warm custard; garnish servings with toasted coconut.

**Date custard:** Use 2 tablespoons sugar; add ½ cup chopped dates before serving.

**Eggnog custard:** Omit vanilla and add 1 tablespoon rum, brandy, or whiskey.

**Floating island:** Use 2 egg yolks and 1 whole egg in custard; beat 2 egg whites until stiff, add gradually 3 tablespoons sugar, ½ teaspoon vanilla. Drop meringue from large spoon onto surface of hot water in flat baking dish; bake in slow oven at 300° F. for 25 minutes. Put chilled custard in attractive bowl, transfer meringues on top. Vary by coloring meringues or sprinkling with colored coconut. Floating island is easy to make and delightful to look at. It is one of my favorite desserts.

**Lemon custard:** Omit vanilla and ¼ cup fresh milk; increase sugar to ½ cup. When custard has chilled, add ¼ cup lemon juice and 1 teaspoon grated lemon rind.

**Orange custard:** Omit vanilla; add orange coloring, 1 teaspoon orange flavoring, and/or grated rind of 1 or 2 oranges. This is a delicious custard.

Whenever I think of baked custards, I chuckle at a ridiculous scene which occurred when I was testing the following recipes. Three of us, all reasonably good cooks and certainly experienced ones, would pierce the custard with a knife, gaze at the knife earnestly and seriously, then argue violently about the degree of doneness. If we disagreed, surely other women would do likewise. When it dawned on me to let the meat thermometer solve the problem, we were unanimous in saying perfection had been attained. Since the custard continues to cook while it is cooling, the texture is easily ruined by slight overbaking.

## BAKED CUSTARD

Combine and beat slightly:

| | |
|---|---|
| ¼ cup sugar stirred with | 3 whole eggs or 6 yolks |
| ½ cup powdered milk | ½ cup fresh milk |
| ⅛ teaspoon salt | 1 teaspoon vanilla |

When mixture is smooth, add and stir:

| | |
|---|---|
| 1½ cups fresh milk | few drops egg coloring |

Pour into a shallow greased baking dish or custard cups; sprinkle with nutmeg; set meat thermometer in 1 cup or insert when custard is almost.

done. Bake in a slow oven at 300° F. for about 40 minutes, or until center of custard is 175° F. and margin is 190° F. If baking dish is used, cut into squares to serve.

*Variations:*

For fluffy custard use whole eggs, fold in stiffly beaten whites sweetened with 2 tablespoons sugar; serve hot.

To shorten baking time, heat 1½ cups milk to lukewarm; add to other ingredients.

Use 2 tablespoons each sugar and blackstrap or dark molasses; add 4 to 8 tablespoons wheat germ with ¼ teaspoon salt; or add ½ cup broken nuts, chopped dates, raisins, or shredded coconut.

Cover bottom of baking dish or custard cups with sweetened fresh or canned peaches, apricots, pears, or well-drained pineapple slices; decrease vanilla to ¾ teaspoon. Vary custard with pears by omitting vanilla and adding 3 tablespoons diced candied or preserved ginger.

Omit vanilla; use 2⅓ cups milk; add ½ teaspoon almond flavoring and ⅓ cup soy grits.

My sisters and I were brought up to be extremely thrifty (my mother's maiden name was McBroom). Whenever stale bread accumulated, bread pudding was served so inevitably that our name for it became "Duty." I suspect other families feel much the same about this somewhat plebeian but nevertheless delicious dish.

## BREAD PUDDING

Combine and beat until smooth:

| | |
|---|---|
| ⅓ cup sugar stirred with | ½ cup fresh milk |
| ½ cup powdered milk | 2 whole eggs or 4 egg yolks |
| ⅛ teaspoon salt | 1 teaspoon vanilla |

When smooth, add:

| | |
|---|---|
| 4 or 5 cups diced stale whole-wheat bread | 2½ cups fresh milk few drops egg coloring |

Pour into baking dish brushed with oil or melted fat; sprinkle top with nutmeg, cinnamon, or sugar. Bake at 325° F. for 45 minutes, or until temperature, taken by inserting meat thermometer in center, is 175° F. Serve with sauce of sweetened diced fresh or canned fruit.

*Variations:*

Stir into pudding before baking ½ cup of any of the following: raisins, chopped dates, shredded coconut, broken walnuts or pecans; or use 3½ cups fresh milk and add ½ cup soy grits.

**Carrot pudding:** Omit vanilla; use 2 cups fresh milk; instead of bread use 2 cups shredded raw carrots; add ⅓ cup dark or blackstrap molasses, 1 teaspoon cinnamon, and ½ teaspoon each salt, nutmeg, allspice. Bake as in basic recipe.

**Cottage cheese bread pudding:** Omit vanilla; beat 1 cup cottage cheese with eggs; add grated rind of 1 lemon, ¼ teaspoon lemon extract, 2 tablespoons lemon juice.

**Date-nut bread pudding:** Add ½ cup each chopped dates and broken walnuts or pecans.

**Molasses bread pudding:** Use 2 tablespoons sugar; add ¼ cup dark molasses and grated rind of 1 lemon; sprinkle with raisins or coconut.

**Peanut-butter bread pudding:** Before cutting bread into cubes spread generously with peanut butter.

## RICE PUDDING

Combine and beat until smooth:

| | |
|---|---|
| ⅓ cup sugar stirred with | ½ cup fresh milk |
| ½ cup powdered milk | 2 whole eggs or 4 yolks |
| ¼ teaspoon salt | 1½ teaspoons vanilla |

Add and stir well:

| | |
|---|---|
| 2 cups fresh milk | 2 cups cooked brown or all-vitamin rice |

Pour into an oiled baking dish; sprinkle with nutmeg. Bake in slow oven at 325° F. for 30 minutes, or until temperature in center of pudding, taken with a meat thermometer, is 175° F. Stir once or twice during baking.

*Variations:*

Add ½ cup of one or more of the following: raisins, chopped dates, shredded coconut, broken walnuts or pecans; or add ¼ to ½ cup wheat germ or soy grits and use ½ teaspoon salt.

Use 3 tablespoons each sugar and dark molasses or omit sugar and sweeten with ⅓ cup molasses.

Poor-man's rice pudding: Omit eggs; use ½ cup uncooked rice and 3 or 4 cups fresh milk; bake in a slow oven at 300° F. for 3 hours. Stir occasionally during baking. Sweeten with sugar or molasses. Add raisins or nuts as desired.

## APPLE BETTY

Mix together:

| | |
|---|---|
| 1 cup whole-wheat-bread crumbs | 3 tablespoons melted butter-flavored fat |
| ½ cup wheat germ | |

Core and slice:

3 or 4 juicy unpeeled apples

Add to apples and mix:

| | |
|---|---|
| ½ to ¾ cup brown sugar | 1 teaspoon cinnamon |
| pinch of salt | |

Fill buttered casserole with alternate layers of apple mixture and crumbs. If apples are dry, add:

¼ cup water or water and lemon juice

Sprinkle top with **nutmeg;** cover casserole and bake in moderate oven at 375° F. for 30 minutes; remove cover and bake 10 minutes longer, or until brown. Serve with top milk.

*Variations:*

Add ½ cup raisins or broken walnuts, pecans, or roasted almonds; or add soy grits and 1 teaspoon black-walnut flavoring or ½ teaspoon almond extract.

Instead of apples use 1½ cups fresh or canned apricots, sliced peaches, pears, or pitted stewed prunes; add ¾ cup water or fruit juice; decrease sugar to 2 tablespoons if sweetened canned fruit is used. Bake uncovered 25 minutes.

Use 2 cups sliced apples, 1 cup steamed pitted prunes, ½ cup prune juice; bake as in basic recipe.

**Apple crisp:** Spread sliced apples on an oiled flat baking dish; add ¼ cup water; combine ¼ cup each white and brown sugar, whole-wheat pastry flour, wheat germ or quick-cooking rolled oats, and melted fat; crumble and sprinkle over top of apples with 1 teaspoon cinnamon.

The trick of whipping evaporated milk easily is to chill it in an ice tray until it is partially frozen.

## MARSHMALLOW CREAM

Beat until stiff:

½ cup chilled evaporated milk

Add and beat slightly:

¼ cup powdered milk                  2 tablespoons each sugar and
1 teaspoon vanilla                   lemon juice

Cut into eighths with wet scissors and drop into whipped milk:

10 or 12 marshmallows

Add:

1 cup drained crushed pineapple      6 quartered maraschino or candied
½ cup broken walnuts or pecans       cherries

Stir until all ingredients are combined; place in sherbet glasses; garnish each with a whole cherry or nut meat. Prepare no earlier than 2 hours before serving. This is an excellent dessert to prepare when time is limited.

*Variations:*

Omit cherries and add ¼ cup shredded coconut, toasted soy grits, raisins, chopped dates, or diced banana.

Instead of pineapple use 1 cup of any of the following: diced bananas; fresh sliced or canned apricots or peaches; fresh or frozen berries; thick applesauce or prune pulp; use peanuts with applesauce or prune pulp; omit sugar if sweetened canned or frozen fruit is used.

**Rice cream:** Use ¼ cup sugar; instead of marshmallows add 1 cup cooked brown or all-vitamin rice to basic recipe or any variation.

## JUNKET

Combine and beat or shake until smooth:

½ cup fresh milk                     1 teaspoon vanilla
⅓ cup powdered milk                  pinch of salt
3 tablespoons sugar                  1 drop food coloring

Add and heat until these ingredients are lukewarm, or 110° F.:

**1½ cups fresh milk**

Meanwhile dissolve 1 rennet, or junket, tablet in 1 tablespoon water; add dissolved tablet to warm milk, stir no longer than 10 seconds, and pour immediately into sherbet glasses; do not move glasses until junket is firmly set, or about 10 minutes.

Chill; sprinkle with **shredded coconut, finely diced citron, or broken nuts.**

*Variations:*

Use 2 tablespoons sugar and 1 tablespoon dark or blackstrap molasses; add ½ teaspoon maple, rum, brandy, or black-walnut flavoring; or omit sugar and sweeten to taste with molasses.

Omit vanilla and flavor to taste with almond, raspberry, strawberry, banana, lemon, maple, or other extracts; vary food coloring with flavorings.

Before adding junket tablet stir into milk ½ cup grapenuts or graham-cracker crumbs.

Since the fillings for meringue-cream pies (p. 534), chiffon-cream pies (p. 504), fresh-fruit pies (p. 535), and ten-minute pies (p. 536) can also be served as puddings, only one pudding recipe is given here.

The less nutritious prepared puddings have gained popularity because of their simplicity and deliciousness. If you use these puddings, increase their nutritive value by adding powdered milk.


## PREPARED PUDDINGS

Mix well *in a metal utensil:*

**1 package prepared pudding          ½ cup powdered milk**

Add a small amount at a time and stir until smooth:

**2½ cups fresh milk**

Cook slowly over direct heat, stirring constantly until mixture is thick, or about 4 minutes; remove from heat, cool slightly, and add:

**1 teaspoon vanilla (optional)**

Pour into serving dishes and chill.

*Variations:*

Stir ½ cup broken walnuts, pecans, or other nuts into pudding after removing from heat.

Beat 1 or 2 eggs slightly with other ingredients before cooking; do not allow pudding to boil.

Fold ½ cup whipped evaporated milk into pudding when cooled.

**Cake filling:** Make pudding with 2 cups fresh milk; add 1 tablespoon each sugar and margarine or butter. Use as filling between layers of cake and/or as substitute for icing. Add diced bananas, chopped dates, sweetened fresh fruit, or nuts as desired.

**Fruit pudding:** Prepare vanilla pudding with 1½ cups fresh milk; after cooling add ½ to 1 cup drained crushed pineapple, sliced strawberries, or sweetened apricots or peaches.

**Pie filling:** Add 2 egg yolks to pudding; do not boil; pour into crumb crust or baked pastry shell; make meringue (p. 533) of egg whites.

**Yogurt pudding:** Prepare pudding with 1½ cups fresh milk; cool and stir in 1 cup thick yogurt.

## MARSHMALLOW SPONGE

Heat to simmering in a *covered, metal utensil:*

**1 cup fresh milk**                          **pinch of salt**

Cut into quarters with wet scissors and drop into milk:

### 1 pound (about 40) marshmallows

Stir until marshmallows are dissolved, or about 2 minutes; remove from heat, *cover*, and cool, stirring occasionally; do not chill.

Meanwhile place **graham-cracker crumbs** ¼ inch deep in flat baking dish, ice tray, square mold, or 9-inch pie pan; sprinkle generously with **cinnamon.**

Whip until stiff:

### 1 cup chilled evaporated milk

Add and whip slightly:

**½ cup powdered milk**                    **2 teaspoons vanilla**
**2 tablespoons lemon juice**

Fold whipped milk into cooled marshmallow mixture and pour into mold; sprinkle with **graham-cracker crumbs and cinnamon.**

Chill, cut into squares or wedges, and serve.

The usual variety of sponges in which flavored gelatins are beaten after they have started to congeal offer almost no nutritive value. The sponges made by folding beaten uncooked egg whites into the whipped gelatin probably cause egg allergies, skin rashes, and unrecognized biotin deficiencies. If both evaporated and powdered milk are used in making sponges, the equivalent of a quart or more of fresh milk may be added, yet the flavor remains delicious.

A friend who "simply couldn't stand the taste of evaporated milk" acted as the final judge of all desserts containing this valuable product. Although some of the recipes had to be changed to please her, she pronounced each final product delicious and the flavor of the milk completely disguised.

## STRAWBERRY SPONGE

Combine and stir well:

1 cup boiling water                    1 package strawberry gelatin

Cool by adding:

¾ cup cold water

Chill until gelatin starts to congeal. Meanwhile beat until stiff:

¾ cup chilled evaporated milk

Add and beat slightly:

2 tablespoons lemon juice              ½ teaspoon strawberry flavoring
½ cup powdered milk                       (optional)

Fold whipped milk into gelatin with 1 cup sliced and sweetened fresh or frozen strawberries. Pour into mold and chill until set.

*Variations:*

Omit strawberries from sponge; pour sponge into ring mold; unmold and fill center with sliced and sweetened or frozen strawberries.

Use raspberry gelatin; fold in fresh, canned, or frozen raspberries; if canned berries are used, substitute juice for part of the water.

**Banana sponge:** Use lemon gelatin; fold in with whipped milk 1 cup mashed bananas; add 2 tablespoons sugar.

**Gelatin chiffon pies:** Prepare basic recipe or any variation; pour into pie plate brushed with soft margarine or butter and sprinkled with cereal, cracker, or cookie crumbs; sprinkle top with crumbs. Or mold gelatin in a 9-inch baked-crumb or pastry shell.

**Lemon sponge:** Use lemon gelatin; instead of ¾ cup water cool with ½ cup lemon juice; whip 1½ cups (1 large can) evaporated milk and fold in powdered milk; sprinkle square mold or buttered 9-inch pie plate with cereal, cookie, or cracker crumbs; pour gelatin over crumbs and sprinkle top with crumbs; cut into cubes or wedges and serve.

**Lime-pineapple sponge:** Use lime gelatin; stir in 1 cup well-drained crushed pineapple with whipped milk; use juice from pineapple to cool gelatin instead of part of the water.

**Orange sponge:** Use orange gelatin; add grated rind of 1 orange and/or 1 teaspoon orange flavoring; fill center of ring mold with sweetened orange sections.

**Yogurt sponge:** Omit evaporated milk and lemon juice; fold into gelatin 1 cup thick, or commercial, yogurt; prepare as in basic recipe or any variation. Yogurt is particularly delicious with the crushed-pineapple variation.


## ORANGE WHIP

Put into saucepan:

| | |
|---|---|
| ½ cup strained orange juice | 1 tablespoon unflavored gelatin |

Soak 5 minutes, dissolve by heating slowly; cool slightly and add:

| | |
|---|---|
| ½ cup sugar | grated rind 1 large orange |
| 2 tablespoons lemon juice | 1¼ cups strained orange juice |

Chill until gelatin starts to congeal. Meanwhile beat until stiff:

¾ cup chilled evaporated milk

Add to this and beat slightly:

½ cup powdered milk

Fold milk into gelatin; pour into square mold, chill, cut into cubes, and serve with sweetened diced oranges; or pour into ring mold and serve with center filled with sweetened orange sections or diced mixed fruits.

*Variations:*

Omit powdered and evaporated milk; beat congealed gelatin before pouring into mold; serve with five-minute custard (p. 493).

Omit orange rind; just before folding in whipped milk add 1 cup of any of the following: diced bananas, sliced fresh and sweetened or canned peaches, pears, or apricots, diced fresh California persimmons, or drained crushed pineapple.

Omit orange rind; instead of orange juice use 1¾ cups of any of the following juices: canned pineapple, apricot, purple plum, Concord grape (this is my favorite), raspberry, or any berry juice. If sweetened juices are used, decrease or omit sugar.

**Gelatin chiffon pies:** Brush serving pie plate generously with soft fat, sprinkle liberally with crumbs; pour mixture of basic recipe or any variation over crumbs; sprinkle top with crumbs; or pour gelatin into a baked crumb or pastry shell.

Bavarian cream is often thought of as being difficult and expensive to prepare. The following Bavarian cream, which I think you'll agree is delicious, can be made in a few minutes at little cost. It supplies the equivalent of 2½ quarts fresh milk, no small amount when protein, riboflavin, and calcium requirements are often difficult to meet.

## BAVARIAN CREAM

Make five-minute custard (p. 493) using 1½ cups fresh milk; add to hot custard:

**1 tablespoon unflavored gelatin     ½ cup cold milk
soaked in**

Chill custard until gelatin starts to congeal; whip:

**¾ cup chilled evaporated milk**

Fold milk into custard after adding to it:

**¼ cup sugar                              2 teaspoons vanilla**

Pour into mold; chill until firmly set.

*Variations:*

Line square baking dish with graham-cracker crumbs and sprinkle generously with cinnamon; pour Bavarian cream over crumbs; sprinkle top with crumbs and cinnamon. Cut in cubes to serve.

Before folding in whipped milk add 1 cup of any of the following: diced banana; fresh sliced and sweetened or canned and drained peaches, pears, or apricots; drained, crushed or sliced canned pineapple; frozen or sweetened fresh strawberries, raspberries, or boysenberries; canned black cherries; diced fresh California persimmons; leftover cooked rice.

Add ½ cup of any of the following: walnuts, pecans, or other nuts; shredded or ground coconut; raisins, chopped dates, diced drained pitted prunes, or ground soft figs; or add ¼ cup each nuts and coconut, dried fruit, or soy grits.

**Almond cream:** Omit vanilla and add 1 teaspoon almond extract and ¼ cup chopped toasted almonds or ¼ cup soy grits.

**Caramel cream:** Omit 2 tablespoons sugar and add 2 tablespoons dark or blackstrap molasses and ½ teaspoon maple, rum, or brandy flavoring; or omit sugar and ¼ cup of fresh milk and sweeten to taste with molasses. Add nuts and/or coconut as desired.

**Eggnog pie:** Omit vanilla and add 2 tablespoons rum or brandy; pour into 9-inch serving pie plate brushed with fat and sprinkled with crumbs or into baked crumb or pastry shell; sprinkle with nutmeg. This pie is truly delicious.

**Gelatin chiffon pies:** Mold basic recipe or any variation in 9-inch baked crumb or pastry shell or in serving pie plate brushed with fat and sprinkled with crumbs; sprinkle top with crumbs, coconut, or ground nuts.

**Lemon cream:** Omit vanilla and ¼ cup fresh milk, making custard with 1¼ cups fresh milk; add to chilled custard grated rind of 1 lemon, ¼ cup lemon juice, and yellow coloring if needed.

**Orange cream:** Omit vanilla; add grated rind of 1 large orange and/or 1 teaspoon orange flavoring, and 2 drops orange coloring.


## ICE CREAM

I have tried many commercial ice-cream mixes, and to my way of thinking none can compare in deliciousness or in texture with the ice creams you can prepare in a few minutes. Moreover, the price asked for such concoctions, which supply only inexpensive colorings, flavorings, sugar, and thickening, distresses my Scotch soul. If you want to spend money on ingredients for ice cream, buy cream itself. Although one can make delicious ice milk and milk sherbets, for genuine ice cream the richer the cream, the more delectable the flavor.

There is no excuse for anyone's serving icy, or gritty, ice cream, even when the freezing is done in a refrigerator tray. When the recipe contains junket, gelatin, or cooked eggs, there is little tendency for large crystals to form unless the mixture is overfrozen before it is beaten. Ice cream should be frozen slowly; fast freezing causes the texture to be coarse. The more often it is beaten during the freezing, the smoother it is. If it should become icy and hard, let it melt to a mush, and break up the crystals by beating vigorously. Since few people are so fortunate as to have ice-cream freezers these days, I have included only recipes designed for freezing in the refrigerator.

The variations on page 507 can be used with any of the three basic recipes.

## ICE CREAM MADE WITH GELATIN

Stir together thoroughly in a freezing tray, preferably a deep one:

| | |
|---|---|
| ⅔ cup sugar | ¼ cup powdered milk |
| 1 tablespoon unflavored gelatin | pinch of salt |

Add:

1 cup top milk or cream

Let soak 10 minutes, stirring occasionally; heat slowly and stir until gelatin and sugar have dissolved, or about 4 minutes; cool and add:

| | |
|---|---|
| 2 teaspoons vanilla | few drops egg coloring or other food |
| 2 cups cream or | coloring |
| 1 cup each cream and evaporated milk | |

Stir well, set in freezing compartment, and freeze slowly to a soft mush. Remove from freezing compartment and beat; if deep tray is used, whip with rotary beater or electric mixer without removing from tray, dipping cream from sides of tray to center with a spoon; continue freezing slowly to a firm mush; if particularly smooth ice cream is desired, beat again. Freeze until solid.

## JUNKET ICE CREAM

Stir together thoroughly in a freezing tray, preferably a large one:

⅔ cup sugar                          pinch of salt
¼ cup powdered milk

Add:

3 cups top milk or cream or          2 teaspoons vanilla
2 cups top milk and 1 cup evapo-     few drops egg coloring or other food
   rated milk                           coloring

Stir constantly while heating to lukewarm, or 110° F. Meanwhile dissolve:

1 rennet, or junket, tablet in       1 tablespoon water

Add dissolved tablet to the lukewarm milk; stir no longer than 10 seconds. Do not move junket until firmly set, or about 10 minutes.

Freeze and beat as directed for ice cream made with gelatin.


## CUSTARD ICE CREAM

Combine in *metal* saucepan and stir well:

⅔ cup sugar                          ⅛ teaspoon salt
¼ cup powdered milk

Add and beat until smooth:

½ cup top milk or cream              few drops egg coloring
1 or 2 whole eggs or 2 to 4 egg yolks

Add and stir slightly:

1 cup top milk or cream

Cook over direct heat about 3 minutes; stir constantly until custard coats spoon, or reaches 175° F. Do not allow the custard to boil. Remove from heat and cool by adding:

1½ cups cream or evaporated milk    2 teaspoons vanilla

Pour into freezing tray; freeze and beat as directed for ice cream made with gelatin.

*Variations:*

Substitute for vanilla any of the following flavorings: almond, banana, black walnut, maple, orange, peach, pineapple, strawberry, raspberry, or oil of peppermint, clove, or cinnamon; add colorings to correspond to flavorings.

**Apricot or peach ice cream:** Omit vanilla; add 1 or 2 cups sweetened apricot or peach purée, using mashed or beaten fresh, canned, or cooked dried fruit.

**Banana ice cream:** Mash 3 or 4 bananas with 2 tablespoons lemon juice; sweeten to taste; add after ice cream is partly frozen; omit vanilla.

**Berry ice cream:** Omit vanilla; mash and sweeten to taste 2 cups strawberries, raspberries, or other fresh or frozen berries; stir in after ice cream is partly frozen.

**Caramel ice cream:** Use ½ cup sugar and add 2 tablespoons dark or blackstrap molasses, ½ teaspoon maple or rum flavoring, and ½ cup coconut meal or ground nuts. If flavor of molasses is enjoyed, omit sugar and sweeten ice cream to taste with molasses, particularly if it is to be served to children.

**Coconut ice cream:** Omit vanilla or decrease to ½ teaspoon; add 1 cup coconut meal or shredded coconut.

**Hawaiian ice cream:** Omit vanilla; add ¾ cup each shredded coconut, drained crushed pineapple, and mashed banana, and a few sliced maraschino cherries.

**Ice milk:** Instead of cream use 2 cups milk with other ingredients of basic recipe; freeze to a soft mush; whip 1 cup chilled evaporated milk until stiff, add partly frozen milk mixture, beat until velvety; return to freezing compartment and freeze slowly to a firm texture.

**Mock-nut ice cream:** Soften ½ cup soy grits (p. 196) and add 1 teaspoon black walnut flavoring or ½ teaspoon almond flavoring; if time permits, allow grits to stand overnight so that flavoring will penetrate well. To make pistachio-nut ice cream, use almond-flavored grits and add 2 or 3 drops green coloring to basic recipe made with junket or gelatin.

**Nut ice cream:** Add 1 cup ground or very finely chopped black or English walnuts, hazelnuts, or toasted, unsalted almonds.

**Orange ice cream:** Add 2 drops orange coloring, 1 teaspoon orange flavoring, and/or grated rind of 1 or 2 oranges.

**Yogurt ice cream:** Prepare plain, junket, or custard ice cream using 2 cups cream; when partly frozen, stir in 1 cup thick, or commercial, yogurt; use as in basic recipe or any variation. Berry and pineapple variations of yogurt ice cream are especially delicious.

## ORANGE SHERBET

Soak for 5 minutes:

**2 teaspoons gelatin in**                    **½ cup orange juice**

Heat until the gelatin is dissolved; cool by adding:

**1½ cups orange juice**

Freeze slowly to a soft mush, then beat until stiff:

**1 cup chilled evaporated milk**

Add and beat until velvety:

**frozen juice**                        **2 drops orange coloring**
**grated rind of 1 orange**

Sweeten to taste; return to freezing compartment; freeze only to a firm texture.

*Variations:*

Instead of orange juice use 2 cups of any of the following juices: purple plum; Concord grape; strawberry, raspberry, or other berry juice; pineapple; apricot; black cherry. Omit orange rind and coloring. When juices from heavily sweetened canned fruits are used, such as juice from commercially canned raspberries, dilute with water or any unsweetened juice; otherwise it is very difficult to freeze them.

Omit orange rind and coloring; instead of orange juice use 2 cups of any of the following fresh, frozen, canned, or cooked dried fruits: bananas, peaches, apricots, purple plums, prunes, California persimmons, crushed pineapple; raspberries, strawberries, youngberries, boysenberries, blueberries, or other berries; applesauce. Dice fruit fine, mash, or make into a purée by beating with rotary beater. Add 1 teaspoon cinnamon or grated lemon rind to applesauce sherbet, 2 drops red coloring with cinnamon; add 2 tablespoons lemon juice to mashed bananas, strawberries, and crushed pineapple; sweeten all fruits or juices to taste. Dissolve gelatin in water when no fruit juice is available.

Make sherbet by using 1 cup each of the fruits in the following combinations: mashed bananas and crushed pineapple; prune pulp and puréed apricots or peaches or applesauce with 1 teaspoon cinnamon or grated lemon rind; crushed strawberries and mashed bananas or crushed pineapple; puréed dried apricots and orange juice. Sweeten to taste. These are delicious sherbets.

**Fruit ices:** Omit evaporated milk; beat partially frozen juice or fruit until velvety; use any fruit or juice or combination of fruits suggested on page 508. Serve with meat or as dessert.

*Cranberry ice:* Drop 2 cups washed cranberries into 1 cup boiling water; boil slowly 10 minutes, or until quite soft; mash through a strainer; freeze; sweeten to taste after beating; add grated rind of 1 orange or lemon as desired. Serve with turkey.

*Mint ice:* Add mint flavoring and green coloring to unsweetened pineapple or grapefruit juice; proceed as for fruit ice. Serve with lamb or mutton.

**Yogurt sherbet:** Instead of evaporated milk add 1 or 2 cups thick yogurt to partially frozen juice or fruit. Prepare as in basic recipe or any variation. Yogurt sherbets are particularly delicious made with strawberries, raspberries, crushed pineapple, or Concord-grape juice.

Few recipes offer such an opportunity to work black molasses into the menu as do Indian pudding and gingerbread. If made of blackstrap, these foods are outstanding sources of iron, calcium, and other minerals and of the heat-stable B vitamins. Indian pudding is an old recipe which was used in New England before refined sugar was available. If you have developed a genuine appreciation of black molasses, you will enjoy this recipe.

### INDIAN PUDDING

Heat:

1½ cups fresh milk

Combine and add to milk, stirring rapidly:

| | |
|---|---|
| 1 cup fresh milk | ½ cup yellow corn meal |

Cook until slightly thick; remove from heat; add and stir well:

| | |
|---|---|
| 1 tablespoon cooking fat | ⅓ to ½ cup blackstrap or dark molasses |
| ¼ teaspoon salt | |
| ½ teaspoon cinnamon or ginger (optional) | |

Pour into casserole brushed with oil; bake in slow oven at 325° F. for 30 minutes; serve with top milk.

*Variations:*

Beat or shake with corn meal and fresh milk, ½ cup powdered milk, and 1 tablespoon or more debittered brewers' yeast.

If pronounced flavor of molasses is not enjoyed, use 3 tablespoons each molasses and sugar.

Add 2 finely diced unpeeled apples or ½ cup raisins, chopped dates, or broken nuts; or add ½ cup each soy grits and fresh milk.

It is indeed unfortunate that the commercial gingerbread mixes prepared with soda and refined flour have gained wide popularity, especially when gingerbread of outstanding nutritive value can be made in a few minutes.

When soda is used in making gingerbread, it not only destroys much of many of the B vitamins but partially breaks down gluten, or wheat protein. It is this breakdown of gluten which gives bakery products containing soda the softness of texture. When gingerbread is made with baking powder, any unnecessary stirring, which would develop the toughness of the gluten, must be carefully avoided to prevent a coarse bready texture from resulting. Gingerbread made with yeast is the most healthful variety and, to my way of thinking, the most delicious.

## GINGERBREAD

Cream together:

| | |
|---|---|
| ⅓ cup soft shortening | ⅓ cup sugar |

Add and stir well:

| | |
|---|---|
| 1 egg | ¾ cup sour milk, buttermilk, or yogurt |
| ⅔ cup blackstrap or dark molasses | |

Sift into moist ingredients:

| | |
|---|---|
| 1 cup sifted whole-wheat pastry flour | 3 teaspoons double-acting baking powder |
| ¼ cup powdered milk | 1 teaspoon ginger |
| ½ cup wheat germ or wheat-germ flour | 1 teaspoon cinnamon |
| | ½ teaspoon salt |

Combine ingredients with no more than 20 strokes. Oil ring mold or 8-inch square loaf pan and dust with flour. Pour batter into pan and bake in moderate oven at 350° F. for 45 minutes, being particularly careful not to overbake. Remove from oven as soon as dough no longer adheres to toothpick or cake tester.

*Variations:*

Instead of ½ cup whole-wheat flour use ½ cup rice polish or soy, peanut, or cottonseed flour. Since these products contain no gluten, they are excellent for making baking-powder gingerbread.

Omit 2 to 4 tablespoons flour and add 2 to 4 tablespoons debittered brewers' yeast; the yeast cannot be tasted.

Use 3 tablespoons shortening; cream ⅓ cup peanut butter with shortening and sugar.

Add 1 teaspoon each maple and vanilla flavoring or 1 teaspoon crushed coriander seeds.

**Applesauce gingerbread:** Add to moist ingredients ¾ cup chilled, thick applesauce; stir well before sifting in dry ingredients; bake as in basic recipe.

**Date-nut gingerbread:** After sifting in but before stirring dry ingredients add ½ cup each chopped dates and broken walnuts.

**Filled gingerbread:** Bake gingerbread in 8- by 14-inch loaf pan at 375° F. for 20 minutes; cut into three equal portions and arrange in layers with cheese filling (p. 524).

**Fruit gingerbread:** Add to dry ingredients before mixing ½ cup raisins or soft dried or well-drained cooked figs or pitted prunes.

**Mincemeat gingerbread:** Add to sifted ingredients before stirring ¾ cup fresh mincemeat.

**Nut gingerbread:** Add to dry ingredients before stirring ½ cup broken walnuts, pecans, or other nuts; or add ½ cup softened soy grits (p. 196) and 1 teaspoon black-walnut flavoring.

**Persimmon gingerbread:** Stir well into moist ingredients ¾ cup mashed persimmon pulp; bake as in basic recipe.

**Upside-down gingerbread:** Cover bottom of baking pan with sliced persimmons, canned apricot halves, sliced canned or fresh and sweetened peaches, sliced pineapple, or thinly sliced and sweetened apples; pour gingerbread batter over fruit.

**Yeast gingerbread:** Omit baking powder; mix 1 or 2 packages or crumbled cakes of bakers' yeast into moist ingredients; stir in dry ingredients, let rise in mixing bowl 3 or 4 hours or longer, stirring down when double in bulk; pour into loaf pan and let rise in warm place 25 to 30 minutes; bake as in basic recipe.

## PLUM PUDDING

Sift into mixing bowl:

⅔ cup sifted whole-wheat pastry
    flour
¾ cup sugar
1½ teaspoons cinnamon
1 teaspoon nutmeg

2 teaspoons double-acting baking
    powder
½ cup powdered milk
¾ teaspoon salt
2 tablespoons debittered brewers'
    yeast (optional)

Add and stir well:

½ cup wheat germ
2 tablespoons dark or blackstrap
    molasses
1 cup each finely ground raw un-
    peeled carrots and potatoes

1 cup raisins
½ cup broken pecans, walnuts, or
    toasted almonds

Brush 2 pint-size tin cans with oil; put pudding in cans and tie wax
paper securely over tops; place in cooking utensil in water 2 inches deep;
cover utensil and boil slowly 2 hours. Serve hot with hard sauce; reheat
in oven.

*Variations:*

Instead of wheat germ use ½ cup rice polish or soy, peanut, or cottonseed flour.

Add ½ cup of any one or more of the following: chopped dates; finely
diced citron; dried currants; diced raw apple or persimmon; ground dried
apricots or peaches; beat batter with 50 strokes if more than 2 cups fruit
are to be added.

Omit baking powder; mix 1 to 3 packages or crumbled cakes of bakers'
yeast into ground vegetables; stir well and set in a warm place while
measuring other ingredients.

**Date pudding:** Omit raisins and nutmeg; add 2 cups chopped dates.

The usual varieties of hard sauce are so rich that only a few
bites can be enjoyed without discomfort. The following sauce is
not only more nutritious but extremely delicious. The powdered
milk absorbs the brandy so readily that the sauce can have a great
deal more flavor without becoming runny than it does when only
powdered sugar is used. While it is certainly delightfully sweet, it
is not nauseously so.

## HARD SAUCE FOR PLUM PUDDING

Mix together:

3 tablespoons soft margarine or
butter
4 tablespoons powdered sugar

4 tablespoons powdered milk
1½ tablespoons brandy or rum

Serve chilled on steaming hot pudding.

For the millions of protein-starved Americans, few desserts surpass cheese cakes in nutritive value. Certainly they are delicious and easily prepared. The uncooked cheese cake, or pasha, is a modification of the famous Russian Easter cake. Persons who have not been lucky enough to eat it are unfortunate indeed.

## UNCOOKED CHEESE CAKE, OR PASHA

Press through a sieve or strainer:

2 pounds hoop cheese, or dry, unsalted cottage cheese

¼ pound sweet, or unsalted, butter

Add and stir well:

¼ cup powdered milk
1¼ cups sugar
1 cup top milk or cream
2 tablespoons vanilla or 1 tablespoon grated vanilla bean

½ small citron, finely chopped
1 cup chopped, blanched almonds
⅛ teaspoon almond flavoring

Cover colander with clean cloth; pour cheese mixture over cloth and place a small inverted plate on top as weight; set colander on cake pan and let stand in refrigerator overnight.

Turn cake onto large plate, remove cloth, slice, and serve.

*Variations:*

Add any of the following: 1 cup seedless raisins, ½ cup finely chopped candied orange peel; 4 tablespoons candied cherries cut into quarters; 3 cooked egg yolks, sieved with cheese; 1 tablespoon grated lemon rind.

If it is impossible to obtain hoop cheese, use farmer-style cottage cheese and omit top milk or cream.

## BAKED CHEESE CAKE

Combine in a mixing bowl:

| | |
|---|---|
| 1 pound (2 cups) cream-style cottage cheese | 3 egg yolks |
| 1 cup evaporated or top milk | ¼ cup whole-wheat pastry flour |
| 1 cup sugar | grated rind of 1 lemon |
| ½ cup powdered milk | 3 tablespoons lemon juice |
| | 2 teaspoons vanilla |

Beat until stiff:

| | |
|---|---|
| 3 egg whites | ⅛ teaspoon salt |

Set egg whites aside and beat cheese mixture with rotary eggbeater until it is smooth and cheese is in small particles. Fold egg whites into cheese mixture.

Brush a deep 9-inch pie pan or spring-form cake tin with soft margarine or cooking fat; sprinkle generously with graham-cracker or cereal-flake crumbs. Pour cheese mixture into pan and sprinkle top with crumbs; bake at 300° F. for 1 hour. Watch temperature carefully so that it does not go above 300° F.

*Variations:*

Instead of cottage cheese use 1 pound hoop cheese, or dry, unsalted cottage cheese; press hoop cheese through a sieve.

Use 1 cup cottage cheese and 2 packages cream cheese.

## BAKING CAKES

The two important factors in cakemaking are stirring and baking. The purpose of stirring is to develop elasticity in the gluten of the flour so that bubbles of air and carbon dioxide are held in during baking. If the batter is beaten too little, the gluten is underdeveloped, the cake flat, its texture coarse, and the crust sugary. If it is beaten too much, the gluten becomes too firm, and the cake has a bready, coarse texture. Although directions for baking cakes usually advise that the batter be beaten for a certain number of minutes, no two persons beat at the same rate of speed, nor does one person beat at the same rate on two different occasions. The only accurate method by which cakes may be made uniform in texture is to count the number of strokes, or complete revolutions around the mixing bowl. If a small amount of sugar is used in proportion to the flour, as in a molasses cake or gingerbread, the particles of gluten readily stick together, and there is great danger of overbeating. The larger the proportion of sugar to flour used, the more the grains of sugar prevent bits of gluten from sticking together. In this case much beating is necessary.

Even though a cake has been carefully combined, it can be easily ruined in the baking. The oven must be sufficiently hot to form a soft but elastic crust almost immediately. Like the gluten, such a crust holds in the carbon dioxide liberated during the baking, as well as the expanding air incorporated when the cake was stirred and the eggs were beaten; yet it allows the cake to rise. If the oven is not hot enough, no crust is formed, the air and carbon dioxide escape, and the cake is flat and heavy. If the oven is too hot, a brittle crust lacking elasticity is formed quickly; as the air expands from heat and the carbon dioxide is formed, such a crust cracks; the dough bubbles up through the cracks, forming a two-layered effect and a lopsided cake. If the cake is to be light and tall, the oven must be preheated to the temperature specified in the recipe, and the temperature checked with an upright oven thermometer placed so that the bulb is on the same level as the cake.

The tendency of an amateur is to overbake cakes. If you want your cake to be moist and delicate and to have a soft, velvety texture, err on the side of underbaking rather than overbaking it. As the end of the baking period draws near, watch the cake carefully. Take it from the oven the minute it meets the three tests for doneness: first, when a toothpick or wire cake tester inserted in the center of the cake can be withdrawn without dough adhering to it; second, when the cake starts to shrink from the sides of the pan; third, when the surface, touched lightly with a finger, springs back into place, or becomes elastic. If a layer of cake can be picked up with one hand without falling apart, the cake has certainly been overbaked.

If you have not used whole-wheat flour for cakes, try the apricot, date-nut, or applesauce variations of the following recipe before trying the basic recipe itself.

## QUICK LAYER CAKE

Set shortening to warm to room temperature.
Combine in flour sifter:

| | |
|---|---|
| 1½ cups sifted whole-wheat pastry flour | 3 teaspoons double-acting baking powder |
| 1 cup sugar | ½ teaspoon salt |
| | ½ cup powdered milk |

Sift over:

| | |
|---|---|
| ½ cup shortening at room temperature | 4 drops butter-flavoring |

Add:

| | |
|---|---|
| ½ cup wheat germ | ½ cup fresh milk or half the fruit suggested under variations |
| 2 unbeaten eggs | |

Mix until dry ingredients are moistened. Beat exactly 1 minute on an electric mixer at slow speed or 100 strokes by hand.
Add:

½ cup milk or rest of liquid suggested under variations

Blend and then beat exactly 2 minutes on an electric mixer or 200 full strokes by hand. Stir in:

| | |
|---|---|
| 1 tablespoon vanilla | ½ to 1 cup broken nuts (optional) |

Pour into 2 greased and lightly floured 8-inch layer-cake pans.
Spread batter evenly to sides of pan. Bake in preheated oven at 350° F. for 30 to 35 minutes. Remove cake from pans and cool on wire rack. Cover with double-boiler frosting.

*Variations:*

Instead of vanilla use 2 teaspoons lemon extract or 1 teaspoon almond, banana, black walnut, or other flavoring; or combine 1 teaspoon lemon, maple, or pineapple flavoring with 2 teaspoons vanilla.

Instead of wheat germ sift with dry ingredients ½ cup rice polish or soy, peanut, cottonseed, or wheat-germ flour.

Use basic recipe or any variation and bake as cupcakes in moderately hot oven at 375° F. for 15 minutes.

Use 1 cup tightly packed brown sugar instead of white or add 1 tablespoon dark or blackstrap molasses.

**Almond cake:** Omit vanilla; add 1 cup blanched ground almonds and 1 teaspoon almond flavoring. Blanch almonds by steaming 5 minutes in 2 tablespoons water; cool and remove skins. Do not soak.

*Mock almond cake:* Simmer ½ cup soy grits in ½ cup hot water for 8 minutes, or until all moisture is absorbed; dry on paper towels; add to batter with ½ to 1 teaspoon almond flavoring.

**Applesauce cake:** Omit vanilla; instead of milk use 1 cup thick sweetened applesauce; sift with dry ingredients 1¼ teaspoons cinnamon and ¾ teaspoon nutmeg; stir in 1 cup raisins with nuts; bake 35 to 40 minutes.

**Apricot cake:** Omit vanilla; instead of milk use 1 cup thin sweetened apricot purée prepared from cooked dried apricots, beaten until smooth; put steamed, well-drained, sweetened dried apricots between layers and over cake; cover with uncooked icing.

**Banana cake:** Omit vanilla; mash with 2 tablespoons lemon juice enough bananas to make 1 cup; use instead of milk; add 1 teaspoon lemon flavoring. Or use basic recipe, slice bananas between layers and over top, and spread with two-minute icing flavored with lemon.

**Boston cream pie:** Put custard filling (p. 534) between layers; cover cake with whipped cream.

**Butterscotch tort:** Drop 5 tablespoons of batter into each of four 9-inch layer-cake pans, making 4 thin layers. Bake at 400° F. for 10 minutes. Prepare butterscotch cake filling (p. 500) and put between layers. Cover tort with whipped cream. Vary by coloring layers with different colors or make filling of vanilla pudding; divide pudding into three portions, and flavor one with lemon, one with almond, one with orange or maple. Add different food colorings to correspond with flavorings.

**Date-nut cake:** Stone and cut into small pieces enough dates to make 1 cup when tightly packed; heat to simmering in 1 cup milk; cool and use instead of milk as the liquid in the recipe. Use 1 cup nuts.

**Doughnuts:** Omit vanilla; decrease fat to ¼ cup and double the amounts of flour and wheat germ. Add 2 teaspoons each cinnamon and nutmeg. Combine all ingredients and stir thoroughly. Chill dough. Roll ¼ inch thick, cut, and brown both sides in fat at 360° F. Makes 36 doughnuts.

**Orange cake:** Omit vanilla; add 2 teaspoons grated orange rind or orange flavoring and 2 drops orange coloring.

**Pineapple cake:** Instead of fresh milk use 1¼ cups crushed pineapple with juice; decrease vanilla to 1 teaspoon; add 1 cup shredded coconut; omit nuts.

**Prune-nut cake:** Omit vanilla; instead of milk use 1 cup thin prune purée; increase nuts to 1 cup; add 1¼ teaspoons cinnamon and ¾ teaspoon nutmeg.

**Upside-down cake:** Melt 2 tablespoons margarine or butter in 9-inch loaf-cake pan; cover bottom with sliced fresh persimmons or canned or cooked and sweetened dried apricots, prunes, peaches, pears, or well-drained pineapple; or combine sliced pineapple and maraschino cherries or apricots and prunes in attractive designs; sprinkle with ⅓ cup brown sugar; add nuts if desired. Pour cake batter on fruits, bake at 350° F. for 50 minutes.

### MAPLE-MERINGUE CAKE

Sift together 5 times onto paper plates:

| | |
|---|---|
| ¾ cup sifted whole-wheat pastry flour | ½ cup sugar |
| | ¼ cup powdered milk |

Combine in a large mixing bowl:

| | |
|---|---|
| 1 cup (8 or 10) egg whites | ¼ cup cold water |
| ¼ teaspoon salt | 1 teaspoon maple flavoring |
| 1 teaspoon cream of tartar | 1 teaspoon vanilla |

Beat until egg whites are stiff; add 2 tablespoons at a time during beating:

½ cup sugar

Add flour mixture in 4 portions, folding in each portion with no more than 15 strokes.

Pour batter into ungreased 9-inch tube pan. Insert knife in batter and circle twice to cut air pockets.

Bake in preheated slow oven at 300° F. for 50 minutes, or until cake starts to shrink from sides of pan. Invert pan and cool thoroughly about 2 hours before removing cake. Sprinkle with **powdered sugar** or cover with **caramel icing.**

*Variations:*

Omit maple flavoring and add 1 teaspoon almond or lemon extract; add 1 drop green coloring with almond, yellow coloring with lemon. For superelegance, fold in ⅓ cup thinly sliced candied cherries with flour in almond-meringue cake; cover with pink frosting flavored with almond.

To mix cake with an electric mixer, beat egg whites with salt at high speed until foamy; add cream of tartar and beat about 2 minutes before adding water. When whites stand in peaks, turn to slow speed and add sugar and flavoring. Fold in flour by hand.

**Black-walnut meringue cake:** Omit maple flavoring; fold in with flour ½ cup chopped black walnuts or add 1 teaspoon black walnut flavoring.

**Butterscotch-meringue cake:** Instead of white sugar use 1 cup tightly packed brown sugar; maple flavoring may be omitted.

**Chocolate-meringue cake:** Sift with dry ingredients 3 tablespoons cocoa; flavor with 1 teaspoon vanilla and ½ teaspoon lemon extract. Cover with pink peppermint icing (p. 524).

**Nut-meringue cake:** Fold in with flour ½ cup chopped or ground pecans, English walnuts, or almonds; add ½ teaspoon almond extract with almonds.

**Orange-meringue cake:** Omit water and vanilla and maple flavoring; add 4 tablespoons orange juice, 2 teaspoons grated orange rind or 1 teaspoon orange flavoring, and 2 drops orange coloring; cover with orange icing (p. 524).


## MOLASSES-SPICE CAKE

Cream together:

½ cup soft cooking fat                    ¾ cup sugar

Add and beat slightly:

2 egg yolks

Add a little at a time and stir well:

1 cup sweet or sour milk, butter-          ½ cup dark or blackstrap molasses
milk, or yogurt                            1 teaspoon maple flavoring

Combine and sift in:

1 cup sifted whole-wheat pastry            ½ cup powdered milk
flour                                      ½ teaspoon salt
½ cup sifted soy flour                     2½ teaspoons baking powder
¼ cup wheat-germ flour or wheat            1 teaspoon each cinnamon and
germ                                          nutmeg

Fold in dry ingredients with no more than 25 strokes. Beat until stiff:

2 egg whites                               2 tablespoons water

Fold in egg whites with no more than 15 strokes.

Brush cake pan with soft cooking fat and dust lightly with flour.

Bake in preheated oven at 350° F. 40 to 45 minutes if loaf pan or 9-inch tube pan is used, 25 to 30 minutes if two 8-inch layer pans are used.

*Variations:*

Add to batter with dry ingredients ½ cup raisins, chopped dates, broken nuts, or well-drained chopped steamed figs, apricots, or prunes; or add ¼ cup soy grits, 1 teaspoon black-walnut flavoring.

Instead of soy flour use ½ cup rice polish or peanut or cottonseed flour; or omit soy flour and use ¾ cup wheat-germ flour.

Add ½ teaspoon each allspice and cloves.

**Coconut-molasses cake:** Add with dry ingredients 1 cup shredded coconut; cover cake with double-boiler frosting sprinkled with coconut.

**Devil's food cake:** Omit spices and ¼ cup of flour; sift ⅓ cup cocoa with dry ingredients; add 1 tablespoon vanilla. Cover with double-boiler frosting flavored with peppermint.

**Ginger cake:** Omit cinnamon and nutmeg and add ½ teaspoon ginger.

Although little has been said about the value of nuts, they are an excellent source of protein and the B vitamins. Use them in as many desserts as your budget allows, particularly if there are growing children in your family. The quantity of nuts used in the following tort makes it of outstanding nutritive value. Regardless of its contribution to health, my husband claims that walnut tort is the most delicious of all desserts.

I have used soy grits in hundreds of recipes, but in no instance has the lowly soybean been made so delicious or so completely disguised as in the mock almond tort. Dozens of persons to whom I have served this tort firmly believed it was made of almonds until told otherwise.

### WALNUT TORT

Line bottoms of two 8-inch layer-cake pans with heavy paper; brush with soft cooking fat.

Stir together thoroughly:

| | |
|---|---|
| 1 cup sugar | ½ cup powdered milk |

Add and stir slightly:

| | |
|---|---|
| 3 egg yolks | ½ cup wheat germ |
| 2 cups ground walnuts | |

Beat stiff and fold 6 egg whites into above ingredients.

Pour batter into pans, spread evenly to edges, and bake in slow oven at 325° F. for 30 minutes. Turn out of pans and remove paper immediately.

Prepare filling by mixing thoroughly:

**⅓ cup sugar**                                    **⅓ cup powdered milk**

Add and stir well:

**3 egg yolks**                                    **½ cup top milk**

Cook slowly over direct heat until thick, stirring constantly; do not boil.

Remove from heat and add:

**1 cup ground walnuts**

Spread between layers of tort.

*Variations:*

Instead of walnuts use ground pecans, Brazil nuts, or hazelnuts; or use half black walnuts and half English walnuts.

Use 1 cup tightly packed brown sugar instead of white, or add 1 tablespoon dark or blackstrap molasses.

Omit nuts from filling, cool, and add 1 cup well-drained crushed pineapple or sliced bananas or ½ cup chopped dates.

Simmer ¾ cup soy grits in ¾ cup water for 8 minutes, or until all water is absorbed; turn out on paper towels; measure after cooking and use 1 cup cooked grits in tort instead of 1 cup walnuts; add 1 tablespoon black-walnut flavoring. Use remaining cooked grits in filling instead of ½ cup walnuts; cool and add ½ teaspoon black-walnut flavoring.

**Almond tort:** Use ground blanched almonds instead of walnuts in tort; add ½ teaspoon almond flavoring to tort, ¼ teaspoon to filling. Or use 1 cup ground almonds in tort, ½ cup in filling, and supplement nuts with soy grits cooked as directed above. Blanch almonds by steaming 3 minutes in 2 tablespoons boiling water; cool and remove skins.

**Mock almond tort:** Cook 1½ cups soy grits as directed above; measure again after cooking and use 2 cups cooked grits in tort instead of walnuts; add 1 teaspoon almond flavoring. Use remaining grits, or about 1 cup, in filling; cool and add ½ teaspoon almond flavoring; or cover tort with any soft icing to which almond flavoring, remaining cooked grits, and food coloring are added.

## CAKE ICINGS

Of the many recipes I have worked on with the idea of improving nutritive value without sacrificing flavor, I believe I am most proud of the cake icings. Dozens of persons who have tasted these icings and many friends who are using the recipes tell me they find them even more delicious than the usual variety of icing. When icings are made of powdered milk, they take only a few minutes to prepare and there is no problem of their being overcooked, sugary, too thick, or too thin. To facilitate even blending, it is important to stir in the flavoring and coloring before adding the powdered milk.

The quantities suggested in the following recipes are sufficient to cover a large loaf cake, a 9-inch cake baked in a tube pan, or two 8- or 9-inch layers.

Since the variations are the same regardless of the type of icing, the variations on pages 523-524 can be used with any of the four icings.

### UNCOOKED ICING I

Combine:

⅔ cup sweetened condensed milk       2 tablespoons soft margarine or but-
2 teaspoons vanilla                              ter (optional)
1 drop food coloring

Stir slightly and add:

⅔ cup powdered milk

Beat until smooth. Spread over cake.

### UNCOOKED ICING II

Combine:

2 tablespoons fresh milk               3 tablespoons soft margarine or but-
2 or 3 teaspoons vanilla                  ter
1 drop food coloring                       ⅔ cup sifted powdered sugar
                                                      ⅔ cup powdered milk

Beat until creamy. Spread over cake.

## TWO-MINUTE ICING

Combine and boil slowly for exactly 2 minutes:

¾ cup sugar                                2 tablespoons margarine or butter
½ cup milk

Cool completely and then beat in:

1 cup powdered milk                        any nuts or food coloring desired
1 tablespoon vanilla

Spread on cake.

## DOUBLE-BOILER ICING

Combine in top of double boiler:

½ cup sugar                                1 teaspoon vinegar
4 tablespoons water                        1 unbeaten egg white
⅛ teaspoon salt

Set over boiling water; beat with rotary beater for 5 minutes; remove
and chill; when cold, add:

1 tablespoon vanilla                       1 cup powdered milk
1 drop food coloring

*Variations of any of the foregoing icing recipes:*

Omit vanilla and add ½ teaspoon of one of the following extracts:
maple, rum, peppermint, almond, banana, black walnut, strawberry, or
brandy; use food colorings to correspond to flavorings.

Just before spreading on cake add any one of the following: ½ cup
finely chopped dates, figs, walnuts, pecans, almonds; ¼ cup peanut butter, chopped candied cherries, candied pineapple, or candied cherries and
pineapple or citron; combine ½ cup each chopped dried or candied fruits
and chopped nuts.

Use juice from maraschino cherries instead of part of the milk in uncooked icing II or two-minute icing; add ¼ cup drained quartered maraschino cherries to any icing.

Mix 1 tablespoon cinnamon with powdered milk; spread icing over hot
yeast rolls.

**Caramel icing:** Use tightly packed brown sugar instead of white in
double-boiler or two-minute icing, or add 1 tablespoon dark or blackstrap
molasses to either uncooked frosting. The sugar will cause the milk to
curdle in two-minute icing, but an even texture will result after beating.

**Cheese filling:** Blend with half the icing 1 package (3 ounces) cream cheese; add 2 teaspoons grated orange or lemon rind. Put between layers of cake; use remaining icing for top.

**Coconut icing:** Spread icing on cake and sprinkle generously with fresh or slightly toasted coconut; color coconut by mixing with a few drops of water to which coloring has been added.

**Icing for banana cake:** Slice bananas lengthwise and spread over layers; brush bananas lightly with lemon juice; cover with icing flavored with ½ teaspoon each lemon and banana flavorings.

**Lemon icing:** Instead of vanilla add 1 teaspoon grated lemon rind and/ or lemon flavoring and 1 drop yellow coloring.

**Maple icing:** Use maple syrup instead of milk or water in two-minute, double-boiler, or uncooked icings; or add 1 teaspoon maple flavoring to any icing. Maple is especially good with ½ cup walnuts.

**Orange icing:** Instead of vanilla add 1 teaspoon grated orange rind and/or orange flavoring and 1 drop orange coloring.

**Peppermint icing:** Add 1 teaspoon peppermint flavoring or few drops oil of peppermint and 1 drop pink coloring; use for chocolate-meringue cake.

**Pineapple icing:** Use crushed pineapple and the juice instead of milk or water in double-boiler icing, two-minute icing, and uncooked icing II; add ¼ cup diced candied pineapple to uncooked icing I; to all pineapple icings add ½ to 1 teaspoon pineapple flavoring. Pineapple is particularly delicious combined with brown sugar or dark molasses as directed for caramel icing.

### CAKE FILLINGS

Since cake fillings require less sugar and contain larger amounts of milk, eggs, fruits, and nuts than do the usual variety of icings, they should be used in preference to icings. They offer the advantage of keeping the cake moist for many days. Commercial puddings (p. 500) and fillings for meringue-cream pie (p. 534) and for ten-minute pie (p. 537) may be used as cake fillings. Cake fillings may be spread over the entire surface of any cake to be served with a fork.

### PIES

When pie dough is made entirely of wheat flour, it contains so much gluten that it becomes tough if stirred or kneaded. Since rice polish and soy, peanut, and cottonseed flour contain no gluten, they are excellent to use in making crisp pie crusts. Although wheat germ and wheat-germ flour contain the same amount of gluten as did the wheat from which they came, they make especially delicious crusts having a rich nutty flavor. It has been a joy to have many persons who have not used whole-wheat flour, wheat germ, or the highly nutritious flours declare that pie crusts made with these flours were the best they have ever tasted.

Pie dough can be easily handled if rolled on a lightly floured canvas with a child's knitted stocking pulled over the rolling pin. The canvas should be small enough to be easily inverted over the pie tin, or about half the size usually sold. If you do not have this equipment, roll the dough on a sheet of floured wax paper.

One often hears women declare that they cannot make flaky pie crusts. Anyone can make flaky crusts provided he understands what makes the crust flake. Four rules must be carefully observed. First, the fat must be as cold and firm as possible. Second, the fat must be cut into the flour only until the pieces of fat are the size of large garden peas. Third, the water used must be cold in order not to soften the fat. Fourth, the oven temperature must be sufficiently high so that the crust will bake before the "peas" of fat have time to melt and penetrate evenly throughout the flour. Check the oven temperature with an upright oven thermometer and know that it is correct before putting the pie in to bake. The bits of cold, firm fat, mashed into layers when the crust is rolled, prevent flour in one part of the crust from sticking to the flour in other parts of the crust, and flakiness results. If the fat is warm or soft before the dough is made, if it is warmed by mixing with the hands or by adding warm water, if the oven temperature is low, a flaky crust cannot possibly be obtained. Crusts made by the hot-water or beaten method can be delicious and crisp but they can never be flaky.

Any type of crust can be made more crisp by being thoroughly chilled or frozen after it has been rolled but before it is baked. The chilled water in the dough has a greater expansion when it is changed into steam during baking than when it is warm. If you have a freezing unit, prepare several single-crust pie shells at one time, keep them frozen until you need them, and then bake them.

To my way of thinking, no shortening can compare with lard for making flaky pie crusts. Since lard is not whipped, it has more shortening power per volume than hydrogenated cooking fats have. Chilled lard is more firm at a given temperature than are other inexpensive shortenings. When I purchase lard, I let it become quite soft and stir into it 20 drops of butter-flavoring per pound, or 2 cups. This procedure takes only a minute and gives the lard the delightful flavor and appearance of butter. I have even had friends eat it on hot biscuits without discovering the difference.

## FLAKY PIE CRUST

To make two single-crust 9-inch pies or one double-crust pie, sift together into mixing bowl:

1 cup whole-wheat pastry flour        1 teaspoon salt

Add and stir well:

1 cup wheat germ                      ⅔ cup other butter-flavored short-
½ cup chilled butter-flavored lard      ening
or

Cut lard into dry ingredients with pastry cutter or two knives until particles of fat are the size of large peas; do not touch with hands. Add:

**4 tablespoons cold water, preferably ice water**

Mix only enough to moisten ingredients. Turn dough onto floured canvas or wax paper. If crust is to be baked without filling, divide into two equal parts; for a two-crust pie, use a slightly larger amount of dough for lower crust. Pat dough quickly into a flat, round "ball," dust top lightly with flour, and roll ⅛ inch thick, using a circular motion of the rolling pin to give a perfect circle of dough; turn canvas or wax paper during rolling; avoid touching the dough if possible.

Turn pie tin upside down over dough; pick up canvas or wax paper and invert over pan; remove canvas or paper; if a single crust is being prepared, trim and flute edges and make perforations with a fork at ½-inch intervals. See page 528 for preparing and baking double-crust pies.

Bake single crusts in hot, preheated oven at 425° F. for 8 to 10 minutes. Wheat germ burns quickly at this temperature; hence watch the baking time carefully.

*Variations:*

If crisp but not flaky crust is desired, all ingredients must be at room temperature; use 3 or 4 tablespoons water, depending on softness of fat, combine ingredients with fingertips if desired. Bake at 350° F. for 18 to 20 minutes.

Instead of ½ cup wheat germ use ½ cup rice polish or soy, peanut, or cottonseed flour; use 5 tablespoons water with soy, peanut, or cottonseed flour. The crusts made with rice polish and cottonseed flour are quite dark but very delicious.

If wheat germ is not available, use 2 cups whole-wheat pastry flour; increase lard to ⅔ cup.

Use 1 cup wheat-germ flour instead of wheat germ; sift with whole-wheat flour; or omit whole-wheat flour and use 1 cup rice polish or soy, peanut, or cottonseed flour with 1 cup wheat-germ flour. Combine ingredients with 25 strokes to develop gluten. Use ⅓ cup, or 6 tablespoons, water with 1 cup soy, peanut, or cottonseed flour.

**Beaten pie crust:** Use ½ cup and 1 tablespoon soft hydrogenated cooking fat; beat with electric mixer or rotary eggbeater until creamy; add water 2 tablespoons at a time and beat until it is taken up. Fold dry ingredients into fat with spoon, using no more than 25 strokes. Bake at 350° F. for 18 to 20 minutes. This method is not successful when lard is used.

**Boiling-water pie crust:** Bring water to boiling; add and melt fat; remove from heat, stir in dry ingredients with no more than 15 strokes; chill thoroughly before rolling. Bake at 350° F. for 18 to 20 minutes. Use this method for basic recipe or any variation. This is an easy and foolproof procedure for making crisp crusts.

I have tried dozens of recipes for crumb crusts and regardless of ingredients have found them crumbly and difficult to work with. For gelatin chiffon pies and any fillings which will hold their shape without needing the support of a crust, I merely brush the serving pie plate generously with soft margarine or butter and sprinkle it liberally with crumbs. This procedure is such an easy and satisfactory substitute for crumb crust that I heartily recommend it.

In case you wish to bake a crumb crust, keep your eye on it unless you have a range with an alarm clock on it. I don't know of any food that seems to burn so easily. More than once I've prepared two crusts, one to burn and one to eat. Of course the telephone was really to blame.

## CRUMB CRUST

Toast and pass through the meat grinder, using smallest knife:

**4 or 5 slices stale whole-wheat bread**

Sift crumbs and measure; combine:

**⅔ cup fine whole-wheat-bread crumbs**
**¼ cup wheat germ**

**¼ cup powdered milk**
**½ to ¾ teaspoon cinnamon (optional)**

Stir dry ingredients together thoroughly; add:

**⅓ cup melted butter-flavored lard or cooking fat**

Mix until fat is evenly distributed; add and blend well:

**1 tablespoon dark or blackstrap molasses, corn syrup, or maple syrup**

Brush 9-inch serving pie pan generously with soft shortening, being particularly careful to grease the rim. Press crumbs firmly against pan to form crust ⅛ inch thick, making the margin first.

Bake in a moderate oven at 350° F. for 10 minutes, or add filling and bake as meringue cooks.

*Variations:*

Use crumbs from any of the following: bran flakes; whole-wheat-cereal flakes; stale cookies of any kind; toasted slices of stale cake; whole-wheat zwieback; graham crackers.


## FRUIT PIES

Prepare dough for two-crust pie; line 9-inch pie pan with dough; chill while filling is being prepared.

Mix together:

**3 to 4 cups fresh sliced fruit or 2 cups canned fruit and ½ cup juice**
**½ to ⅔ cup sugar, depending on sweetness of fruit**

**2 or 3 tablespoons whole-wheat pastry flour**
**pinch of salt**

Spread filling over lower pie shell. Roll dough for top crust ⅛ inch thick; make attractive feather design in dough with blunt edge and end of silver knife, making holes through which steam can escape; moisten edges of lower shell with small amount of juice; pick up canvas or wax paper upon which dough has been rolled, invert it over pie, and remove cloth or paper; press down dough firmly around edges; trim and flute edges by pinching with thumbs and forefingers.

If juicy uncooked fruit is used, such as cherries, rhubarb, or berries, make small cones of heavy paper 3 inches square; fasten together with pins or paper clips; insert in holes in upper crust to prevent juice from spilling during baking.

Bake in hot oven at 425° F. for 8 minutes; lower heat to 325° F. and continue baking 30 to 35 minutes for uncooked fruit pies, or 20 minutes for mince pie or canned-fruit fillings.

*Variations:*

If flaky crust is not desired or if beaten or boiling-water crust is used, bake pie at 350° F. for 45 to 50 minutes.

**Apple pie:** Slice 4 to 6 tart apples; mix 1 teaspoon nutmeg or cinnamon with sugar and flour. If apples lack flavor, add 1 tablespoon each margarine and lemon juice, ½ teaspoon grated lemon rind; if dry, add 2 to 4 tablespoons sweet or sour cream; if apples are a variety which will not cook readily, slice and steam for 8 minutes in ½ cup water; chill before mixing with other ingredients.

**Apricot or peach pie:** Use sliced fresh, canned, or partially cooked dried fruit; decrease sugar to ⅓ cup if sweetened canned apricots or peaches are used; proceed as in basic recipe.

**Berry pies:** Use blackberries, strawberries, raspberries, currants, gooseberries, blueberries, or other berries; sweeten fresh currants or gooseberries with 1 cup sugar; add 1 tablespoon lemon juice to blueberries or loganberries; proceed as in basic recipe. Prepare paper cones as directed above and insert in upper crust to prevent juice from spilling.

**Cherry or grape pie:** Use pitted pie cherries or Concord grapes; increase sugar to 1 cup if uncooked fruit is used or decrease to ⅓ cup with sweetened canned grapes, pie cherries, or black cherries.

**Mince pie:** Omit sugar, flour, and salt; most prepared mincemeat is improved by adding 1 or 2 finely diced unpeeled apples; prepare and bake as in basic recipe.

**Pineapple pie:** Use canned crushed pineapple, omitting sugar or decreasing to 2 tablespoons; prepare as in basic recipe or cook pineapple with flour until thick, pour into baked shell or crumb crust, and top with meringue (p. 533).

**Rhubarb pie:** Use diced fresh rhubarb; increase flour to 4 tablespoons, sugar to 1 cup.

**Prune or raisin pie:** Use steamed raisins, steamed and pitted prunes; omit sugar if seeded raisins are used; add **1 tablespoon lemon juice or ½ teaspoon grated rind;** prepare and bake as in the basic recipe or mix flour, salt, and sugar with **1 cup prune or raisin juice,** cook until thick, add lemon rind and **½ cup chopped nuts;** pour into baked shell or crumb crust, cover with meringue (p. 533).

There are numerous suggestions for preventing the crust of a custard pie from becoming soggy: brush the crust with fat or egg white; bake the crust 10 minutes before pouring the custard into it; and many similar precautions. I spent an entire day testing every such recommendation I could find, and although there were degrees of sogginess, not by any stretch of the imagination could any crust be called crisp.

To my way of thinking there is only one way to bake a custard pie. Bake the shell first; while it is baking, prepare the custard; removed the baked shell from the pan and pour the custard into the same pan; lower the oven temperature and bake the custard. Immediately before the pie is to be served, slip the custard onto the crust. This method works like a charm. A properly baked custard settles into the crust so beautifully that only the closest observer would notice the two had not been baked together. The contrast between the soft yet firm custard and the crisp, flaky crust so delights the palate that to bake a custard pie by another method seems a gastronomic crime.

### CUSTARD PIE

Prepare a 9-inch flaky pie crust (p. 526); bake in pan with circular knife if available; while it is baking, combine:

⅓ to ½ cup sugar                        pinch of salt
½ cup powdered milk

Stir dry ingredients well; add:

½ cup fresh milk                        1 teaspoon vanilla
3 eggs

Beat until smooth and add **1½ cups fresh milk**

Take baked pie shell from oven; slip shell onto serving plate; without washing the pan, grease it generously and pour custard into it; sprinkle top with nutmeg.

Lower oven temperature to 325° F.; bake custard 25 to 30 minutes, or until barely firm; cooking will continue as custard cools.

Immediately before serving, loosen custard with spatula or knife attached to pie pan; slip carefully into crust; serve hot or cold. The crust can become soggy about 30 minutes after the custard is put into it; combine the two just before pie is to be eaten.

*Variations:*

Substitute for vanilla ½ to 1 teaspoon of any of the following flavorings: banana, black walnut, lemon, maple, rum, or brandy; grated rind of 1 lemon or orange.

Make custard of 2 whole eggs and 2 yolks; use ¼ cup sugar; prepare a meringue of 2 egg whites, sweeten with ⅓ cup sugar; bake filling 10 minutes; cover with meringue, being careful not to allow meringue to touch the sides of the pan; bake 20 to 25 minutes longer.

Bake shell 8 minutes at 425° F. while preparing custard; remove from oven and brush generously with fat. Pour custard into shell and bake as directed above. Serve hot.

Add ¼ cup each milk and soy grits to basic recipe or any variation.

Use ⅓ cup sugar and add 2 tablespoons dark or blackstrap molasses with ½ teaspoon each vanilla and maple flavoring.

**Almond-custard pie:** Omit vanilla and nutmeg; add ½ teaspoon almond flavoring, ¼ cup each soy grits and fresh milk.

**Apple-custard pie:** Use 1 cup each thick applesauce and fresh milk; omit vanilla; add grated rind of 1 lemon. This is a delicious pie.

**Banana-custard pie:** Omit vanilla; add ½ teaspoon lemon extract or grated rind of 1 lemon to custard; immediately before serving slice 2 bananas over crust; slip custard over bananas.

**Coconut-custard pie:** Add ¼ cup shredded coconut to custard; sprinkle top of filling with ¼ cup before baking.

**Date-custard pie:** Use ⅓ cup sugar in custard; sprinkle ½ cup chopped dates over bottom of pan before adding custard; use ½ cup broken walnuts or pecans with dates as desired.

**Lemon-custard pie:** Omit vanilla; use 1¾ cups fresh milk; stir gradually into custard ¼ cup lemon juice, grated rind of 1 lemon.

**Orange-custard pie:** Omit vanilla; add 1 teaspoon orange flavoring or grated rind of 1 orange, 1 drop orange coloring. This is my favorite custard pie.

**Pineapple-custard pie:** Omit vanilla; add ½ teaspoon lemon extract to custard; put crushed pineapple in strainer, squeeze out as much juice as possible; immediately before serving sprinkle ½ to 1 cup drained crushed pineapple over pie crust, cover with custard.

**Pecan pie:** Sprinkle ¾ cup broken pecans over pie pan before pouring custard.

**Pumpkin or squash pie:** Combine custard ingredients, using 1 cup fresh milk; add 1 cup steamed and mashed or canned pumpkin or squash, 3 tablespoons dark or blackstrap molasses, ½ teaspoon ginger and cinnamon; increase salt to ¼ teaspoon. If fluffy pie is desired, beat egg whites until stiff and fold into custard just before baking.

**Raisin-nut pie:** Sprinkle ½ cup each raisins and broken walnuts or pecans over bottom of pan before pouring custard into it.

You can consistently make beautiful meringue pies if you bear two facts in mind: first, that hard-cooked eggs are firm; second, that high heat causes protein to shrivel and become tough. If the meringue is baked long enough for the egg white to be hard-cooked, it cannot fall. It must be baked at a low temperature if it is to stay tender and mountainous. Always check the oven temperature with a thermometer before putting a meringue in to bake.

When water is added to egg whites, the surface tension is increased and the eggs will whip to a much larger volume than if no water is used.

The taste and texture of a meringue are greatly improved if a generous amount of sugar is beaten into the egg whites. To prevent the pie from becoming too sweet, little sugar should be used in the filling. All meringues are more delicious when a small amount of flavoring is added to them. A drop of coloring added to the meringue used for apricot and orange pies is particularly delightful.

Chiffon-cream pies in which the egg whites are stirred into the filling seem to me even more delicious and more easily prepared than are meringue pies. The success of this type of pie depends entirely upon having the sweetened cream sauce boiling slowly while the eggs are being folded into it. If the sauce is not boiling, the eggs remain undercooked and the filling is runny; if the sauce is allowed to boil too hard or too long, the egg whites overcook and the texture becomes curdly. The eggs are cooked largely by low heat during the cooling process. If the directions are followed, pitfalls can easily be avoided.

Chiffon-pie fillings make delicious puddings which, if properly cooked, will hold their shape when molded.

## MERINGUE-CREAM PIE

Mix well in a *metal* saucepan:

⅓ to ½ cup sugar                    ¼ cup whole-wheat pastry flour
½ cup powdered milk                 pinch of salt

Add and beat well:

½ cup fresh milk                    2 egg yolks

When batter is smooth, add and stir:

1½ cups fresh milk

Cook over moderate heat, stirring constantly, about 8 minutes, until custard becomes quite firm; remove from heat and add:

**1 tablespoon margarine or butter     2 teaspoons vanilla**

Pour into a 9-inch crumb crust or baked pastry shell; cover with meringue.

## MERINGUE

Combine:

**2 egg whites                       ½ teaspoon vanilla
2 tablespoons water**

Beat until egg whites are stiff; add 2 tablespoons at a time:

¼ cup sugar

Spread meringue over pie and bake in a slow oven at 300° F. for 30 minutes.

*Variations:*

Instead of vanilla add ½ teaspoon of the following flavorings to filling, ¼ teaspoon to meringue: almond, black walnut, banana, lemon, maple, strawberry, rum, or brandy; or omit 2 tablespoons milk from custard, add 2 tablespoons rum or brandy before pouring into crust.

**Almond pie:** Omit vanilla and 2 tablespoons flour from filling; add ¼ cup soy grits, ¾ teaspoon almond flavoring. Follow same procedure in using soy grits with black-walnut flavoring.

**Banana pie:** Slice 2 or 3 bananas into crust and cover with filling and meringue, or add sliced bananas to filling before pouring into crust.

**Cake filling:** Increase sugar in filling to ½ cup; omit meringue; use the basic recipe or any variation for cake filling.

**Coconut pie:** Add ½ cup shredded or ground coconut to filling; sprinkle coconut over top of meringue before baking.

**Chiffon-cream pies:** Use a 2-quart saucepan; combine ingredients of filling, omitting egg yolks; beat egg whites without water; after sugar is added, drop egg yolks into meringue and beat only until evenly blended; set meringue aside. Cook filling immediately, stirring constantly; when filling boils, add flavoring, margarine, coloring and nuts or fruit suggested under variations; lower heat and fold in meringue while filling continues to boil slowly for 1 minute. Pour immediately into pie crust; omit baking. Use for basic recipe or any variation.

**Date-nut pie:** Just before pouring filling into crust add ½ cup each chopped dates and broken walnuts or pecans. Vary by cooking ½ cup raisins in filling or adding ½ cup drained prune pulp. Or add ¼ cup soy grits and 1 teaspoon black-walnut flavoring with dates.

**Fruit-cream pies:** Prepare filling, using 2 tablespoons sugar, 1 cup fresh milk; just before pouring filling into crust or folding in meringue add 1 cup fresh sweetened or canned berries, sliced peaches, apricots, or crushed pineapple and juice.

**Fruit-meringue pies:** Omit cream filling; prepare fruit filling as directed on pages 528-529, using half the sugar; cook fruit with flour, sugar, salt until thick; spread over crust, cover with meringue; add yellow and orange coloring to meringue for peach or apricot pies, red coloring for berry pies.

**Lemon pie:** Omit vanilla; use ½ cup sugar, 1½ cups fresh milk in filling; before pouring filling into pie add ½ cup lemon juice, grated rind of 1 lemon; add 1 teaspoon grated rind to meringue.

**Maple-nut pie:** Add 1 tablespoon dark or blackstrap molasses, ½ teaspoon maple flavoring, ½ cup broken walnuts or pecans; or omit sugar and ⅓ cup fresh milk from filling, add and ⅓ cup maple syrup.

**Puddings:** Increase sugar in filling to ½ cup; use 3 tablespoons flour, 1 or 2 whole eggs; omit meringue. Pour into sherbet glasses while warm. Serve the basic recipe or any variation as pudding.

*Chiffon-cream pudding:* Prepare as for chiffon-cream pie; pour into sherbet glasses or into wet ring mold. Unmold before serving.

**Orange pie:** Omit vanilla; add to filling grated rind of 1 orange, 1 teaspoon orange flavoring, 1 drop orange coloring; add to meringue ½ teaspoon each grated orange rind and flavoring, 1 drop orange coloring.


## GELATIN CHIFFON PIES

An almost endless variety of chiffon pies may be prepared by using as fillings any of the gelatin sponges (pp. 502, 503) or Bavarian creams (p. 504). Allow the gelatin to become sufficiently set to pile well. Brush a 9-inch serving pie plate generously with butter-flavored fat, being careful to grease the rim; sprinkle with ½ cup crumbs. Pour gelatin over crumbs or into a 9-inch baked crumb or pastry shell. Sprinkle top with crumbs if desired. I prefer toasted whole-wheat-bread crumbs to other varieties because they retain their crispness and are less rich.


## FRESH-FRUIT PIES

Mix in small saucepan:

| | |
|---|---|
| ⅔ cup sugar | pinch of salt |
| 3 tablespoons whole-wheat pastry flour | |

Add:

1½ cups small fresh berries, sliced apricots, or diced peaches

Stir well to mash fruit; cook 10 minutes; chill.
Put into 9-inch baked crumb or pastry pie shell:

2 cups berries or sliced apricots or peaches

Whip until stiff:

½ cup chilled evaporated milk

Stir into whipped milk:

| | |
|---|---|
| ¼ cup powdered milk | 1 tablespoon lemon juice |

Combine whipped milk with chilled cooked fruit; pour over uncooked fruit in crust. Keep chilled until served.

*Variations:*

Pour chilled cooked fruit over uncooked fruit without adding whipped milk; whip ½ cup heavy cream, add powdered milk, ½ teaspoon vanilla sweeten to taste; spread over top of pie.

Use strawberries, boysenberries, raspberries, loganberries, youngberries, mulberries, or blueberries.

**Cake filling:** Omit evaporated milk; chill cooked fruit, blend in fresh fruit; use basic recipe or any variation as a cake filling.

A friend who by careful vigilance maintains a magnificent figure views rich and nauseously sweet desserts with such disdain that she calls them "glop." Although there are times when I share her disdain, the following pies are my idea of "glop" put on an intelligent plane. Compared with pies of similar variety, these pies contain far less sugar and fat and supply the equivalent of a glass of milk per slice; yet they are delicious and amazingly easy to make.

It is wise to keep a can of evaporated milk in the refrigerator at all times, ready to whip at a moment's notice. If friends drop in for dinner unexpectedly, you can quickly prepare a crust, stir up the filling, and have a delicious dessert with little effort.

When the following pies are held as long as 24 hours, the filling dries and becomes the texture of cheese cake. For this reason the recipe is planned for a 7-inch crust. The pies should not be prepared earlier than 8 hours before serving.

My name for this kind is "the milk, milk, and milk" pie.

### TEN-MINUTE BERRY PIE

Combine:

½ cup sweetened condensed milk      pinch of salt
⅓ cup lemon juice      1 or 2 drops food coloring (optional)
½ cup powdered milk

Stir well and add:

1 cup fresh sweetened, frozen, or well-drained canned raspberries, boysenberries, strawberries, or other berries

Whip stiff and fold in:

### ½ cup evaporated milk

Pour into a 7-inch baked pastry shell or crumb crust. Chill 15 minutes before serving. Keep in refrigerator.

*Variations:*

Instead of berries use 1 cup of any of the following sweetened fruits: well-drained crushed pineapple; thick applesauce or drained stewed apples; sliced fresh, canned, or steamed dried apricots or peaches; well-drained purple plums; pitted black cherries; sliced or diced bananas; sliced fresh or frozen California persimmons (this persimmon pie is food for a king); diced peeled guavas; add grated rind of 1 lemon to pineapple, apple, banana, persimmon, and guava pies; sprinkle apple pie with nutmeg; add ¼ teaspoon vanilla to peach pie.

**Almond or black-walnut pie:** Omit berries; cook ¼ cup soy grits in ¼ cup water for 5 minutes, or until all water is absorbed; chill and add ½ teaspoon almond or black-walnut flavoring; fold into pie with whipped milk. Use chopped blanched almonds or broken walnuts with or without grits if desired.

**Cake filling:** Use basic recipe or any variation for cake filling if to be eaten within 8 hours; let filling chill 15 minutes before spreading on cooled layers.

**Date-nut pie:** Instead of berries add ½ cup each chopped dates, broken walnuts or pecans; vary by adding 2 tablespoons rum or brandy.

**Hawaiian pie:** Instead of berries add 1 cup well-drained crushed or cubed pineapple, ¼ cup shredded coconut, 2 tablespoons quartered maraschino cherries, ¼ teaspoon lemon flavoring or grated rind of 1 lemon.

**Lemon pie:** Use ⅔ cup condensed milk, ½ cup lemon juice; add 1 drop yellow coloring, grated rind of 1 lemon, ½ teaspoon lemon extract; omit berries.

**Orange pie:** Use ⅔ cup condensed milk, ½ cup lemon juice; add 1 drop orange coloring, grated rind of 1 orange, ¾ teaspoon orange flavoring; omit berries.

**Pear pie:** Use 1 cup diced canned pears instead of berries; add ½ teaspoon ground ginger or 3 tablespoons finely diced preserved or candied ginger. This pie is particularly delicious with preserved ginger. Add 1 drop green coloring if desired.

**Pudding:** Prepare basic recipe or any variation; put in sherbet glasses and chill.

## COOKIES

Since cookies are often eaten between meals or carried in box lunches, they should be made to contribute as many nutrients as possible. Cookies made with powdered milk, wheat germ or wheat-germ flour, rice polish, or soy, peanut, or cottonseed flour are more crisp and have a much higher vitamin, mineral, and protein content than those made with wheat flour only. When soy grits and walnut or almond flavoring are added to cookies, the taste and texture are much the same as when nuts are added.

## DROP SUGAR COOKIES

Mix well together:

| | |
|---|---|
| ½ cup butter-flavored shortening | 1 tablespoon vanilla or grated |
| ¾ cup sugar | lemon rind |
| 2 eggs | 3 tablespoons evaporated or fresh |
| | top milk |

Sift in:

| | |
|---|---|
| 1 cup sifted whole-wheat pastry flour | ½ cup powdered milk |
| | ½ teaspoon salt |
| ½ cup wheat germ or wheat-germ flour | 2 teaspoons double-acting baking powder |

Stir only enough to mix well; drop from teaspoon onto baking sheet brushed with oil; sprinkle lightly with sugar.

Bake in a moderate oven at 350° F. no longer than 8 minutes.

*Variations:*

Omit vanilla and add 1 or 2 tablespoons poppy, caraway, or anise seeds or the grated rind of 2 oranges.

Use ¾ cup whole-wheat flour and add 3 tablespoons debittered brewers' yeast, 1 teaspoon each nutmeg, cinnamon, allspice.

Instead of ½ cup whole-wheat flour use ½ cup rice polish or soy, peanut, or lima-bean flour; or omit whole-wheat flour and use 1 cup rice polish or soy, peanut, or lima-bean flour.

Add ½ to 1 cup soy grits, 1 teaspoon black-walnut or almond flavoring; or add ½ cup each soy grits and chopped nuts with or without flavoring.

Sprinkle top of cookies with any of the following: raisins; chopped candied cherries, pineapple, or citron; chopped or ground nuts; shredded coconut; anise, poppy, sesame, or caraway seeds; cinnamon and sugar or colored sugar (p. 553); press lightly into dough before baking.

**Apricot cookies:** Omit vanilla; instead of fresh milk use ½ cup well-drained cooked dried apricots; beat apricots with an eggbeater until smooth.

**Banana cookies:** Omit fresh milk and add ½ cup mashed bananas; use grated lemon rind for flavoring.

**Coconut cookies:** Add ½ to 1 cup shredded coconut and/or drop dough from teaspoon into a dish of shredded coconut, toss coconut over top, and transfer to the baking sheet with a spatula. Color coconut by mixing with a few drops of water to which coloring has been added.

**Cream-cheese cookies:** Instead of ¼ cup shortening use 1 package cream cheese; increase lemon rind to 2 tablespoons; add ½ cup raisins, soy grits, or chopped nuts as desired. Vary by dropping into ground walnuts or pecans before placing on baking sheet; garnish center with candied cherry.

**Lemon cookies:** Omit vanilla; add 2 teaspoons lemon extract with grated lemon rind, 1 drop yellow coloring.

**Mincemeat cookies:** Omit fresh milk and add 1 cup mincemeat.

**Oatmeal cookies:** Omit ½ cup flour and add 1½ cups rolled oats, 1 teaspoon each cinnamon and nutmeg. Vary by adding ½ cup each raisins and soy grits; or add to basic recipe ½ cup each rolled oats, chopped nuts, soy grits, shredded coconut or raisins.

**Peanut-butter cookies:** Use 2 tablespoons shortening; cream ½ cup peanut butter with sugar and shortening; use half whole-wheat flour and half peanut flour. Proceed as in basic recipe. Flatten cookies with prongs of fork, crossing at right angle.

*Peanut-butter-banana cookies:* Prepare as peanut-butter cookies except to omit milk and add ½ cup mashed bananas.

**Pineapple cookies:** Omit flavoring and fresh milk; add 1 cup very well drained crushed pineapple.

Cookies made of blackstrap molasses, powdered milk, and wheat germ are superior nutritionally to any other variety. I make mine entirely of wheat-germ flour, as I do waffles, muffins, pie dough, and many other products, but I have not specified it in the recipes because wheat-germ flour is not widely distributed.

I recently saw an 8-year-old child who was extremely thin. I gave his mother the following cookie recipe and advised her to allow the youngster to eat as many cookies as he desired. He made a gain of six pounds the following month!

## MOLASSES DROP COOKIES

Cream together:

½ cup shortening                        ⅓ cup sugar

Add:

**1 egg**                                    ¼ cup evaporated or fresh milk
½ cup blackstrap or dark molasses

Sift in:

½ cup sifted whole-wheat pastry        2 teaspoons double-acting baking
flour                                    powder
½ cup sifted rice polish or soy,        ½ teaspoon salt
peanut, or cottonseed flour             ½ teaspoon each cinnamon, gin-
½ cup powdered milk                      ger, and nutmeg or cloves
½ cup wheat germ or wheat-germ
flour

Stir only enough to mix well, or about 25 strokes; drop from a teaspoon
to a baking sheet brushed with oil.
Bake in moderate oven at 350° F. for 12 to 15 minutes.

*Variations:*

Use ⅛ cup whole-wheat flour and add 3 tablespoons debittered brewers'
yeast; increase spices to 1 teaspoon each.

**Coconut-molasses cookies:** Add 1 cup shredded coconut; sprinkle coconut over top.

**Fruit cookies:** Add ½ to 1 cup raisins, chopped dates, or figs to molasses
cookies or spice cookies.

**Gingersnaps:** Increase ginger to 1½ teaspoons; add ½ cup more whole-
wheat flour, turn onto floured wax paper, make into small rolls, and chill
overnight; slice ⅛ inch thick and bake 8 minutes.

*Gingerbread men:* Use gingersnap dough; chill overnight; roll ¼ inch
thick, cut with figure cutter; use raisins or candied cherries for buttons
and eyes.

**Maple-nut cookies:** Omit spices; add 1 teaspoon maple flavoring, ½
cup each walnuts or pecans and soy grits.

**Mock nut cookies:** Omit spices; add 2 teaspoons black-walnut flavoring, 1 cup soy grits.

**Nut cookies:** Add 1 cup broken English or black walnuts, pecans, almonds, or peanuts; or drop dough from teaspoon into a dish of ground nuts before transferring to baking sheet.

**Refrigerator cookies:** Add ½ cup more whole-wheat or soy flour to the basic recipe or any variation; turn onto floured wax paper, make into a roll 2 inches in diameter, wrap in wax paper; chill overnight in ice compartment; slice ⅛ inch thick and bake 8 to 10 minutes at 350° F.; or bake half the recipe as drop cookies; stir ¼ cup flour into the other half and bake later as refrigerator cookies.

**Spice cookies:** Increase spices to 1 teaspoon each ginger, cinnamon, and nutmeg and ¼ teaspoon each cloves and allspice.

I have purposely made the recipe for refrigerator cookies unusually large. After the dough is prepared, it may be divided and nuts, fruits, bran, oatmeal, soy grits, colorings, and flavorings added, thus making a wide variety of cookies at one time. The dough can be kept frozen indefinitely and baked at any time you are in the cookie mood.


### REFRIGERATOR COOKIES

Cream together:

| | |
|---|---|
| 1 cup butter-flavored shortening | 1½ cups sugar |

Add and mix well:

| | |
|---|---|
| 2 eggs | 1 tablespoon vanilla |

Sift together and add:

| | |
|---|---|
| 1 cup whole-wheat pastry flour | ½ cup powdered milk |
| 1 cup rice polish or soy or peanut flour | 2 teaspoons baking powder |
| 1 cup wheat germ or wheat-germ flour | ½ teaspoon salt |

Stir only enough to mix well, or about 30 strokes. Turn out on wax paper, form into a roll; slice and bake immediately or wrap in the wax paper and chill or freeze overnight or longer.

Cut into ⅛-inch slices and bake on oiled baking sheet in moderate oven at 350° F. for 8 to 10 minutes.

*Variations:*

Instead of whole-wheat flour increase wheat germ, rice polish, or soy, peanut, or wheat-germ flour to 2 cups.

Omit vanilla and add 1 or 2 tablespoons poppy, caraway, or anise seeds.

Instead of white sugar use 1½ cups tightly packed brown sugar or 1 cup brown sugar with ½ cup white; add 1 teaspoon cinnamon.

Add ½ to 1 cup of any of the following: soy grits; coconut meal; ground walnuts, pecans, almonds, peanuts, raisins, currants, dates, or figs. Add 1 teaspoon maple flavoring with walnuts or pecans, ½ teaspoon each almond and lemon extract with almonds, 1 teaspoon black-walnut or almond flavoring with soy grits; or divide dough and add different nuts or fruits to each portion.

**Bran cookies:** Add 1 cup bran flakes, 1 tablespoon grated orange rind; omit or use vanilla.

**Butterscotch cookies:** Use tightly packed brown sugar instead of white; add 1 cup ground walnuts or pecans.

**Lemon cookies:** Omit vanilla; add 1 tablespoon grated lemon rind or 2 teaspoons lemon extract.

**Oatmeal cookies:** Use tightly packed brown sugar instead of white; add 2 cups quick-cooking rolled oats, 1 cup ground raisins, 1 teaspoon each cinnamon and nutmeg.

**Peanut-butter cookies:** Use ½ cup shortening and ¾ cup each white and tightly packed brown sugar; cream 1 cup peanut butter with shortening and sugar; proceed as in basic recipe.

**Rainbow cookies:** Divide dough into two parts; color one half; roll out each half separately, then place one on top of the other, and press firmly together; roll, slice, and bake. Vary by making several colors as desired.

**Spice cookies:** Add 1½ teaspoons ginger or 1 teaspoon cinnamon and ½ teaspoon each nutmeg and allspice; add ground nuts, soy grits, and raisins as desired.

## BUTTERSCOTCH BROWNIES

Melt: `

    ¼ cup butter-flavored shortening

Add:

| | |
|---|---|
| 1 tablespoon dark or blackstrap molasses | 2 eggs |
| | 2 teaspoons vanilla |
| ⅞ cup sugar | |

Stir well; sift in:

| | |
|---|---|
| 2/3 cup soy, peanut, or wheat-germ flour | 1/2 teaspoon baking powder |
| 1/2 cup powdered milk | 1/4 teaspoon salt |

Add before stirring:

### 1/2 cup broken walnuts or pecans

Stir only enough to blend, or no more than 20 strokes. Spread in 8-by-8-inch pan completely covered with wax paper. Bake in moderate oven at 350° F. for 30 minutes. Turn out of pan; remove paper immediately. Cut into squares or bars while hot.

*Variations:*

Instead of vanilla add 1 teaspoon cinnamon or use 1/2 teaspoon maple or rum flavoring or ground coriander or cardamom with vanilla.

Add 1 teaspoon black-walnut flavoring, 1/2 cup soy grits; bake 25 minutes.

Add to dough 1/2 to 1 cup of any of the following or sprinkle over top and press in firmly: shredded coconut; diced citron; chopped candied pineapple and shredded coconut or candied cherries; raisins, currants, chopped dates or figs, or ground dried apricots.

**Chocolate brownies:** Add to hot melted fat 2 squares (2 ounces) unsweetened cooking chocolate; let chocolate melt while gathering dry ingredients; or sift 1/4 cup cocoa with dry ingredients; prepare as in basic recipe; 1 tablespoon debittered brewers' yeast may be added. This recipe cannot be recommended nutritionally, but people will continue making chocolate brownies and these are certainly superior in both nutrients and flavor to the usual variety.

**Coconut-fruit brownies:** Add 1/2 cup coconut and 1/4 cup each diced candied pineapple and citron.

**Date-nut brownies:** Add 1/2 cup chopped dates with 1 cup walnuts or pecans; or add with dates 1/2 cup soy grits and 1 teaspoon black-walnut, maple, rum, or brandy flavoring; if soy grits are used, bake 25 minutes.

**Spice brownies:** Use 3/4 cup sugar and add 1/4 cup dark or blackstrap molasses, 2 teaspoons cinnamon, 1/4 teaspoon each allspice and nutmeg, 2 tablespoons brewers' yeast, 1 cup raisins or 1/2 cup each raisins and shredded coconut or soy grits.

**Wheat-germ brownies:** Instead of flour use 1 cup wheat germ or wheat germ and middlings. The texture is somewhat coarse but the flavor is delicious.

## COCONUT CHEWS

Combine:

| | |
|---|---|
| ⅔ cup sweetened condensed milk | ¼ cup powdered milk |
| 2 teaspoons vanilla | ¼ cup wheat germ |
| ⅛ teaspoon salt | |

Stir until thoroughly blended; add:

### 1½ cups shredded coconut

Mix well. Drop from a teaspoon onto baking sheet lined with greased heavy paper. Bake in moderate oven at 325° F. for 12 to 15 minutes. Remove from paper while hot.

*Variations:*

Instead of ¾ cup coconut add ¾ cup broken walnuts, pecans, or other nuts; bran flakes; ground dried apricots or chopped dates; or ⅓ cup soy grits. If soy grits are used, let batter stand 20 minutes before dropping onto baking sheet.

*Omit coconut in the following variations.*

**Almond chews:** Omit vanilla; add 1½ cups ground blanched almonds, ½ teaspoon almond extract. Vary by using 1 cup ground almonds, ⅓ cup soy grits, ¾ teaspoon almond extract. If soy grits are used, let batter stand 20 minutes before dropping on baking sheet.

**Apricot chews:** Omit vanilla; add 1 cup ground dried apricots, ½ cup chopped or broken peanuts, walnuts, or other nuts.

**Date chews:** Add 1½ cups chopped dates or ¾ cup each chopped dates and broken walnuts or pecans; increase wheat germ to ⅓ cup.

**Fruit chews:** Add 1½ cups seedless raisins or ground seeded raisins, currants, or ground dried figs; or use 1 cup dried fruit, ½ cup broken nuts or soy grits.

**Nut chews:** Add 1½ cups broken walnuts, pecans, coarsely chopped peanuts, or other nuts. Vary by using ¾ cup nuts, ⅓ cup soy grits.

**Soy chews:** Add ⅔ cup soy grits; vary by omitting vanilla and adding 1 teaspoon almond or black-walnut flavoring. Before dropping onto baking sheet let batter stand 20 minutes or longer so that grits will become soft. Soy chews are the most inexpensive and most nutritious of all chews.

**Oatmeal chews:** Add ⅓ cup steel-cut oats, ½ cup raisins; let batter stand 20 minutes or longer for oats to soften before dropping onto baking sheet.

# CHAPTER 25

## CANDIES AND CANDY SUBSTITUTES

Few foods cause so much ill-health as do the usual varieties of candy, although the harm they do is largely indirect. Since most candies are made principally of refined sugar which contains no vitamins, minerals, or proteins, they cannot build health. Any concentrated sweet destroys the appetite to such an extent that the person who eats many sweets rarely eats sufficient other foods to meet his body needs. Furthermore, a type of bacteria, known as bacillus acidophilus, thrives in the mouth on sugar, breaking it down into lactic and pyruvic acids. These acids combine with the calcium in the teeth and cause them to decay or erode. Tooth decay has been produced in children who were formerly immune to decay in as short a time as six weeks when a single piece of candy was given to them daily. Whether the teeth of your children decay or stay beautiful depends largely upon the amount of sweets allowed them.

Despite the fact that some 96 per cent of our population suffers from tooth decay, and that the examination of teeth in gathering the army for World War II revealed that the actual number of teeth decayed had doubled in twenty years, candy will probably always be eaten. It is for the persons who wish to serve candy with the greatest nutritional value possible that candy recipes have been included in this book. If you wish to make candy, see that it contains health-building ingredients and can contribute its part toward meeting the daily requirements.

Honey has often been recommended by people posing as nutrition specialists; yet it contains an insignificant amount of vitamins and is almost lacking in minerals. It appears to bring about tooth decay as quickly as does refined sugar. One tablespoonful of honey has more calories than a tablespoonful of refined sugar.

Although blackstrap molasses is by far the most nourishing sweet one can use, its taste is so pronounced that few people would enjoy candies made of it. I have therefore most frequently used dark rather than blackstrap molasses in the candy recipes, hoping that you will change to blackstrap as its flavor becomes appreciated. Experiments in which blackstrap molasses has been given to children show that although the amount of tooth decay has not lessened, at least it has not increased. This molasses is rich in pantothenic acid, a B vitamin which, although best known for helping to prevent graying of hair, appears to protect teeth against decay. Any molasses, however, is so sweet that it can readily destroy the appetite.

The detrimental effect of sweets upon the teeth can be overcome partly by adding generous amounts of calcium to candy and other foods containing much sugar. When the calcium supply is more than adequate, the saliva contains sufficient calcium to neutralize the acid formed by the bacterial breakdown of sugar; calcium is therefore not removed from the teeth. It is for this reason that I have included powdered milk in many candy recipes. Only spray-processed milk of the best quality should be used; if it is fresh and has been kept sealed from moisture, it does not alter the taste of the candy. Candies made of powdered milk, however, dry out quickly and should not be held for several days.

Serve candy substitutes rather than candies, especially if there are children in the family. Keep every variety of dried fruits on hand: dates, figs, raisins, peaches, prunes, and particularly apricots. Serve popcorn, salted soybeans, or soy nuts, peanuts, and other nuts as candy substitutes. Nuts are rich in protein and the B vitamins and tend to destroy the appetite far less readily than do candies. If candies are to be made, add generous amounts of fruits and nuts to them.

Most of the following recipes were created by Mrs. Mabel Garvey. Her samples were convincing proof that delicious candies can be made to contribute substantially to health without sacrifice of taste appeal.

## STUFFED DRIED FRUIT

Wash and dry fruit; stone dates; cut opening in figs which have not been pressed; use soft uncooked prunes or steam until tender before stoning; press halves of soft uncooked or partly steamed apricots or peaches together with filling between. Fill with any of the following:

Broken pecans, English or black walnuts, butternuts
Salted peanuts or almonds
Whole or chopped Brazil nuts
Marshmallows halved or quartered
Candied cherries, pineapple, or citron
Peanut-butter candy, fondant, or any soft candy

## FRUITIES

Put through the meat grinder, using medium knife, and measure after grinding:

1 cup dates              ½ cup walnuts or pecans
½ cup graham-cracker crumbs

Add and stir well:

3 tablespoons orange or pineapple    4 tablespoons powdered milk
juice                              8 chopped marshmallows

Press firmly on wax paper or buttered pan to thickness of ¾ inch; cut into squares or mold into balls or rolls. Chill. After chilling, roll in ground nuts, powdered sugar, coconut, or graham-cracker crumbs.

*Variations:*

Instead of dates use 1 cup ground dried figs or ¾ cup soft uncooked or partly steamed dried apricots; if fruit is moist, add more graham crackers or powdered milk.

Omit marshmallows and cracker crumbs. Combine the following groups of ingredients with powdered milk and juice: ½ cup each dates and figs, 1 cup English walnuts; ¾ cup each raisins and walnuts; ¾ cup each pecans and dried apricots; ½ cup each pecans, walnuts, dates, and figs or apricots; ½ cup each dried apricots, dates, walnuts; add ½ cup coconut to any variation.

**Fruit-filled bars:** Prepare fondant (p. 554); roll ⅛ inch thick, cover with ground fruit pressed ½ inch thick; cover fruit with another layer of fondant; press together. chill, and cut into bars.

**Fruit rolls:** Form fruit into small rolls 2½ inches long, ¾ inch thick; cover surface with whole pecans or large peanut halves.

**Spiced fruit bars:** Add to basic recipe or any variation 1 teaspoon cinnamon, ⅛ teaspoon nutmeg; when flavor of fruit is prominent, add 1 to 3 teaspoons debittered brewers' yeast.

## POPCORN

Pop ½ cup popcorn by shaking slowly in dry covered frying pan over moderate heat until popping begins; shake rapidly until popping stops. Remove from heat and prepare in any of the following ways. Makes 6 cups.

**Buttered popcorn:** Melt 3 or 4 tablespoons margarine, butter, or butter-flavored cooking fat; pour over popcorn and stir until evenly coated; sprinkle generously with salt.

**Cheese popcorn:** Sprinkle hot popcorn with grated American cheese, using 1 cup cheese to 4 cups popcorn; salt to taste. If popcorn is cold, put in flat pan, sprinkle with cheese, and set in a slow oven until cheese melts; stir well and salt; vary by using part pimento cheese or Roquefort.

## POPCORN BALLS

Combine:

| | |
|---|---|
| 1 cup dark molasses | 1 tablespoon vinegar |
| ½ cup sugar | ¼ teaspoon salt |

Boil, stirring constantly, to 270° F., or until brittle when tried in cold water; add:

**1 tablespoon butter or margarine**

Pour over:

| | |
|---|---|
| 6 cups popcorn | ½ to 1 cup salted peanuts |

Stir gently until evenly coated; when popcorn is cool enough to handle, press into balls.

*Variations:*

Use 4 cups popcorn and 2 cups large peanuts or 1 cup each peanuts and puffed wheat.

**Taffy:** Prepare basic recipe, cooking to 260° F.; pour on sheets of well-buttered wax paper; when taffy is cool enough to handle, pull until light brown.

**Peanut brittle:** Cook molasses slowly to 280° F., being extremely careful not to burn it; add 2 cups unsalted peanuts; cover wax paper generously with butter and lay over flat pan; pour brittle on paper; when candy is cool enough to handle, break into small pieces; set in refrigerator to keep candy from becoming sticky.

**Puffed-wheat bars:** Add to basic recipe with butter 3 cups puffed wheat, ½ to 1 cup peanuts; stir until wheat is well coated; cover wax paper with thick layer of butter and pour puffed wheat onto paper; press firmly to thickness of ¾ inch; cool slightly and cut into bars.

The texture of soy nuts varies so widely with the age and variety of the beans used that it is impossible to give a recipe which will be equally successful with all types of beans. Some beans need only to be soaked, then browned, and salted; others require varying amounts of precooking. When the beans have soaked or cooked until their texture is that of fresh peanuts, care must be taken that they are not dried out as they are fried. Since few foods are so excellent for growing children as are soy nuts, a little experimentation with the type of beans you have is worth while. Whenever preparing soybeans as a meat substitute, add 1 cup to be made into soy nuts.

### SOY NUTS

Soak in ice tray for 2 hours or longer:

1 cup soybeans     1 cup water

Freeze for 2 hours or preferably overnight. Drop into:

½ cup hot water

Simmer for 30 minutes; taste and cook longer if soybeans are not as tender as salted peanuts; remove lid of utensil and let water evaporate. Cool beans.

Heat until smoking hot:

¼ cup vegetable oil

Add beans and cook quickly to a delicate brown, or about 1 or 2 minutes; remove from heat at once; add:

1 teaspoon salt

*Variations:*

When fresh green soybeans are available, omit soaking and precooking; fry as in basic recipe; salt to taste.

Fry a few beans after soaking 1 or 2 hours or after soaking and freezing; if moisture content of the beans is high, they will not require precooking.

## PINEAPPLE KISSES

Combine and stir well:

| | |
|---|---|
| 2 tablespoons melted margarine or butter | 1 cup tightly packed brown sugar<br>½ cup well-drained crushed pineapple |

Boil slowly 2 minutes, or until sugar is melted; remove from heat, cool thoroughly, and add:

**¾ to 1 cup powdered milk or enough to give firm, creamy consistency**

Beat until smooth; drop from teaspoon onto buttered wax paper; chill 1 hour or longer, or until easily handled.

*Variations:*

Add any one of the following before adding powdered milk: ½ teaspoon ground ginger or 1 to 3 tablespoons finely chopped candied ginger; dash of salt, 4 tablespoons each wheat germ and chopped nuts; ½ to 1 cup shredded or ground coconut; ½ to 1 cup chopped walnuts, almonds, pecans, or other nuts; ¼ cup or more diced candied cherries.

Use white sugar instead of brown in basic recipe or any variation; add ⅛ teaspoon lemon extract. This candy is particularly delicious with chopped candied cherries or preserved ginger.

**Coconut drops:** Prepare candy as in basic recipe; drop from teaspoon into dish of shredded coconut, toss coconut over top, and transfer to oiled wax paper; before adding powdered milk add ½ cup coconut if desired and/or color coconut by mixing with a little water and food coloring.

**Pecan roll:** Chill candy 1 or 2 hours after powdered milk is added; flour hands with powdered milk, form candy into rolls 4 inches long and ¾ inch thick; cover entire surface with pecan halves; serve whole or cut into slices.

**Wheat-germ fudge:** Before adding powdered milk stir in ½ cup each wheat germ and walnuts, ¼ teaspoon salt, 1 teaspoon vanilla; press ¾ inch thick on buttered pan or wax paper; cut into cubes.

# DIVINITY

Beat until stiff:

**1 egg white**

Set egg aside; combine and stir:

**3 tablespoons water**              **1 cup sugar**
**1 teaspoon vinegar**

Boil slowly 2 minutes, or until sugar is melted; begin to count time when bubbles cover entire surface. Pour boiling syrup over egg white and beat 2 or 3 minutes; cool.

When egg mixture is cold, add:

**2 or 3 teaspoons vanilla**         **1 to 1¼ cups powdered milk, or**
**½ to 1 cup broken walnuts or**        **enough to give consistency de-**
**pecans**                               **sired**

Push from teaspoon onto buttered wax paper; cool 1 hour or longer.

*Variations:*

Before adding powdered milk stir in 2 or 3 drops food coloring.

If candy is to be held a week or longer, add only ¾ cup powdered milk; chill 2 hours before dropping onto paper.

Use brown sugar instead of white; decrease or omit vanilla.

Add ½ to 1 cup of one or more of the following: raisins; chopped dates; ground dried apricots; or add ¼ cup quartered candied cherries or chopped candied pineapple.

# FUDGE

Stir together:

**⅓ cup fresh milk**                 **2 tablespoons margarine or butter**
**1 cup sugar**

Boil 2 minutes; begin to count time when bubbles cover entire surface. Remove from heat, cool thoroughly, and add:

**2 teaspoons vanilla**              **½ to 1 cup walnuts**
**2 or 3 drops food coloring**          **⅔ to ¾ cup powdered milk**
**(optional)**

Stir until smooth and creamy; turn onto buttered wax paper or pan

*Variations:*

Instead of walnuts add ½ cup or more shredded coconut, broken pecans, hickory nuts, hazelnuts, peanuts, or other nuts; or add shredded coconut or chopped candied cherries with nuts.

Omit vanilla and nuts; add 3 drops orange or yellow coloring, 1 or 2 teaspoons orange or lemon flavoring. Use red coloring and add a few drops clove or peppermint oil or 1 teaspoon strawberry flavoring. Use green coloring and add 1 teaspoon almond flavoring or a few drops oil of wintergreen. Add 1 teaspoon black-walnut, rum, brandy, maple, or any fruit flavoring and corresponding coloring.

Use any fudge recipe; boil ingredients 2 or 3 minutes, chill, and add powdered milk to give consistency desired.

Add 2 tablespoons peanut butter, or omit fat and add 4 tablespoons peanut butter; decrease or omit vanilla; add ½ to 1 cup broken peanuts if desired.

**Maple fudge:** Boil 1 or 2 cups maple syrup 5 to 8 minutes; add 2 to 4 tablespoons margarine or butter; chill; stir in enough powdered milk to give consistency desired; turn onto buttered wax paper and cut into squares; add walnuts or pecans as desired.

**Panocha fudge:** Instead of white sugar use 1 cup tightly packed brown sugar; prepare as in basic recipe. Vary by adding 2 to 4 tablespoons peanut butter or ½ cup coconut, pecans, or other nuts.

Since children enjoy making their own candies, it seemed wise to Mrs. Garvey and me to stress uncooked varieties. Although the sugar must be melted in nut creams and the potato cooked for the modeling fondant, the procedure in each case is that of uncooked candy.

Cooked potato holds moisture in candy, keeping it fresh, and is used commercially in many delicious imported candies. The potato used in the modeling fondant gives it a wonderfully smooth texture, making it easy to handle without being sticky. No other fondant recipe, I believe, can compare with this one.

If you want to give a party which I'll guarantee will be a success regardless of the age of your guests, prepare a supply of modeling candy; furnish food colors and small brushes. I use tiny lipstick brushes. It is likely that your guests will promptly declare that they can neither model nor paint, will start by timidly making carrots and pears, and end up not only by making pigs, giraffes, and caricatures of each other but also by forgetting to go home.

## MODELING FONDANT

Peel, quarter, steam, and mash through a sieve or wire strainer·

**1 medium potato**

Measure carefully:

**¼ cup mashed potatoes**

Add and stir well while potato is still warm:

**1 teaspoon almond flavoring          2 tablespoons margarine or butter**

Sift together and add:

**1 cup powdered sugar          ½ cup powdered milk**

Stir well and chill. After chilling, knead in enough powdered milk to handle well.

Shape into tiny melons, fruits, and vegetables. Use cloves for apple and pear stems, green-tinted coconut for other stems; paint with food colorings. Use cinnamon or cocoa for potatoes and bananas; roll strawberries in tinted sugar; model and paint leaves on strawberries, peaches, plums, and ears of corn. Knead orange coloring into a portion of the fondant to be used for oranges, carrots, pumpkins; red for radishes, apples, tomatoes, strawberries; yellow coloring for lemons, pears, and bananas. Use toothpick to make depression on cantaloupes and pumpkins.

*Variations:*

Omit almond flavoring, divide into portions, and add vanilla, lemon, banana, orange, or oil of peppermint, clove, or wintergreen to taste. Use different food colorings for each portion; blend colorings to give colors desired.

Shape candy into balls, roll in cinnamon, crushed nuts, colored coconut, or colored sugar. Color sugar or coconut by mixing food coloring with ½ teaspoon water; moisten coconut or sugar, spread on paper, and let dry.

Use fondant for stuffing dates, figs, prunes; or press between halves of walnuts, pecans, apricots, or dried peaches; or surround pieces of nuts or candied fruits with fondant and roll in colored sugar.

**Tricolored fudge:** Roll fondant of one color ⅛ inch thick; add second and third layers of different colors; put a drop of water between layers to hold candy together; press firmly and cut into squares or rectangles. Or make two outer layers of same color, center layer of contrasting color. Or use two colors, roll, and cut as pinwheels.

## NUT CREAMS

Combine in top of double boiler:

½ cup brown sugar                    2 tablespoons margarine or butter
½ cup sweetened condensed milk

Heat over boiling water for about 10 minutes, or until sugar is melted. Remove from heat, cool thoroughly, and stir in:

⅔ to ¾ cup powdered milk, or enough to give consistency desired

Drop from teaspoon onto buttered wax paper; put a walnut half on top of each cream.

*Variations:*

Stir in any of the following before adding powdered milk: ½ to 1 cup coconut, broken walnuts, pecans, almonds, hickory nuts, or other nuts; ¼ cup diced candied cherries and/or candied pineapple; 2 tablespoons peanut butter; press on wax paper to thickness of ½ inch.

**Pecan fudge:** Before adding powdered milk stir in 1 cup broken pecans; spread on wax paper and cut into squares.

**Pecan pralines:** Drop candy from tablespoon onto wax paper; press 6 or 8 pecan halves into each praline.

**Walnut-date creams:** Stir in ½ cup each broken walnuts and ground or finely chopped dates; vary by using pecans, hickory nuts, or almonds.

## UNCOOKED FONDANT

Combine and stir thoroughly:

⅔ cup sweetened condensed milk      2 teaspoons vanilla

Sift together and add:

1 cup powdered milk                 ¼ cup powdered sugar

Turn on wax paper sprinkled with powdered sugar and knead gently until firm enough to handle, adding more powdered sugar if needed.

Divide into portions and add a different food coloring to each portion; flavor to taste with banana, peppermint, strawberry, orange, almond, rum, brandy, black walnut, vanilla, or lemon.

Use for stuffing dates, figs, prunes; or press between nut or apricot halves; or surround pieces of nuts or fruit with fondant.

Shape into balls, roll in cinnamon, coconut, or ground nuts.

*Variations:*

Add any of the following: 1 cup coconut meal or shredded coconut; ½ cup peanut butter, chopped walnuts, pecans, or other nuts; ½ cup each nuts or peanut butter and coconut; press to thickness of ½ inch and cut into squares or rectangles.

Roll fondant ⅛ inch thick; put between similar layers of contrasting color and flavor; press together firmly and cut into rectangles.

## UNCOOKED PEANUT-BUTTER CANDY

Combine and stir well:

| | |
|---|---|
| ½ cup smooth or crunchy peanut butter | ½ cup strained or cream honey ¾ to 1 cup powdered milk |

Turn on buttered wax paper and press to thickness of ¾ inch; cut into cubes.

*Variations:*

Add any of the following: ½ cup broken walnuts, small peanuts, chopped blanched almonds, pecans, hazelnuts, or Brazil nuts.

Add ½ to 1 cup shredded coconut and 1 teaspoon vanilla; make into balls, roll in coconut, powdered sugar, or crushed nuts.

Use for stuffing prunes, dates, figs; or press between halves of dried apricots, peaches, or nuts.

Make into rolls; chill and cut into slices.

Use ¼ cup each blackstrap molasses and honey.

## MARZIPANS, OR UNCOOKED ALMOND CANDIES

Blanch by steaming over hot water 5 minutes:

½ pound almonds

Remove skins, dry well, and pass through meat grinder 3 or 4 times, using small knife; add and mix well:

| | |
|---|---|
| ½ teaspoon almond extract | 1 cup powdered sugar |
| ½ cup sweetened condensed milk | ½ to ¾ cup powdered milk |

Turn on wax paper sprinkled with powdered milk and knead until smooth.

Shape into tiny apples, peaches, bananas, carrots, potatoes, strawberries, and other fruits and vegetables; use whole cloves for stems; color
by painting with food colorings; use cinnamon for potatoes and bananas;
roll strawberries in tinted sugar.

*Variation:*

Roll ¼ inch thick and cut into fancy shapes with small cookie cutters;
or use to stuff dates, figs, prunes, or apricots.

**Mock marzipans:** Use uncooked fondant or modeling fondant; add 1
teaspoon almond extract; shape into miniature fruits and vegetables.

The wheat germ and molasses candies which follow can scarcely
be dignified by the name of candy; yet it is almost impossible to
conceive of any food which contains such a concentration of vitamins, minerals, and protein as do these two foods. Since the taste
may not be enjoyed at first, the candy should be served when a
person is most hungry. Almost everyone who has used either of
the candies has become enthusiastic about the gains in health
which followed. Mothers of young children have found these foods
particularly satisfactory as a substitute for other sweets.

## UNCOOKED MOLASSES CANDY

Mix together:

| | |
|---|---|
| ½ cup dark or blackstrap molasses | 1 cup powdered milk |
| ½ cup crunchy peanut butter | ½ cup raisins |

Turn on wax paper sprinkled with powdered milk and knead until
consistency of pie dough; pat ½ inch thick and cut into small squares.

*Variations:*

Add 1 tablespoon debittered brewers' yeast with milk; gradually increase amount as flavor becomes familiar.

Add ½ cup peanuts, coconut, broken walnuts, or other nuts; or flavor
with 1 tablespoon cinnamon or ½ teaspoon nutmeg.

**Wheat-germ candy:** Omit powdered milk; use 2 tablespoons peanut
butter and add 2 cups slightly toasted wheat germ; knead on wax paper
sprinkled with ¼ cup powdered sugar; press ¾ inch thick; cut into cubes.
Add coconut or nuts as desired.

# CHAPTER 26

## REVISING AND CREATING RECIPES

Probably every homemaker has her own pet recipes which she especially enjoys using. She can improve almost every recipe by changing the method of preparation and by substituting or adding more nutritious ingredients than those called for. Often only slight revisions bring about tremendous improvements. For example, if you wish to substitute wheat germ for part of the flour called for in a recipe in order to increase your family's intake of vitamin $B_1$, you also increase the supply of ten or more B vitamins, vitamins E and K, protein, iron, copper, and a variety of other minerals. The substitution or addition of any nutritious food likewise brings multiple improvements. Should you alter a cooking procedure slightly in order to retain vitamin C, you probably retain larger amounts of some fifteen minerals and other vitamins. Make it a rule, therefore, to try to improve each recipe you use.

Learn to be critical of recipes you read or about which you hear. This morning, for example, my newspaper gave a recipe for stuffing bell peppers, excerpts from which are as follows: "Wash 6 green peppers and remove seeds; soak peppers in water half an hour and drain off water; cover with cold water and bring to a boil; drain well; stuff peppers . . . bake 1 hour."

This recipe advises one to extract and throw away as much vitamin C alone as could be obtained from 3 glasses of fresh orange juice, to say nothing of other vitamin and mineral losses. By substituting ripe peppers for green ones and by revising the recipe, the amount of vitamin C equal to that in 6 glasses of fresh orange juice could probably be retained, a saving by any standard.

Study each recipe carefully before you use it. Could procedures of handling and cooking be improved to retain nutritive value? Could less sugar be used or could dark or blackstrap molasses be substituted for the sugar? Could milk, fruit juice, or soup stock

557

be used in place of water? Could undiluted canned milk be used instead of fresh milk, or could powdered milk be added? Could baking powder be substituted for soda, or yeast for baking powder? Might the cooking time be shortened, or might an entirely different method of cooking be used in order to shorten the cooking time? Could the temperature be lowered to protect the B vitamins, or could the initial heating be speeded up to increase the retention of vitamin C? Could wheat germ, rice polish, or some high-protein flour be substituted for part of the flour called for? Could cheese be added to improve both taste and nutritive value? If, with these questions in mind, you revise each recipe you use, you will find not only that you produce greater health in yourself and your family but that you will enjoy cooking more than before. You will have discovered that cooking is truly a creative art.

After you have learned the general rules for scientific cookery, originate your own recipes. This habit will bring delight and will satisfy your creative impulses. Since refrigerated ships and quick-freezing units are now realities, many new foods will probably appear on the market. There will be no recipes at first to guide you in preparing such foods. In general, follow recipes of a familiar food which is similar to the new food in variety and texture. For example, if you plan to cook a new tuber, try preparing it in all the ways you would cook potatoes; if you wish to serve a new type of greens, add them to salads and cook as you would spinach or chard; add a tropical fruit to fruit appetizers, fruit cup, fruit salads, ice cream, and gelatin desserts. When you arrive at an especially successful recipe, do not keep it to yourself; send it on to your newspaper or to a women's magazine and let others enjoy it.

The woman who follows recipes blindly, without revision or creation, has not yet discovered the fun of cooking.

## CHAPTER 27

# WHERE TO BUY FOODS NOT YET ON THE MARKET

My particular pet peeve is the comment I hear almost every time a little-known food of unusual nutritive value is discussed, "I can't buy it." Every food product mentioned in this book can be located and purchased by anyone with very little persistence.

Not long ago I had a fan letter from a Mrs. Ruth Hoffmann of Oklahoma City; it was a charming letter which sparkled with the personality of the writer. A few weeks later when I was passing through her city, I had the pleasure of being her guest. Any number of health-building foods were new to her, and I knew nothing about the market in Oklahoma City. Mrs. Hoffmann, however, is one of those fine women who get things done, not tomorrow, but now. After perhaps a half-hour on the telephone she had located each product. A miller had told her where she could purchase soy and whole-wheat flour, where she could write to obtain peanut and cottonseed flour. A dairyman had directed her to a source of powdered milk and yogurt. The leading brewery told her where she could purchase dried brewers' yeast. She located blackstrap molasses at a bakery and a health-food store. She not only obtained these products for herself but also for a large group of friends who were eating intelligently. The service which she rendered to her community you can render to yours.

Let us suppose you live in some isolated spot where there are no classified telephone books. You can obtain the names and addresses of milling companies from packages of flour and cereal in your local store. Get a dozen penny postcards and write to one or more of the milling companies, asking where you can purchase unrefined rye flour, 100 per cent whole-wheat flour, wheat germ, unground wheat, whole buckwheat, whole soybeans, soy grits, and buckwheat, peanut, cottonseed, or soy flours. In the same way

559

get the addresses of firms which produce macaroni, spaghetti, and noodles, and ask them for the whole-wheat or soy products. If the names of the leading dairies and breweries are not familiar to you, get them from advertisements in magazines or from the labels on packaged cheese and beer bottles; they can direct you to sources of powdered milk, yogurt, and brewers' yeast. The label on a bottle of dark molasses will give you an address which can bring information about blackstrap molasses. Firms which package flavorings and spices can tell you where to write for information about any herbs, food coloring, unusual flavorings, and aromatic seeds you may wish to purchase. Do not worry if you do not have the street address of the firms you write to. A letter recently reached me addressed merely to "Los Angeles Somewhere."

If you have a health-food store in your community or have the address of such a store, communicate with it first. Such stores usually carry all the products of outstanding nutritive value.

There are two sources of information which I have never known to fail anyone: the chamber of commerce in any large city, whose purpose it is to foster commerce; and the public-service departments of our leading newspapers. If you wish to purchase rice polish, all-vitamin rice, or cottonseed or peanut flour, for example, write to the chamber of commerce or the newspapers in leading cities in states where rice, cotton, and peanuts are grown.

If you live in or near a town large enough to produce its own ice cream and bread, you can usually obtain spray-processed powdered milk from the baker or the factory where the ice cream is made. If such firms are not willing to share their supply, they can tell you where they purchase it. Most bakers use blackstrap molasses because it is cheaper than other varieties of dark molasses; often they will sell you a gallon or more. You may insult the baker, however, if you ask him for blackstrap molasses. Many people associate blackstrap with stock-feeding and wrongly think of it as unclean. Be tactful and ask him only for dark molasses. A few brands of blackstrap molasses are sold at grocery stores and may be differentiated from ordinary dark molasses by the iron content given on the label. If the label states that the molasses contains 7 milligrams or more of iron per tablespoon, the molasses is blackstrap.

If you live in a city where there are bakery, creamery, or confectionery supply houses, find out what products they have to sell. By purchasing in quantity and sharing your purchase with friends, you can save a considerable amount of money. An acquaintance of mine, for example, purchases 50 pounds of peanuts at a time from a confectionery supply house and shares them with her club members who have growing children. I purchase not only powdered milk and blackstrap molasses from these sources, but delicious black walnuts and pecans, vanilla by the quart, gelatin by the pound, and many other products which would cost three or four times as much if purchased in the usual channels.

Powdered brewers' yeast is sold at most drugstores, but at present it costs about eight times more than that obtained directly from the large breweries where it is dried. When bakers' or brewers' yeast which is fresh, that is, has not been dried, is eaten, it grows in the intestines. Yeast requires vitamins to grow, but does not produce vitamins itself. When live yeast grows in the intestines, the question arises, "Who gets the vitamins, you or the yeast?" When live yeast is first eaten, some of the B vitamins are probably absorbed from it. As it continues to grow, however, there is the possibility that it uses our vitamin supply which we have obtained from other foods. Dried brewers' yeast has been pasteurized and cannot grow under any circumstances.

Any flour mill which produces white flour has wheat germ or wheat germ and middlings as a by-product. In every book I have written, I have stated repeatedly that wheat germ may be purchased at your nearest flour mill. Despite that fact I receive thousands of letters asking me where wheat germ can be obtained. I patiently answer them and say, "At your nearest flour mill." The smaller the mill, the cheaper the wheat germ usually is. Any number of small mills sell it for 5 cents per pound; yet in retail stores wheat germ which is not one iota better is often priced at a dollar a pound. If your budget is limited, locate a small mill.

In case little-known foods of outstanding nutritive value are not on general sale, ask your grocer to order them for you. If he does not, ask him again and again. Get as many women as you can to do the same. Health-building foods will become available to all as soon as you and other women demand their sale.

Only a few enterprising women will make the effort to obtain foods not generally on the market. After they have located a source of supply or the food is put on sale because of their efforts, other families soon use the food, and the health of the community is improved accordingly. Hugh Black has said, "The purpose of life is to serve, not to be served; to give, not to get; to love, not to be loved; and to the giver comes the wonder of it, and the joy."

# CHAPTER 28

## YOUR REWARD

The health of yourself and your family is a mirror which reflects your intelligence, your efficiency, and your cooking methods. If you purchase your foods wisely, plan your menus carefully, prepare meals with minimum nutritive loss, and see that each body requirement is supplied to every member of your family daily, then you, your children, and your husband can probably possess vibrant, buoyant health. With this degree of health come beauty, clear thinking, co-operativeness, cheerfulness, and freedom from bickering and quarreling, as well as freedom from illnesses and infections.

To the mother of such a family come pride of accomplishment and deep satisfaction of a job well done. To her comes ego-gratification infinitely more satisfying than she may once have obtained from such trivialities as preparing fluffy-textured cake or devitalized white bread. When she hears her physician praise the beauty of her children, when she sees her husband, young beyond his years, succeeding because of his energies, when she feels the surge of vibrant health in her own body, she will realize that she is largely responsible. She has shouldered her tasks and has seen to it that good health has come from good cooking.

# NOTES AND OTHER RECIPES

# NOTES AND OTHER RECIPES

# NOTES AND OTHER RECIPES

# NOTES AND OTHER RECIPES

# NOTES AND OTHER RECIPES

# NOTES AND OTHER RECIPES

# NOTES AND OTHER RECIPES

# NOTES AND OTHER RECIPES

# NOTES AND OTHER RECIPES

# NOTES AND OTHER RECIPES

# NOTES AND OTHER RECIPES

# NOTES AND OTHER RECIPES

# NOTES AND OTHER RECIPES

# NOTES AND OTHER RECIPES

# NOTES AND OTHER RECIPES

# NOTES AND OTHER RECIPES

# NOTES AND OTHER RECIPES

# NOTES AND OTHER RECIPES

# NOTES AND OTHER RECIPES

# NOTES AND OTHER RECIPES

# NOTES AND OTHER RECIPES

# INDEX

Acetic acid, use in body, 23
"Acid-forming" foods, 405
Acids, effect of protein on, 422
 effect on enzymes, 482
 in "strong-flavored" vegetables, 381
 value in aiding digestion, 23; in cooking meats, 50, 86, 142; in mineral absorption, 23
Acorn squash, baked, 414
 broiled, 414
 mashed, 415
 sautéed, 415
 steamed, 415
 stuffed, 415
Acrolein in garlic, onions, 26
Age of animal, relation to tenderness, juiciness, and flavor of meat, 55–57
"Alkaline-forming" foods, 405
Allergies, relation of vitamin C to, 31
Almond Bavarian cream, 504
 cake, 517; mock, 517
 candy, 555
 chews, 544
 custard, 493
 -custard pie, 531
 pie, 534, 537
 rolls, spiced, 427
 tort, 521
Aluminum cooking utensils, advantages of, 31
Amino acids, in eggs and cheese, 238; glandular meats, 110; muscle meats, 110; soybeans, 193
 lack in meat substitutes, 193
Anemia, relation to faulty food preparation, 31
Appetizers, 256–266
 artichoke, 339

Appetizers (Cont.)
 citrus fruit, 259–260; grapefruit halves with oysters, 259; orange-apricot, 259; orange with cherries, 260; orange-pear, 260; persimmon-grapefruit, 260
 contribution to health, 256–258
 enrichment of, 257
 fish, 265
 fresh juices, commercially prepared, 257
 frozen juices or purées, 262–263; applesauce, 263; apricot, 263; juice with decorative cubes, 264; nectarine, 263; pear or peach, 263; persimmon, 263; pineapple juice, with purée cubes, 263; strawberry, 263; yellow-tomato, 262; youngberry, 263
 glandular meats, brain, 116, 266; kidney, 266; liver, 266; sweetbread, 266
 melon, 260–261; cantaloupe baskets, 261; cantaloupe-raspberry, 260; mixed melon, 261
 mixed fruit, 261; apricot-grape, 261; guava, 261; loquat, 261; papaya, 261; persimmon-pear, 262; raspberry-peach, 261
 nutritive value of, 256
 sea food, 265
 shrimp, 265
 tomato juice, 258; with grapefruit juice, 258; sauerkraut juice, 259
 yellow-tomato juice, 262
Apple betty, 497
 crisp, 497
 -custard pie, 531
 juice, 264, 456; directions for canning, 475

585

CPSIA information can be obtained
at www.ICGtesting.com
Printed in the USA
BVHW030048260820
587163BV00002B/144